Aphasia
REHABILITATION
Clinical Challenges

Patrick Coppens
SUNY Plattsburgh Communication Sciences and Disorders
Plattsburgh, New York

Janet Patterson
VA Northern California Health Care System
Martinez, California

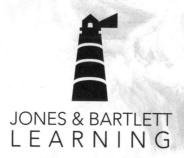

JONES & BARTLETT
LEARNING

World Headquarters
Jones & Bartlett Learning
5 Wall Street
Burlington, MA 01803
978-443-5000
info@jblearning.com
www.jblearning.com

Jones & Bartlett Learning books and products are available through most bookstores and online booksellers. To contact Jones & Bartlett Learning directly, call 800-832-0034, fax 978-443-8000, or visit our website, www.jblearning.com.

Production Credits

VP, Executive Publisher: David D. Cella
Executive Editor: Matt Kane
Acquisitions Editor: Laura Pagluica
Editorial Assistant: Mary Menzemer
Senior Vendor Manager: Sara Kelly
Associate Marketing Manager: Alianna Ortu
VP, Manufacturing and Inventory Control:
  Therese Connell
Composition and Project Management:
  Cenveo® Publisher Services
Cover Design: Michael O'Donnell
Rights & Media Specialist: Jamey O'Quinn
Media Development Editor: Troy Liston
Cover Image: © VLADGRIN/Shutterstock
Printing and Binding: Edwards Brothers Malloy
Cover Printing: Edwards Brothers Malloy

Library of Congress Cataloging-in-Publication Data
Names: Coppens, Patrick, 1944- editor. | Patterson, Janet L., 1955- editor.
Title: Aphasia rehabilitation : clinical changes / [edited by] Patrick
  Coppens and Janet Patterson.
Other titles: Aphasia rehabilitation (Coppens)
Description: Burlington, MA : Jones & Bartlett Learning, [2018] | Includes
  bibliographical references and index.
Identifiers: LCCN 2016044794 | ISBN 9781284042719 (pbk. : alk. paper)
Subjects: | MESH: Aphasia—rehabilitation | Aphasia—therapy
Classification: LCC RC425 | NLM WL 340.5 | DDC 616.85/5206—dc23
LC record available at https://lccn.loc.gov/2016044794

6048

Printed in the United States of America
21 20 19 18 17   10 9 8 7 6 5 4 3 2 1

DEDICATION

To Noé: Dream big.

To Anthony: Believe in yourself.

CONTENTS

Chapter 4 Agrammatic Aphasia 101

Yasmeen Faroqi-Shah and Angela Lea Baker

Chapter 5 Echophenomena in Aphasia: Causal Mechanisms
and Clues for Intervention. 143

Marcelo L. Berthier, Guadalupe Dávila, and María José Torres-Prioris

Chapter 6 Stroke-Related Acquired Neurogenic Stuttering. 173

Luc F. De Nil, Catherine Theys, and Regina Jokel

PREFACE

Clinical aphasia rehabilitation is a multifaceted and complex enterprise. Clinicians must possess knowledge and skills that take years to acquire, develop, refine, and adapt. To get this process started, the beginning clinician acquires, in a relatively short period of time, a substantial amount of basic but critical information about aphasia and aphasia rehabilitation from a broad-based aphasiology textbook. From such a source, clinicians-in-training study how language is lateralized and organized; how to differentially diagnose the various aphasia types; which assessment tools to use; how to treat major aphasia symptoms, such as comprehension impairment and anomia; and how to involve the patient and family in therapy planning, among many other clinical skills. However, these new clinicians quickly realize that patient variability and symptom inconstancy render the clinical interaction more unpredictable and fluid than they had anticipated. In other words, many clinical situations they face were not discussed in their textbook, at least not in enough clinical detail for a clinician to face these situations with confidence and aplomb. In this volume, we have attempted to remedy those lacunae. Many of the topics appear here as a separate overview chapter for the first time.

The impetus for this volume was to concentrate on clinically useful information that tends to be overlooked or only summarily covered in contemporary aphasiology textbooks. This rationale led us to focus on two types of topics: (a) specific aphasia symptoms and (b) particular features of the clinical interaction. This distinction represents the basic organization of the chapters into two parts.

Part One of this volume contains our selection of the symptoms that clinicians encounter regularly in their clinical responsibilities but that are typically not treated as discrete topics. In Chapter 1, Jacqueline Stark provides a thorough overview of the nature of perseveration and suggests clinical strategies to minimize this behavior. Chapter 2, authored by Michael de Riesthal, offers creative suggestions on how to reduce the frequency of paraphasias. In Chapter 3, Jane Marshall focuses on jargon and offers clinical solutions to address the problem. In Chapter 4, Yasmeen Faroqi-Shah and Angela Lea Baker discuss the nature of agrammatism and how to remedy this symptom clinically. Marcelo Berthier, Guadalupe Davila, and María José Torres-Prioris review the interesting challenge of echo phenomena in Chapter 5 and consider how it can be overcome. Finally, in Chapter 6, Luc De Nil, Catherine Theys, and Regina Jokel examine the issue of the nature and rehabilitation strategies associated with acquired neurogenic stuttering.

Part Two of this volume assembles a variety of topics that have historically received little attention but that are nevertheless crucial to the rehabilitation process. In Chapter 7, Patrick Coppens and Janet Patterson offer some suggestions on how to facilitate stimulus and response generalization in aphasiology rehabilitation. In Chapter 8, Sarah Wallace provides insights on how to combine various modalities to maximize therapy effects. Authored by Janet Patterson, Anastasia Raymer, and Leora Cherney, Chapter 9 defines the various components of therapy intensity and provides guidance for clinicians. In Chapter 10, Jacqueline Hinckley discusses the best options to combine various rehabilitation strategies to maximize therapy outcomes. In Chapter 11, Janet Patterson and Patrick Coppens address the issue of evidence-based practice and offer some useful suggestions on how to seamlessly insert those strategies into clinical aphasiology. In Chapter 12, Mike Biel, Leslie Nitta, and Catherine Jackson provide original information on what we know about patient motivation and how to promote it. Finally, in Chapter 13, Patrick Coppens and Nina Simmons-Mackie discuss informal assessment and its effective clinical application.

We believe that, as a scientific field, aphasiology rehabilitation makes advances thanks to the reciprocal interactions between theory and clinical practice. As such, each chapter in this volume contains important theoretical information as well as practical clinical applications. The latter is brought to life in each chapter by a case illustration that highlights the logic of the clinical process, as informed by the background theoretical issues.

We are extremely grateful that such an international "dream team" of colleagues accepted the difficult challenge we posed to write about these clinically important topics. Each chapter author possesses the highest theoretical and clinical expertise in the topic covered. Their competence and hard work shines through the pages. We are deeply indebted to all of them for the time and expertise they each committed to this book. We sincerely hope that clinicians will benefit from this collective effort.

—Patrick Coppens and Janet Patterson, Editors

Challenging Symptoms

CHAPTER 1

Perseveration: Clinical Features and Considerations for Treatment

Jacqueline Stark

INTRODUCTION

In the category of repetitive verbal behaviors, perseveration is different from echolalia, recurring utterances, or speech automatisms (i.e., verbal stereotypy), and palilalia. Stark (2011a) defines perseveration as "a phenomenon whereby the subject unintentionally produces or "gets stuck" on an information unit, i.e., a particular linguistic form or action unit, which he/she has previously produced or at some level has heard, i.e., auditorily processed, or seen, i.e., visually processed" (p. 136) in place of the correct response. Linguistically speaking, the perseverated unit can be a phoneme, word, phrase, syntactic structure, semantic feature, or an idea. In addition to the perseveration of linguistic units, action units (as observed in apraxic disorders), or gestures, as well as features or single elements in drawing, can also be affected. The perseverative response can be the immediate repetition of a linguistic unit or it can be separated by several intervening correct or incorrect responses resulting in a complex pattern of responses. The unit perseverated can be a correct response to a former item or an incorrect one, that is, a paraphasia. However, within the context of a specific deficit, it is not predictable *if* and *when* a person with aphasia (PWA) will produce a perseveration instead of a correct response, a paraphasia, or no response at all. Given the complexity of the phenomena subsumed under the heading of perseveration, it is comprehensible that perseveration, in particular verbal perseveration, continues to be a challenge for clinicians working with PWA in a therapeutic setting.

Over the past decades, clinicians and researchers have advanced our understanding of the complex perseverative phenomena in terms of the origin of the errors and have proposed explanations and models for the source of their occurrence. Still, there have been few studies directly addressing the treatment of verbal perseveration in PWA. In particular, few case studies discuss providing therapy to PWA who have a moderate to severe tendency to perseverate. This leaves clinicians with little guidance on how to recognize and treat perseveration in PWA.

This chapter provides an overview of the various aspects of perseveration with the goal of preparing the reader for meeting the challenges when confronted with a PWA who shows a moderate to severe tendency to perseverate. The following questions are addressed:

- What type of cognitive/linguistic deficit is perseveration?
- What accounts have been put forward regarding the origin or cause of perseverative responses?
- Do perseverative responses produced by PWA share common mechanisms with nonperseverative errors produced by healthy subjects?
- Which factors have been cited to trigger a perseverative response?
- Which types of verbal perseveration exist at the various linguistic levels?
- How does perseveration manifest itself in the various aphasia types?
- Which other repetitive symptoms can co-occur with perseveration?
- In the context of the overall impairments in a PWA, how can perseveration be treated?
- Why does a PWA produce a perseverative response and not a paraphasia or no response at all?

THEORETICAL BACKGROUND

In the literature on verbal perseveration, various classifications of the types of perseveration are proposed. Each one is based on the theoretical assumptions of the authors. The standpoint taken in this chapter is that the types of perseveration are an expression of the specific language processing deficits observed in each case. Thus, the types of perseveration are to be characterized in terms of the linguistic units (e.g., phonemes, grammatical morphemes, etc.), levels (e.g., phonological, lexical, syntactic, discourse), and the modalities (e.g., oral vs. written) affected in each case of aphasia.

Despite its elusive nature, the occurrence rate of perseveration reported in aphasia studies is high, and this underlines the clinical importance of this symptom and its analysis according to aphasia type, severity, and affected linguistic units. The reported frequency of perseveration varies from 50 to 93% in the cases reported in the literature (Basso, 2004; Helm-Estabrooks, Albert, & Nicholas, 2013; Santo-Pietro & Rigrodsky, 1982, 1986; Yamadori, 1981). Moreover, the frequency of perseverative responses does not seem to vary with aphasia type, but rather is related to aphasia severity (Basso, 2004; Helm-Estabrooks, Ramage, Bayles & Cruz, 1998).

Types of Perseveration

In the aphasia literature, the most widely used taxonomy of perseverative responses is that of Sandson and Albert (1984; Albert & Sandson, 1986; Sandson, 1986; Yamadori, 1981), which is very similar to Liepmann's (1905) original typology of *tonic, clonic,* and *intentional* perseveration discussed in the classical literature. Sandson and Albert's tripartite classification consists of the following types of perseveration which are differentiated in terms of their clinical features, processes, and neuroanatomy:

1. *Continuous*: the inappropriate repetition or prolongation of an activity without interruption due to a motor output deficit caused by damage to the basal ganglia (e.g., the continuous drawing of loops in a drawing task).

2. *Stuck-in-set*: the inability to switch from one task or response strategy that results in inappropriate maintenance of a current category or framework due to a deficit in executive functioning stemming from a lesion in the frontal lobe. This type can also be termed *task perseveration.* For example, when asked to count from 1 to 10 and then to recite the days of the week, the PWA continues to count.

3. *Recurrent*: the unintentional repetition, after cessation, of a previously emitted response—either immediate or delayed—to a subsequent stimulus. This is caused by damage to the posterior left hemisphere.

These three types refer to how the system responds and breaks down when performing a specific task in correlation with the level of complexity required for achieving that task. The *recurrent* type is most prevalent in PWA and is the main type discussed in the literature on perseveration, particularly in discussions of perseverative behavior on oral confrontation naming tasks, picture descriptions, and in conversational speech.

Linguistic Context

Perseveration can be observed at all linguistic levels starting with conceptual information and ideas or thoughts, to syntactic constructions in tasks requiring the production of a single-word response (e.g., confrontation naming, repetition), or text (e.g., picture description or retelling of a story). The severity of the specific deficit(s) is a determining factor for the occurrence of any type of perseveration. Examples for the various types are described here and listed in **TABLE 1.1**.

- *Phonological level*: distinctive features, phonemes, and consonant clusters are perseverated within items; for example, within a syllable, across syllables, or across items (Table 1.1, examples 1 to 16).

TABLE 1.1 Examples of perseveration at the various linguistic levels.

Linguistic level	#	Target Form (origin of error underlined) (error in bold italics)	Feature Perseverated	Task
Phonological Level				
Distinctive features				
Intramorphemic	1	Danke ("thank you") → *Dante*	[+ alveolar]	Spontaneous speech
	2	Hundehütte ("dog house") → *Hundehutte*	[+ back]	Naming
	3	Giesskanne ("watering can") → *Giesskange*	[+ back]	Naming
Phonemes				
Within item intramorphemic	4	Meine Mutter sitzt im *Rorstuhl* (for "Rollstuhl") ("My mother is sitting in a wheelchair")	[- lateral] or phoneme /r/	Spontaneous speech
Interitem	5	1) Stift ("writing utensil") + 2) Schlacht ("battle") → *Schlaft*	Phoneme /f/	Repetition
Interitem	6	1) Fleisch ("meat") + 2) Messer ("knife") → **Fesser...Vesser**	Phoneme /f/	Repetition
Within item, intermorphemic	7	Fleischpreissteigerung ("increase in meat price") → *Fleischpreissteiberung*	[+ frontal] (Labial) or phoneme /b/	Repetition
Within sentence, sentential	8	merke ich gar (→ *ger*) nicht ("I don't notice at all")	[- low] [+high] or phoneme /e/	Spontaneous speech
Within sentence	9	"...als er zu ihr im *Finster* (for Fenster) geschaut hat" ("...when he looked at her in the window")	[+ high] or phoneme /i/	Picture description

			a) Consonant cluster /bl/ b) Phoneme /u/	
Intermorphemic	10	Blinde Kuh ("Blind man's bluff") → *Blinde Bluhe* ... *Blunde Kuh*	a) Consonant cluster /bl/ b) Phoneme /u/	Picture description
Intermorphemic	11	*/ no smok / → / no *smok* /	Phoneme /n/	Spontaneous speech
Within item, intermorphemic	12	Schillingstück ("Schilling piece" = coin) → *Schillingstücking*	Assimilated phonemes / ng/ → ŋ Phoneme / ŋ/ or [ŋ]	Spontaneous speech
Sentence level	13	Jetzt ein Taucher mit 'n **Tisch** [table] (for "Fisch'") ("Now a diver with a fish")	Phoneme /t/	Picture sequence
Sentence level	14	Priester beten *träglich* (for täglich) ("Priests pray daily")	Phoneme /r/	Repetition
Intersentential	15	Ein Bauer hat einen Esel. Diesen Esel hat er in ein **Bell** (for "Fell") ("The farmer has a donkey. This donkey he has [put] in a fur")	Phoneme /b/	Story retelling
Intersentential	16	"Der Mann nimmt den Buben beim *Flock …beim Spo…beim *Spock- beim Haar Schopf- beim Schopf und das zweite Bub hat sich verst- hat sich ver- hat sich *verstopft* [clogged] (for "versteckt") ("The man takes the boy by the *flock [paraphasia] …by the spo- by the *spock [paraphasia] by the hair tuft- by the tuft and the second boy has hi- has hi- himself – has hidden himself")	Vowel /o/ plus affricate /pf/	Picture description

(Continues)

TABLE 1.1 Examples of perseveration at the various linguistic levels. (Continued)

Linguistic level	#	Target Form (origin of error underlined) (error in bold italics)	Feature Perseverated	Task
Morphological Level				
Derivational morphology				
Intersentential	17	1. Schnellbremsung ("emergency braking") 2. Lokomotivführer (= "engine driver") → *Lokomotivführung*	Morpheme –ung	Story retelling
Intersentential	18	1. Die Mutter ist entrüstet ("The mother is outraged") 2. erzürnt ("angry") (→ *entzürnt*)	Unseparable prefix morpheme ent-	Picture description
Intersentential	19	Es ging so weit gut, bis eines Tages einer- einer der den- die Mut hatte den Esel zu das Fell des Esels zu bewachen oder zu *bemuten* (for "belauern") ("It went pretty well, until one day one- one who had the- the courage to watch over or to" [neologism for stalk])	Morpheme (= word)	Story retelling
Inflectional morphology				
Intersentential	20	"Der Bub schaut der schlafenden Katze zu und er tut was ich nicht mit meiner Katze *tut*" (for "tue") ("The boy is watching the sleeping cat and he does what I don't with my cat")	third person singular -t	Picture sequence
Intersentential	21	"Tochter schaut zu und bemerkt aber dann auch wahrscheinlich, dass *sie* (for er) stürzen wird" ("The daughter is watching and notices then also probably that he will fall down")	Gender: +feminine	Cookie Picture description

			Participle	Picture description
Intersentential	22	"Und entsetzlich hat die Mutter geschrieen. Um Gottes Willen ihr habt das Geschirr heruntergeschmissen und … Den Krug, die Milch und die Teller. Alles ist heruntergeschrieen" (for "heruntergefallen") (And terrible the mother has screamed. For God's sake you have thrown down the dishes and… The jug, the milk, the plates. Everything has fallen down)	Participle	Picture description
Lexical (Whole Word) Level				
Interitem	23	1) Ein kleines rotes Auto ("A small red car"); 2) Ein großes weißes **Auto** (for "Haus") ("A big white house")	Whole word	Story Completion Test (Goodglass et al., 1972)
Interitem	24	1) Zwetschenknödel ("plum dumplings") 2) Blechlöffel ("metal spoon") 3) Topfenstrudel ("cream cheese strudel") 4) Fleischpreissteigerung ("increase in meat price") → *Fleischpreisknödel*	Whole word, part of compound word	Repetition
Intrasentential	25	Das *Eichhörnchen* knabbert ein *Eichhörnchen* (for "Nuss") ("The squirrel is nibbling on a nut")	Whole word	Oral sentence production to a picture stimulus

(Continues)

TABLE 1.1 Examples of perseveration at the various linguistic levels. (Continued)

Linguistic level	#	Target Form (origin of error underlined) (error in bold italics)	Feature Perseverated	Task
Semantic Level				
Interitem	26	1) Er wird arbeiten (He will work) ... 3) Soldat - Unteroffizier (→ **Arbeiter** – **Chef**)	Semantic feature: relationship between subordinate and superordinate	Story Completion Test (Goodglass et al., 1972)
Interitem	27	1) Stiefel ("boots") 2) Gans ("goose") ... rote **Stiefel** (for "Füße" [feet])	Semantic feature: having to do with feet	Naming
Interitem/intertextual	28	1) Teller fallen ("Plates fall down") 2) ... **kalte Teller** ("cold plates") (for Schneebälle [snowballs])	Semantic feature: + round (Plates, snowballs)	Picture description
Interitem	29	1) Birne ("pear") 2) Katze ("cat") → *Kapfel (/k/ + "apple")	Semantic category: fruit (Initial phoneme /k/ is correct but the resulting production is a nonword)	Naming
Interitem	30	1) When naming the picture "Auto" ("car"), the PWA counted the four wheels: "1, 2, 3, 4" 2) Elefant → **Auto**	Associative perseveration: Car: 4 wheels Elephant: 4 legs	Naming

Syntactic Level

Interitem—form	31	1) Trink die Milch! Trink sie! Trink sie damit du gesund bleibst! (Drink the milk! Drink it! Drink it so that you stay healthy!) 2) [Stimulus to be completed: "A baby has a toy. I take the toy away. What will happen?"] Das Baby weint. **Spiele nicht mit dem Spielzeug!** ('The baby cries. Don't play with the toy!")	Imperative construction	Story Completion Test (Goodglass et al., 1972)
Intersentential –Form/ Content	32	Ich habe Radio gehört... Fernsehen **gehört** (for geschaut) (I have listened to the radio.... watched TV)	Structure + content	Spontaneous speech

Ideational Level

Interitem /Intertextual	33	Context: The PWA and the clinician had a prior conversation about the weather and gardening (trees and plants). Then, the PWA described a picture about children playing (a boy pulls on the table cloth and the dishes fall onto the floor). 'Also ein größeres und zwei kleinere ah... also laufen mit und ... einen.. einen Krug der dürfte runterfallen und die **Blätter sind von den Bäumen heruntergefallen** ... und das große Mädchen ("an older and two younger ... and the leaves fell from the tree") [Clin: What fell down?]. Also die **Blätter** ("the leaves")	Idea of gardening: leaves and trees; Association triggered by the verb 'to fall down'	Picture description: Blind man's bluff

(*Continues*)

TABLE 1.1 Examples of perseveration at the various linguistic levels. (Continued)

Linguistic level	#	Target Form (origin of error underlined) (error in bold italics)	Feature Perseverated	Task
Interitem /Intertextual	34	1) Picture description: a child falls down. 'Diese Mädchen oder die Mutter schreit da heraus und sagt, dass das Kind herausgefallen ist [paraphasia: hingefallen] .. und der läuft daher. [Clin: Was sagt die Frau?] Frau wird sagen, der Bub ist **herausgefallen** [fell out]" (the mother screams that the child has fallen…and runs towards it. [Clin: What does the woman say?] The woman says that the child has fallen). 2) Questions after retelling of another story: Child playing on train tracks, trips and falls down. A train is approaching. The engine driver uses the emergency brakes, gets off the train, picks up the child, and hands it to her mother. [Clin: Wo liegt das Kind?] "Vor dem Zug." [Clin: Wie ist es dort hingekommen?] "Es ist **herausgefallen**. Es ist aus dem Zug **herausgefallen**." ([Clin: Where is the child lying?] "In front of the train." [Clin: How did it get there?] "It fell out. It fell out of the train.")	Idea of child falling down Association triggered by the verb 'stürzen' = 'to fall down'	1) Picture description 2) Story retelling: Child on the train tracks

Interitem	35	1) Uhr ("watch")	Perseveration of the time or of the idea of telling time and also verbal and semantic paraphasias and also lexical perseveration	Naming + Answering questions about picture stimuli
		[Clin: What time is it?] 12:30		
		2) Tür ("door") → Tisch [paraphasia] ("table") [Th: What about it? (= door is open)] "Mit dem *Tisch. Da ist es 12:30*" ("With the table. It is 12:30")		
		3) Hase ("rabbit") → Eichhörnchen [paraphasia] ("squirrel")		
		4) Auto ("car") ↓ [Clin: What color is it?] "It is blue"		
		5) Flugzeug oder Flieger ("Airplane or plane") "Aber ich weiss es nicht, *wie spät es darauf ist* ("But I do not know what time it is on it")		
		6) Balloon (for Bälle) ("balls")		
		[Clin: Where are they?] "Sie sind in einem *Flieger*. (for "Netz" ["net"] [perseveration]) ("They are in an *airplane*.")		

- *Morphological level*: bound and free morphemes are perseverated. Both derivational and inflectional morphology are affected by perseveration (Table 1.1, examples 17 to 22).

- *Lexical perseverations*: lexical items, parts of words, and whole words that are not semantically related can be perseverated (Table 1.1, examples 23 to 25).

- *Semantic perseverations*: include the perseveration of semantic features, semantically related words and more complex associations. For example, visual-perceptive and form features. A semantic perseveration can usually be distinguished from a semantic paraphasia, since in the case of a perseverative response, the feature perseverated is apparent from the context and is often inappropriate; for example, for a plate the form "round" is perseverated in a following picture description and the word "cold plates" is produced for the target word "snowballs" (Table 1.1, examples 26 to 30).

- *Syntactic level*: perseverations encompass syntactic form and content. Either a syntactic construction as such (e.g., wh- question, imperative construction, auxiliary and adjective, perseveration of a prepositional phrase) or the content or meaning of a syntactic phrase can be perseverated (Table 1.1, examples 31 to 32).

- *Text or discourse level*: with regard to the text level, ideational perseverations are observed within a text and from one text to another (Table 1.1, examples 33 to 35).

On the various linguistic levels, a perseverative response can be clear cut or simple in its structure whereby single phonemes, parts of words, whole words, and semantic features are perseverated. In more complex examples, several types of perseverative responses can be interlaced and can co-occur with paraphasias. The phonological, morphological, lexical, and semantic types of perseverative responses are the most common types (Stark, 1984). These errors are striking and easier to detect in the speech flow or in written samples from PWA than subtler and more complex perseverative responses. In particular those related to the perseveration of an idea or thought, can at first glance be difficult to detect.

Ideational Perseveration

An *ideational* or *idea* perseveration refers to a perseverative response in which an idea or parts of an idea are perseverated to new items (e.g., from a first question to a second question in conversation, or to a subsequent picture description, or from one picture description to another). An ideational perseveration can result from a syntactic perseveration of form or content or a semantic perseveration (e.g., semantic features). The meaning or idea(s) of the following utterance(s) is/are uncertain or not discernable, or the meaning of the utterance is in contradiction to real-world knowledge (e.g., in picture descriptions) or to the assertions made in previous utterances. An ideational perseveration is usually produced within lengthier language samples (i.e., picture descriptions, retellings of stories, or a combination of tasks). Examples of complex perseverations across test and therapy sessions separated by days have been observed (Stark, 2007b).

An idea can persist without a new question being posed or without presentation of another stimulus item and the PWA then continues his or her response with uncalled-for, additional responses to items (e.g., in a naming task) that actually require only a single-word response. An interesting example of an ideational perseveration is example 35 in Table 1.1: After the clinician asked the PWA what time was shown on the watch in the picture, she perseverated both *the concept of time* and *what time it is* over the next several items. For the next item, she produced a semantic paraphasia: (open) door → table. In an attempt to elicit the correct response, the clinician asked, "What about it?" referring to the fact that the door was open. The PWA added, "With the *table* it is 12:30." Then, following two other items, after naming an airplane correctly, she continued her response with, "but I do not know what time it is on it" (i.e., on the airplane). Idea perseverations have been reported in other disorders including right hemisphere stroke, traumatic brain injury, and dementia.

Factors Influencing the Occurrence of a Perseverative Response

In the publications on perseveration, various factors have been put forward that are assumed to trigger or induce a perseverative response in the context of the specific processing difficulties a PWA reveals. In general, linguistic variables that have been found to influence language performance in healthy subjects, also apply to the tendency to perseverate in PWA.

The linguistic factors that may influence or play a role in triggering a perseverative response include:

- *Phonological relatedness*: similar or identical phonological form in the onset, nucleus, or coda of a word
- *Semantic relatedness*: similar or overlapping semantic features
- *Syllable or word structure*: same syllable structure or word form and word length
- *Lexical/word frequency*: less frequent words have a greater tendency to be perseverated.
- *The overall level of difficulty*: of the individual task, test, or individual items and the order of the tasks

Task demands such as the presentation rate can influence a person's response (Muñoz, 2011, 2014). A faster presentation rate and a very brief or no interval between the presented stimuli can lead to a breakdown in the PWA's ability to process the stimuli. The ordering of the individual tasks in assessing the PWA as well as the ordering of the individual stimuli can also influence the response. Other general factors that are discussed in the classical and recent literature include fatigue, attention deficits, memory disorders, and the difficulty of the task to be performed. Although certain tasks, such as repetition priming, have been shown to improve word retrieval abilities, repeating the presented stimuli several times may increase the tendency to perseverate an item upon presentation of the following stimulus.

Classical Theories of Perseveration

Classical works written by the most famous aphasiologists such as Wernicke, Broca, and Pick, have been translated into English. However, numerous classical works on perseveration are only available in German and French. In particular, the German classical aphasia literature from the 1880s to the 1930s abounds in discussions of perseveration. These studies may not always follow the rigorous structure of recent publications, but their theoretical merit is undisputed.

Excluding the classic Greek and Latin literature, the first actual use of the term *perseveration* dates back to 1894 when Neisser responded to a patient presentation by Arnold Pick at the 65th meeting of the East German Psychiatrists in Breslau (Neisser, 1895). Neisser recommended that the term "perseveration" should be applied instead of the term "pseudo-apraxia" for a patient's "getting stuck on the impressions." Neisser suggested that the phenomenon Pick called pseudo-apraxia was appropriate for the particular case in question, but that this symptom was found in very different conditions. For this reason, he asserted that it is necessary to have a term that can be applied to all the conditions; namely, "perseveratory response" or "perseveration."

From 1890 to 1931 three explanations for the occurrence of perseveration in brain damaged individuals were put forward in the German publications, all of which remain relevant today. These accounts differ in their view of perseveration as a primary or secondary symptom.

1. ***Deficit account*** (Heilbronner, 1895, 1897, 1906; Lissauer, 1890): Perseveration is considered a symptom secondary to the primary language deficit. According to this account, a perseverative response is produced, for example, when a PWA experiences difficulty retrieving and producing a target word in a naming task. The gap produced by the primary word-finding difficulty is filled by the perseverative response. Thus, the perseverative response mirrors the underlying word-finding impairments (Basso, 2004; Moses, Nickels, & Sheard, 2004; Stark, 1984).

2. ***Overactivation account*** (von Sölder, 1895, 1899): Perseveration is seen as the primary symptom. Increased activation of a previously produced unit—a phoneme, word, phrase, sentence, idea—results in the production of a perseverative response. The correct target does not have a chance of being produced due to the ongoing overactivation in the language processing system of the just-produced item.

3. ***Underactivation*** or ***Weakened Activation account*** (Pick, 1892, 1900, 1902, 1903, 1906, 1931): According to this account perseveration is a secondary symptom. The PWA produces a perseverative response because his/her overall activation level is too weak. The to-be-produced target response does not receive sufficient activation to reach production.

Contemporary Accounts of Perseveration

According to Yates (1966), brain damage results in three types of symptoms/deficits. His trifold hierarchical differentiation encompasses the following types:

> Type-a: "... a general deterioration in all aspects of functioning"; but will also produce
> Type-b: "... differential (group) effects, depending on the location, extent, etc. of the damage," and will produce
> Type-c: "... highly specific effects if it occurs in certain highly specified areas of the brain." (Yates, 1966, p.122).

Stark (1984) analyzed an extensive database encompassing language data produced by 20 PWA with different aphasia types (6 anomic, 5 Broca's, 4 Wernicke's, 1 transcortical sensory, 4 global) in response to various language tasks tapping all linguistic levels. In that study, the author put forward two working hypotheses regarding the nature of verbal perseveration:

> Hypothesis 1. Verbal perseveration is to be characterized as a non-specific indicator of brain damage and, for that reason, the same type(s) of perseveration will be observed in all people with aphasia, regardless of aphasia type.
> Hypothesis 2. Verbal perseverative responses reflect the specific language impairment and, therefore, are not generalized across every aspect of language processing. Verbal perseverative responses are to be characterized as Type-b effects, according to Yates (1966).

These two hypotheses derive from the neuropsychological literature on cognitive deficits, in which the symptoms of brain damage are divided into localizing (or specific) versus nonlocalizing (or nonspecific) symptoms. Goodglass and Kaplan (1979) consider perseveration to be a nonspecific effect or nonlocalizing symptom. Other nonspecific deficits include behaviors such as slowing and "stickiness" of ideational processes, stimulus boundedness, and reduced scope of attention. In contrast, agrammatism or paragrammatism are considered specific impairments of grammar and syntax. It is interesting to note that paraphasia is cited as a lateralizing and localizing deficit, although—just as is the case with perseverative responses—the types of paraphasic errors differ according to the PWA's specific deficits. Not all types of paraphasia will be produced by a single PWA, and the origin will differ depending on the functional locus of the underlying impairment(s). One possible reason for Goodglass and Kaplan considering perseveration to be a nonspecific deficit, is that a nonspecific disorder may affect all areas of performance.

Hypothesis 2 is concordant with Yates' (1966) Type-b effects, which capture the essence of the different forms of perseveration observed in PWA with various lesions more adequately than the twofold dichotomy of Goodglass and Kaplan (1979). Stark's (1984) analyses of the language data from the 21 PWA provided evidence for Hypothesis 2, namely that the perseverative errors observed in the PWA diagnosed with the main aphasia types reflected their respective primary language processing deficits. Perseverative responses were observed in those language processing domains that were affected and not in an across-the-board fashion. Only in the case of a severe overall language breakdown (e.g., in the late phase of a progressive degenerative disease such as Creutzfeldt-Jacob), will perseveration be observed in all language tasks.

Recent Accounts of Perseveration

Reminiscent of the classical accounts, several proposals regarding the mechanisms involved in the production of perseverative responses have been put forward in recent years. These accounts are mainly based on connectionist, spreading activation models of language processing (Cohen & Dehaene, 1998; Gotts, della Rochetta, & Cipolotti, 2002; Gotts & Plaut, 2004; Martin & Dell, 2004, 2007).

Cohen and Dehaene (1998) provide the most detailed theoretical and analytical account on the origin of perseveration, and they document their findings with formulas for determining the presence and severity of the tendency to perseverate in terms of a *lag distribution analysis* and *perseveration probability analysis*. The perseverative responses produced by three PWAs with naming difficulties due to a functional lesion at different stages of language processing provide evidence in support of their innovative statistical account.

According to their account, perseverative responses are the result of persistent activity unmasked by deficient input. That is, a perseverative response is produced when a given processing level does not receive the input it normally requires and activity from a previous trial persists. Cohen and Dehaene also maintain that another possible source for perseveration is that previous responses remain activated at an abnormally high level, due to impairment of some inhibitory mechanism or check-off mechanism. According to their account, a single mechanism operating at different stages of speech production can be considered to explain the occurrence of various perseverative responses.

With regard to the duration of perseveration on any processing level, Cohen and Dehaene (1998) refer to the term *exponential decay*, which states that the probability that a perseverative response is produced decreases in accordance with the lag between the two trials. These authors have developed an algorithm for determining the presence and duration of perseverative responses, that is, the lag distribution analysis and perseveration probability analysis (see **TABLE 1.2**). An exponentially decaying internal level of activation is assumed to be responsible for the recurrence of perseverations.

In the framework of their serial position model, Dell, Burger, and Svec (1997) postulate that perseveration occurs because a current target item is weakly activated. The previous utterances that are residually activated intrude into the current utterance. The perseverative response correlates with the functional locus of the deficit(s). In recovery, the proportion of perseverative errors decreases, and an increase in anticipatory errors is observed as calculated by an *anticipatory perseverative ratio*.

According to their account of word production, at any one point in time there is competition between the past, present, and future elements to be produced. In the context of

TABLE 1.2 Quantifying perseverative behavior in PWA.

Authors	Description	Measure
Helm-Estabrooks et al. (2013)	Picture stimuli from the BDAE (2nd ed.): 7 semantic categories objects, letters, geometric forms, actions, numbers, colors, body parts	Divide the number of items that elicited a perseveration by 38; then multiply by 100. < 5% = minimal 5% to 19% = mild 20% to 49% = moderate > 49% = severe
Muñoz (2014)	Items from Boston Naming Test (Kaplan, Goodglass, & Weintraub, 1983)	Percentage of items for which a perseveration was produced
Cohen and Dehaene (1998)	*Lag distribution analysis:* • Used for revealing local perseverations and their duration • For each perseverative response the clinician looks backward in the protocol to the first production of the response perseverated. • The number of trials separating the two responses is noted. Each immediate recurrence = 1. • The frequency distribution of the lags is plotted for the entire corpus.	Observed distribution for *x* errors: Lag, number of matches, and number of remaining non-matches
	Lag perseveration probability analysis PP(L): • Captures the temporal aspects such as several recurrences of the same response • This method links each error to all preceding trials and takes into account multiple matches of each error with previous trials. • "If a patient produces an error on Trial *T*, *PP(L)* provides an estimate of the probability that this error matches the response produced on trial *T-L*" (p.1644).	Ratio: perseveration probability (*PP(L)*): $$\frac{M(L)}{N(L) + M(L)}$$ For each lag *L*, the number of matches *M(L)* and the number of non-matches *N(L)* at this lag is calculated

a mechanism that maintains serial order in speech production, Martin and Dell (2004) postulate that perseverations and anticipations produced by PWA result from the malfunctioning of one of the three components of that mechanism: (1) a means to turn off past utterances, (2) a means to activate the present utterance, or (3) a means to prime the future utterance.

In a later study, Martin (2011) characterized similarities and differences between perseverative and nonperseverative errors in aphasia from a theoretical and clinical perspective. She applied the account of perseveration put forward in Martin and Dell (2007), which postulates that word and sound perseverations result from the same mechanisms as nonperseverative errors, namely, a slowed activation of the intended utterance and the linguistic similarity between the target and the produced error.

Extending a connectionist modeling approach, Gotts and colleagues (2002) provide a neurophysiological account of recurrent perseveration in terms of a cholinergic deficit hypothesis (or deafferentation; Buckingham & Buckingham, 2011; McNamara & Albert, 2004; Sandson & Albert, 1984). In an earlier report, Sandson and Albert (1984) suggested that recurrent perseverations result from low levels of acetylcholine and cholinergic deficits. In accordance with that proposal, Gotts and colleagues (2002) put forward the following neural mechanisms to account for the underlying perseveration in general and with regard to data from a single-case study (EB):

> "Under a cholinergic deficit, the normal suppression of intrinsic and feedback projections is removed and cells are somewhat less excitable overall. One potential impact of this is that neural activity will sustain itself for longer through the undamped intrinsic/feedback projections. This will require that new stimuli override persistent activity at even longer delays. Perseverations will be more likely, particularly to stimuli with low frequency names, because afferent input contributes proportionately less to processing, making it harder to override sustained activity" (p. 1944).

In sum, recent accounts further illustrate the complexity of the perseverative behavior and provide evidence for the specific nature of the perseverative responses revealed by the different language processing system deficits of each PWA. The terminology used in the recent accounts for the two aspects of processing which can be affected in isolation or in combination are *activation level* and *decay rate*. In one scenario, the system in general is affected; it is underactivated, and the target item does not reach the threshold needed for it to be retrieved and in turn produced (i.e., Pick's account). Alternatively the activation level, which should return to its resting state, instead remains activated or overactivated and the new target does not have a chance of being retrieved and produced (i.e., von Sölder's account). The final possibility is that the overall system is affected in combination with an ongoing activation of a previously produced item. The decay rate is compromised in this case, that is, the previously activated unit reveals a very slow decay rate. Ultimately, it seems that perseveration is closely related to the specific language processing system deficits of each PWA.

The Role of Executive Processes

Any attempt to address the topic of perseveration must consider the fundamental role of executive functions including activation, inhibition, attention, and monitoring in performing any activity. Most often the role of activation or facilitation is emphasized. However, without inhibitory processes interference would be a constant disruptive factor and a necessary balance could not be achieved. Although activation and inhibition are considered opposites, they actually are oppositional only in their results. In both cases, for all neurophysiological processes they both require nervous activity to attain the desired results. Dempster (1991) draws attention to the relevance of inhibitory processes in relation to intelligence. He states that "inhibitory processes appear to define a basic cognitive dimension that enters into a broad spectrum of intellectual processes" (p. 167) which are necessary for suppressing task-irrelevant information that would otherwise interfere with effective performance. Attention is also a key component in the processing of information. Under normal conditions, being able to attend to a stimulus enables more adequate processing. However, when this basic capacity is impaired, information processing will be adversely affected.

Monitoring one's own speech is an important factor in the ongoing speech production process and important for treating perseverative behavior. Producing an error is the first half of the process, and recognizing and in turn correcting the incorrect response is the second half. When a PWA produces a specific error—i.e., a paraphasia or a perseveration—and immediately attempts to correct it, his or her monitoring can be considered to be intact for that particular type of error. If however, specific types of errors remain unrecognized and no attempts at correction are made, monitoring is impaired. In these cases making a person aware of a particular error is more difficult than when monitoring is successful. In any case, the clinician should not repeat the incorrect response; this would only reinforce it. If a PWA recognizes and corrects certain types of errors (e.g., phonological but not semantic paraphasias) his or her monitoring is differentially affected and the impairment is more severe. Thus, monitoring is another key component in the processing of information.

Perseveration Observed in the Main Aphasia Types

The perseverative responses produced by a PWA must be analyzed within the context of the PWA's overall language performance. However, it may be possible to associate general patterns of perseveration with particular aphasia types. Indeed, Stark (1984) classified the perseverative errors produced by PWA based on aphasia types as well as linguistic levels.

Anomic Aphasia
In anomic aphasia ($N = 6$), perseverations were found when word-finding difficulties were apparent in oral confrontation naming, and in particular in the more difficult tasks requiring semantic processing such as reactive naming, providing opposites, finding shared features to pairs of words, and providing definitions of words. Nouns and verbs were perseverated, for example, when defining professions:

1. "A shoemaker *repairs* shoes" (correct)
2. "A gardener *repairs* gardens" (incorrect)

Perseverative responses were also found in spontaneous conversational speech, oral sentence production, picture descriptions, and retelling stories in the context of word-finding difficulties. Few perseverations were observed in repetition tasks and these errors were immediately self-corrected. Phonemic and morphological perseverations were seldom produced. In most cases, the person with anomic aphasia was aware of his or her errors and in turn tried to correct them.

Broca's Aphasia

In Broca's aphasia (*N* = 5), the perseverative responses were observed on the morpho-syntactic and the phonological levels, that is, (a) in agrammatic sentence production with impaired morphosyntactic processing, and/or (b) in the production of phonological units. The main perseverative responses were observed in word and sentence repetition tasks in the form of perseveration of single phonemes and consonant clusters intra-syllabically, intersyllabically, within a phrase or a sentence, between task items, and between successive and more remotely produced sentences. Lexical perseverations were also common; however, few semantic perseverations were observed. Several perseverations of syntactic form were produced particularly by severely impaired individuals with Broca's aphasia. Specific sentence constructions were repeatedly used, although they were less adequate as responses.

Wernicke's Aphasia

People with Wernicke's aphasia (*N* = 4) predominantly produced phonological or semantic errors, or a mixture of these two types. Individuals with moderate to severe Wernicke's aphasia perseverated on all oral production tasks and produced phonological, morphological, semantic, syntactic, as well as ideational perseverations. In conversational speech, the ideational perseverations manifested themselves as the continuation of a response that was adequate for the previous question. Impaired auditory comprehension may also play a role. For example:

> P: "I really have to have something to eat."
> Clinician: "Where do you live?"
> P: "I didn't get anything!"

Individuals with neologistic jargon were not included in the study. Although these patients' productions abound with perseverative responses, their severe comprehension difficulties prevented them from understanding the instructions to the assessment tasks. Buckingham and colleagues (Buckingham, 1985, 1987; Buckingham & Kertesz, 1976) provide elaborate descriptions of perseverative behavior in people with neologistic jargon aphasia.

The phonemic perseverations produced by individuals with Wernicke's and conduction aphasias were more complex in their structure, with the exception of the responses to compound words. In compound words, the first component was better retained and the second component included more semantic and phonemic paraphasias. For example, in a word repetition task, *"Hausbau"* ("house building") was correctly repeated and then appeared three items later for the item *"Bootshaus"* ("houseboat"); the PWA responded **"Bau, Baus, na da is ein Bau, Baus net Bau sondern ein Bau net Bau sondern Boot, Boots."** ("building, building+s, no that is a building, building+s not building rather a building not building rather a boat, boat+ s"). Perseverative responses affecting one component of a compound word were also observed in people with Broca's aphasia.

Global Aphasia

Because of the severe nature of global aphasia (*N* = 4), perseverative responses were found in all tasks requiring an oral or written response. Single phonemes or consonant clusters, parts of words, and sentences—insofar as these can be produced at all—were perseverated. For example, in response to test item 1, the target word cannot be immediately produced; however, it is produced in response to item 5. Perseveration is already observed when producing serial speech (e.g., days of the week, counting) and even more pronounced when switching from days of the week to months of the year.

　　In summary, the perseverative responses produced by people with fluent aphasia—Wernicke's, conduction, mild anomic—are characterized by a predominance of phonemic errors, whereas people with anomic aphasia seldom produce phonemic perseverations and if they do, they most often self-correct. The conduite d'approche behaviors of the individuals with conduction aphasia often result in moving away from the target word. The individuals with nonfluent aphasias (i.e., Broca's, global) differ in particular with regard to the monitoring of their own perseverative responses. Individuals with global aphasia tend not to be aware when producing an error, whereas the person with Broca's aphasia produces approximations that may or may not be perseverations in an attempt to arrive at the correct pronunciation of the target item.

Simple Versus Complex Forms of Perseverations

In the aphasia literature, analyses of perseverative responses are usually based on language data from oral and written naming, writing to dictation, or from repetition tasks. In these cases, single-word responses are required. Buckingham and colleagues' (1978; Buckingham, 1985) analyses of perseverative behavior from text-level samples from individuals with neologistic jargon are a notable exception. When examining language data from tasks requiring a single-word response, the perseverative responses are readily detectable and can be characterized as "simple." The most common perseverative response is observed in confrontation naming tasks, in which an item is either correctly named or the original response is a paraphasia. For the immediately following item or after a few intervening items, the same name is produced. A "simple" example from an oral confrontation naming task is:

　　Item 1. book → [correct]
　　Item 2. table → **book** or Item 3. +; Item 4. +; Item 5. **book**

The response to item 2 is an example of an immediate perseverative response and the response to item 5 is a delayed recurrent perseveration with correct responses in the interval.

However, when examining extended speech production consisting of spontaneous speech produced in a semistandardized interview or narrative production (e.g., picture description, story generation or retelling), the task of detecting perseverations can become more difficult. The resulting examples of perseveration are more complex in their overall structure. Further, the aforementioned ideational perseveration can result in an entanglement or interlacing of several different items from various types of tasks. Because in many publications, the analyzed corpora consist of single-word errors, the question remains unsettled as to whether the assumption of shared mechanisms holds for all types of perseverative behavior, in particular for extended speech production.

Simple perseverative responses are rarely observed in non–brain-damaged subjects. When analyzing extended passages of language production, the complexity of the perseverative responses actually produced by a PWA makes it difficult to assume that a healthy subject would produce such utterances. Such complex examples span several utterances (intra- and intertextual) and often consist of a blend of several parts of those utterances. The temporal duration can range from seconds up to several days. However, the longer the time passed, the more difficult it will be to consider a response to be perseverative since the contextual information may be lacking. Temporally speaking, the clinician may not have been present when the original occurrences were produced by the PWA, further complicating identification of a perseverative response.

The following examples of complex verbal perseveration were produced by MH—a person with transcortical sensory aphasia. A lengthy discussion of MH's perseverative responses is provided in Stark (1984, 2007b). MH's main deficits were impaired word retrieval with the production of semantic paraphasias, impaired comprehension, inability to monitor her own production for semantic anomalies, echolalia, and a severe tendency to perseverate. The most interesting aspect of her perseverative responses is that, although her productions were almost always syntactically correct, they were semantically incorrect and consisted of words and phrases perseverated from several task items and extended over several days. For this reason, Stark (2007b) postulated that based on her analysis of the responses produced by MH a clear dissociation between syntactic and semantic processing could be discerned. That is, syntactically speaking, MH's utterances were grammatically correct, but semantically anomalous. The syntactically correct utterances consisted of words from various sentences resulting in semantically anomalous and incorrect utterances.

Example 1. Picture description—Blind Man's Bluff (translation from German)
Content: The children are playing blind man's bluff. The blindfolded boy thinks that he is holding a girl's skirt in his hand, but he is pulling the tablecloth from the set table and the dishes are falling on the floor. In the background the mother is raising her arms in desperation.

MH: "**Here an accident is happening. Something is breaking and the mother is unhappy about it.... The mother, the son and the child and the daughter.... The daughter // f-//** it happens to the daughter that something is falling down and the mother is unhappy about it and ... **Th//the mother (dative case) she is happy about it that the daughter is unhappy.** (Ex.: What does the mother say?) **The mother says be careful** *that nothing falls over you.*

Example 2. Examples from Story Completion Test (SCT) (Goodglass, Gleason, Bernholtz, & Hyde, 1972) (translation from German) (Task administered following the above picture description)

Ex. 1a) Target: "Sit down!" → "**Be careful so that nothing happens to you!**"
Ex 1b) Target: "Come in! → **Follow me so that nothing happens to you!**"
Ex. 2a) Target: "Drink your milk" → "Drink it so that you stay healthy!"
Ex. 2b) Target: "Mow the lawn!"/ "Cut the grass!" → "Cut the lawnmower **so that nothing happens to you!**
Ex. 3a) Target: "The baby cries/will cry" → "**Don't play with the toy or else something will happen to you.**"

In further examples from the Story Completion Test, MH produces correct responses intervening with perseverative responses and incorporates parts of three SCT items into a semantically incorrect response:

> Target: "He will work again" → **Where have you put Peter's toy?**
> "**Where (= Test item 7a), have you put Peter's (= Test item 8b), toy (= Test item 7b).**"

Echolalia and Recurring Utterances

Although the various types of repetitive verbal behaviors are distinguishable, they can be difficult to differentiate at times (Lebrun, 1993). In addition to perseverative responses, echolalic and stereotypical utterances can be also found back-to-back in successive responses. Christman, Boutsen, and Buckingham (2004) suggest that the salient features constituting the overall performance of a PWA must be considered to distinguish between related repetitive phenomena. These include the overall speech fluency, the inventory of available utterances, the nature of the task being administered, and the content of the response.

Echolalia is one form of repetitive behavior that is often also present in PWA who reveal a more severe tendency to perseverate (see Chapter 5, this volume). However, the two phenomena can be differentiated upon analysis of the source of utterances produced.

Stereotypical responses, automatisms, and *recurring utterances* are considered in the literature by some authors to represent the same phenomenon. Other authors consider stereotypies as the overproduction of single words or phrases, for example, "of course," "naturally," "so-so," "and so on," which can be appropriate in certain contexts. However, their extreme overuse makes them stereotypical. Recurring utterances are by far the most persistent type of repetitive oral behavior and, thus, most easily distinguishable from the other types of repetitive verbal behavior. They consist of the production of a single-phoneme combination (i.e., a real word or a neologism) each and every time a PWA spontaneously produces a response. The most famous case is Paul Broca's client "Monsieur Leborgne" who produced the recurring utterance "tan tan" (Broca, 1861).

The symptoms *recurring utterances, speech automatisms,* or *stereotypies* are present in individuals with severe language impairment—predominantly global aphasia. In this case, the PWA is only able to produce the same single word, phrase, or meaningless sound combination every time communication is attempted. Recurring or recurrent utterances (RUs) are defined by Blanken and colleagues (1988) as highly stereotyped and repetitively used utterances that are produced without phonological control. They constitute a highly complex and persistent production deficit in people with predominantly nonfluent, and in particular global aphasia. Wallesch (1990) and Code (1982) reported that real word recurring utterances (RWRU) result from activity of the right hemisphere. The functional lesion for non-meaningful recurring utterances (NMRU) is considered to be at the "bottom of the formulation apparatus" and may be indicative of basal ganglia damage.

For the clinician working with PWA, recurring utterances are the most severe repetitive deficit and also the most difficult to treat. Breaking through recurring utterances, that is, getting a PWA to produce words other than his/her recurring utterance(s) is very difficult. In the context of such a severe language production deficit, the symptoms of perseverations and recurring utterances overlap. For example, patient KB consistently produced two recurring utterances: the nonword *"unterfiat"* and the real word *"the greatest"* (English translation; Stark, 2014). In this context, novel perseverative responses can be considered an improvement. In one instance, KB perseverated a target word for the next item (instead of using one of the recurring utterances) and in another, KB produced a word that had been practiced the week before. Such perseverative responses are an indication that at some stage they were processed by KB and are still "active." KB also exhibited perseverations in his drawing of objects to be named. Helm-Estabrooks and colleagues (2013) provide interesting examples of perseveration in drawing, as drawing of the objects to be named is included in their Treatment of Aphasic Perseveration program.

ASSESSING VERBAL PERSEVERATION

In the clinical setting, it is seldom the case that a PWA will present with a "pure" deficit for which an exact procedure can be readily and directly applied and measurable changes in language performance achieved quickly. In the literature, most PWA are in the chronic stage and reveal multiple and severe deficits that require specific, intensive treatment over a longer period of time. Perseveration is one of the striking symptoms that requires the clinician's utmost attention. The clinician needs to understand that the observed perseverative behavior is a reflection of the PWA's underlying deficits. Thus, perseveration must be treated in the overall context of the individual's language impairment. It must be stressed that there is no specific assessment tool for assessing perseveration. In the process of administering standardized language tests and selected nonstandardized tasks that allow the clinician to assess specific aspects of language processing not included in the standardized procedures or to evaluate them in depth, the clinician observes the PWA's overall language performance and in particular documents the type of tasks (e.g., confrontation naming, picture description) where perseverations are present as well as their frequency.

Thus, a traditional in-depth language assessment of a PWA's abilities is required to reveal the PWA's strengths and weaknesses in various aspects of language processing and in turn to aid the clinician in developing the most adequate therapy approach for the PWA. The results from such an assessment will also bring to light the presence and severity of the perseverative behaviors in each language domain assessed. The clinician will then be able to combine language therapy goals and approaches with specific objectives and strategies to address the perseverative behaviors.

On the one hand, with regard to verbal perseveration, a comprehensive understanding of the PWA's language processing difficulties and the assumed functional locus/loci of the deficits will allow the clinician to treat the specific difficulties more adequately and target the cause(s) of the perseverative responses directly, as the perseverative responses result from the primary language deficit(s). On the other hand, an analysis of the evolution of a PWA's perseverative responses over time can help the clinician evaluate how the PWA is responding to the therapy being administered. If the administered treatment addressing the underlying language deficits is successful, the clinician will observe a concomitant reduction of perseverative responses and in some cases their total elimination.

The starting point for any therapeutic intervention to target verbal perseveration is a comprehensive understanding of the PWA's intact abilities, specific deficits, and their degree of severity. Formal, standardized tests or assessment materials preferred by the clinician can be used (e.g., Boston Diagnostic Aphasia Examination [BDAE]; Goodglass, Kaplan, & Barresi, 2001; Western Aphasia Battery-Revised [WAB-R], Kertesz, 2007), and informal assessment performed (see Chapter 13, this volume). The communicative experiences of the PWA (i.e., speaking, writing, hearing, reading) immediately prior to the appointment with the clinician may represent significant information for assessment purposes because any specific error could be a perseverative response. Without that information, responses may be classified as paraphasia, although they may actually be perseverative in nature. In this case, any information of prior communication may be of use to the clinician, but a complete record of the PWA's verbal communicative activities outside the therapy room is unlikely to be compiled.

In the process of conducting an interview or administering the language assessment tasks to determine the PWA's specific language difficulties, the reappearance of an immediately or recently produced language unit (i.e., phoneme, word, phrase, semantic feature, sentence, or idea) should be documented as a perseverative response. Oral and written confrontation naming tasks also provide valuable information regarding the tendency to perseverate phonemes and/or lexical items. Further it is important to evaluate word-finding for nouns and verbs further in the production of larger language units (i.e., sentences and texts) both orally and in writing. This will allow the clinician to determine whether the observed difficulties at the single-word level are more or less evident at the syntactic and discourse levels and in which modality they are observed.

Since the repertoire of language assessment tools at the clinician's disposal is dependent on the purpose of the language evaluation and his or her preferences, a prescribed set of specific tests or tasks for assessing perseveration is neither available nor necessary. The important issues are when, where, and how much a PWA responds with a perseveration.

As stated previously, the severity of perseverative behaviors can be described using several continuums:

1. *Frequency*: amount or percentage of perseverations per unit of language

2. *Persistence of perseverations*: PWA perseverates on multiple consecutive stimuli, possibly with a correct response in-between (= severe, but simple in form)

3. *Delay between source and perseveration*: PWA perseverates after a longer temporal or stimulus interval with correct items in-between

4. *Combination of perseveration types*: PWA perseverates using several stimuli resulting in an interlacing or blending of features (severity due to complexity of form)

In the first continuum, the mere frequency of perseverations determines the level of severity. In the second continuum, when a PWA continues to perseverate the same form (e.g., phoneme(s), whole word, etc.) over several consecutive items and then perseverates another response also for several items (even if it is only a single phoneme or word), the tendency to perseverate is to be characterized as severe. The most serious form of this type of repetitive behavior is a recurring utterance. In the third continuum, the PWA is able to correctly name or produce paraphasias for the target items. However, the perseverated word remains activated and fills the gap when the next lexical retrieval difficulty arises. In the fourth continuum, the perseverative behavior is to be characterized as severe due to the complexity of the response: components or parts of several responses are interlaced resulting in more complex perseverative responses. All of these continuums should be considered when evaluating perseverative behavior in PWA.

In the literature, various measures are described for calculating the severity of perseveration in a PWA as well as the candidacy for a specific therapy method targeting perseverative behavior. These measures are summarized in Table 1.2. The two perseveration measures advocated by Cohen and Dehaene (1998) require statistical analyses to compute chance values. This process requires a time commitment and some knowledge of statistical procedures.

TREATING VERBAL PERSEVERATION

Moses and colleagues (2004) examined recurrent perseveration in PWA and suggested possible directions for intervention. After diagnosing presence, type, and severity of perseveration, they recommended that the clinician should:

- *Increase the activation of the target.* By providing specific cues that are adequate for the PWA (e.g., semantic, phonemic, etc.), the clinician can increase the activation level for the target word, which should result in the production of the correct name. This suggestion is in line with the view that the activation of the target word is insufficient.

- *Avoid adding more activation to the perseveration.* The clinician should avoid using the perseverated word and should not produce it when providing the PWA with feedback or assistance. The clinician's use of the word would draw more attention to the perseveration, which would thus receive more activation.

- *Provide alternative communicative strategies.* If the clinician cannot elicit the target word by providing one or more cues to the PWA, then the clinician should resort to other strategies, such as providing a circumlocution or gesture to elicit the target word or instructing the PWA to acknowledge that he or she does not know the word.

- *Encourage self-monitoring.* One aim of therapy should be to develop the PWA's ability to self-monitor and self-correct errors. The authors suggested that the clinician encourage the PWA to stop and think before producing a response, in the hope that the PWA will produce the target word or, possibly, state that he or she does not know the answer.

- *Educate family members and caregivers about perseveration.*

The overall suggestions notwithstanding, the authors nevertheless conclude that the clinician should focus on treating the underlying language impairment rather than treating perseverative errors as an isolated problem, since perseveration is symptomatic of the specific underlying language impairment. This illustrates the two possible approaches to remediating perseverative behaviors in PWA: *targeting perseverations* and *targeting the underlying language impairment.* These two alternatives are discussed in detail next.

Treatment Targeting Perseveration

This approach considers perseverations as the root cause of the problem and posits that perseverations block the retrieval of a target word. According to this hypothesis, the clinicians should use general strategies to prevent the blockage such as increased stimulus interval or extended pause time. This approach is related to the overactivation account (von Sölder, 1895, 1899). However, the proponents of this approach also usually provide concomitant therapy for naming, which transforms this technique into a hybrid approach.

In theory, this approach focuses on specific aspects of therapy administration and requires that the clinician immediately respond to a client who perseverates. The strategies used in this approach aim at breaking through the tendency to perseverate by (a) asking the client to take a deep breath, (b) using a hand gesture to stop the client from responding too quickly, (c) pausing by conversing with the PWA briefly about something entirely different, or (d) presenting the task items with more than the usual amount of time between each one. These suggestions may seem like common sense but they often succeed because they interrupt the PWA from continuing to speak or write. The short interruption allows the (over)activated language units to return to their resting state or to a lower activation level. This allows the PWA to start again and possibly overcome the specific difficulties, for example, of finding a specific word. In such an instance, the brief interruption in producing speech may positively influence the word retrieval process.

The aforementioned strategies are important for treatment planning as well as for administering therapy to PWA who reveal a tendency to perseverate. For a PWA whose oral language production consists mainly of perseverative responses, targeting the specific language deficits as well as the perseverative behavior will be difficult. Initially, the manner in which the clinician is able to break through the severe perseverative tendency is crucial for the therapy process. Only when the frequency of the perseverations decreases will it be possible to administer the planned specific language treatment. In the case of a PWA with milder symptoms, a judicious selection of the stimuli may have a heightened contribution to reducing the frequency of perseverative responses. For example, words that are very different phonologically or semantically will tend to minimize the risk of perseveration, whereas selecting minimal pairs or phonologically similar words or lexical items from the same semantic category will tend to increase the tendency to perseverate.

In the context of this approach targeting perseverations directly, two therapy programs have been published to date: *Treatment of Aphasic Perseveration* (TAP; Helm-Estabrooks, Emery, & Albert, 1987; Helm-Estabrooks et al., 2013) and *Reducing Aphasic Perseveration* (RAP; Muñoz, 2011, 2014).

Treatment of Aphasic Perseveration (TAP)

The first published therapy approach for explicitly and directly treating perseveration is the TAP therapy protocol (Helm-Estabrooks, 1987), which was revised in Estabrooks et al. (2013). The authors state that nonperseverative responses can be achieved by bring-ing perseverative responses, which block the production of the correct ones, under con-trol. The intent of their approach is to bring "perseverative behavior to the individual's level of awareness and help him or her suppress perseverative responses" (p. 264) and in turn to produce correct responses. Thus, the functional goal of their program is to reduce recurrent verbal perseverations that block retrieval and production of the correct target words by bringing perseverative responses under control.

Based on results from a pretest, the best candidates for the TAP program are PWA who reveal a moderate to severe tendency to perseverate, but are fully alert, have moderately preserved auditory comprehension and memory skills, and are able to name some objects. To determine a person's candidacy for the program, a two-step procedure is followed. The PWA must score at least 20% on the Perseveration Severity Rating, which is calculated by dividing the number of perseverative responses in the visual confrontation naming and word discrimination tasks of the Boston Diagnostic Aphasia Examination (BDAE; Good-glass et al., 2001) by the number of total responses (see Table 1.2). The TAP approach follows an ABAB therapy design alternating TAP therapy periods with standard language therapy periods. Each phase consists of five sessions: TAP—standard treatment—TAP—standard treatment—TAP. After each phase, progress is charted by the changes (a) in the number of correctly named objects and (b) the percentage of perseverative responses. The scoring system ranges from 0 for no perseveration up to 4 for a perseverative response produced after three cues have been given.

Before administering the program, a hierarchy of semantic categories (taken from the categories assessed by the BDAE in the confrontation naming task) is established for each PWA based on his or her test performance. In the actual therapy the PWA is required to name pictured and real objects. The clinician may provide up to 3 of the following 10 specific strategies, which are selected for each PWA based on the diagnosed symptoms (described later here). A list of 38 TAP stimuli to be used with all patients is also provided by the authors.

The authors provide four general strategies that are applied with each PWA participat-ing in the program. These include:

1. *Explain and alert to perseveration.* Before initiating the TAP program, the clinician explains to the PWA what perseveration is and the purpose of TAP.

2. *Establish task sets.* Before proceeding to the next item to be named, the PWA should be made aware that it is a new item.

3. *Bring perseveration to the level of awareness.* The clinician makes the PWA aware that he or she is perseverating, for example, by writing down the perseveration on a piece of paper and then ripping it up and leaving the pieces of paper on the table and pointing to them when the PWA perseverates again.

4. *Monitor presentation pace.* Allow at least a 5-second break before presenting the next item stimulus to be named.

Furthermore, the authors propose 10 specific strategies to be used for cueing in the TAP approach. They are ranked according to the amount of assistance provided by the clinician from minimal to maximal assistance:

1. *Time interval* (TI): A 5- or 10-second interval is imposed before the PWA can respond.

2. *Gestural cue* (GC): A pantomime associated with the object to be named is provided.

3. *Drawing* (D): A picture of the object is drawn and the PWA says the name as soon as he or she recognizes the object, or the clinician asks the PWA to draw the object.

4. *Descriptive sentences* (DS): The object or its function is described by the clinician.

5. *Sentence completion*: An open-ended sentence for the PWA to complete is provided.

6. *Graphic cue* (GC): The first (two) letter(s) of the target word is (are) written down and the PWA is asked to complete writing it and then read the word aloud.

7. *Phonemic cue* (PC): The initial phoneme of the target word is provided. ("This is a(n) /initial phoneme/.")

8. *Oral reading* (OR): The PWA is asked to read aloud the target word written down by the clinician.

9. *Repetition* (R): The PWA is asked to repeat the target word.

10. *Unison speech or singing* (US): The PWA is asked to say or sing the target word with the clinician. (p. 271)

The authors stress that the selection of the order of the strategies is based on the individual needs of each PWA and can be modified if needed.

Since the introduction of the TAP approach in 1987, Helm-Estabrooks and her colleagues have administered it successfully to numerous clients and have also refined the technique. In summary, even though the TAP approach is designed to directly treat perseveration, by means of the TAP procedure of general strategies the authors are also actually providing therapy for the underlying functional naming deficit(s). Although TAP is subsumed under the first approach, that is, to treat perseverative behavior, it actually adheres to both approaches: applying general strategies for targeting perseverations and therapy for underlying word-finding difficulties.

Reducing Aphasic Perseveration (RAP)

Another treatment focusing directly on perseverative behaviors is Reducing Aphasic Perseveration (RAP; Muñoz, 2011, 2014). Muñoz (2011) summarizes a therapy study that is specifically aimed at reducing perseverative responses in a Spanish-speaking PWA (SC) presenting with moderate to severe receptive-expressive aphasia with severe naming deficits. The theory behind RAP stems from Cohen and Dehaene's (1998) and Martin and Dell's (2007) account of the origin of perseverative responses: persistent activation of a previous response in combination with weak activation of the new target word. The treatment protocol targets the overactivation of the perseverative response and the underactivation of the correct target response by systematically manipulating the interstimulus interval (ISI) between items in a picture naming task. The time interval before presenting the next picture was increased or decreased depending on whether a perseveration was or was not produced. Between stimuli an ISI of 20 seconds was used and it was reduced by 2 seconds if a perseverative response was not produced regardless of the accuracy of the response. If a perseveration was produced, the interval for the next picture stimuli was increased by 2 seconds. As a second component of the therapy, the Semantic Feature Analysis (SFA) protocol (Boyle & Coelho, 1995) was administered in which SC was asked to identify attributes of the items that were incorrectly named by providing their function and physical properties.

The therapy resulted in a decrease in perseverative responses. However, naming accuracy showed only a minor improvement on trained and untrained stimuli, possibly due to the short duration of the therapy. The author notes an observed increase in the PWA's overall verbal output, as well as an increase in his communicative effectiveness as judged by the PWA and his family. At follow up, his decreased tendency to perseverate was maintained. Muñoz claims that the results of her study suggest that the language therapy provided to SC successfully reduced perseveration and increased verbal output.

Muñoz (2011, 2014) designed RAP to reduce the occurrence of perseverative responses on trained and untrained picture stimuli using a naming paradigm by systematically manipulating the time between the presentation of each item and increasing the activation of the target. The RAP method is for PWA who frequently perseverate—on the order of 30% or more (see Table 1.2). The author emphasizes that the goal of the therapy protocol is not to increase the PWA's naming accuracy, although that may occur. For this reason, this method is considered to be representative of the first approach. Under the second approach, the clinician would expect naming accuracy to improve, since the treatment target would be to improve naming and this would result in a reduction of perseverative responses.

Before therapy is initiated the clinician administers a naming task and records a spontaneous speech sample (interview and picture description). Then the PWA and caregivers are instructed about what perseveration means. RAP itself consists of a two-part treatment cycle: (1) Manipulation of the interstimulus interval (ISI) between the presentation of each picture stimulus from a confrontation naming task, and (2) SFA. The therapy itself consists in administering SFA (Boyle & Coelho, 1995) to those items incorrectly named in the first part of the cycle. This cycle is repeated for each item and the ISI is adjusted to the needs of the PWA. The homework involves practicing the trained words using the pictures from therapy.

Although the stated emphasis of both TAP and RAP is to treat perseverative behavior directly, it must be noted that both also include structured naming tasks. Thus, in both protocols the clinicians are also addressing the specific deficits of the PWA, which is the main tenet of the second approach to treating perseverative behaviors by administering therapy targeting the specific deficits.

Treatment Targeting the Underlying Language Impairment

In the second rehabilitation approach, the clinician targets the specific language deficits in therapy. This approach posits that perseverations are a reflection of the primary language deficits of the PWA in accordance with the Deficit Account (Heilbronner, 1895, 1897, 1906; Lissauer, 1890). This explains why a PWA will display perseverative behaviors in the impaired language domains. For example, if a word cannot be retrieved (i.e., anomia), the gap is automatically filled by an available (i.e., previously activated) item. In this instance, the perseveration is secondary to the word-finding problem and the therapy should focus on the underlying anomia problem. It is anticipated that the administered therapy will result in a reduction of perseverative responses. In this case, perseverations are treated by directly treating the specific underlying language deficits of a PWA and thereby eliminating the source for perseverative behavior. This perspective is reflected in some patient studies on perseveration (Basso, 2003, 2004; Moses et al., 2004; Papagno & Basso, 1996; Stark, 1984, 2007a, 2007b, 2011b; Stark, Kristoferitsch, Graf, Gelpi, & Budka, 2007).

Basso (2003, 2004) and Papagno and Basso (1996) are proponents of this approach focused on treating the underlying language impairment. Basso (2004) analyzed language data collected from 50 consecutive PWA from her clinic to determine the occurrence of perseveration in an unselected group. In that study she also described the language therapy administered to two PWA who showed a high rate of perseveration. Treated Subject 1 (cited as TS1, AB, or BA in various publications) displayed transcortical sensory aphasia—resulting from a gunshot wound—with a severe impairment of the lexical-semantic system and relatively well preserved sublexical processing. He perseverated in all production and comprehension tasks, except for repetition, reading aloud, and writing to dictation. He also perseverated in drawing objects. The therapy concept developed for him targeted his impairments in the lexical-semantic system, because perseverations were produced only when TS1 was unable to produce the correct response (Papagno & Basso, 1996). The therapy administered to this PWA focused on semantic processing (Basso, 1993, 2004) and consisted of the following tasks:

1. Categorization

2. Odd-one-out

3. Picture verification tasks

For the categorization tasks, two categories were targeted: clothing and food. Initially he was unable to perform the odd-one-out task, which consisted of five pictures, four of which were animals and one was from a distant category (furniture). The authors report that targeting whole semantic categories was not successful for this patient. For this reason, in a second therapy attempt, single concepts were targeted, starting with the category of tools. The procedure consisted of several steps:

1. A picture of a hammer was shown to him and after being unable to name it, he was asked to copy it.

2. Discussion of all the parts of a hammer and explanation of its use.

3. Demonstration of use of the hammer. With the picture in view, he was asked to pretend to use it.

4. The next step was for him to pretend to use it without the picture being visible and then to draw the object from memory.

It took a great deal of therapy for the PWA to achieve a recognizable drawing of a hammer. When this was achieved, a new concept was introduced and the same procedure was followed. Two other categories were worked on: kitchen utensils and clothing. The perseverative responses first disappeared in pointing tasks, followed by written naming tasks. The authors reported "TS1 showed a slow but progressive improvement and simultaneous reduction of semantic errors and perseverations" (p. 383). Therapy was administered for 2 years, and at the last control he revealed mild Wernicke's aphasia with rare semantic errors, perseverations, and word-finding difficulties.

Treated Subject 2 (TS2) had mild Wernicke's aphasia with agraphia. She also revealed a functional deficit at the level of the semantic system that expressed itself as semantic errors in oral naming. TS2's more severe writing impairment was ascribed to a deficit in the output buffer. She perseverated in all writing tasks. TS2 received treatment for her output buffer deficits (according to the cognitive-neuropsychological model; Whitworth, Webster, & Howard, 2005) that resulted in a striking reduction of perseverative responses in writing. Summarizing the two case studies, Basso (2004) maintains that treatment should vary according to the underlying deficit (as proposed by Moses et al., 2004 and Stark, 2011b). By treating the underlying deficits the clinician should observe a reduction in the PWA's perseverative behavior. Moreover, "... besides having a hypothesis about when perseverations occur, we should know the mechanisms responsible for the appearance of perseverations" (p. 388). After locating the deficit, a theoretically based treatment *must* be administered for language in general, which will result in a reduction of perseveration, if the hypothesis underlying the therapy concept is valid.

CONCLUSION

Perseveration is one of the most challenging symptoms for a clinician to deal with in the clinical setting. The claim being made throughout this chapter is that a PWA's perseverative behavior is a reflection of his or her underlying deficits. For this reason, the perseverative behavior must be treated in the context of the individual's language deficit(s). The therapy goals developed to treat the PWA's specific language impairment(s) are paramount. The clinician also should implement general strategies necessary for the provision of any therapy protocol such as appropriate cueing, feedback, and reinforcement. However, particular emphasis should also be placed on reducing the occurrence of perseverative responses by selecting and applying strategies shown to reduce perseverations, such as pausing, increasing interstimulus delays, etc. Although there is no single assessment for perseveration, in-depth assessment of a PWA's language abilities is required to arrive at an overall picture of the nature and extent of the perseverative behavior and, in turn, to conceptualize the most appropriate therapy approach for that client with a tendency to perseverate.

With regard to verbal perseveration, a comprehensive understanding of the PWA's language processing difficulties will allow the clinician to treat the specific difficulties more adequately and at the same time treat perseveration directly, as the perseverative responses result from the primary deficit(s). In addition, analysis of a PWA's perseverative responses will provide the clinician with more information regarding the assumed functional locus/ loci of the deficits and also how the therapy is proceeding. Most importantly, under the assumption that the perseverative tendency will decline when the administered treatment targeting the underlying deficits is successful, the clinician will observe a reduction of perseverative responses and in some cases total elimination.

CASE ILLUSTRATION

Another example illustrating the second approach is the case illustration of MV. She is a 69-year-old, German-speaking pharmacist 7 months post CVA presenting with moderate Wernicke's aphasia. Extensive language testing revealed a moderate tendency to perseverate nouns and verbs in various oral and written naming tasks, and other production tasks, including sentence and discourse tasks. When MV could lead the conversation and was not required to produce a specific single target word, her language production was generally more coherent and adequate. Initially, she frequently produced phonemic and semantic paraphasias as well as neologisms, and she revealed self-correcting behaviors in conversational speech, confrontation naming, and repetition tasks. Her successive approximations often resulted in perseverative responses.

In **FIGURE 1.1** the results are given for the first Aachen Aphasia Test (AAT; Huber, Poeck, Weniger, & Willmes, 1983) administered pre-therapy at 7 months post onset.

Initially MV was most impaired on the naming subtests of the AAT (59/120) that required the production of simple and compound nouns and color names and sentences. For the repetition subtest in which phonemes, words, and sentences were repeated, her score was 108 out of 150. For the other subtests of the AAT: Token Test, written language, and auditory and written comprehension of words and sentences, she was mildly impaired. She produced recurrent perseverations mainly in confrontation naming of nouns, compound nouns, and color names on the AAT and also for items on the Boston Naming Test (BNT; Kaplan, Goodglass, & Weintraub, 1983) and the Action Naming Test (ANT; Obler & Albert, 1979).

MV's pretherapy score on the BNT was 11/60 correct (18%) and on the ANT 44/63 correct (70%). It must be stressed that MV was allowed ample time to respond. On all tasks she produced multiple responses; however, in most cases her attempts resulted in phonological and semantic paraphasias.

For example, MV produced the following perseverative responses on the AAT:

1. Word repetition:
   a) ***Kn**irps* (umbrella) → [correct]
      Zwist (dispute) → ***kn**ick-**kn**icks- swis*
   b) Püre (mashed potatoes) → [correct]
      Pilot → pire

2. Sentence repetition (translated from German):
   "He picked his mother with a new ***car*** from the train station up" → He picked my mother from a –ah with the ***car*** from the ***car*** up

3. Sentence naming to picture stimuli:
   Item 3: "The man fished/caught a boot" The man fished/caught a boot That is the ah- ah /flos/ and /lof/ he has led a pair of shoes instead a ***/fusch/- /fusch/*** [for /fish/] …
   Item 6: "The policeman is arresting the criminal" → Here is the /po-poliziden/ poli-police is holding him ah-ah backwards with the ***fish*** [for the target: handcuffs].

In these examples phonemes and phoneme clusters as well as whole words were perseverated.

Based on the data from the language assessments, the clinician designed the therapy protocol to target MV's difficulties in retrieving and producing nouns and verbs, particularly in the context of oral and written sentence to picture stimuli. The assumption behind the therapy protocol conceived for MV was to reduce or eliminate her word retrieval and production difficulties that often resulted in perseverative behavior by directly targeting her noun and verb retrieval deficits in the context of oral sentence production with extensive retrieval practice and recall of the treated items. Moreover, as her auditory comprehension was relatively intact for single words and sentences, she was considered a good candidate for the ELA-Syntax program (ELA= Everyday Life Activities; Stark, 2005). It was assumed that she would benefit from the structure of the protocol requiring her to retrieve the nouns and verbs depicting relevant everyday activities and to stick with the first semantically adequate sentence produced to a picture stimulus, as well as to answer questions about the constituents of the produced sentences.

AATP for Windows
Assessment Program for the Aachen Aphasia Test
T-Value Profile of the Subtests

Patient: MV
Address: Vienna
Patient ID: 1
Test number: 1

Date of birth (d/m/yr): 05/06/1924
Age: 69
Aphasia begin (d/m/yr): 01/12/1993
Months post onset: 6

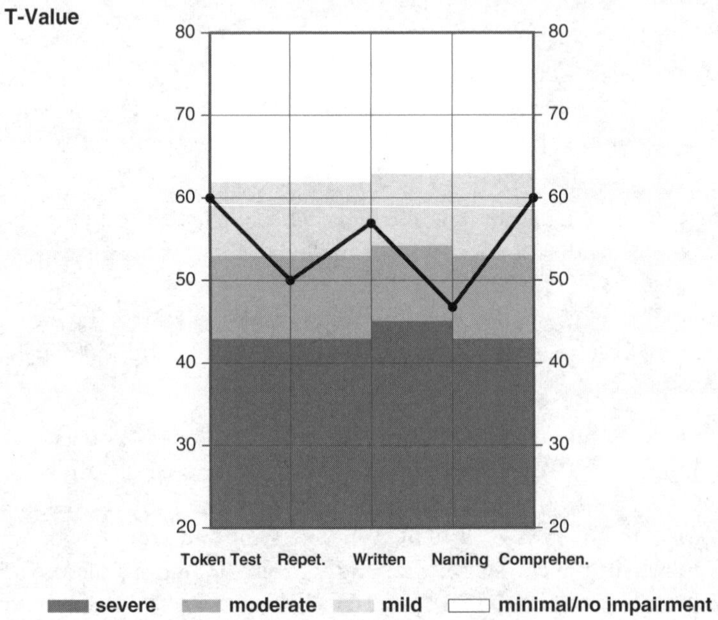

T-Value

Token Test   Repet.   Written   Naming   Comprehen.

■ severe   ■ moderate   ■ mild   ☐ minimal/no impairment

Single case diagnostic results:

	NAMING	REPET.	WRITTEN	COMPREHEN.	TOKEN TEST
	(47)	(50)	(57)	(60)	(60)

FIGURE 1.1 Results from the pre-therapy language assessment for the Aachen Aphasia Test (AAT) at seven months post onset

Three trial sessions were administered to introduce the overall structure of the program to MV and for the clinician to acquaint herself with the most adequate way of providing feedback to MV. She then received 60 hourly therapy sessions. The therapy protocol consisted of a sequence of steps that was held constant for the 60 sessions and the therapy was provided three to four times per week. The overall structure of the ELA protocol is in accordance with the principles of experience-dependent neuroplasticity (Kleim & Jones, 2008) with a main focus on oral sentence production to picture stimuli depicting everyday life activities. Following a brief conversation, the steps for each session included:

1. Recall of the sentences worked on in the previous session

2. Sentence production to picture stimuli from last session ("old cards")

3. Sentence production to new picture stimuli (N = 12) ("new cards")

4. Questions about the constituents of the sentence
   (Steps 3 and 4 done consecutively for each stimulus)

5. Auditory sentence comprehension check

6. Second trial of sentence production to new picture stimuli

7. Recall of the sentences worked on in the actual session

Intensive feedback was provided for steps 2 to 6. Multiple repetitions and production of the correct sentences in unison resulted in a steady improvement, and in turn, fewer perseverative responses. The homework assignment consisted of writing down the sentences worked on in therapy from memory.

In the first therapy session examples of MV's perseverations included:

1. *Stimulus card 1.* Das Mädchen **putzt** sich die Ohren ["The girl is cleaning her ears"] (After multiple attempts and feedback from the clinician MV finally produces the whole sentence correctly.)
   Stimulus card 2. Der Bub stellt den Wecker ab ["The boy is turning off the alarm clock"] → Der Bub will **sich die Ohren** [persev.] ... Der Bub buz- **putzt** [persev.] ["The boy wants to his ears ~ ~ The boy is ~ clean—cleaning"]

2. *Stimulus card 4.* Das Mädchen föhnt seine Haare ["The girl is blow drying her hair"]. She also produced "das Fräulein" [paraph.] ["the young lady"] for girl.
   Stimulus card 5. "Die Frau raucht eine Zigarette" ["The **woman** is smoking a cigarette"] → Das **Fräulein [persev.]** pfeunt [neologism] mit der .. ah zeunt [neologism] mit der Zigarette" ... Sie fennt -... sie **föhnt** [persev.] sich gerade die Zigarette auf. ["She blow dries just now a cigarette on/up"]

Several instances of perseveration were observed for single phonemes and consonant clusters affecting both the verbs and nouns in the produced sentences. Each stimulus required multiple attempts before MV was able to produce a correct response which upon repetition was either correct, a perseveration, or a paraphasia. MV's self-monitoring ability, that is, her awareness of the produced errors improved over time. Initially, she revealed less self-corrective behavior, which is one indication that she was not aware of them. Her responses to questions pertaining to single components of the sentences were often correct, but she also produced phonological and semantic paraphasias and neologisms and semantically inadequate responses. She also perseverated verbs in her home practice assignment: The verb "give" was perseverated for three sentences.

a. "Der Bub gibt [paraph.] (Target: "nimmt") einen Teller aus dem Kasten" ["The boy is **giving** (Target: "taking") a plate out of the cupboard]

b. "Die Frau **gibt** [persev.] (Target: "steckt … ein") den Stecker in die Steckdose" ["The woman is **giving** (Target: "putting … in") the plug into the outlet"]

c. "Der Mann **gibt** [persev.] (Target: "schenkt … ein") aus der Flasche ein Glas Wein" ["The man is **giving** (Target: "pouring … in") from the bottle a glass [of] wine"]

The first verb was incorrectly produced as "give" in place of "take." In sentences to the following picture stimuli, she perseverated the verb "give" in the third person singular form. In one case "give" would be an adequate verb as a less specific formulation for "steckt … ein" ("put … in").

It is important to note that during the assessment MV produced a mixture of errors and perseverative responses were among them. However, in the initial phase of therapy her retrieval and production difficulties became more pronounced and she produced more perseverative responses. However, as therapy progressed MV's ability to retrieve the correct nouns and verbs improved steadily. Initially, during home practice, MV was able to recall 7 of the 10 sentences worked on in therapy, although her written productions exhibited paraphasias and perseverations. In later therapy sessions, she recalled all of the sentences with minor spelling errors. As therapy progressed, it became apparent that interrupting MV's attempts to retrieve and produce the correct verb were successful in breaking through the perseverative tendency. For this reason, the clinician added having MV take a deep breath and pausing whenever she perseverated. This general strategy carried over so well to everyday life that a relative thought MV had difficulties breathing! Initially the clinician had MV stop speaking and listen to the correct production and only then had her repeat it. This interruption sufficed until she produced a perseverative response; then it became necessary to introduce the "breathing pause."

As a proponent of the importance of qualitatively analyzing language data from therapy sessions as a realistic indicator of a PWA's performance, the transcripts from the 1st and 60th therapy sessions were analyzed. In **TABLE 1.3** a comparison of MV's language performance in the 1st and 60th therapy sessions revealed a marked reduction in the number of errors on the variables which related to her language deficits.

The second AAT, administered following the 60 therapy sessions at 12 months post onset, revealed improved performance on the subtests that were initially most impaired (**FIGURE 1.2**): mild impairment for the naming and repetition subtests and minimal to no impairment on the other subtests.

MV's scores improved on the BNT and ANT: 37/60 (67%) and 52/63 (82.5%), respectively. Thus, MV's post-therapy performance on the BNT revealed an increase in 49% correct and for the ANT an increase in 12.5% correct. A carryover of therapy effects from oral sentence production—the modality worked on in therapy—to the untrained modality of written sentence production (= home practice assignment in which she also perseverated) was also observed. Thus, by specifically treating MV's lexical retrieval difficulties in a systematic, linguistically structured manner in combination with general strategies to minimize perseveration, perseveration was no longer an issue for her.

TABLE 1.3 Comparison of MV's language performance in the 1st and 60th therapy sessions for selected variables.

Analyzed Variables	1st Therapy Session	60th Therapy Session
Perseveration	40	1
Phonological paraphasia	45	4
Neologisms	37	1
Semantic paraphasia	18	0
Successive approximations (incorrect) (conduite d'approche)	33	1
Self-correction	13	17
Incorrect verbs	18	1

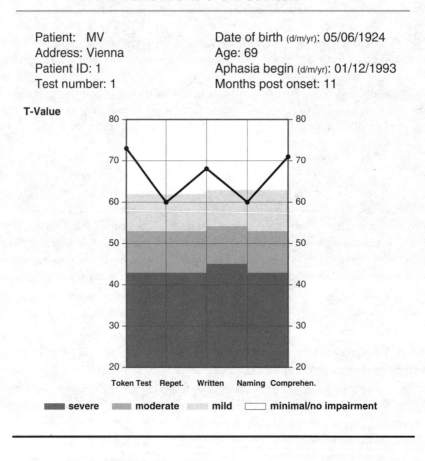

FIGURE 1.2 "Results from the post-therapy language assessment for the Aachen Aphasia Test (AAT) at 12 months post onset Aachen Aphasia Test.

REFERENCES

Albert, M. L., & Sandson, J. (1986). Perseveration in aphasia. *Cortex, 22,* 103–115.

Basso, A. (1993). Two cases of lexical-semantic rehabilitation. In F.-J. Stachowiak (Ed.), *Developments in the assessment and rehabilitation of brain-damaged patients.* Tübingen: Gunter Narr Verlag, pp. 259–262.

Basso, A. (2003). *Aphasia and its therapy.* New York: Oxford University Press.

Basso, A. (2004). Perseveration, or the Tower of Babel. *Seminars in Speech and Language, 25,* 375–389.

Blanken, G., Dittmann, J., Haas, J.-C., & Wallesch, C.-W. (1988). Producing speech automatisms (recurring utterances): Looking for what is left. *Aphasiology, 2,* 545–556.

Boyle, M., & Coelho, C. A. (1995). Application of semantic feature analysis as a treatment for aphasic dysnomia. *American Journal of Speech-Language Pathology, 4,* 94–98.

Broca, P. (1861). Perte de la parole: Ramollissement chronique et destruction partielle du lobe antérieur gauche du cerveau. *Bulletins de la Sociéte d'anthropologie, 1ère série, 2,* 235–238.

Buckingham, H. W. (1985). Perseveration in aphasia. In: S. Newman & R. Epstein (Eds.), *Current perspectives in dysphasia* (pp. 113–154). Edinburgh: Churchill Livingston.

Buckingham, H. W. (1987). Phonemic paraphasia and psycholinguistic production models for neologistic jargon. *Aphasiology, 1,* 381–400.

Buckingham, H. W., Avakian-Whitaker, H., & Whitaker, H. A. (1978). Alliteration and assonance in neologistic jargon aphasia. *Cortex, 14,* 365–380.

Buckingham, H. W., & Buckingham, S. S. (2011). Is recurrent perseveration a product of deafferented functional systems with otherwise normal post-activation decay rates? *Clinical Linguistics and Phonetics, 25* (11–12), 1066–1073.

Buckingham, H. W., & Kertesz, A. (Eds.). (1976). *Neologistic Jargon Aphasia.* Amsterdam: Swets & Zeitlinger.

Christman, S., Boutsen, F. R., & Buckingham, H. W. (2004). Perseveration and other repetitive verbal behaviors: Functional dissociations. *Seminars in Speech and Language, 25*(4), 295–307.

Code, C. (1982). Neurolinguistic analysis of recurrent utterances in aphasia. *Cortex, 18,* 141–152.

Cohen, L., & Dehaene, S. (1998). Competition between past and present assessment and interpretation of verbal perseverations. *Brain, 121,* 1641–1650.

Dell, G. S., Burger, L. K., & Svec, W. L. (1997). Language production and serial order: A functional analysis and a model. *Psychological Review, 104,* 123–147.

Dempster, F. N. (1991). Inhibitory processes: A neglected dimension of intelligence. *Intelligence, 15,* 157–173.

Goodglass, H., Gleason, J. B., Bernholtz, N. A., & Hyde, M. R. (1972). Some linguistic structures in the speech of a Broca's aphasic. *Cortex, 8,* 191–212.

Goodglass, H., & Kaplan, E. (1979). Assessment of the cognitive deficit in the brain-injured patient. In: M. S. Gazzaniga (Ed.), *Handbook of behavioral neurobiology,* Volume 2 neuropsychology (pp. 3–22). New York: Plenum Press.

Goodglass, H., Kaplan, E., & Barresi, B. (2001). *Boston Diagnostic Aphasia Examination* (3rd ed.). Philadelphia, PA: Lippincott Williams & Wilkins.

Gotts, S. J., della Rochetta, A. I., & Cipolotti, L. (2002). Mechanisms underlying perseveration in aphasia: Evidence from a single case study. *Neuropsychologia, 40,* 1930–1947.

Gotts, S. J., & Plaut, D. C. (2004). Connectionist approaches to understanding aphasic perseveration. *Seminars in Speech and Language, 25*(4), 323–334.

Heilbronner, K. (1895). Krankenvorstellung (Fall von "Asymbolie"). *Allgemeine Zeitschrift für Psychiatrie, 51,* 1014–1015.

Heilbronner, K. (1897). Über Asymbolie. *Psychiatrische Abhandlungen, 3 und 4*, 1–60.

Heilbronner, K. (1906). Über Haftenbleiben und Stereotypie. *Ergänzungsheft der Monatsschrift für Psychiatrie, 18*, 293–371.

Helm-Estabrooks, N., Albert, M. L., & Nicholas, M. (2013). *Manual of aphasia and aphasia therapy* (3rd ed.). Austin, TX: Pro-Ed.

Helm-Estabrooks, N., Emery, P., & Albert, M. L. (1987). Treatment of Aphasic Perseveration (TAP) program. A new approach to aphasia therapy. *Archives of Neurology, 44*, 1253–1255.

Helm-Estabrooks, N., Ramage. A., Bayles. K. A., & Cruz, R. (1998). Perseverative behavior in fluent and non-fluent aphasia. *Aphasiology, 12*, 7–8.

Huber, W., Poeck, K., Weniger, D., & Willmes, K. (1983). Aachener Aphasie Test (AAT). Göttingen: Verlag für Psychologie.

Kaplan, E., Goodglass, H., & Weintraub, S. (1983). *Boston Naming Test*. Philadelphia, PA: Lea & Febiger.

Kertesz, A. (2007). *Western Aphasia Battery-Revised*. San Antonio, TX: Psychological Corporation.

Kleim, J. A., & Jones, T. A. (2008). Principles of experience-dependent neural plasticity: Implications for rehabilitation after brain damage. *Journal of Speech, Language, and Hearing Research, 51*, S225–S239.

Lebrun, Y. (1993). Repetitive phenomena in aphasia. In G. Blanken, J. Dittmann, H. Grimm, J. C. Marshall, & C.-W. Wallesch (Eds.), *Linguistic disorders and pathologies: An international handbook* (pp. 225–238). Berlin, Germany: Walter deGruyter.

Liepmann, H. (1905). *Ueber Störungen des Handelns bei Gehirnkranken*. Berlin: Karger.

Lissauer, H. (1890). Ein Fall von Seelenblindheit, nebst einem Beitrag zur Theorie derselben. *Archiv für Psychiatrie und Nervenkrankheiten, 21*, 222–270.

Martin, N. (2011). Similarities and differences between perseverative and non-perseverative errors in aphasia: Theoretical and clinical implications. *Perspectives on Neurophysiology and Neurogenic Speech and Language Disorders, 21*(4), 166–174.

Martin, N., & Dell, G. S. (2004). Perseverations and anticipations in aphasia: Primed intrusions from the past and future. *Seminars in Speech and Language, 25*(4), 349–362.

Martin, N., & Dell, G. S. (2007). Common mechanisms underlying perseverative and non-perseverative sound and word substitutions. *Aphasiology, 21*(10/11), 1002–1017.

McNamera, P., & Albert, M. L. (2004). Neuropharmacology of verbal perseveration. *Seminars in Speech and Language, 25*(4), 309–321.

Moses, M., Nickels, L., & Sheard, C. (2004). That dreaded word perseveration! Understanding might be the key. *Acquiring Knowledge in Speech, Language and Hearing, 6*, 70–74.

Muñoz, M. L. (2011). Reducing aphasic perseverations: A case study. *Perspectives on Neurophysiology and Neurogenic Speech and Language Disorders, 21*(4), 175–182.

Muñoz, M. L. (2014). *The clinician's guide to reducing aphasic perseveration*. Fort Worth, TX: Recipe SLP.

Neisser, C. (1895). 65. Sitzung des Vereins ostdeutscher Irrenärzte zu Breslau den 1. Juli 1894, Krankenvorstellung (Fall von Asymbolie). *Allgemeine Zeitschrift für Psychiatrie, 51*, 1016.

Obler, L. K., & Albert, M. L. (1979). *Action Naming Test. Experimental Edition*.

Papagno, C., & Basso, A. (1996). Perseverations in two aphasic patients. *Cortex, 32*, 67–82.

Pick, A. (1892). Beiträge zur lehre von den störungen der sprache. *Archiv für Psychiatrie, 23*, 896–918.

Pick, A. (1900). Über die bedeutung des akustischen sprachzentrums als hemmungsorgan des sprachmechanismus. *Wiener Klinische Wochenschrift, 37*, 823–827.

Pick, A. (1902). Beiträge zur lehre von der echolalie. *Jahrbuch für Psychiatrie und Neurologie, 21,* 282–293.

Pick, A. (1903). Etude clinique sur les troubles de la conscience dans l'état postépileptique. *Annales Médico-psychologiques, 17,* 18–54. (Extrait: Janvier-Févier, 1903: Reprint of journal article used for quotation, pp. 1–37.)

Pick, A. (1906). Rückwirkung sprachlicher Perseveration auf den Assoziationsvorgang. *Zeitschrift für Psychologie und Physiologie der Sinnesorgane, 42,* 241–257.

Pick, A. (1931). Aphasie von Arnold Pick. In A. Bethe, G. v. Bergmann, G. Embden, & A. Ellinger (Eds.), *Handbuch der normalen und pathologischen Physiologie, 15/2* (pp. 1416–1524). Berlin, Germany: Springer.

Sandson, J. (1986). *Varieties of perseveration.* (Unpublished PhD thesis). Cornell University, Ithaca, NY.

Sandson, J., & Albert, M. L. (1984). Varieties of perseveration. *Neuropsychologia, 22*(6), 715–732.

Santo-Pietro, M. J., & Rigrodsky, S. (1982). The effects of temporal and semantic conditions on the occurrence of the error response of perseveration in adult aphasics. *Journal of Speech and Hearing Research, 25,* 184–192.

Santo-Pietro, M. J., & Rigrodsky, S. (1986). Patterns of oral-verbal perseveration in adult aphasics. *Brain and Language, 29,* 1–17.

Stark, J. (1984). *Verbale Perseveration bei Aphasie: Ein neurolinguistischer Ansatz.* (Unpublished doctoral dissertation). University of Vienna, Vienna, Austria.

Stark, J. (2005). Analyzing the therapy process: The implicit role of learning and memory. *Aphasiology, 19*(10/11), 1074–1089.

Stark, J. (2007a). A review of classical accounts of verbal perseveration and their modern-day relevance. *Aphasiology, Special Issue Verbal Perseveration, 21*(10/11), 928–959.

Stark, J. (2007b). Syntax detached from semantics: Qualitative analysis of examples of verbal perseveration from a transcortical sensory aphasic. *Aphasiology, Special Issue: Verbal Perseveration, 21*(10/11), 1114–1142.

Stark, J. (2011a). Verbal perseveration in aphasia: Definitions, historical perspective, origins. *Perspectives on Neurophysiology and Neurogenic Speech and Language Disorders, 21*(4), 136–151.

Stark, J. (2011b). Treatment of verbal perseveration in persons with aphasia. *Perspectives on Neurophysiology and Neurogenic Speech and Language Disorders, 21*(4), 152–166.

Stark, J. (2014, May). *Recurring utterances - Targeting a breakthrough.* Paper presented at the 52nd Academy of Aphasia Conference, Miami, FL. doi:10.3389/conf.fpsyg.2014.64.00087

Stark, J., Kristoferitsch, W., Graf, M., Gelpi, E., & Budka, H. (2007). Verbal perseveration as the initial symptom in a case of Creutzfeld-Jakob disease. *Aphasiology, Special Issue: Verbal Perseveration, 21*(10/11), 1079–1113.

von Sölder, F. (1895). Über Perseveration. Vortrag in der Prager Wanderversammlung des Vereines für Psychiatrie und Nervenheilkunde in Wien am 5. Oktober 1895, ref. *Neurologisches Centralblatt, 14,* 958.

von Sölder, F. (1899). Über Perseveration, eine formale Störung im Vorstellungsablaufe *Jahrbücher für Psychiatrie und Neurologie, 18,* 479–525.

Wallesch, C.-W. (1990). Repetitive verbal behavior: Functional and neurological considerations. *Aphasiology, 4,* 133–154.

Whitworth, A., Webster, J., & Howard, D. (2005). *A cognitive neuropsychological approach to assessment and intervention in aphasia.* Hove, England: Psychology Press.

Yamadori, A. (1981). Verbal perseveration in aphasia. *Neuropsychologia, 19,* 591–594.

Yates, A. (1966). Psychological deficit. *Annual Review of Psychology, 17,* 111–144.

Paraphasias

Michael de Riesthal

INTRODUCTION

All individuals who produce spoken and written language make errors in naming or word retrieval. The reasons for these errors differ and may result in specific types of errors. For individuals with aphasia, these errors—referred to as *paraphasias*—occur more frequently and can have a significant impact on the efficiency and effectiveness of communication. The term *paraphasia* means "a substitution in speech." These substitutions often share some feature(s) with the target word—form, meaning, or both—although other substitutions may be unrelated to the intended word. The substitutions may result in a real word or a nonword. The presence of these features permits placing the errors into categories or types of paraphasia. Typically, the types of paraphasia are separated into "lexical paraphasias," including semantic paraphasia, formal paraphasia, and mixed paraphasia, which result in a substitution of a whole word, and "sublexical paraphasias," including phonemic paraphasia and neologism, which result in substitution of phonemes or syllables. This chapter focuses on describing the different types of paraphasias, providing a theoretical model for why these errors occur, and discussing the principles for assessing and treating these errors.

NAMING ERRORS IN PEOPLE WITH AND WITHOUT APHASIA

Naming difficulty is the most common symptom in aphasia. It may be evident in both speaking and writing and may result in the production of several types of errors. Naming errors have also been noted in individuals without aphasia; however, evidence suggests that the errors produced by individuals with aphasia are quantitatively and qualitatively different. Duffy, Duffy, and Pearson (1975) and Duffy and Duffy (1981) each administered an oral-naming test to individuals with aphasia and individuals without neurological injury or damage. In each investigation, performance was significantly poorer than performance of individuals without aphasia. Moreover, performance within the aphasia group was more variable than the performance within the non-aphasia group. Similarly, Dell, Schwartz, Martin, Saffran, and Gagnon (1997) examined aphasic and non-aphasic performance on the Philadelphia Naming Test (PNT; Roach, Schwartz, Martin, Grewal, & Brecher, 1996). Results indicated that the individuals with aphasia produced a significantly greater number of errors and more variable errors on the PNT than the individuals without aphasia. Further, Dell and colleagues (1997) noted that the type of errors differed among groups. The participants without aphasia tended to produce semantic and mixed (semantic and phonemic) errors. In contrast, the participants with aphasia produced various types of errors, including semantic paraphasias, formal paraphasias, mixed paraphasias, neologisms, and unrelated errors. These findings suggest that oral-naming difficulty in aphasia is not simply an increase in the number of typical naming errors made by individuals without aphasia, but also an increase in qualitatively different types of errors.

TYPES OF PARAPHASIA

Lexical Paraphasias

Semantic Paraphasia

Semantic paraphasia is the most common type of lexical paraphasia and refers to the substitution of a whole word that is related by meaning to the target word intended for communication. The relationship between the two words may vary across errors. Buckingham (2011) describes several ways words may be associated and those that are most commonly observed in semantic paraphasias, such as associations based on similarity of meaning (semantic coordinates, e.g., "fork" for "spoon"), functional continuity (semantic associates, e.g., "hammer" for "nail"), and spatial contiguity (semantic associates, e.g., "ring" for "diamond"). Models of word production that describe the interaction between semantic representations and phonology and orthography in lexical access have been examined to account for these errors (Caramazza & Hillis, 1990; Dell et al., 1997) and will be discussed in more detail later in this chapter. In general, there is evidence that semantic errors may arise from inefficiencies at various levels of lexical access in these models (e.g., impaired access to semantic representations or phonological representations) and result in a different constellation of error types.

Formal Paraphasia

Formal paraphasia refers to word errors that are phonologically similar to their intended targets, but are not associated by meaning (e.g., "rabbit" for "rapid"). When these types of errors occur in individuals without aphasia, they are referred to as malapropisms. There is debate in the literature as to whether malapropisms and formal paraphasias have the same origin. Individuals with aphasia who produce formal paraphasias also frequently produce neologisms—nonword errors that may be phonologically related to the target (see further description later). The percentage of formal paraphasias tends to be significantly lower than the production of neologisms in the language of individuals with aphasia. This finding has been used to suggest that formal paraphasias may result from neologisms that produce a real word error by chance (Buckingham, 1980; Nickels & Howard, 1995). Other studies, however, have found a lexical bias for formal paraphasias, which may suggest that they reflect, in part, word substitutions and not necessarily chance production of a real word (Best, 1996; Blanken, 1990; Gagnon, Schwartz, Martin, Dell, & Saffran, 1997; Martin, Dell, Saffran, & Schwartz, 1994).

Mixed Paraphasias

Mixed paraphasias are errors that are both semantically and phonologically related to the target (e.g., "rat" for "cat" or "cow" for "cat"). This type of error is believed to result from the influence of both semantic and phonological activation of the word during production.

Sublexical Paraphasias

Phonemic Paraphasia

Phonemic paraphasia refers to word and nonword naming errors that share some phonemic feature with the target word (e.g., "lelophone" for "telephone"). In individuals without aphasia, these errors are often referred to as "slips of the tongue." Buckingham (1992) used Crystal's (1987) classification of error types during slips of the tongue to describe the types of phonemic paraphasia observed in individuals with aphasia, because there are certain characteristics that are consistent across phonemic paraphasias and slips of the tongue. First, they occur primarily in content words and follow phonotactic constraints (Buckingham & Kertesz, 1976). Second, the phonemes involved in the paraphasic error are always a part of the speaker's language. Third, errors maintain their structural position in the word, for example, onsets move to onset position, codas move to coda positions, and vowels move to vocalic positions (Blumstein, 1973; Lecours & Lhermitte, 1969). Models of word production (discussed in the next section) suggest that phonemic paraphasias result during the encoding of the word when it is retrieved from the lexicon.

Neologisms

Neologisms are nonword errors that may be phonemically related to the target (e.g., /aɪ dau/for "eyebrow") or phonemically unrelated to the target (abstruse neologism; e.g., /les mə-tan/for "eyebrow"). Neologisms occur more frequently when the target is a low frequency compared to a high frequency word (Kay & Ellis, 1987). Target-related neologisms tend to maintain the stress pattern and number of syllables of the target word. There is general agreement that neologisms occur during the process of mapping the lexical representation to the specified phonological representation.

Unrelated Errors

Unrelated word errors are real words that are neither semantically nor phonemically related to the target word (e.g., "lamp" for "dog").

Phonemic Paraphasia Versus Apraxia of Speech

For some individuals with aphasia, it may be difficult to determine whether an error in word production is due to inefficiencies in the language system or speech mechanism. This issue is most significant in the distinction between phonemic paraphasia and apraxia of speech (AOS) errors. AOS is a phonetic-motoric disorder of speech production that results in distortions of the temporal and spatial characteristics of phonemes, syllables, and words (McNeil, Robin, & Schmidt, 2009). The errors associated with AOS and phonemic paraphasia differ in their origins—AOS from impairment to motor networks and phonemic paraphasia from impairment to the language system. However, it is possible that one can hear an error and not know whether it derived from AOS or a phonological paraphasia. In particular, the presence of sound substitution errors as a characteristic of both AOS (motor speech impairment) and phonemic paraphasia (language impairment) makes the distinction between the two more challenging. For example, an error such as "dart" for "tart" may reflect a phonemic, sound substitution error consistent with a paraphasia or a phonetic, voicing error consistent with AOS. In addition, it is possible that the two disorders coexist. Several researchers have identified the common diagnostic features of AOS that separate it from phonemic paraphasia. These include the presence of slow rate, sound distortions, distorted sound substitutions, errors that are consistent in type and location, and prosodic abnormalities (McNeil et al., 2009; Wambaugh, Duffy, McNeil, Robin, & Rogers, 2006). The notion that consistency in type and location of errors may be used to differentiate AOS from phonemic paraphasia has been challenged recently. Haley, Jacks, and Cunningham (2013) found no difference between individuals with AOS and those with aphasia with phonemic paraphasia in terms of error variability. The authors suggest removing this factor as a common diagnostic feature that separates the two disorders.

MODELS OF PARAPHASIC ERRORS

A Theoretical Model

In order to understand the nature of paraphasic errors in the language of individuals with aphasia, it is necessary to examine the breakdown in the language system that causes these errors. Psycholinguistic and connectionist models of lexical access have been proposed to account for the errors produced in the language of speakers with and without aphasia. While there is overlap regarding the basic structure of many of these models, there is considerable disagreement in the literature regarding the specific functionality of these models in accounting for each type of error. In the next section, a two-step model of lexical access proposed by Dell and colleagues (Dell, 1985, 1986; Dell et al., 1997) is described to provide a foundation for conceptualizing how damage to the language system may result in specific paraphasic errors.

Like most models of lexical access, Dell and colleagues propose the need for two steps from concept to production. These steps occur within an interactive connectionist network that is organized into three levels—semantic, word, and form—and within each level, additional lexical information is selected, leading toward the production of a word (see **FIGURE 2.1**). The connections between the levels are bidirectional, meaning that while there is feed-forward activation from concept to word selection to phonological encoding, there is also feedback activation from downstream levels.

Semantic Level

The semantic level is where the stage of lexical concept selection occurs. Each concept is represented by a set of nodes that are associated with the features of the concept. For example, for the concept DOG, the nodes may include animal, four legs, with fur, with tail, barks, etc. Concepts that are similar, for example CAT, will have overlapping nodes, as well as distinct nodes that separate the concepts. The target concept and associated concepts will receive activation, but only the concept with the highest activation will be selected.

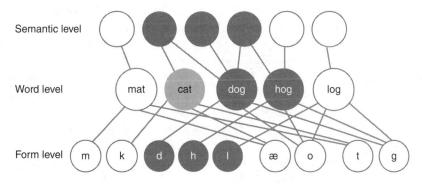

FIGURE 2.1 Model of lexical access

Word Level

The word level is where the stage of lemma selection occurs. A *lemma* is a semantically and syntactically specified lexical representation. When a semantically specified lexical concept activates its lemma to the degree that it can be selected, the lemma makes its syntactic features available for retrieval. Specifically, the lemma will make available several important syntactic features, for example, lexical category, number, person, tense, and aspect. Activation of the lemma occurs after the lexical concept from the semantic level has been selected. As previously discussed, when a lexical concept is activated, it spreads its activation to all semantically related concepts. All of the activated concepts (e.g., the target concept and semantically related concepts) spread some of their activation to their individual lemmas in the word level. The degree of activation for the lemma of the target concept is higher than that of the lemmas for the semantically related concepts. Therefore, there is a greater probability that the lemma for the target concept will be selected.

Form Level

The form level is where the stages of morphological encoding, phonological encoding, and phonetic encoding occur. Once a lemma has been selected in the word level, the next step is the retrieval of its word form for spoken production. For the lemma that is selected, retrieval of the word form occurs including morphophonological encoding, syllabification, and phonetic encoding.

Paraphasic Errors in This Model

As previously mentioned, Dell and colleagues (1997) propose that, within the model, there are connections in both top-down and bottom-up directions. Thus, while activation spreads from concept (semantics) to lemma (word) to form (phonemic and phonetic encoding), it also spreads in the opposite direction. This structure permits accounting for the number and type of paraphasias observed in individuals with aphasia. In this model, *semantic paraphasias* occur when the nodes for the target concept do not receive sufficient activation and an associated concept is selected in its place (e.g., CAT selected in place of DOG). This type of error may also occur due to "noise" in the activation levels of the model. *Formal paraphasias* may result from an error within the word level or form level. In the word level, lemma activation is driven by feed-forward activation from the semantic level, as well as feedback activation from the form level. The feedback from the form level results in activation of lemmas (or word nodes) that share phonemes with the target lemma. Errors occur when the incorrect lemma is selected based on feedback activation from the form level. Because a lemma is a syntactically specified lexical representation, it has been suggested that form errors that occur at lemma access will likely maintain the grammatical features of the target lemma (i.e., a noun will be substituted for a noun— LOG selected in place of DOG). In the form level, a form-related error may occur due to incorrect selection of a phoneme that results in production of a real word. Because the lemma has already been selected and the only change is at the phoneme level, the error will not necessarily maintain the grammatical features of the target word (e.g., JOG selected in place of DOG). *Mixed semantic-formal paraphasias* (HOG for DOG) occur due to the interactive, bidirectional nature of the lexical system, which suggests that semantic and phonological information are active simultaneously. While the top-down processes result in activation of semantically related associates, the bottom-up processes activate phonologically related associates. Activation of words that are both semantically and phonologically associated with the target will be increased relative to other competitors and, therefore, more likely to be selected in error. *Phonemic paraphasias*, which are nonword errors that share similar phonemes to the target (e.g., GOG for DOG), occur within the form level during phoneme selection. The correct lemma (or word node) is selected, but the selection of phonemes and placement into the appropriate slot (e.g., onset, vowel, and coda) is impaired. *Neologisms* that are related to the target (e.g., stress pattern, number of syllables) result from impaired phonological access. Abstruse neologisms likely result from significant impairments at the level of phonological access or both lemma and phonological access. Similar to neologisms, *unrelated errors* may occur within the word level, form level, or both. In the word level, the unrelated error may occur due to selection of a lemma that is not related to the target. In the form level, it is possible that significant deficits in phonological access may result in the selection of phonemes that create a real word that is unrelated, independent of whether or not the correct lemma was selected.

A Neuroanatomical Model of Paraphasic Errors

In addition to theoretical models explaining the origins of paraphasic errors, neuroanatomical models of language and lesion studies suggest that the different types of paraphasia may result from damage to specific parts of the brain. Damage to the brain may occur due to acquired brain injury (e.g., stroke, tumor, or trauma) or progressive disease (e.g., primary progressive aphasia). Hickok and colleagues (Hickok, 2012; Hickok, Houde, & Rong, 2011; Hickok & Poeppel, 2007) present a dual-stream model for the processing and production of single words, which provides a framework for conceptualizing the association between neuroanatomy, language function, and error types. In particular, the model proposes that the localization of the conceptual semantic system is widely distributed throughout both hemispheres of the cerebral cortex. Drawing from the widely distributed semantic network, the association between semantic representations and phonologically encoded lexical items occurs in the left posterior middle and inferior temporal gyri. Phonological processing, including the encoding of the phonological word form occurs along the left superior temporal sulcus. The model's most significant contribution to understanding speech production is its account of the role of auditory and somatosensory targets associated with the phonological word. It suggests that these targets make predictions about the future state of the motor articulators and the sensory consequences of the predicted actions. These predictions permit the individual to detect errors in speech production and make corrections more quickly. In the proposed model, this feed-forward mechanism is mediated by area Spt, which stands for sylvian, parietal, and temporal, located at the junction of the posterior parietal and temporal lobes. Finally, there is activation of the frontal articulatory network, including the left posterior inferior frontal gyrus, premotor cortex, and anterior insula to execute the production of the word.

Hickok and colleagues suggest that posterior temporal areas, especially middle temporal gyrus, bilaterally, but with a weak left hemisphere bias, are implicated in semantic deficits in comprehension and production. In addition, there is evidence that anterior temporal lobe areas may be involved in semantic processing. Cloutman and colleagues (2009) examined the semantic naming errors in 196 individuals with acute onset of aphasia due to stroke. Diffusion-weighted imaging and perfusion-weighted imaging studies were completed for comparison with naming data. Participants with semantic deficits who made purely semantic paraphasias presented with hypoperfusion and/or infarct in the left superior temporal lobe (Brodmann's area [BA] 22) and the left posterior middle temporal lobe (BA 21). Similarly, participants who made semantic errors due to lexical access deficits, presented with hypoperfusion and/or infarcts in the left inferior temporal gyrus (BA 37). These findings are consistent with the site for the association between semantics and phonologically encoded lexical items in the Hickok model. The production of mixed errors (semantic and phonemic) was associated with fairly large areas of hypoperfusion and/or infarct in the left frontotemporal cortex. The production of phonemic paraphasias has been associated with left posterior perisylvian cortical lesions (Buckingham, 2011).

Individuals with aphasia are often classified into a specific type or category of aphasia. The most common types include Broca's, transcortical motor, global, mixed transcortical, anomic, conduction, Wernicke's, and transcortical sensory. Semantic, formal, phonemic, mixed, and/or neologistic errors may be present in any type of aphasia; however, there are types for which certain paraphasias are more common. For example, individuals with conduction aphasia tend to produce more phonemic paraphasic errors, and, despite being aware of their errors, tend to have more difficulty self-correcting. Their multiple attempts to self-correct, which do not necessarily result in closer approximations to the target, are often referred to as *conduites d'approche* (Ueno & Lambon Ralph, 2013). Individuals with Wernicke's aphasia may produce semantic and phonemic paraphasias, as well as neologisms. Those who present with a more severe Wernicke's aphasia are often described as having "jargon aphasia" due to the presence of a significant percentage of neologisms in their oral expressive language (see Chapter 3, this volume). Unlike conduction aphasia, individuals with Wernicke's aphasia do not demonstrate the same ability to self-monitor and, thus, tend not to attempt repairs of incorrect utterances. In addition to types of aphasia, there is evidence that severity of naming difficulty is associated with a higher incidence of certain types of errors. Dell and colleagues (1997) found that individuals with a more severe aphasia produced more formal paraphasias, unrelated words, and non-word errors than individuals with a less severe aphasia. Semantic errors and mixed errors occurred to the same degree across all severity levels. Studies examining the evolution of naming errors during recovery have found that as individuals with more severe aphasia improve, there is a shift from errors that are unrelated to the target toward errors that bear a semantic or phonemic relationship with the target (Basso, Corno, & Marangolo, 1996; Crary & Kertesz, 1988).

VARIABLES TO CONSIDER DURING ASSESSMENT AND TREATMENT

In conceptualizing the remediation and compensatory techniques used in the treatment of paraphasias, it is important to understand the differences between naming errors across modalities, including speaking and writing, and the influence of modality of stimulus input on performance. Understanding these differences will inform the assessment of naming errors, including paraphasias, and the determination of the best approach to elicit naming responses and facilitate accurate production.

Dissociation Between Spoken and Written Naming in Aphasia

Early theories of language production suggested that in order to write the name of an object the semantic representation of the object and its phonological word form must be retrieved before the written word form could be generated (Hier & Mohr, 1977). Therefore, to write a word, the phonological representation of the word should be translated into written letters. Based on these early theories, the written naming ability of an individual with aphasia must be either equal to or inferior to his or her spoken naming ability. If access to the phonological representation is impaired, then writing will be equally impaired. However, if the translation of the phonological representation to writing is impaired, written naming will be poorer than spoken naming. Current theories of naming, however, suggest that the generation of spoken names and written names result from two separate mechanisms (Bub & Kertesz, 1982; Deloche et al., 1997; Hier & Mohr, 1977; Hillis, Rapp, & Caramazza, 1999; Miceli, Benvegnu, Capasso, & Caramazza, 1997). According to these current theories, once a semantic representation is retrieved, encoding occurs independently for the phonological word form and the written word form. Thus, written naming performance may be inferior, superior, or equal to spoken naming performance.

The distinction between the mechanisms involved in spoken and written naming is represented in a model of lexical processing that frequently appears in the literature. This model provides a schematic representation of the relationships among the cognitive processes involved in lexical tasks (see **FIGURE 2.2**) and suggests that spoken and written responses result from two independent processes. The phonological output lexicon encodes the phonological word forms for spoken responses and the orthographic output lexicon encodes the orthographic word forms for written responses. Both output lexicons receive activation from a common semantic system, but they are activated independent of each other. The activation of a representation within the semantic system will activate independent lexical representations in the phonological and/or orthographic output lexicons.

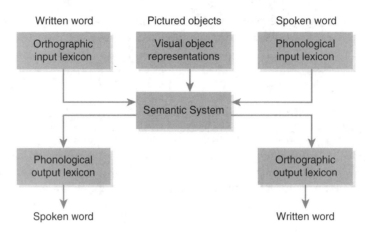

FIGURE 2.2 Example of a lexical processing model

Thus, it is hypothesized that individuals with aphasia who have damage to the semantic system may demonstrate relatively equal deficits in speaking and writing, because both independent output lexicons receive input from a shared semantic system. However, individuals with aphasia who have damage to each output lexicon may demonstrate unequal deficits in speaking and writing, because the output lexicons function independently and, therefore, may differ in the degree to which they are damaged in aphasia.

Several investigators have reported cases of individuals with aphasia with superior performance in written naming compared to spoken naming. Hier and Mohr (1977) described a patient with Wernicke's aphasia (AF) who was unable to provide a spoken name when shown pictures of objects from two vocabulary lists, but was 24% and 52% accurate in providing a written name when shown pictures of objects from the same two lists. Similarly, Caramazza and Hillis (1990) described the performance of a patient with aphasia (RGB) who produced numerous semantic errors in spoken naming (e.g., "socks" for "mittens") but made no semantic errors in written naming when presented with the same stimuli. Spelling errors were noted in many of RGB's written responses (e.g., "dokey" for "donkey"); however, fewer errors were made compared to spoken naming.

Conversely, several investigators have described individuals with aphasia with superior spoken naming compared to written naming. Hillis and colleagues (1999) reported a patient (RCM) with anomic aphasia who was 100% accurate in spoken naming on a picture naming task, but was only 53% accurate, producing primarily semantic errors, in written naming using the same stimuli. The dissociation between spoken and written naming demonstrated by these cases suggests that spoken and written output may result from independent processes. Moreover, it suggests that, following current theoretical views, written naming may be superior, inferior, or equal to spoken naming performance in individuals with aphasia.

As it relates to error types, Basso and colleagues (1996) examined spoken and written naming errors in 84 individuals with aphasia at two points in time to determine the evolution of error types during spontaneous recovery. Errors were coded in 1 of 10 categories (i.e., no response, word-finding difficulty, semantic paraphasia, unrelated error, phonemic/orthographic paraphasia, neologism, paraphasic jargon, phonemic/neologistic jargon, stereotypy, and other). The results indicated that the participants made significantly fewer no response errors in both spoken and written naming and fewer neologisms in spoken naming when comparing the first and second assessments. There was an increase in the number of phonemic/orthographic paraphasic errors, with a larger increase observed on the written versus spoken naming tasks. Thus, while there are differences in spoken versus written output in individuals with aphasia, there may also be a change in error types that occurs during recovery.

Influence of Input Stimulus on Naming

The model proposed by Caramazza and Hillis (1990) indicates that spoken and written output may be influenced by the mode of stimulus presentation. In their model, the independent stimulus input modes are connected to the independent response output modes via a common semantic system. The relationship among three stimulus modes—auditory (spoken words), printed (written words), and pictorial (pictured object)—is shown in Figure 2.2. Based on this model, individuals who have difficulty processing information from a specific stimulus mode, for example spoken words, will demonstrate naming deficits in all response modalities when spoken words are presented. However, while isolated deficits based on stimulus mode are possible, most individuals with aphasia do not demonstrate an isolated deficit. Typically, naming deficits are evident in all stimulus modes, but the severity of the deficit may differ among modes. Several early studies on the influence of a stimulus on spoken naming performance in a group of individuals with aphasia examined sensory modality (i.e., auditory, visual, tactile) stimulus context within a modality (i.e., sentence completion, naming to definition) on spoken naming performance. Results indicated that individuals with aphasia may exhibit poorer spoken naming to stimuli presented in one modality compared to another (Spreen, Benton, & Van Allen, 1966). In addition, results suggest that individuals with aphasia, as a group, were more accurate in naming when presented with a sentence completion task than with a picture naming or object description task. However, as demonstrated in other studies, individual variability was noted, suggesting that not all individuals with aphasia demonstrate the same task hierarchy in naming performance (Gardner & Brookshire, 1972).

In addition to the mode of stimulus presentation, there are variables associated with the selected stimulus items that may influence naming. For example, word frequency has been shown to influence naming in aphasia (Kittredge, Dell, Verkuilen, & Schwartz, 2008). In general, errors occur more often in lower frequency words, including the production of paraphasias. Variables such as imageability, word length, and age of acquisition may also influence word retrieval in aphasia, with shorter, more imageable words, acquired at a younger age being easier to name.

Assessment Approach

Determining the best approach for addressing naming errors in individuals with aphasia begins with a detailed assessment to identify the types of errors the individual is producing and the location of the breakdown in the language system. The assessment may include formal measures that examine picture naming, such as the Boston Naming Test (Kaplan, Goodglass, & Weintraub, 2001), Philadelphia Naming Test (Roach et al., 1996), and the Action Naming Test (Obler & Albert, 1986). More importantly, given the characteristics that may influence naming performance, it is necessary to examine differences in performance across input modes (e.g., auditory, visual-object, visual-printed) and output modalities (e.g., speaking, writing, and gesture). These differences will help identify the locus of damage in the language system and provide a target for focusing treatment. Formal measures, such as the Psycholinguistic Assessment of Language Processing Abilities (Kay, Coltheart, & Lesser, 1992), exist to examine performance across lexical tasks that require processing information through different input modalities and generating a response via spoken, written, and gesture. In the absence of formal measures, a clinician may perform an informal assessment using a variety of input and output tasks (**TABLE 2.1**) (see Chapter 13, this volume).

TABLE 2.1 Tasks that may be used to assess breakdown in the language system as a function of different input modes and output modalities.

Output Tasks	Input Tasks
Oral picture naming	Auditory word to picture matching
Written picture naming	Written word to picture matching
Oral naming to spoken definition	Semantic associates matching
Written naming to spoken definition	Auditory lexical decision
Oral word reading	Written lexical decision
Writing to dictation	Category sorting
Name to tactile object	Auditory word to picture matching
Name to environmental sounds	
Gesture to command	
Gesture to viewed objects	

In addition to assessing potential linguistic deficits, it is also important to consider an individual's ability to self-monitor errors. Several studies of individuals with aphasia have found differential ability to detect and repair semantic errors as compared to phonemic errors (Marshall, Rappaport, & Garcia-Bunuel, 1985; Stark, 1988). If an individual is able to recognize an error, he or she may be able to correct it. In fact, awareness of errors may be indicated by an individual's attempts at overt repair or self-correction of a spoken utterance, which suggests recognition of the error. More challenging to identify are the covert repairs that occur when the individual recognizes that the word they are about to produce will be incorrect. This often manifests as an interruption to the flow of speech and a restart during connected speech (Levelt, 1989). In a single-word naming task, the presence of false starts may reflect error detection. There is a question regarding whether the ability to recognize errors in naming is associated with auditory comprehension in individuals with aphasia. While a deficit in auditory comprehension may contribute to difficulty in detecting naming errors, several studies with individuals with aphasia have suggested that the detection and self-correction of semantic and phonemic errors is not associated with comprehension (Nickels & Howard, 1995; Nozari, Dell, & Schwartz, 2011). In a recent study, Nozari and colleagues (2011) proposed a conflict-based account of error detection, which suggests that the ability to detect semantic and phonemic errors in spoken language is mediated by a domain-general monitoring system that compares the actual response (produced word) with the internally generated predicted response (intended word). The authors suggest that this process involves frontal brain structures, including the anterior cingulate cortex. For individuals with aphasia who produce paraphasic errors, determining whether they can recognize their errors and attempt to correct them during and/or after production will provide a potential target for treatment.

REHABILITATION STRATEGIES

In the next section we will examine the rehabilitation strategies that are designed to address paraphasias produced by individuals with aphasia. Few treatments have been designed specifically to correct paraphasic errors; however, many treatments for naming have been applied to individuals who produce paraphasias and have been successful in reducing the number of paraphasias produced and improving overall naming performance. Therapy approaches designed to remediate paraphasic errors target the area of breakdown in the language system that is responsible for the errors, for example, the semantic and/or phonological systems. These techniques manipulate the mode of input to the system (e.g., auditory, printed, visual object) and may utilize alternative output modalities (e.g., writing and gesture) to cue accurate verbal production or to provide another means of communication. In the next section, we examine the literature regarding treatments for semantic and phonological naming deficits in aphasia. In particular, four general approaches will be examined: cueing hierarchies, semantic network treatments, alternative modality (e.g., writing and gesture) facilitation techniques, and developing self-awareness of errors.

Cueing Hierarchies

One method for improving naming in individuals with aphasia who produce paraphasic errors is to provide a cue to facilitate accurate production. The cue may provide information related to the semantic representation of the word, its phonemic makeup, or both. Cueing hierarchies have been used in therapy to improve naming performance in individuals who experience breakdown at various levels of the language system. One of the first published cueing hierarchies (Linebaugh & Lehner, 1977), described by Linebaugh, Shisler, and Lehner (2005), included both semantic and phonemic/phonetic cues that were designed to promote self-cueing by the patient and provide cues from the clinician, as needed. The treatment employed a 10-step cueing hierarchy progressing from minimal to maximum external cues. Initial cues required the patient to generate semantic information associated with the word via semantic description and gesture, followed by semantic and phonemic cues presented by the clinician. Semantic cues included a description of the target item, pantomime of how the item is used, and sentence completion tasks. Phonemic/phonetic cues for a treated word included silent articulation of the first sound, presentation of the first sound, presentation of the first two sounds, and presentation of the entire word for repetition. The patient first proceeded down the hierarchy until the picture was named and then worked back up the hierarchy. Linebaugh and colleagues (2005, 1977) reported implementation of the cueing hierarchy improved naming performance with fewer cues required to retrieve the object name.

While the hierarchy developed by Linebaugh and colleagues (2005, 1977) included both semantic and phonemic cues, many recent studies have utilized separate semantic and phonemic cueing hierarchies in order to examine the benefits of one versus the other in patients with naming deficits localized to specific areas of the language system (e.g., primarily semantic vs. primarily phonologic impairment). Raymer and colleagues (1993) employed a phonemic cueing hierarchy that included presentation of a word that rhymes with the target, a phonemic cue, and repetition. Three of the participants presented with lexical-semantic–level deficits and one participant had primary phonological-level deficits. Improvement was reported in the naming of treated items for all participants and results were maintained post-treatment in two of the four participants. Wambaugh and colleagues (2001) examined the application of a semantic-level cueing treatment (SCT) and a phonological-level cueing treatment (PCT) to three individuals with aphasia based on their level of lexical processing impairment—predominantly semantic (semantic paraphasias), predominantly phonological (phonemic paraphasias), or mixed (semantic and phonemic paraphasias). Both the semantic and phonemic cueing hierarchies provided cues with increasing information. SCT included cues such as verbal description, semantically nonspecific sentence completion, semantically loaded sentence completion, and repetition. PCT included non-real word rhymes, first sound phonemic cue, sentence completion phrase that includes the rhyme, and repetition. All participants responded positively to both treatments, though degree of response varied. The subject with the semantic-level deficit responded similarly to both treatments; the subject with the mixed deficit reached criterion on both phases of PCT but only on the first phase of SCT; the subject with the phonological-level deficit responded better to SCT in that he achieved higher levels of accuracy with fewer sessions with SCT compared to PCT. All participants demonstrated an overall decrease in number of paraphasic errors across types as evidenced by an increase in accuracy to at least 83% for treated items. Wambaugh, Cameron, Kalinyak-Fliszar, Nessler, and Wright (2004) further examined PCT and SCT on the ability to retrieve action names/verbs. The participants made significantly more semantic paraphasias than phonemic or mixed paraphasias at the onset of treatment. Both treatments improved verb naming, though not to the consistent degree they induced improvement in noun naming seen in previous studies (Wambaugh et al., 2001). Similarly, Raymer and Ellsworth (2002) compared the relative effects of three types of verb retrieval treatments (semantic cueing, phonologic cueing, and repetition cueing) on the individual with aphasia's ability to name actions and produce sentence-level utterances. At baseline, over 70% of errors were semantically related to the target. All three treatments resulted in an improvement in accuracy of both verb naming and sentence production for the treated items. Maintenance of treatment effects was present and significant at 1 month post-treatment. Cameron and colleagues (2006) utilized a combined semantic/phonologic treatment cueing hierarchy to ameliorate incorrect productions of target words in the context of a story retell procedure that included the treatment stimuli. The cueing hierarchy included the use of "wh-" questions to facilitate story retell, semantically nonspecific sentence completion, semantically loaded sentence completion with and without first phoneme cue, verbal model, and integral stimulation. Participants included individuals with anomic aphasia, conduction aphasia, and Broca's aphasia. Outcome was indexed in terms of information units (IUs) from the story retell procedure (Doyle et al., 2000). Overall, the participants improved in their retrieval of the targeted IUs, but there was little generalization to untrained stories.

Semantic Network Treatment

Semantic feature analysis (SFA) is based on the theory of spreading activation in semantic processing. That is, an individual may improve the ability to produce a specific word by strengthening the connections among its semantic descriptors and associates. The clinician facilitates the patient's completion of a semantic map that includes information regarding category membership, location, action, properties, and associations. The participant attempts to name a target picture, and then completes the semantic map information about the target word. The semantic features are written in the appropriate locations on the chart for future reference. If the patient is not able to name the picture after completing the map, the clinician provides the name of the item and the patient repeats it and reviews its associated features. Boyle and Coelho (1995) applied SFA treatment to a patient with agrammatic aphasia and significant difficulty naming. Patient performance improved for treated items and these effects generalized to untreated pictures, but not to connected speech. Treatment effects were maintained for 2 months post-therapy. SFA has also been applied to individuals with fluent aphasias, including anomic and Wernicke's, with noted improvements in picture naming and measures of discourse (e.g., correct information units [CIUs] and CIUs/minute; Boyle, 2004; Peach & Reuter, 2010). Moreover, it has been shown to be effective when applied during group treatment (Antonucci, 2009). During group treatment, SFA was incorporated into connected speech tasks using a modified-PACE protocol to elicit responses. Participants utilized pocket-sized SFA charts to aid their descriptions during conversation. Improvements were noted in discourse, including number of words, CIUs, percent CIUs, and percent of retrieved nouns. Several studies have examined changes in types of paraphasias and other word-finding errors after SFA. Boyle (2004) described two participants with aphasia. Participant 1 presented with an anomic aphasia and produced predominantly semantic paraphasic errors in confrontation naming. Participant 2 produced semantic and phonemic paraphasias, as well as reformulations, repetitions, and empty words. Following treatment, participant 1 demonstrated no difference in frequency of type of paraphasic errors, while participant 2 demonstrated a decrease in semantic paraphasias and a slight increase in number of phonemic paraphasias. Neither of these differences was statistically significant. Hashimoto (2012) compared a modified semantic feature treatment that included only three features per word—group (category), physical sensory properties, and association—with a phonological-based feature approach that included three features associated with the sound of the word—rhyme, first sound, and number of syllables. The two participants with aphasia performed differently in each treatment based on their relative strengths and weaknesses in the semantic and phonological systems. For example, the participant who responded best to the semantic feature treatment demonstrated a significant reduction in "no response" errors and an increase in semantic paraphasias, thought to be a reflection of an improved, though still impaired, semantic system.

Facilitation with Other Modalities

Some individuals with aphasia benefit from the inclusion of alternative input modes and output modalities to improve naming performance. In particular, reading, writing, and gesture may serve as a salient cue to facilitate the correct spoken production of a word (see Chapter 8, this volume).

In an early study, Boyle (1989) examined the use of reading within a cueing hierarchy to reduce the occurrence of phonological paraphasic errors in an individual with conduction aphasia. The treatment consisted of the participant reading lists of words that progressed from one to three syllables, presented both as single words, and within phrases and sentences. The cueing hierarchy first required the participant to think about how the word sounded before reading it again, which incorporated an element of self-monitoring that may support reduction of paraphasic errors. Other cues included repetition of a model presented by the clinician. The participant experienced a decrease in the number of phonemic paraphasias and revisions in connected speech and maintained these effects at the 6-week follow up.

Wambaugh and Wright (2007) examined the benefit of adding orthographic forms of targeted action names (verbs) to semantic cueing treatment (SCT) and phonologic cueing treatment (PCT) in an individual who had shown limited benefit from either SCT or PCT alone. The participant was an individual with moderate to severe Wernicke's aphasia and significant word retrieval deficits. The typical SCT and PCT protocols (Wambaugh et al., 2001) were adapted to include the orthographic word form during presentation of treatment trials that included either SCT or PCT. Participants improved on both treatments, which was significantly different from the treatment response associated with SCT or PCT alone. Treatment effects were maintained at 2- and 6-weeks post-treatment.

Wright, Marshall, Wilson, and Page (2008) examined the effects of a written cueing treatment program on verbal naming ability in two adults with aphasia. Treatment involved using a written cueing hierarchy that was modeled after Copy and Recall Treatment (CART; Beeson, 1999) and included both spoken and written naming components. Stimuli used in treatment were black and white pictures representing English nouns (Snodgrass & Vanderwart, 1980). A total of 40 pictures scored as incorrect in a baseline naming probe were selected as target words. These were randomly assigned to four 10-word lists: three treated and one untreated. Both participants improved their verbal naming ability for the target items over the course of treatment, but they responded differently to treatment. One participant maintained verbal naming performance for the treated items 4 weeks after treatment and also generalized to untreated items; the other did not. Results support and extend previous findings that treating in one modality improves performance in a different modality. Underlying differences in participants' deficits may account for why they responded differently to the treatment.

Raymer and colleagues (2006) examined the benefits of pairing a gesture (pantomime) with verbal production of a word in improving noun and verb retrieval in individuals with aphasia. The participants were trained to produce both the word and associated gesture for the treated items in each category (nouns and verbs). Both gesture and naming improved for the treated nouns and verbs, and there was no significant difference in performance between categories. There was modest improvement in gestural performance for untrained nouns and verbs. The authors concluded that a combined gesture and verbal treatment can facilitate improvement in gesture and lexical retrieval for both nouns and verbs, and may also lead to increased use of spontaneous gesture for untrained stimuli; this may be of particular benefit to increase use of nonverbal communication for individuals with severe anomia.

Rodriguez, Raymer, and Rothi (2006) examined the effects of two treatments on verb retrieval—gesture plus verbal production and semantic-phonologic—in individuals with chronic aphasia. Two participants had mixed semantic and phonologic impairments, one had a primary phonologic impairment, and one had a primary semantic impairment. The gesture plus verbal treatment trained the simultaneous production of a pantomime and spoken production of the target word. The semantic-phonologic treatment required the participant to respond to four yes/no questions about semantic and phonologic characteristics of the picture. In both treatments correct responses are reinforced and incorrect responses are corrected and modeled by the clinician. Overall, there was no significant difference between gesture plus verbal and semantic-phonologic treatment, although some differential effects were observed across participants. The participant with phonologic impairment demonstrated a better response to treatment than any of the others with semantic impairments; however, both treatments may affect lexical representations during word retrieval.

Rose and Sussmilch (2008) compared the effects of semantic, gesture, repetition, and combined semantic and gesture treatments for verb retrieval deficits associated with chronic Broca's aphasia. Two participants had a primarily phonological-level (word form) verb retrieval deficit, and one participant had a semantic (abstract lexical representation) deficit. The semantic and combined semantic and gesture treatment protocols were based on semantic feature analysis methods. For each error item, participants were asked to say, or say and produce a gesture of an associated object, movement (body part), and location (where the action is carried out). If they could not spontaneously generate the information, they were provided with verbal models. If the semantic feature training failed to elicit the correct verb or gesture response, a spoken or spoken and gesture model was then provided. The gesture-only protocol involved production of an iconic gesture. In the repetition-only protocol, participants were provided with the spoken word to imitate in the presence of the picture. Results indicated that, similar to Rodriguez and colleagues (2006) the two participants with phonological-level verb retrieval impairment showed good acquisition of trained items, use of these items in picture description and conversation tasks, and some small amount of untreated item generalization. However, the results were poor for the participant with a more semantic-based impairment. The authors suggested that this may be due to the participant's overall poor baseline performance, which included an extreme paucity of any noun or verb output. Similarly, they suggested that the differential effect of the combined treatment on the participants with phonological-level impairment was due to differences in error types produced by each participant for the word lists used in this condition. That is, the participant with the less consistent response in the combined condition, made more "no response" errors, while the participant with more robust gains made more paraphasic errors. Making a paraphasic error is evidence for partial activation of semantic or phonologic information of a word, which may mean that it is more responsive to facilitation via external cues. The authors suggest that this should be a variable that is explored in future studies.

Developing Self-Awareness

As previously discussed, the ability of individuals with aphasia to recognize an error is key to them being able to correct the error. Marshall and Tompkins (1982) examined self-correction behaviors in individuals with nonfluent and fluent aphasia. The results indicated that across both groups and across six different types of aphasia, individuals with aphasia were able to recognize and attempt to correct at least 50% or more of their errors (paraphasias and apraxic/dysarthric errors). In contrast, the ability to successfully correct the error was influenced by severity. The individuals with milder nonfluent and fluent aphasias were more successful in their self-correction attempts than the individuals with a more severe aphasia. When it comes to treatment, some individuals with a more severe fluent aphasia, such as Wernicke's aphasia, may respond to alternative approaches to treatment. Individuals with Wernicke's aphasia often produce a variety of paraphasic errors (semantic, phonemic, formal, and mixed) and neologisms in connected speech. Marshall (2008) describes several strategies that may facilitate successful communication and improve the patient's language performance. First, he describes the importance of establishing the communication context (i.e., the topic or theme of conversation) by which the individual's verbal output may be interpreted. Within this context, the clinician may train the individual with aphasia to improve self-monitoring of errors and self-correction by using a "stop" strategy—a signal to the individual with aphasia that an error has been made and encouraging self-correction. In addition to encouraging self-monitoring and self-correction, individuals with aphasia may benefit from the clinician translating their utterance and model the correct production of a word produced as a paraphasia. In doing so, the clinician is able to verify the portion of the message that was conveyed successfully by the individual with aphasia, while also providing a model to facilitate a successful correction of the utterance. Although described as an approach for individuals with a severe fluent aphasia, it may be applied also to individuals with a less severe aphasia.

CONCLUSION

Individuals with aphasia produce naming errors, including paraphasias, which may have a significant impact on the efficiency and effectiveness of communication. For the practicing clinician, it is essential that she or he understand the theoretical basis for these errors to inform assessment procedure, diagnosis, and treatment decisions. While there are few treatments designed specifically to address paraphasias, techniques and strategies developed to improve naming, in general, often target the areas of weakness within the language system (e.g., semantics, phonology) that result in paraphasias. These treatments may reduce the occurrence of paraphasias in addition to other types of naming errors. In addition, individuals who produce paraphasias may benefit from the use of alternative communication modalities, such as writing and gesture. Developing compensations is important, because, while naming performance will improve, some residual deficit will likely persist.

CASE ILLUSTRATION

JD was a 61-year-old male, 4 weeks post-onset of aphasia secondary to an embolic stroke. He had a history of coronary artery disease, status post coronary bypass surgery, as well as chronic atrial fibrillation and hypertension. Magnetic resonance imaging (MRI) showed an infarct in the posterior left middle cerebral artery territory, predominantly affecting the temporal lobe. Prior to being referred for an outpatient speech-language assessment and therapy, the patient received two weeks of therapy at an inpatient rehabilitation facility. During the initial interview with the patient and his wife, they both indicated that JD's communication had improved since the onset of aphasia, but that he still had difficulty with naming, generating meaningful sentences, understanding what he hears and reads, and writing. His wife reported the presence of phonemic errors and occasional nonsense words. She and the family tried using writing and drawing to help facilitate communication. The patient and his wife indicated that the primary goal for treatment is to improve his overall communication skills.

JD was administered the Western Aphasia Battery-Revised (WAB-R; Kertesz, 2006), Boston Naming Test (BNT; Kaplan et al., 2001), and Pyramid and Palm Trees Test (PPT; Howard & Patterson, 1992). The testing results at initial testing and two other points during his treatment program are shown in **TABLE 2.2**.

TABLE 2.2 Language assessment data for patient JD at initial assessment and after 3 and 6 months of treatment.

Tests	Pretreatment	3 months	6 months
Western Aphasia Battery			
Spontaneous speech	12	17	18
Fluency	7	8	8
Information content	5	9	10
Auditory verbal comprehension score	7.6	9	9
Repetition score	4.2	7.6	7.8
Naming and word-finding score	6.3	7.6	8.9
Reading score	14.2	15.8	17.8
Writing score	12.0	14.6	17.0
Aphasia Quotient	60.2	82.4	87.4
Language Quotient	63.9	80.6	87.5
Boston Naming Test	23/60		
Pyramids and Palm Trees Test	42/52		

Overall, JD's performance on the WAB-R revealed a moderately severe fluent aphasia (aphasia quotient = 60.2, language quotient = 63.9) characterized by mostly fluent speech with some grammatical organization, marked word-finding difficulty (phonemic paraphasias, semantic paraphasias, unrelated word errors, and nonsense word errors), and auditory comprehension deficits. Regarding his auditory comprehension, his yes/no response was fairly reliable for personal information and his auditory word recognition was a relative strength, although he had specific difficulty with letters and numbers, and at times, confusion of left and right. He had more difficulty processing sequential commands as they increased in length and complexity. Word retrieval deficits were noted on confrontation naming, generative naming, sentence completion, and responsive speech tasks. On the WAB-R, he was able to name 14/20 items without any cueing and 3/6 remaining items with semantic or phonemic cueing. On the BNT, he correctly named 23/60 items spontaneously and an additional 8 items with a phonemic/phonetic cue. He did not benefit from the semantic cue. In fact, he generated several semantic descriptions of his own that did not facilitate correct word retrieval. JD's errors were predominantly phonemic paraphasias (e.g., "caper pin" for "paper clip"; "coom" for "comb") and he was mostly aware of his incorrect productions. He benefitted from repetition and phonemic cueing to produce the correct word. On the WAB-R, the client was able to read and comprehend fairly well at the simple, single-sentence and short, two-sentence paragraph level, but had more difficulty with longer, more complex material. He performed very well on single-word written to picture matching. He demonstrated more significant deficits in writing. He was able to write his name and most of his address, but any communicative writing was limited to single words and the spelling of single words was often incorrect. Number writing was also a relative strength. JD did not demonstrate any significant limb or oral-nonverbal apraxia.

Based on the assessment, it was determined that JD had a good prognosis for recovery. He was approximately 4 weeks post-onset and had made significant improvement in that time. He was motivated to improve and had a very supportive family and community. In addition, he demonstrated the ability to learn and to generalize skills learned in the clinic to the home environment and community.

A primary focus of the treatment program was to reduce the number of paraphasic errors produced during specific naming tasks and in conversation, because these errors were having a significant influence on JD's communicative effectiveness. For the purposes of this chapter, the description will be limited to treatments targeting word retrieval and sentence production. To address JD's tendency to produce phonemic and semantic paraphasic errors, three treatment approaches were implemented—a combined semantic and phonological cueing hierarchy, semantic feature analysis, and the training of alternative modalities to cue spoken naming or serve as a compensatory communication strategy. The cueing hierarchy, which included a combination of semantic and phonological cues, similar to Cameron and colleagues (2006), was used to target a set of functional vocabulary that was decided upon by the patient, family, and clinician. In addition to improving the production of the treatment stimuli, the clinician attempted to develop the patient's self-monitoring skills by having JD rate the accuracy of his production after each attempt. Semantic feature analysis (SFA) was implemented to improve JD's ability to produce functional vocabulary; however, it also served to develop circumlocution as a strategy to compensate for the patient's word retrieval difficulty. Recall that during the assessment, the patient generated some semantic information related to pictures he could not name, but the self-generated semantic cue did not facilitate word retrieval. The choice to include SFA was based on the need to provide JD with a structure for generating semantic descriptions during word retrieval difficulty. Finally, single-word writing was trained via copy and recall treatment (CART) to develop a corpus of written words for communication and to target spoken word production similar to Wright and colleagues (2008). In addition to targeting word retrieval in single-word tasks, the patient's ability to retrieve words during sentence production was targeted via response elaboration training (RET; Kearns, 1985). RET is a loose training paradigm that uses "wh-" questions and clinician modeling to expand the length and meaningfulness of utterances in an individual with aphasia. Outcome for the spoken naming and written naming tasks were indexed in terms of number correct and percent accuracy. Improvement during RET was indexed in terms of correct information units (CIUs) and percent CIUs (%CIUs).

The patient was scheduled for treatment two times per week for 6 months. During this time, he made significant improvements in word retrieval, sentence production, and overall communication. As seen in Table 2.2, the patient's performance on the WAB-R improved significantly across language domains from initial testing to discharge. Most notable was the significant reduction in phonemic paraphasic errors on the WAB-R picture naming subtest. He produced 13 paraphasic errors on the task (8 of which he self-corrected) during the initial assessment, compared to no paraphasic errors on the task during the final assessment. On specific word retrieval tasks, the patient met the targets of 80% accuracy over three sessions for each set of treatment stimuli included in the cueing hierarchy and CART. There was no generalization to untrained items, which were defined as sets of stimuli that were being monitored for baseline performance and eventually included in treatment. In addition, the patient was able to utilize the structure of the semantic web trained in SFA to develop his skill at circumlocution and use writing to compensate for word retrieval issues. Finally, the patient demonstrated improvement in sentence production, increasing from 5.2 to 9.4 CIUs per sentence on a picture description task. In addition, the percent CIUs per sentence increased from 66% to 87%.

The improvement made by JD in his therapy program is consistent with the research evidence that suggests word retrieval can and will improve in individuals with aphasia. In addition, it highlights the significant impact paraphasic errors can have on functional communication and how improvement in word retrieval can influence performance on naming tasks, as well as measures of discourse.

REFERENCES

Antonucci, S. M. (2009). Use of semantic feature analysis in group aphasia treatment. *Aphasiology, 23*, 854–866.

Basso, A., Corno, M., & Marangolo, P. (1996). Evolution of oral and written confrontation naming errors in aphasia. A retrospective study on vascular patients. *Journal of Clinical and Experimental Neuropsychology, 18*(1), 77–87.

Beeson, P. M. (1999). Treating acquired writing impairment: Strengthening graphemic representations. *Aphasiology, 13*, 767–785.

Best, W. (1996). When racquets are baskets but baskets are biscuits, where do the words come from? A single-case study of formal paraphasic errors in aphasia. *Cognitive Neuropsychology, 3*, 443–480.

Blanken, G. (1990). Formal paraphasias: A single case study. *Brain and Language, 38*, 534–554.

Blumstein, S. E. (1973). *A phonological investigation of aphasic speech*. The Hague, The Netherlands: Mouton.

Boyle, M. (1989). Reducing phonemic paraphasias in the connected speech of a conduction aphasic subject. In T. E. Prescott (Ed.), *Clinical aphasiology* (18, 379–393). Boston, MA: College-Hill.

Boyle, M. (2004). Semantic feature analysis treatment for anomia in two fluent aphasia syndromes. *American Journal of Speech-Language Pathology, 13*(3), 236–249.

Boyle, M., & Coelho, C. (1995). Application of semantic feature analysis as a treatment for aphasic dysnomia. *American Journal of Speech-Language Pathology, 4*(4), 94–98.

Bub, D., & Kertesz, A. (1982). Evidence for lexico-graphic processing in a patient with preserved written over oral single word naming. *Brain, 105*, 697–717.

Buckingham, H. W. (1980). On correlating aphasic errors with slips-of-the-tongue. *Applied Psycholinguistics, 1*, 199–220.

Buckingham, H. (1992). The mechanisms of phonemic paraphasia. *Clinical Linguistics and Phonetics, 6*, 41–63.

Buckingham, H. (2011). Semantic paraphasia. In J. S. Kreutzer, J. DeLuca, & B. Caplan (Eds.), *Encyclopedia of clinical neuropsychology* (pp. 2248–2250). New York, NY: Springer.

Buckingham, H. W., & Kertesz, A. (1976). *Neologistic jargon aphasia*. Amsterdam, The Netherlands: Swets & Zeitlinger.

Cameron, R., Wambaugh, J., Wright, S., & Nessler, C. (2006). Effects of a combined semantic/phonologic cueing treatment on word retrieval in discourse. *Aphasiology, 20*(2), 269–285.

Caramazza, A., & Hillis, A. (1990). Where do semantic errors come from? *Cortex, 26*(1), 95–122.

Cloutman, L., Gottesman, R., Chaudhry, P., Davis, C., Kleinman, J. T., Pawlak, M., ... Hillis, A. E. (2009). Where (in the brain) do semantic errors come from? *Cortex, 45*(5), 641–649.

Crary, M., & Kertesz, A. (1988). Evolving error profiles during aphasia syndrome remission. *Aphasiology, 2,* 67–78.

Crystal, D. (1987). *The Cambridge encyclopedia of language.* Cambridge, England: Cambridge University Press.

Dell, G. S. (1985). Positive feedback in hierarchical connectionist models: Applications to language production. *Cognitive Science, 9,* 3–23.

Dell, G. S. (1986). A spreading activation theory of retrieval in sentence production. *Psychological Review, 93,* 283–321.

Dell, G. S., Schwartz, M. F., Martin, N., Saffran, E. M., & Gagnon, D. A. (1997). Lexical access is aphasic and nonaphasic speakers. *Psychological Review, 104,* 801–838.

Deloche, G., Hannequin, D., Dordain, M., Metz-Lutz, M.-N., Kremin, H., Tessier, C., ... Pichard, B. (1997). Diversity of patterns of improvement in confrontational naming rehabilitation: Some tentative hypotheses. *Journal of Communication Disorders, 30,* 11–22.

Doyle, P. J., McNeil, M. R., Park, G., Goda, A., Rubenstein, E., Spencer, K., ... Szwarc, L. (2000). Linguistic validation of four parallel forms of a story retelling procedure. *Aphasiology, 14,* 537–549.

Duffy, R. J., & Duffy, J. R. (1981). Three studies of deficits in pantomimic expression and pantomimic recognition in aphasia. *Journal of Speech and Hearing Research, 46,* 70–84.

Duffy, R. J., Duffy, J. R., & Pearson, K. L. (1975). Impairment of pantomime recognition in aphasics. *Journal of Speech and Hearing Research, 18,* 115–132.

Gagnon, D. A., Schwartz, M. F., Martin, N., Dell, G. S., & Saffran, E. M. (1997). The origins of formal paraphasias in aphasic's picture naming. *Brain and Language, 59,* 450–472.

Gardner, G., & Brookshire, R. H. (1972). Effects of unisensory and multisensory presentation of stimuli upon naming by aphasic subjects. *Language and Speech, 15,* 342–357.

Haley, K. L., Jacks, A., & Cunningham, K. T. (2013). Error variability and the differentiation between apraxia of speech and aphasia with phonemic paraphasia. *Journal of Speech, Language, and Hearing Research, 56,* 891–905.

Hashimoto, N. (2012). The use of semantic- and phonological-based feature approaches to treat naming deficits in aphasia. *Clinical Linguistics & Phonetics, 26,* 518–553.

Hickok, G. (2012). Computational neuroanatomy of speech production. *Nature Reviews Neuroscience, 13,* 135–145.

Hickok, G., Houde, J., & Rong, F. (2011). Sensorimotor integration in speech processing: Computational basis and neural organization. *Neuron, 69,* 407–422.

Hickok, G., & Poeppel, D. (2007). The cortical organization of speech processing. *Nature Reviews Neuroscience, 8,* 393-402.

Hier, D. B., & Mohr, J. P. (1977). Incongruous oral and written naming. *Brain and Language, 4,* 115–126.

Hillis, A. E., Rapp, B. C., & Caramazza, A. (1999). When a rose is a rose in speech but a tulip in writing. *Cortex, 35,* 337–356.

Howard, D., & Patterson, K. E. (1992). *The Pyramids and Palm Trees Test: A test of semantic access from words and pictures.* London, England: Thames Valley Test Company.

Kaplan, E., Goodglass, H., & Weintraub, S. (2001). *Boston Naming Test.* Austin, TX: Pro-Ed.

Kay, J., Coltheart, M., & Lesser, R. (1992). *Psycholinguist Assessment of Language Processing in Aphasia.* London, England: Psychology Press.

Kay, J., &. Ellis, A. W. (1987). A cognitive neuropsychological case study of anomia: Implications for psychological models of word retrieval. *Brain, 110*, 613–629.

Kearns, K. P. (1985). Response elaboration training for patient initiated utterances. In R. H. Brookshire (Ed.), *Clinical Aphasiology* (pp. 196–204). Minneapolis, MN: BRK.

Kertesz, A. (2006). *Western Aphasia Battery–Revised* (WAB-R). San Antonio, TX: Pearson.

Kittredge, A. K., Dell, G. S., Verkuilen, J., & Schwartz, M. F. (2008). Where is the effect of frequency in word production? Insights from aphasic picture-naming errors. *Cognitive Neuropsychology, 25*(4), 463–492.

Lecours, A. R., & Lhermitte, F. (1969). Phonemic paraphasias: Linguistic structures and tentative hypotheses. *Cortex, 5*, 193–228.

Levelt, W. J. M. (1989). *Speaking: From intention to articulation.* Cambridge, MA: MIT Press.

Linebaugh, C. C., & Lehner, L. H. (1977). Cueing hierarchies and word retrieval: A therapy program. In *Clinical Aphasiology Conference* (pp. 19–31). Minneapolis: BRK Publishers.

Linebaugh, C. W., Shisler, R. J., & Lehner, L. H. (2005). Cueing hierarchies and word retrieval: A therapy program. *Aphasiology, 19*, 77–92.

Marshall, R. C. (2008). Early management of Wernicke's aphasia: A context-based approach. In R. Chapey (Ed.), *Language intervention strategies in aphasia and related language disorders* (pp. 507–529). Baltimore, MD: Lippincott Williams & Wilkins.

Marshall, R. C., Rappaport, B. Z., & Garcia-Bunuel, L. (1985). Self-monitoring behavior in a case of severe auditory agnosia with aphasia. *Brain and Language, 24*, 297–313.

Marshall, R. C., & Tompkins, C. A. (1982). Verbal self-correction behaviors of fluent and nonfluent aphasic subjects. *Brain and Language, 15*(2), 292–306.

Martin, N., Dell, G. S., Saffran, E. M., & Schwartz, M. F. (1994). Origins of paraphasias in deep dysphasia: Testing the consequences of a decay impairment to an interactive spreading activation model of lexical retrieval. *Brain and Language, 47*, 609–660.

McNeil, M. R., Robin, D. A., & Schmidt, R. A. (2009). Apraxia of speech. In M. R. McNeil (Ed.), *Clinical management of sensorimotor speech disorders* (pp. 249–268). New York, NY: Thieme.

Miceli, G., Benvegnu, M., Capasso, R., & Caramazza, A. (1997). The independence of phonological and orthographic lexical forms: Evidence from aphasia. *Cognitive Neuropsychology, 14*, 33–70.

Nickels, L., & Howard, D. (1995). Phonological errors in aphasic naming: Comprehension, monitoring and lexicality. *Cortex, 31*, 209–237.

Nozari, N., Dell, G. S., & Schwartz, M. F. (2011). Is comprehension necessary for error detection? A conflict-based account of monitoring in speech production. *Cognitive psychology, 63*(1), 1–33.

Peach, R. K., & Reuter, K. A. (2010). A discourse-based approach to semantic feature analysis for the treatment of aphasic word retrieval failures. *Aphasiology, 24*(9), 971–990.

Obler, L. K., & Albert, M. (n.d.) Action Naming Test. Retrieved August 22, 2016, from the Boston University, Department of neurology, Language in the Aging Brain Project: http://www.bu.edu/lab/action-naming-test/

Raymer, A. M., & Ellsworth, T. A. (2002). Response to contrasting verb retrieval treatments: A case study. *Aphasiology, 16*, 1031–1045.

Raymer, A., Singletary, F., Rodriguez, A., Ciampitti, M., Heilman, K., & Gonzalez-Rothi, L. (2006). Effects of gesture+verbal treatment for noun and verb retrieval in aphasia. *Journal of the International Neuropsychological Society, 12*, 867–882.

Raymer, A. M., Thompson, C. K., Jacobs, B., & LeGrand, H. R. (1993). Phonological treatment of naming deficits in aphasia: Model-based generalization analysis. *Aphasiology, 7*, 27–53.

Roach, A., Schwartz, M. F., Martin, N., Grewal, R. S., & Brecher, A. (1996). The Philadelphia Naming Test: Scoring and Rationale. *Clinical Aphasiology, 24*, 121–133.

Rodriguez, A. D., Raymer, A. M., & Rothi, L. J. G. (2006). Effects of gesture+verbal and semantic-phonologic treatments for verb retrieval in aphasia. *Aphasiology, 20,* 286–297.

Rose, M., & Sussmilch, G. (2008). The effects of semantic and gesture treatments on verb retrieval and verb use in aphasia. *Aphasiology, 22,* 691–706.

Snodgrass, J. G., & Vanderwart, M. (1980). A standardized set of 260 pictures: Norms for name agreement, image agreement, familiarity, and visual complexity. *Journal of Experimental Psychology: Human Learning and Memory, 6*(2), 174–215.

Spreen, O., Benton, A. L., & Van Allen, M. W. (1966). Dissociation of visual and tactile naming in amnesic aphasia. *Neurology, 16,* 807–814.

Stark, J. (1988). Aspects of automatic versus controlled processing, monitoring, metalinguistic tasks, and related phenomena in aphasia. In W. Dressler & J. Stark (Eds.). *Linguistic analyses of aphasic language* (pp. 179–223). New York, NY: Springer-Verlag.

Ueno, T., & Lambon Ralph, M. A. (2013). The roles of the "ventral" semantic and "dorsal" pathways in conduite d'approche: A neuroanatomically-constrained computational modeling investigation. *Frontiers in Human Neuroscience, 7,* 1–7.

Wambaugh, J., Cameron, R., Kalinyak-Fliszar, M., Nessler, C., & Wright, S. (2004). Retrieval of action names in aphasia: Effects of two cueing treatments. *Aphasiology, 18*(11), 979–1004.

Wambaugh, J. L., Duffy, J. R., McNeil, M. R., Robin, D. A., & Rogers, M. A. (2006). Treatment guidelines for acquired apraxia of speech: Treatment descriptions and recommendations. *Journal of Medical Speech-Language Pathology, 14,* xxxv–lxvii.

Wambaugh, J. L., Linebaugh, C. W., Doyle, P. J., Martinez, A. L., Kalinyak-Fliszar, M., & Spencer, K. A. (2001). Effects of two cueing treatments on lexical retrieval in aphasic speakers with different levels of deficit. *Aphasiology, 15,* 933–950.

Wambaugh, J., & Wright, S. (2007). Improved effects of word-retrieval treatments subsequent to additional of the orthographic form. *Aphasiology, 21,* 633–642.

Wright, H. H., Marshall, R. C., Wilson, K. B., & Page, J. L. (2008). Using a written cueing hierarchy to improve verbal naming in aphasia. *Aphasiology, 22,* 522–536.

CHAPTER 3

Therapy for People with Jargon Aphasia

Jane Marshall

INTRODUCTION

Jargon aphasia describes an acquired language impairment in which speech is fluent and easily articulated, but largely unintelligible. It is associated with Wernicke's and transcortical sensory aphasia and usually follows left hemisphere posterior brain lesions, for example in the region of the supramarginal gyrus, the inferior parietal lobe, and the posterior portion of the first temporal gyrus (Kertesz, 1981). The motor cortex is often spared, leaving the person without motor impairments.

Manifestations of jargon aphasia vary. A defining characteristic is the production of jargon, or largely meaningless speech, which can take different forms (see definitions and examples in **TABLE 3.1**). Semantic jargon is composed mainly of real words, albeit in very anomalous combinations. Neologistic jargon contains frequent neologisms, or nonword errors, which are typically embedded in empty, but syntactically structured phrases. Phonemic, or undifferentiated jargon is composed almost entirely from nonwords. These different manifestations, in part, reflect the severity of the condition, with semantic jargon being the least and phonemic jargon the most impaired. Evidence for this view comes from longitudinal studies showing that nonword errors typically reduce as speech recovery occurs (Eaton, Marshall, & Pring, 2011; Simmons & Buckingham, 1992).

Errors in jargon aphasia are profuse and diverse, even within the same speaker. They may bear a semantic or phonological relationship to the target or be entirely unrelated.

TABLE 3.1 Definition of terms and examples

Term	Definition	Example
Semantic jargon	Fluent but unintelligible speech that is constructed mainly from real words, but with frequent semantic errors and verbal paraphasias (real word errors that are unrelated to the target)	"foot, nose, feets, shoe feets, shoe, the shoe itself, but the knife seems more strenuous than anything else" (RG naming a picture of a foot; from Marshall, Chiat, Robson, & Pring, 1996)
Neologistic jargon	Fluent but unintelligible speech that contains frequent nonword errors	"and looks like the lugyburgers. It says oh we're gonna to pick a ligyburger that we want to get our liggyburgers. And so they, the . . . the king say or the so the men the uh the pigyburger say ah well here's the bigyburger and bloblah and all the rest of it" (FF retelling the Cinderella narrative; from Bose & Buchanan, 2007)
Phonemic/ undifferentiated jargon	Fluent but unintelligible speech, containing very few recognizable real words	"he /spɪtæl ˈdʒɒlɪtə/ erm his, erm /ˈvɛdɪʃən ˈhalɪʃ wɪz ʃɜm/ it er /raɪʧ/ with /ˈaɪdrɒɪtɪn ˈtɛlɪ tɛlˈradədʒɪn/" (LT responding to a question about his son in America; from Robson, Pring, Marshall, & Chiat, 2003)

Neologisms or nonword errors are present in almost all speakers. These are varyingly defined. Some researchers classify all nonword errors as neologisms (e.g., Bose & Buchanan, 2007), while others reserve the term for abstruse errors containing less than 50% of the target phonology (e.g., Kohn, Smith, & Alexander, 1996; Moses, Nickels, & Sheard, 2004).

Another common symptom in jargon aphasia is perseveration. This may involve the repetition of whole words, or word fragments (Bose & Buchanan, 2007; Eaton, Marshall, & Pring, 2010; Moses et al., 2004; Pitts, Bhatnagar, Buckingham, Hacein-Bey, & Bhatnagar, 2010). FF's sample in Table 3.1 is illustrative, with neologisms constructed around a repeated and minimally changing phonological form. There is some evidence that perseveration is a marker of severity in jargon aphasia. For example, it is associated with poor recovery over time (Kohn et al., 1996) and with the overall number of speech errors produced by individuals (Goldman, Schwartz, & Wilshire, 2001).

Logorrhea is a further possible symptom (Caspari, 2005). Also referred to as a "press of speech," this involves the use of incessant talking that is difficult to inhibit. The rate of speech may also seem abnormally fast, although this may be an impression arising from the unintelligible content.

In the face of so many speech impairments it is worth reflecting on what is intact in jargon aphasia. A speaker of jargon can usually signal whether he or she is asking a question or making a statement. It will also be clear whether the speaker is pleased, puzzled, sad, or annoyed. We might even know if he or she is telling us a joke or recounting something serious. These elements can be conveyed largely because the paralinguistic properties of speech, such as intonation and stress, are typically intact. Indeed, one jargon speaker known to me was able to mimic the accents of her care staff (in jargon) for the guilty amusement of her visitors.

Most people with jargon aphasia also obey the phonological constraints and phonotactic rules of their language, even if they produce virtually no real words. So, they only use their native speech sounds and combine these into legal syllables (Hanlon & Edmondson, 1996; Robson et al., 2003). Many speakers also display elements of preserved syntax (although see Butterworth & Howard, 1987, for evidence of syntactic impairments). Perhaps most striking is the finding that even abstruse neologisms may be correctly inflected, again pointing to a degree of syntactic preservation (Macoir & Beland, 2004; Miller & Ellis, 1987).

This brief introduction shows that speech in jargon aphasia is highly varied, particularly in terms of the errors that are produced. The common features are fluency and a lack of intelligibility, coupled with a retained melodic line, and aspects of phonology and syntax. Thus, in severe cases, speech can be almost entirely unintelligible but sound deceptively "normal," particularly if heard from a distance.

The disorder of speech may be accompanied by a number of additional impairments. Many (but not all) speakers of jargon show signs of anosognosia. This is a lack of awareness of neurological deficit, in this case related to speech (Butterworth, 1979; Cappa, Miozzo, & Frugoni, 1994; Cohen, Verstichel, & Dehaene, 1997; Hanlon & Edmondson, 1996; Hillis, Boatman, Hart, & Gordon, 1999; Marshall et al., 1996; Marshall, Robson, Pring, & Chiat, 1998; Panzeri, Semenza, & Butterworth, 1987; Robson, Pring, Marshall, Morrison, & Chiat, 1998; Robson et al., 2003; Sampson & Faroqi-Shah, 2011; Simmons & Buckingham, 1992; Weinstein, 1981). For example, they do not attempt to correct their speech or show dissatisfaction with it. They may become annoyed or mystified when others fail to understand. These speakers may be equally unaware when they have said something correctly. So, when tested, they may persist with a response even when they have already produced the correct word (see the example from RG in Table 3.1). It seems, therefore, that the mechanisms that monitor speech have broken down in at least some individuals with jargon aphasia.

Many speakers also have impaired auditory comprehension (e.g., Robson, Keidel, Lambon Ralph, & Sage, 2012). Indeed, this problem can be profound, and may manifest as word deafness (Maneta, Marshall, & Lindsay, 2001). Writing problems are also common, and can include jargonagraphia with fluent but meaningless writing (Cappa, Cavalloti, & Vignolo, 1987; Schonauer & Denes, 1994).

The language symptoms associated with Wernicke's aphasia, the syndrome most associated with jargon, may improve over time (Laska, Hellbolm, Murray, Kahan, & von Arbin, 2001). However, there is evidence that the prognosis is worse than for other types of aphasia (Bakheit, Shaw, Carrington, & Griffiths, 2007; Nicholas, Helm-Estabrooks, Ward-Lonergan, & Morgan, 1993). In line with this, it is often argued that jargon is particularly difficult to treat (e.g., Marshall, 2006). A number of factors contribute to this view. First of all, as we have seen, jargon aphasia is not simply an absence of speech. Rather there is a profusion of overt symptoms, such as semantic errors, neologisms, and perseverations. Many speech production tasks will elicit these errors, and so run the risk of reinforcing the very symptoms that we would hope to suppress. The frequent coexistence of impaired auditory comprehension is a further challenge. This generates an additional goal for intervention, and may affect treatment compliance because therapy tasks cannot be understood. Above all, the seeming lack of awareness can inhibit attempts to remediate speech and even lead to the rejection of therapy.

This chapter will review some of the treatment approaches that have been attempted with people who jargon. These have been directed at several levels of the International Classification of Functioning Disability and Health model (World Health Organization [WHO], 2001). Communication activities have been addressed by attempting to remediate the language impairment and by promoting the use of compensations. Participation has also been addressed, either by promoting the transfer of therapy skills to everyday contexts, or through environmental modifications.

The chapter will first consider attempts to remediate the comprehension and monitoring impairments that typically occur in jargon aphasia. It will then turn to production and describe both direct and compensatory attempts to address the impairment. Finally, it will consider the importance of working with those who are in the environment of the jargon speaker.

TREATMENTS OF AUDITORY COMPREHENSION

When auditory comprehension is impaired, this may be an initial focus of therapy because of the likely effects on everyday communication. Disordered comprehension may also impair understanding of the rehabilitation processes, again making it a priority for intervention.

Accounts of comprehension therapy in the literature are often underpinned by cognitive neuropsychological models of word processing (Morris & Franklin, 2017; Whitworth, Webster, & Howard, 2014). The impairment is initially diagnosed by identifying the level of breakdown in the auditory processing system, and this diagnosis motivates the content of therapy. For example, tasks may attempt to remediate the impaired level of processing or engage intact skills to compensate for the problem.

This approach was taken in three single-case accounts of comprehension therapy with jargon speakers. LR (Grayson, Hilton, & Franklin, 1997) had unintelligible speech that combined "English jargon" (p 259), that is semantic jargon, and neologisms. Understanding of speech was also severely impaired. For example, LR was unable to respond accurately to simple yes/no questions. Assessment revealed difficulties with all auditory input tasks, but judgments of meaning were particularly impaired, regardless of modality. For example, LR could not match spoken or written words to pictures, and was impaired on the all-picture version of the Pyramids and Palm Trees Test (Howard & Patterson, 1992), where pictures have to be associated on the basis of their meaning. The authors therefore concluded that a central semantic deficit was core to LR's problems.

LR was given three programs of comprehension therapy delivered over a period of 24 weeks (with breaks for assessment). The regime involved daily sessions, at least initially. The first program entailed semantic therapy, and included spoken word to picture matching, picture categorization, and written word association tasks. In the second program these tasks were augmented by auditory therapy, in which LR had to match words to pictures with rhyming foils. In the final program the stimuli were extended to include sentences. Although the study did not employ an experimental design, each program of therapy was evaluated with relevant assessment tasks. Crucially, gains on these were consistent with the content of therapy. So after the first program, semantic tasks like word to picture matching improved, whereas minimal pair tasks did not. The latter, however, did improve after the second program, which involved the discrimination of very similar sounding words.

PK, the individual in the second single-case study, also produced neologistic jargon and had very impaired understanding of speech (Maneta et al., 2001). In his case the comprehension deficit seemed due to word sound deafness, or an inability to discriminate between speech sounds. In line with this, he was poor on all auditory input tasks including minimal pair judgments; whereas written input tasks were largely intact. The first program of therapy with PK worked directly on his auditory discrimination. He was given a series of tasks in which he had to match spoken stimuli to written words and pictures with similar sounding distractors. For example, the word "man" had to be matched to one of three written words: "man," "tan," and "can." He was supported in these tasks with lip reading information. For example, he was encouraged to watch the clinician's face and was given diagrams illustrating lip to sound correspondences. The clinician also used cued articulation (Passy, 1990), which is a series of hand signals indicating phonemic features, such as the presence or absence of voicing. After 12 sessions of this therapy, delivered twice a week, PK was reassessed on a number of auditory tasks. Unfortunately, there were no significant gains.

The lack of progress prompted the authors to change tack. Rather than attempting to remediate PK's impairment, they decided to employ an indirect, compensatory approach. The second program, again comprising 12 sessions, trained PK's wife to use a number of strategies to assist his understanding. In particular, she was encouraged to use single-word writing alongside speech, to simplify messages, and to check that PK had understood after each exchange. This program of therapy was evaluated through an interactive task, in which PK was asked a number of yes/no biographical questions by his wife. Before therapy he scored virtually at chance, and the task resulted in frequent and extended breakdowns in communication. After therapy he scored 28/30, and there were only four communication breakdowns, which were quickly resolved.

KW, the individual treated in the final case study (Francis, Riddoch, & Humphreys, 2001) had very impaired auditory comprehension alongside phonemic jargon speech. A series of investigations indicated that his difficulties were due to word meaning deafness. Individuals with this impairment can discriminate speech sounds and recognize spoken words. They cannot, however, derive any meaning from the language they hear. Accordingly, KW succeeded on minimal pair and lexical decision tasks, but failed on tasks that required comprehension, such as synonym judgment and word to picture matching. His problems were specific to speech; thus he had no difficulties when the equivalent tasks used written words.

KW was given two programs of therapy, each lasting 3 weeks and each targeting 26 different words. The treatment was largely self-administered via work sheets that KW practiced intensively at home. The first program was called "Implicit Access Therapy" and involved two written tasks. In one task KW had to read definitions of the target words and attempt to fix the meaning in his mind. For example, the definition for "annual" was: "Annual refers to something that occurs every year." After reading the definition, he had to write the target word down several times while thinking about its meaning. In the other task he was given triads of written words, and had to identify the two that were most related in meaning (e.g., "annual," "yearly," and "monthly"). The second therapy program was called "Explicit Access Therapy." This involved very similar tasks. However, now the stimuli were also audiotape-recorded and KW had to listen to the tape while completing the tasks. He was also required to repeat the target words after the definition task, rather than writing them down. The authors argued that auditory processing might be engaged implicitly in the first therapy program during silent reading, whereas this was an explicit feature of the second program. Both treatments exploited KW's strengths in reading comprehension.

Therapy outcomes were assessed by asking KW to define spoken words. Both programs of therapy improved KW's performance on this task, but only with the treated words. The immediate gain was similar after each therapy. However, follow-up assessment showed that the benefits of Explicit Access Therapy were more durable.

It is clear that the therapy practiced with KW improved his understanding of speech. The authors discuss two ways that this may have been achieved. One mechanism was compensatory, which involved KW visualizing the spelling of words so that he could effectively read and understand them. The other mechanism entailed direct remediation of his impairment, or the reconnection of spoken words with their semantic representations. Interestingly, both mechanisms seemed specific to treated words.

The studies reviewed in this section all describe attempts to tackle comprehension failure in jargon aphasia. Change was achieved either by remediating the impairment or by using compensations. For example, Francis and colleagues (2001) encouraged their participant to make compensatory use of his spelling and reading skills in order to "bootstrap" his understanding of speech. In Maneta et al. (2001), compensation was achieved by changing the behaviors of the client's main communication partner.

Studies of comprehension therapy for people with aphasia are few in number (see review in Morris & Franklin, 2017) and are often limited to single-case or small-group designs. Clinicians, therefore, are not provided with a strong evidence base to inform their clinical decisions. Findings from the existing studies are also equivocal, in that not all participants responded positively (e.g., Woolf, Panton, Rosen, Best, & Marshall, 2014) or achieved generalized gains (Francis et al., 2001). If comprehension skills are difficult to restore, working through those who interact with the person with aphasia will be an important aspect of intervention, as was the case in Maneta et al. (2001). We need to make communication partners aware of the comprehension difficulties that typically accompany jargon, and give them strategies for coping with them. Such indirect work is further discussed in the final section of this chapter.

TREATMENTS FOR MONITORING OF SPEECH

The seeming lack of awareness (anosognosia) that often accompanies jargon speech is one of the most striking and puzzling features of the condition. It also poses a clinical challenge. If the person believes their speech is intact, they will not see the need for therapy, or for alternative channels of communication. Clinicians may also worry that confronting a client with their difficulties will cause psychological distress or even a catastrophic reaction (Chriki, Bullain, & Stern, 2006).

Identifying the nature and origin of the awareness deficit in jargon aphasia is challenging. Anosognosia is known to be complex and multidimensional (Prigatano, 2010). For example, it may encompass an inability to detect neurological symptoms, a misattribution of their cause, or an underestimation of their functional consequences. There may also be a discrepancy between explicit and implicit signs of awareness; for example, a patient may assert that he or she can walk, but still refuse to leave his or her wheelchair.

Anosognosia is typically probed by self-reporting measures that are highly dependent on language, such as structured interviews and questionnaires (Jehkonen, Laihosalo, & Kettunen, 2006). Of course such measures are difficult to use with people who have aphasia, and particularly jargon aphasia. For this reason, anosognosic impairments may be under detected in this group (Cocchini, Beschin, Cameron, Fotopoulou, & Della Sala, 2009; Orfei, Caltagirone, & Spalletta, 2009).

Determining the cause of anosognosia in jargon aphasia is a further challenge. An early view attributed the problem to the psychological denial of deficits, stemming from a need to maintain emotional equilibrium and preserve a sense of self (Weinstein, 1981;

Weinstein & Lyerly, 1976). While this may be true for some individuals, it cannot explain all cases, or account for the diverse manifestations of the condition. It is also challenged by evidence that awareness and mood may not correlate (Cocchini, Crosta, Allen, Zaro, & Beschin, 2013). An alternative proposal argues that impairments in cognitive skills, such as attention, memory, and executive function, prevent the person from absorbing new information about their current state. However, this hypothesis struggles to explain modality specific anosognosias, for example where hemiplegia is recognized but aphasia is not (Cocchini et al., 2013). Dissociations within language are even more challenging, for instance where there is differential awareness of speech and writing errors (Marshall et al., 1998).

The final proposal argues that anosognosia can arise from monitoring failures for specific cognitive functions. Thus, in the context of jargon aphasia, there seems to be a breakdown in the system that monitors speech. This in turn, suggests that treatment needs to address monitoring skills.

Treating the monitoring failure in jargon aphasia requires an understanding of how monitoring of speech is normally accomplished. Here there are differing views (Postma, 2000). According to one account, monitoring involves feedback through the auditory comprehension system, in effect enabling a person to listen to his or her own speech (Hartsuiker & Kolk, 2001; Levelt, 1989; Oomen & Postma, 2002; Oomen, Postma, & Kolk, 2001). Feedback can be pre- and post-articulatory. The pre-articulatory feedback route monitors speech before it is produced, thus preventing speech errors from occurring. The post-articulatory route monitors speech after it is produced. This route cannot inhibit errors; but it generates awareness of them, and initiates post-production repairs.

Failure of the feedback monitor is a likely explanation for anosognosia in some speakers with jargon, particularly when there are coexistent deficits in auditory comprehension (e.g., Ellis, Miller, & Sin, 1983; Maneta et al., 2001). However, this view is challenged by evidence of dissociations between comprehension and monitoring (e.g., Maher, Gonzalez-Rothi, & Heilman, 1994). Take RMM as an example (Marshall et al., 1998). She was a speaker with fluent neologistic jargon with no apparent awareness of her speech deficit. She made no overt attempts to self repair, and her speech lacked the hesitancies that might signal covert error detection. Yet her auditory comprehension was surprisingly intact. For example, she scored over 90% correct on tests of minimal pair judgment, auditory lexical decision, and spoken word to picture matching. Thus she could analyze speech sounds and judge the lexical status of words and comprehend speech, yet she failed to recruit these skills in order to monitor her own output. A more recent investigation of five speakers with jargon similarly found that comprehension scores were not predictive of monitoring behaviors (Sampson & Faroqi-Shah, 2011).

It seems that for some jargon speakers a viable auditory system is unavailable for error detection. This could be due to a disconnection in the feedback pathways or could reflect a limitation in processing resources. Employing the feedback monitor requires a speaker to carry out two tasks at once, namely produce speech and scrutinize that speech for errors. Some individuals may lack the capacity for such dual processing.

A number of studies have explored these proposals by asking participants to carry out tasks in which they had to judge the integrity of their own production, while varying the conditions in which the judgments were made (Maher et al., 1994; Marshall et al., 1998; Sampson & Faroqi-Shah, 2011; Shuren, Smith-Hammond, Maher, Rothi, & Heilman, 1995). So, in one task, the person might be asked to name a picture and then immediately judge whether their attempt was correct or not. This condition might be compared to judgments of their tape-recorded responses, judgments made in the context of masking noise, or judgments of responses on different production tasks. A number of findings emerged from these studies. Firstly, some individuals were impaired when making immediate judgments of their speech, but less so when they listened to themselves on tape (Maher et al., 1994; Shuren et al., 1995). It seemed that these individuals lacked the processing resources to carry out a dual task. In other words, monitoring could only be accomplished when it was disconnected from speaking. Sampson and Faroqi-Shah (2011) showed that all but one of their participants were less able to monitor when subjected to masking noise. This showed that these individuals *were* making use of post-articulatory feedback, and when they could no longer hear their own speech, their judgments were impaired. However, this monitoring mechanism was far from perfect, given that many errors were undetected even in normal listening conditions. Finally, there is evidence that, at least for some individuals, monitoring depends on the nature of the production task (Marshall et al., 1998; Sampson & Faroqi-Shah, 2011). So, more errors were detected in a repetition task than in picture naming.

Taken together, these studies suggest that for many speakers with jargon, feedback monitoring is imperfect and varyingly applied. Its concurrent use with speaking, in particular, cannot be assumed. The finding that error detection depends on the nature of the production task is consistent with the existence of a secondary monitor, which is intrinsic to the output rather than the input system (Postma, 2000). This monitor might employ editors that are attached to each level of the production system or may arise from feedback connections that "detect" mismatches between the target and a pending error (see arguments in Marshall et al., 1998). It is assumed that this monitor can only operate when the production system is functioning, at least to some degree. In line with this proposal, there is evidence that rates of error detection correlate with production success (Eaton et al., 2011; Sampson & Faroqi-Shah, 2011).

What are the implications for therapy? It seems that treatment might aim to improve the functioning of two monitoring mechanisms; one of these employs feedback through the auditory comprehension system, while the other is intrinsic to production. An obvious target for the former is to work on auditory input, particularly when there is a coexistent deficit in speech comprehension. So therapy might target phoneme discrimination, word recognition, or access to semantics, depending on the level of impairment. If successful, this should bring about gains in auditory comprehension coupled with improved self-monitoring. However, there are a number of caveats. As we have seen, although there are reports of successful comprehension therapy with jargon speakers (Francis et al., 2001; Grayson et al., 1997), there are also negative accounts (Maneta et al., 2001). It may be, therefore, that achieving change in comprehension skills is challenging. The findings from self-judgment experiments also show that even if auditory input skills recover, these may not be employed successfully for monitoring. In such instances, tasks that promote "dual attention" might be attempted. For example, the person may be asked to judge the quality of their own speech under increasingly demanding conditions. For example, they might first hear the clinician repeat back their responses but later make unaided and immediate judgments. To my knowledge, such a treatment has not been reported.

One study reports a direct attempt to remediate the production monitor (Marshall et al., 1998). CM produced fluent neologistic jargon. Although he did not deny his aphasia, he seemed unable to judge the quality of his speech. For example, he did not try to self-correct and he relied on feedback from his conversation partner to determine whether or not he was making sense. On all spoken input tasks, such as minimal pair judgments, lexical decision, and word to picture matching, CM scored well above chance. Yet he was clearly failing to use these input skills for the purposes of self-monitoring. CM's monitoring skills were investigated through a series of judgment tasks. For example, he had to name a picture and then indicate whether or not his attempt was correct. These showed that he was largely oblivious to his errors in naming, but much more aware of his errors in repetition. The authors concluded that CM's capacity to monitor depended on the nature of the production task. When this required him to access phonology from semantics, as is the case in naming, monitoring broke down. When he could bypass semantics, as is the case in repetition, monitoring was achieved.

This hypothesis was the springboard for therapy. CM was given 6 hours of treatment aiming to improve his production of 40 words. The tasks required him to carry out semantic judgments with the target words; for example, he had to select written words that were related to the target in the presence of distractors. Thus treatment aimed to facilitate the impaired connection between semantics and phonology; if successful, naming should increase coupled with improved monitoring of naming errors.

Treatment was evaluated by asking CM to name the 40 treated words and 40 control items that had not been featured in therapy (items were presented in one block in random order). After each naming attempt CM was asked to signal whether or not he had produced the word correctly. Thus the task yielded a naming and a monitoring score. Results for the former were disappointing. CM produced marginally fewer correct words after therapy than before, with no specific benefit for treated words. Monitoring, however, did improve. CM's judgments of his naming attempts after therapy were significantly better than before, including his detection of neologisms. However, this gain was almost entirely confined to treated words. Neologisms produced for untreated words still passed below his radar. Interpreting this result, the authors concluded that therapy improved semantic processing for treated items only. The gain was insufficient to benefit production, possibly because therapy had required very little spoken output. Treatment did, however, enable the production monitor to kick in, making CM aware of his errors.

The results achieved with CM were theoretically interesting, but clinically disappointing. Treatment had not improved CM's speech, but had made him more aware of its failings. Indeed, such an outcome might even have adverse psychological consequences (although, fortunately, this did not seem to be the case for CM). More positively, improved awareness might stimulate correction attempts or encourage the person to convey their message by alternative means.

Unfortunately, there are few studies of self-monitoring in jargon aphasia, particularly with respect to therapy. It is not clear, therefore, whether the feedback or production monitors can be rehabilitated and therapists are left with little guidance about how to address the communicative consequences of monitoring failure. In the absence of an evidence base, clinicians are likely to make individual decisions, probably following careful consultation with family members and friends. A number of clinical papers allude to "stop" strategies (e.g., making a "sh" gesture), whereby the clinician attempts to inhibit unmonitored and unintelligible speech (Marshall, 2008; Martin, 1981; Strauss Hough, 1993). It is argued that these strategies can help individuals who have logorrhea or press of speech and do not pause to listen. However, some individuals may respond negatively to such inhibitory techniques, or fail to see the rationale for them. As an alternative, individuals with relatively intact comprehension might respond to explicit discussion about the failings in their speech, possibly reinforced by video playback, so that they can observe themselves talking. Others might benefit from consistent feedback during communication exchanges, such as that provided by family members and all rehabilitation staff. For example, this feedback might indicate when speech is not comprehensible and offer suggestions about alternative strategies that might be attempted. Finally, Marshall (2008) stresses that if the person does attempt to correct his or her speech, this should be explicitly reinforced.

Whatever the technique, therapy aiming to improve awareness of jargon should additionally give the person resources for dealing with the problem. In other words, parallel treatments of production should be attempted.

TREATMENTS OF PRODUCTION

Output therapies in jargon aphasia can attempt to remediate the language production impairment or compensate for it. Remediation therapies aim to boost the functioning of the speech production system. Compensations include the use of alternative language modalities, such as writing, or nonverbal techniques, such as gesture and drawing.

Treatment Aimed at Remediation

There is good evidence that the errors in jargon aphasia reflect an underlying impairment in word retrieval (e.g., Bose & Buchanan, 2007; Olson, Romani, & Halloran, 2007; Robson et al., 2003). For example, many studies have demonstrated that neologisms occupy content word positions in connected speech, encouraging the view that they are substituting for words that cannot be accessed (e.g., Buckingham, 1990; Stenneken, Hoffmann, & Jacobs, 2008). Butterworth (1979, 1985) additionally showed that they follow pauses, suggesting that an unsuccessful word search has taken place. Longitudinal studies provide further evidence, showing that when the florid symptoms of jargon subside the residual anomia is typically revealed (e.g., Eaton et al., 2011; Panzeri et al., 1987; Simmons & Buckingham, 1992). Finally, simulation studies have shown that jargon errors can be elicited by lesioning an interactive lexical network (Dell, Schwartz, Martin, Saffran, & Gagnon, 1997).

If a failure in word production underpins jargon, therapy could address that failure. Successful outcomes should be marked by improved word retrieval, coupled with a reduction in the symptoms of jargon. This is a promising avenue, given that a number of word-finding therapies have been developed for people with aphasia, several of which have a good evidence base (e.g., see Carragher, Conroy, Sage, & Wilkinson, 2012; Nickels, 2002). However, evaluations of these treatments with speakers with jargon are rare.

Boyle (2004) conducted Semantic Feature Analysis with two participants who had fluent aphasia. One had a diagnosis of Wernicke's aphasia and produced neologisms in naming tasks. This participant worked on 80 words over two phases of therapy. Treatment required him to attempt naming each word and then access a range of semantic features associated with it, such as its category, use, physical properties, and location. Naming of treated nouns improved as a result of this therapy, with some generalization to untreated probes. There was also improved word retrieval in discourse. The author hypothesized that the treated individual had an impaired semantic system, and that therapy improved his ability to access the semantic features of words, with subsequent benefits for naming.

A different semantic therapy was tested with another individual who had Wernicke's aphasia (Davis, Harrington, & Baynes, 2006). Treatment was highly intensive and involved semantic decision tasks, mainly delivered on a computer. For example, the participant had to answer questions (such as "which one grows on a tree?") by selecting a target picture from among a choice of four. None of the tasks involved production. Despite this, naming of both treated and untreated words improved, and there were gains on noun production in narrative speech. Pre- and post-therapy functional imaging showed that the behavioral gains were accompanied by increased left hemisphere brain activation, particularly in the perilesional and inferior frontal gyrus areas.

These studies suggest that individuals with fluent Wernicke's aphasia may benefit from semantic naming treatments. However, the degree to which jargon was a feature of their presentation is unclear. This was not the case for two investigations of phonological treatment. GF (Robson, Marshall, Pring, & Chiat, 1999) produced unintelligible neologistic jargon, with picture naming scores that were virtually at floor. Despite her severe production impairment, GF's auditory input skills were surprisingly intact. For example she could distinguish minimal pairs and scored 97% correct on spoken word to picture matching. She also demonstrated awareness of her jargon, with frequent comments about her production failures. Further testing confirmed that GF retained semantic knowledge about words, but could not access their phonologies. Therapy therefore adopted a phonological approach. It required GF to make phonological judgments about target words, focusing on their syllabic structure and first phoneme. Stimuli were initially spoken by the clinician, but then only represented with pictures. Once GF had identified the number of syllables and the first phoneme of a word, she was asked to produce it. The program was delivered over 6 months, and comprised 40 sessions each lasting 20 minutes. Fifty words were included in therapy, and GF made significant gains in naming these words as a result of therapy. Encouragingly, untreated words also improved, suggesting that she had recovered general, rather than item-specific access to the phonological lexicon.

The second phonological treatment study adopted a similar approach (Bose, 2013). FF had neologistic jargon aphasia (see example in Table 3.1) and achieved approximately 40% accuracy in tests of picture naming. Like GF, he seemed to have impaired access to the phonological representations of words. Therapy involved Phonological Component Analysis (Leonard, Rochon, & Laird, 2008). First, FF was asked to produce each word in response to a picture. Regardless of his success, he was then required to identify five phonological features related to that target: a rhyming word, the first sound, a first sound associate (i.e., another word with the same first sound), the final sound, and the number of syllables. The word was then presented again for naming. Therapy improved FF's naming of 30 treated words. Generalization to a large set of untreated items was not observed in terms of naming accuracy. However, his errors became more target related and less likely to be nonwords.

These studies show that word retrieval in jargon aphasia may respond to phonological treatment. However, the approach has only been tested with two individuals, and aspects of their presentation might be regarded as atypical. For example, they retained the auditory input and self-monitoring skills required by the therapy tasks. Further evaluations of anomia therapy in jargon aphasia are needed, including explorations of factors that make individuals good (or poor) candidates for therapy. More diverse techniques also need to be tested. One could be errorless learning. This approach does not outperform other treatments of aphasic naming (Fillingham, Sage, & Lambon Ralph, 2006); however, it may particularly benefit speakers of jargon, as it would minimize the production of jargon errors during treatment tasks.

The semantic and phonological treatments described here involved single-word tasks. Some discourse therapies have also been attempted with people who have Wernicke's aphasia. Attentive Reading and Constrained Summarization (ARCS) therapy involves reading passages aloud sentence by sentence, and attempting to summarize the content (Rogalski & Edmonds, 2008). Participants are constrained in that they are not permitted to use pronouns or nonspecific language (such as "thing" or "stuff"). Thus the retrieval of meaningful content words is emphasized. ARCS was attempted with two individuals who had chronic Wernicke's aphasia (Rogalski, Edmonds, Daly, & Gardner, 2013). Both had "empty" discourse, featuring frequent phonemic and semantic errors and nonspecific language. They received 18 treatment sessions over 10 weeks, each session lasting 50 minutes. As a result, one showed marked gains on the Boston Naming Test (Kaplan, Goodglass, & Weintraub, 2001) and on the number of information units produced in discourse production tasks. The other, however, did not improve on these outcome measures, possibly because her aphasia was more severe and of longer duration.

An alternative discourse therapy is AphasiaScripts (Lee, Kaye, & Cherney, 2009). This is a computerized treatment in which the person with aphasia practices a scripted discourse with an avatar clinician acting as their conversation partner. Each discourse is personally developed. For example, it may consist of a conversation about a recent holiday, or a graduation speech for a son. The script is programmed into the computer, so that it can be practiced independently at home. Different levels of cue can be provided. In the most cued condition, the person with aphasia sees the written text and the avatar speaking each section of the discourse. These cues can be faded out, so that by the end of therapy the person with aphasia is producing his or her side of the discourse without any assistance from the computer. One small group trial ($N = 3$) of AphasiaScripts involved a participant with Wernicke's aphasia (Cherney, Halper, Holland, & Cole, 2008). This person made no changes on standard aphasia tests as a result of 9 weeks practice with the program. However, his production of the scripted dialogues did improve, most notably in the percentage of script-related words. The authors comment that this was due to a reduction in empty speech and circumlocutions.

These preliminary findings suggest that working at the level of discourse may be productive for some people with Wernicke's aphasia. It is also encouraging that one individual benefited from a self-administered computerized treatment. However, the studies did not employ controlled experimental designs, and data are available from very few participants. It is also unclear whether these therapies would be suitable for individuals with florid and highly aberrant jargon or for individuals who have poor self-monitoring. Indeed the results from Rogalski et al. (2013) suggest that the severity of impairment may be a negative prognosticator.

Treatment Aimed at Compensation

Rather than attempting to remediate the speech impairment, therapy might aim to exploit an alternative output modality. This option may be taken if speech proves resistant to intervention or if there is a severe monitoring deficit, making it impossible for the people with aphasia to detect or correct their speech errors.

For some individuals, writing may be a potential target for treatment. Although jargon can manifest in writing as well as speech (e.g., Schonauer & Denes, 1994), this is not always the case (Hillis et al., 1999). When writing is relatively preserved, it may offer a means by which communication can be established.

Two single-case studies demonstrate the potential of writing for people with jargon aphasia (Beeson, 1999; Robson et al., 1998). Both participants mastered a written vocabulary through therapy and learned to write words to support communication. One study involved a participant whose jargon had evolved to empty stereotypical speech (Beeson, 1999). This section will focus on the other paper describing RMM. RMM (Robson et al., 1998) produced highly unintelligible phonemic jargon, with virtually no real words. As described previously (Marshall et al., 1998), she seemed unaware of her speech deficit, and often became irate when others failed to understand her. This caused profound difficulties with her care staff and had led her to reject previous speech and language therapy.

RMM's writing was also impaired, with virtually no correct responses on written picture naming tasks. However, the writing impairment was different from the speech impairment. First of all, writing was very effortful and nonfluent. Secondly, it was clearly monitored. RMM was acutely aware of her writing errors. She voiced concern about them and would often strike them out and attempt a correction.

One task particularly revealed the potential of writing. This was delayed copying of words and nonwords. Here, each item was shown to RMM then removed. A 10-second delay was imposed, after which RMM was asked to write down the target. Her responses showed a clear effect of lexicality, with words written more successfully than nonwords. It seemed that the orthographic representations of words were still available to RMM, and were supporting her performance on this task.

Thus a number of factors encouraged the decision to focus on writing in therapy. Speech was profoundly impaired, unmonitored, and difficult to treat. In contrast, RMM was aware of her writing problems and motivated to work on them. She also retained some "latent" knowledge of written forms that might be promoted in therapy.

Three stages of writing therapy were provided for RMM, comprising a total of 59 sessions. All stages involved practicing word sets, with targets represented by a picture. Tasks on each word included: identifying the first letter, anagram sorting, immediate copying, delayed copying, writing the picture name with a first letter cue, and writing the picture name without a cue. The therapy targets were chosen on the basis of their relevance to RMM. In the second and third stages of therapy, the single-word practice was supplemented with tasks that aimed to promote the communicative use of writing. For example, RMM was required to use her practiced words in order to answer a question ("Where did you go this weekend?"), label local landmarks on a map, or using Message Therapy, convey parts of a message (see examples in **FIGURE 3.1**).

Message examples: My blouse needs ironing

                         The laundry is late this week

The written messages were shown to RMM. She had to complete the following tasks

    i)   Relate the messages to one of two given words (**shirt** and *vicar*)
    ii) Relate to messages to one of two given pictures (a picture
         of a **shirt** and a picture of hair); write the picture name
    iii) Write a target word that was related to the given messages

---

FIGURE 3.1 Examples of Message Therapy used with RMM (Robson et al., 1998)

Reproduced from Robson, J., Pring, T., Marshall, J., Morrison, S., & Chiat, S. (1998). Written communication in undifferentiated jargon aphasia: A therapy study. International Journal of Language and Communication Disorders, 33, 305-328.

Therapy outcomes were evaluated by asking RMM to write the names of pictures. After the second and third stages she was also tested on her ability to respond to questions with written words, or to write words in order to convey a message. RMM showed consistent and highly significant gains in written picture naming following each stage of therapy, and these were maintained at follow-up assessments. However, gains were item specific. Unpracticed words did not improve. The question and message tasks also improved, but again only when RMM could use her practiced words. Encouragingly, by the end of therapy RMM started to use writing to resolve some of the communication difficulties that occurred in her everyday life. For example, she wrote "hair" (one of her practiced words) to indicate that a hairdressers appointment clashed with a proposed therapy session.

A follow-up small group study explored whether the therapy approaches used with RMM might benefit others with jargon aphasia (Robson, Marshall, Chiat, & Pring, 2001). The 10 participants in the study had fluent but unintelligible speech, largely composed of neologisms. They also had impaired writing, with poor written naming scores. However, as with RMM, there were some positive prognosticators for writing therapy. All but one were able to monitor their writing errors, and most had at least some skills in delayed copying and anagram sorting.

In this study, six participants progressed to therapy. Twelve sessions were delivered in which they practiced personally chosen sets of words. Tasks were similar to those used with RMM and included: writing the first letter of words, completing words with missing letters, anagram sorting, copying written words, and cued written picture naming. Four of the participants made significant gains on a written picture naming assessment as a result of this therapy. The other two also improved, but only marginally. As with RMM, gains were specific to treated words; so words that had not been featured in therapy did not improve. The participants were also tested on a message assessment. This required them to write a single word that might convey a given message. For example, the message for "newspaper" was "I want a copy of the *Telegraph*." This task did not improve as a result of the first program of therapy, despite the fact that half the messages targeted treated words. Three participants were given a second program of therapy, this time targeting communicative writing. The program consisted of six sessions and involved a communication partner, typically a friend or family member. The tasks required participants to use their practiced words in order to convey information to their partner. For example, one participant had to convey the information that his son had phoned (his son's name was a therapy target). This therapy brought about further gains on the picture naming task. All participants also improved on the message task, although the gain was significant for only one.

An interesting adaptation of writing therapy was conducted with one other individual (Jackson-Waite, Robson, & Pring, 2003). MA produced undifferentiated jargon that was poorly monitored. Previous therapy had attempted to remediate speech and promote alternative communication strategies, such as gesture, but with minimal success. MA also seemed a poor candidate for writing therapy, as she was totally unable to write or even copy words. Her errors included letter reversals, repetitions of letter strokes, and switches between upper and lower case. These pointed to a peripheral dysgraphia, affecting the selection and realization of letter forms. As a result, writing therapy was administered on a Lightwriter, a portable keyboard communication aid. Three stages of therapy practiced different sets of words, using anagram, copying, and picture naming tasks (all on the Lightwriter). After the first two stages, naming of each word set improved very significantly, but with no carryover to communicative tasks. The third stage therefore included tasks in which MA had to use her vocabulary to convey information. This produced gains on a questionnaire measure, but not in an assessment of conversation.

The studies reviewed here show that writing therapy may be useful for a number of people with jargon aphasia. It is striking that only practiced words seem to improve, suggesting that these need to be carefully chosen. It also seems that the use of writing for communication may not occur unless it is specifically promoted in the therapy. The group study showed that gains varied across individuals, with not everyone improving. Therefore further research would be beneficial to explore factors that predict treatment outcomes. Finally, the work with MA showed that therapy might be enhanced with technology. Although this study employed a Lightwriter, many of the mainstream technologies that have since become available offer exciting opportunities here. For example, words might be practiced on tablets and then converted into speech, using speech synthesis software.

Writing is not the only compensatory modality that has been promoted in aphasia therapy. A number of studies have also explored the use of nonlanguage techniques such as drawing (Sacchett, Byng, Marshall, & Pound, 1999) and gesture (Rose, Raymer, Lanyon, & Attard, 2013). For example, it has been shown that people with severe aphasia can learn a "vocabulary" of gestures (Marshall et al., 2012), and improve their interactive communication as a result of gesture and naming therapy (Caute et al., 2013). Most studies of gestural therapy have involved people with nonfluent or global aphasia (see Rose, 2006). An exception is the study by Carlomagno and colleagues (2013) in which two individuals with chronic Wernicke's aphasia were treated using a functional therapy program that incorporated gesture. Tasks were interactive and involved sending and receiving information, for example, to describe pictures or tell a story. When speech failed, participants were encouraged to employ supplementary gestures and thus integrate the modalities to convey information. After 6 weeks of this therapy (approximately 25 hours) one participant demonstrated improved functional communication on the Communicative Abilities in Daily Life test (CADL-2; Holland, Frattali, & Fromm, 1999). Analysis also showed that his gestures were less copious but more informative than prior to therapy, mainly because they combined more meaningfully with his speech. The other participant unfortunately showed no change.

Although the use of compensatory strategies is an obvious solution to some of the problems of jargon aphasia, uptake may be affected by monitoring impairments. In other words, individuals with poor awareness of their jargon may not see the need for such strategies and may resist their adoption. Here interactive therapy approaches, such as PACE

(Promoting Aphasic Communicative Effectiveness; Davis, 2005) may help. PACE has four main principles: (1) therapy tasks should involve the communication of novel information to another person; (2) the clinician and client should participate equally as both the sender and receiver of information; (3) the communication channel is unconstrained, so may involve speech, writing, gesture, or drawing; and (4) feedback reflects communicative success rather than accuracy. PACE offers an ideal medium in which to model and practice communication strategies, and, in the context of jargon aphasia, may demonstrate that a gesture or drawing is effective when speech is not.

This section outlined treatments that address the production problems of jargon aphasia. One approach aims to remediate the word production impairment, with the hypothesis that this will improve speech accuracy and reduce florid jargon errors. There is some evidence to support this view, particularly from studies that have used semantic and phonological naming therapies. However, these are mainly single cases, making it difficult to draw generalized conclusions. A more indirect approach aims to compensate for the impairment by promoting alternative communication strategies. Here writing has been employed with some success, although again the evidence base is weak. Finally nonverbal media were considered, such as drawing and gesture.

WORKING WITH AND THROUGH OTHERS

It is well recognized that the consequences of aphasia are not confined to the individuals with the condition, but also extend to individuals in their immediate environment (e.g., Michallet, Le Dorze, & Tetreault, 2001; Michallet, Tetreault, & Le Dorze, 2003). When asked about the support that they need, family members typically stress the importance of information, for example about the nature of stroke and aphasia and the prognosis for recovery (Avent et al., 2005; Hilton, Leenhouts, Webster, & Morris, 2014). This need is likely to be particularly acute for the relatives of people with jargon aphasia, given the very puzzling symptomatology. The presence of fluent but meaningless speech, coupled with a seeming lack of awareness, is very difficult to understand and may even generate false beliefs. For example, family members may worry that their relative is confused or mentally ill. Some may think that the person has reverted to a previously known foreign language. One relative known to me was convinced that his partner was speaking "in code," and that he needed to crack this in order for communication to be restored. Even when such beliefs are not present, family members will need clear and accessible information about the nature of jargon aphasia, and why the symptoms are occurring.

In addition to information, family members and friends will need new skills. In terms of the ICF model (WHO, 2001), this will help to modify the environment of the person with aphasia and hence promote social participation. As we have seen already (Maneta et al., 2001), relatives may need to adapt their language to make it comprehensible to their partner. They will also need guidance about how to respond to the jargon speech, particularly if it is unmonitored, and strategies for dealing with repair. It is hoped that changes in their behavior will ease everyday interactions and, perhaps more optimistically, help the person with jargon aphasia to modify their output.

There is considerable evidence that the conversation partners of people with aphasia respond positively to training, and that this improves the quality of communication that takes place with the aphasic person (Simmons-Mackie, Raymer, Armstrong, Holland, & Cherney, 2010; Turner & Whitworth, 2006). Training can take a variety of forms. It may be administered in groups, and cover general themes about the nature of aphasia and how to adapt communication when speaking with a person with aphasia (Cunningham & Ward, 2003; Kagan, Black, Duchan, Simmons-Mackie, & Square, 2001; Rayner & Marshall, 2003). Alternatively, training may be individual and focus on the specific needs of one pair. Such training may draw on the insights of conversation analysis, for example to tease out the repair behaviors that are being used and which may be usefully adapted (Beeke, Maxim, & Wilkinson, 2007). Alternatively, it might employ Conversation Coaching (Hopper, Holland, & Rewega, 2002) or Solution Focused Therapy (Boles & Lewis, 2003). These techniques also scrutinize the conversational behaviors that take place between a person with aphasia and his or her partner, typically by using video. The therapist and the couple identify behaviors that facilitate or hinder the conversation, and then attempt to promote the former and reduce the latter, for example by using communication exercises.

Studies of conversation partner training have involved a wide range of participants, leading Simmons-Mackie et al. (2010) to conclude that the effects can be generalized across aphasia types. However, their review identifies no individuals specifically with jargon aphasia and few with a diagnosis of Wernicke's aphasia. They also acknowledge that issues of candidacy need to be further explored. Applications with people who have jargon aphasia may be particularly challenging, because of the multiple communication impairments, and because of reduced insight on the part of the person with aphasia. Nevertheless, the likely consequences of jargon aphasia for communication make partner training a priority.

CONCLUSION

This chapter has reviewed the treatment approaches that have been attempted with people who have jargon aphasia. In so doing, it has presented evidence that the problems of jargon can be mitigated, either through direct remediation of the impairment or through indirect approaches that encourage compensations. The chapter also considered techniques that have barely been tested with people with jargon, but which might be advocated, most notably the training of conversation partners.

In many respects, therapy for speakers with jargon is unexceptional. For example, it will involve the same stages of treatment as for any other person with aphasia. That is, the clinician will typically start with an exploration of the problems and the setting of goals. This will lead to the development of a treatment plan, followed by the administration of therapy and outcome measurement. Yet, each of these stages may be beset with problems if the person has jargon aphasia. Just to take one instance, exploration and goal setting will be very difficult with a client who has minimal awareness of the speech difficulties, and hence no appreciation of the need for therapy.

Some responses to these challenges have been presented, largely drawn from the literature. However, more treatment studies are needed. Ideally these will take different forms. We need experimental evidence to determine which jargon symptoms respond best to which treatments. But we also need qualitative accounts that discuss the detail of how therapy is conducted and how clients respond. Such a combined literature should help clinicians to tease apart the dos and don'ts of therapy for jargon aphasia.

CASE ILLUSTRATION

Sam is a 76-year-old man who experienced a left hemisphere stroke approximately 1 year prior to the current course of treatment. At the time of his stroke he was diagnosed with a Wernicke-type aphasia, severe anomia, and unintelligible speech containing semantic errors, unrelated errors, and neologisms. Sam received in- and outpatient speech and language therapy for 5 months after his stroke. Treatment goals included auditory comprehension of single words; item-specific functional communication, such as a word or gesture for a favorite food; and naming. Although Sam showed progress in all areas, at discharge he was judged to be highly dependent on his communication partner in most conversation exchanges.

Sam lives independently with his wife, Linda, who recently observed some improvement in Sam's communication abilities. Linda has also persuaded Sam to join a weekly stroke group. She is seeking additional speech and language therapy in the hope that this will promote further improvement, and support Sam's participation in the group.

The clinician's initial session with Sam and Linda involved a discussion about Sam's current communication status and what they hoped to achieve in therapy. Sam's speech was observed to be fluent and still largely unintelligible, with semantic errors, unrelated real word errors and neologisms. With prompting from Linda, he occasionally attempted to write. For example, when asked what soccer team he supported, he wrote "LIV" (Liverpool). Linda described everyday communication as "difficult." She was often unable to determine Sam's meaning and said that he rarely attempted to gesture or write when his speech was unintelligible. She felt that Sam could not judge whether his speech was making sense. She also commented that he often misunderstood others, particularly if they spoke quickly.

In terms of goals, Sam indicated that he wanted to improve his speech. Linda agreed that this would be positive. She also wanted Sam to be more aware of his speech errors, and to make better use of other modalities, such as writing. She felt that they needed help with Sam's comprehension difficulties. The clinician asked about communication activities that Sam and Linda wanted to target. They agreed on the following:

- Communicating basic information at home, such as food preferences or choices of leisure activities
- Participating in conversations at the stroke group
- Participating in Skype conversations (internet video communication) with Sam's adult granddaughter

In the light of this discussion, the therapist decided to administer four assessments. The first explored Sam's production, using the 40-item picture naming test from the Psycholinguistic Assessment of Language Processing in Aphasia (PALPA; Kay, Lesser, & Coltheart, 1992). The clinician introduced two modifications to the test. After Sam attempted to say the name of each item, he was asked to judge if his response was correct or not (by pointing to a check mark or a cross). He was then invited to write the name of the picture. Two assessments explored his auditory comprehension: the Spoken Word to Picture Matching and Sentence to Picture Matching subtests of the Comprehensive Aphasia Test (Swinburn, Porter, & Howard, 2004). Finally the clinician administered the all picture version of the Pyramids and Palm Trees Test (Howard & Patterson, 1992).

Sam named only five items correctly in the first test, all other responses being real or nonword errors. However, he judged 60% of his responses to be correct. His written attempts were better, with 12 correct responses and a further 8 in which he achieved at least the first letter. His comprehension of words and particularly of sentences was impaired, although he scored above chance on both tests. He was close to normal limits on the Pyramids and Palm Trees test, showing retained non-verbal semantic knowledge.

Drawing on the initial discussion and the test results the clinician drew up her therapy plan. The regime spanned 4 months, with two, 1-hour sessions per week. There were four components of therapy aiming to meet the activity targets identified by Sam and Linda. These were:

- Vocabulary training
- Awareness training
- Script training
- Supported conversation

Most of the components were administered in parallel, although vocabulary training was provided before script training.

Vocabulary training: Sam and Linda drew up a list of 40 words that would help Sam to convey personally relevant information. Drawing on published naming therapy techniques (e.g., Davis et al., 2006), Sam was invited to make a series of semantic judgments about these words. He was then encouraged to say them and judge whether or not his attempt was correct. Finally he was asked to write the words down, in response to a hierarchy of cues (e.g., see Robson et al., 1998).

Awareness training: The therapist began this therapy component by discussing the awareness problem with Sam, using simple, aphasia-friendly materials. They also viewed videos of Sam talking, so that he could observe his speech difficulties. Linda, his granddaughter, and a stroke group volunteer agreed on a feedback strategy. They used a consistent hand gesture and facial expression to indicate that they had not understood Sam, and encouraged him to use writing or gesture instead. They also discussed when to apply this (so that they were not always giving Sam negative feedback). During production tasks Sam was encouraged to listen to his responses and judge if they were correct. Initially he judged recordings of his speech; later he attempted to judge without a recording.

Script training: This therapy component drew on the principles of AphasiaScripts (Cherney et al., 2008). The clinician, Sam, and Linda developed 10 personally relevant scripts for Sam to practice, all of which integrated at least one item from his vocabulary training. Scripts were designed to convey basic information or support Sam's conversation goals. For example, one was about walking his dog. Practice followed the hierarchy of AphasiaScripts. In addition, Sam was encouraged to write relevant words if his speech production broke down. During practice, the therapist frequently asked Sam to judge whether he had said the target correctly.

Supported conversation: This involved sessions with Sam's main conversation partners to give them skills in supporting Sam's communication. The partners were Linda, a volunteer at the stroke group, and his granddaughter. The sessions covered Sam's comprehension difficulties, how to modify speech to support his understanding, how to elicit output, and how to respond to his errors (see previous discussion). The clinician also drew on the principles of Conversation Coaching (Hopper et al., 2002). Sam was videorecorded in conversation with Linda and his granddaughter. They discussed strategies that worked (and did not work) in the conversation, and attempted to repeat the conversation making more use of the positive strategies. Conversation coaching with the granddaughter took place over Skype, so that strategies suitable for Skype could be promoted.

Sam showed strong item-specific gains from therapy. His naming of practiced vocabulary improved dramatically, both in speech and writing, as did his production of the scripts. Linda reported that Sam made some use of the trained material in everyday interactions, although this was variable. Sam's conversation partners became skilled at using supported communication, and Sam continued to Skype his granddaughter successfully almost every week. He integrated well into the stroke group and the volunteers reported that he was involved in both individual and group conversations. At the end of therapy Sam's speech was still difficult to understand and communication remained difficult with unfamiliar conversation partners. However, Sam showed more awareness of his speech difficulties and became more likely to use writing or gesture when communication broke down.

REFERENCES

Avent, J., Glista, S., Wallace, S., Jackson, J., Nishioka, J., & Yip, W. (2005). Family information needs about aphasia. *Aphasiology, 19*(3–5), 365–375.

Bakheit, A., Shaw, S., Carrington, S., & Griffiths, S. (2007). The rate and extent of improvement with therapy from the different types of aphasia in the first year after stroke. *Clinical Rehabilitation, 21*, 941–949.

Beeke, S., Maxim, J., & Wilkinson, R. (2007). Using conversation analysis to assess and treat people with aphasia. *Seminars in Speech and Language, 28*, 136–147.

Beeson, P. (1999). Treating acquired writing impairment: Strengthening graphemic representations. *Aphasiology, 13*, 9–11, 767–785.

Boles, L., & Lewis, M. (2003). Working with couples: Solution focused aphasia therapy. *Asia Pacific Journal of Speech, Language and Hearing, 8*, 153–159.

Bose, A. (2013). Phonological therapy in jargon aphasia: Effects on naming and neologisms. *International Journal of Language and Communication Disorders, 48*(5), 582–595.

Bose, A., & Buchanan, L. (2007). A cognitive and psycholinguistic investigation of neologisms. *Aphasiology, 21*, 726–738.

Boyle, M. (2004). Semantic feature analysis treatment for anomia in two fluent aphasia syndromes. *American Journal of Speech Language Pathology, 13*, 236–249.

Buckingham, H. (1990). Abstruse neologisms, retrieval deficits and the random generator. *Journal of Neurolinguistics, 5*, 215–235.

Butterworth, B. (1979). Hesitation and the production of verbal paraphasias and neologisms in jargon aphasia. *Brain and Language, 18*, 133–161.

Butterworth, B. (1985). Jargon aphasia: Processes and strategies. In S. Newman & R. Epstein (Eds.), *Current perspectives in dysphasia* (pp. 61–96). Edinburgh, England: Churchill Livingstone.

Butterworth, B., & Howard, D. (1987). Paragrammatisms. *Cognition, 26*, 1–37.

Cappa, S., Cavallotti, G., & Vignolo, L. (1987). Jargonagraphia: Clinical and neuropsychological correlates. *Neuropsychologia, 25*, 281–286.

Cappa, S., Miozzo, A., & Frugoni, M. (1994). Glossolalic jargon after a right hemispheric stroke in a patient with Wernicke's aphasia. *Aphasiology, 8*, 83–87.

Carlomagno, S., Zulian, N., Razzano, C., De Mercurio, I., & Marini, A. (2013). Coverbal gestures in the recovery from severe fluent aphasia: A pilot study. *Journal of Communication Disorders, 46*, 84–99.

Carragher, M., Conroy, P., Sage, K., & Wilkinson, R. (2012). Can impairment-focused therapy change the everyday conversations of people with aphasia? A review of the literature and future directions. *Aphasiology, 26*(7), 895–916.

Caspari, I. (2005). Wernicke's aphasia. In L. LaPointe (Ed.), *Aphasia and related neurogenic language disorders* (3rd ed.; pp. 142–155). New York: Thieme.

Caute, A., Pring, T., Cocks, C., Cruice, M., Best, W., & Marshall, J. (2013). Enhancing communication in aphasia through gesture and naming therapy. *Journal of Speech, Language and Hearing Research, 56*(1), 337–351.

Cherney, L., Halper, A., Holland, A., & Cole, R. (2008). Computerised script training for aphasia: Preliminary results. *American Journal of Speech Language Pathology, 17*, 19–34.

Chriki, L., Bullain, S., & Stern, T. (2006). The recognition and management of psychological reactions to stroke: A case discussion. *Primary Care Companion to the Journal of Clinical Psychiatry, 8*(4), 234–240.

Cocchini, G., Beschin, N., Cameron, A., Fotopoulou, A., & Della Sala, S. (2009). Anosognosia for motor impairment following left brain damage. *Neuropsychology, 23*(2), 223–230.

Cocchini, G., Crosta, E., Allen, R., Zaro, F., & Beschin, N. (2013). Relationship between anosognosia and depression in aphasic patients. *Journal of Clinical and Experimental Neuropsychology, 35*(4), 337–347.

Cohen, L., Verstichel, P., & Dehaene, S. (1997). Neologistic jargon sparing numbers: A category specific phonological impairment. *Cognitive Neuropsychology, 14*, 1029–1061.

Cunningham, R., & Ward, C. (2003). Evaluation of a training programme to facilitate conversation between people with aphasia and their partners. *Aphasiology, 17*, 687–707.

Davis, A. (2005). PACE revisited. *Aphasiology, 19*, 21–38.

Davis, C., Harrington, G., & Baynes, K. (2006). Intensive semantic intervention in fluent aphasia: A pilot study with fMRI. *Aphasiology, 20*(1), 59–83.

Dell, G. S., Schwartz, M., Martin, N., Saffran, E., & Gagnon, D. (1997). Lexical access in aphasic and nonaphasic speakers. *Psychological Review, 104*(4), 801–838.

Eaton, E., Marshall, J., & Pring, T. (2010). 'Like déjà vu all over again': Patterns of perseveration in two people with jargon aphasia. *Aphasiology, 24*(9), 1017–1031.

Eaton, E., Marshall, J., & Pring, T. (2011). Mechanisms of change in the evolution of jargon aphasia. *Aphasiology, 25*(12), 1543–1562.

Ellis, A., Miller, D., & Sin, G. (1983). Wernicke's aphasia and normal language processing: A case study in cognitive neuropsychology. *Cognition, 15*, 111–144.

Fillingham, J., Sage, K., & Lambon Ralph, M. (2006). The treatment of anomia using errorless learning. *Neuropsychological Rehabilitation, 16*(2), 129–154.

Francis, D., Riddoch, M., & Humphreys, G. (2001). Cognitive rehabilitation of word meaning deafness. *Aphasiology, 15*(8), 749–766.

Goldman, R., Schwartz, M., & Wilshire, C. (2001). The influence of phonological context on the sound errors of a speaker with Wernicke's aphasia. *Brain and Language, 78*, 279–307.

Grayson, E., Hilton, R., & Franklin, S. (1997). Early intervention in a case of jargon aphasia: Efficacy of language comprehension therapy. *European Journal of Disorders of Communication, 32*(3), 257–276.

Hanlon, R., & Edmondson, J. (1996). Disconnected phonology: A linguistic analysis of phonemic jargon aphasia. *Brain and Language, 55*(2), 199–212.

Hartsuiker, R., & Kolk, H. (2001). Error monitoring in speech production: A computational test of the perceptual loop theory. *Cognitive Psychology, 42*(2), 113–157.

Hillis, A., Boatman, D., Hart, J., & Gordon, B. (1999). Making sense out of jargon: A neurolinguistic and computational account of jargon aphasia. *Neurology, 53*, 1813–1824.

Hilton, R., Leenhouts, S., Webster, J., & Morris, J. (2014). Information support and training needs of relatives of people with aphasia: Evidence from the literature. *Aphasiology, 28*(4–7), 797–822.

Holland, A., Frattali, C., & Fromm, D. (1999). *Communication Activities of Daily Living–2*. Austin, TX: Pro Ed.

Hopper, T., Holland, A., & Rewega, M. (2002). Conversational coaching: Treatment outcomes and future directions. *Aphasiology, 16*, 745–761.

Howard, D., & Patterson, K. (1992). *The Pyramids & Palm Trees Test*. Bury St Edmunds, England: Thames Valley Test Company.

Jackson-Waite, K., Robson, J., & Pring, T. (2003). Written communication using a Lightwriter in undifferentiated jargon aphasia: A single case study. *Aphasiology, 17*(8), 767–780.

Jehkonen, M., Laihosalo, M., & Kettunen, J. (2006). Anosognosia after stroke: Assessment, occurrence, subtypes and impact on functional outcome reviewed. *Acta Neurologica Scandinavia, 114*, 293–306.

Kagan, A., Black, S., Duchan, J., Simmons-Mackie, N., & Square, P. (2001). Training volunteers as conversation partners using "Supported Conversation for Adults with Aphasia" (SCA): A controlled trial. *Journal of Speech, Language and Hearing Research, 44*, 624–638.

Kaplan, E., Goodglass, H., & Weintraub, S. (2001). *The Boston Naming Test* (2nd ed.). Philadelphia, PA: Lippincott, Williams & Wilkins.

Kay, J., Lesser, R., & Coltheart, M. (1992). *Psycholinguistic assessments of language processing in aphasia*. New York, NY: Routledge.

Kertesz, A. (1981). The anatomy of jargon. In J. Brown (Ed.), *Jargonaphasia* (pp. 63–112). New York, NY: Academic Press.

Kohn, S., Smith, K., & Alexander, M. (1996). Differential recovery from impairment to the phonological lexicon. *Brain and Language, 52*, 129–149.

Laska, A. C., Hellbolm, A., Murray, V., Kahan, T., & von Arbin, M. (2001). Aphasia in acute stroke in relation to outcome. *Journal of International Medicine, 249*, 412–422.

Lee, J., Kaye, R., & Cherney, L. (2009). Conversational script performance in adults with non-fluent aphasia: Treatment intensity and aphasia severity. *Aphasiology, 7*, 885–897.

Leonard, C., Rochon, E., & Laird, L. (2008). Treating naming impairments in aphasia: Findings from a phonological components analysis treatment. *Aphasiology, 22*(9), 923–947.

Levelt, W. (1989). *Speaking from intention to articulation*. Cambridge, MA: MIT Press.

Macoir, J., & Beland, R. (2004). Knowing its gender without knowing its name: Differential access to lexical information in a jargonaphasic patient. *Neurocase, 10*, 471–482.

Maher, L., Gonzalez-Rothi, L., & Heilman, K. (1994). Lack of error awareness in an aphasic patient with relatively preserved auditory comprehension. *Brain and Language, 46*, 402–418.

Maneta, A., Marshall, J., & Lindsay, J. (2001). Direct and indirect therapy for word sound deafness. *International Journal of Language and Communication Disorders, 36*(1), 91–106.

Marshall, J. (2006). Jargon aphasia: What have we learned? *Aphasiology, 20*, 387–410.

Marshall, J., Best, B., Cocks, N., Cruice, M., Pring, T., Bulcock, G., . . . Caute, A. (2012). Gesture and naming therapy for people with severe aphasia. *Journal of Speech, Language and Hearing Research, 55*, 726–738.

Marshall, J., Chiat, S., Robson, J., & Pring, T. (1996). Calling a salad a federation: An investigation of semantic jargon: Paper 2, verbs. *Journal of Neurolinguistics, 9*, 251–260

Marshall, J., Robson, J., Pring, T., & Chiat, S. (1998). Why does monitoring fail in jargon aphasia? Comprehension, judgement and therapy evidence. *Brain and Language, 63*, 79–107.

Marshall, R. (2008). Early management of Wernicke's aphasia: A context based approach. In R. Chapey (Ed.), *Language intervention strategies in aphasia and related neurogenic communication disorders* (5th ed.). Baltimore, MD: Lippincott, Williams & Wilkins.

Martin, A. (1981). Therapy with the jargonaphasic. In J. Brown (Ed.), *Jargonaphasia* (pp. 305–326). New York, NY: Academic Press.

Michallet, B., Le Dorze, G., & Tetreault, S. (2001). The needs of spouses caring for severely aphasic persons. *Aphasiology, 15,* 731–747.

Michallet, B., Tetreault, S., & Le Dorze, G. (2003). The consequences of severe aphasia on the spouses of aphasic people: A description of the adaptation process. *Aphasiology, 17,* 835–859.

Miller, D., & Ellis, A. (1987). Speech and writing errors in 'neologistic jargonaphasia': A lexical activation hypothesis. In M. Coltheart, G. Sartori, & R. Job (Eds.), *The cognitive neuropsychology of language.* Hove, England: Lawrence Erlbaum Associates.

Morris, J., & Franklin, S. (2017). Disorders of auditory comprehension. In I. Papathanasiou & P. Coppens (Eds.), *Aphasia and related neurogenic communication disorders* (2nd ed.; pp. 151–168). Burlington, MA: Jones & Bartlett Learning.

Moses, M., Nickels, L., & Sheard, C. (2004). Disentangling the web: Neologistic perseverative errors in jargon aphasia. *Neurocase, 10,* 452–461.

Nicholas, M. L., Helm-Estabrooks, N., Ward-Lonergan, J., & Morgan, A. R. (1993). Evolution of severe aphasia in the first two years post onset. *Archives of Physical Medicine and Rehabilitation, 74,* 830–836.

Nickels, L. (2002). Therapy for naming disorders: Revisiting, revising, and reviewing. *Aphasiology, 16,* 935–979.

Olson A., Romani, C., & Halloran, L. (2007). Localizing the deficit in a case of jargonaphasia. *Cognitive Neuropsychology, 24*(2), 211–238.

Oomen, C., & Postma, A. (2002). Limitations in processing resources and speech monitoring. *Language and Cognitive Processes, 17,* 163–184.

Oomen, C., Postma, A., & Kolk, H. (2001). Prearticulatory and postarticulatory self-monitoring in Broca's aphasia. *Cortex, 37,* 627–641.

Orfei, M., Caltagrione, C., & Spalletta, G. (2009). The evaluation of anosognosia in stroke patients. *Cerebrovascular Diseases, 27,* 280–289.

Panzeri, M., Semenza, C., & Butterworth, B. (1987). Compensatory processes in the evolution of severe jargon aphasia. *Neuropsychologia, 25,* 919–933.

Passy, J. (1990). *Cued Articulation.* Victoria, Australia: Australian Council for Educational Research.

Pitts, E., Bhatnagar, S., Buckingham, H., Hacein-Bey, L., & Bhatnagar, G. (2010). A unique modality-specific domain for the production of neologisms: Recurrent perseveration and oral reading. *Aphasiology, 24*(3), 348–362.

Postma, A. (2000). Detection of errors during speech production: A review of speech monitoring models. *Cognition, 77,* 97–131.

Prigatano, G. (2010). *Study of anosognosia.* New York: Oxford University Press.

Rayner, H., & Marshall, J. (2003). Training volunteers as conversation partners for people with aphasia. *International Journal of Language and Communication Disorders, 38,* 149–164.

Robson, H., Keidel, J., Lambon Ralph, M., & Sage, K. (2012). Revealing and quantifying the impaired phonological analysis underpinning impaired comprehension in Wernicke's aphasia. *Neuropsychologia, 50,* 276–288.

Robson, J., Marshall, J., Chiat, S., & Pring, T. (2001). Enhancing communication in jargon aphasia: A small group study of writing therapy. *International Journal of Language and Communication Disorders, 36*(4), 471–488.

Robson, J., Marshall, J., Pring, T., & Chiat, S. (1999). Phonological naming therapy in jargon aphasia: Positive but paradoxical effects. *Journal of the International Neurospychological Society, 4,* 675–686.

Robson, J., Pring, T., Marshall J., & Chiat, S. (2003). Phoneme frequency effects in jargon aphasia: A phonological investigation of neologisms. *Brain and Language, 85,* 109–124.

Robson, J., Pring, T., Marshall, J., Morrison, S., & Chiat, S. (1998). Written communication in undifferentiated jargon aphasia: A therapy study. *International Journal of Language and Communication Disorders, 33,* 305–328.

Rogalski, Y., & Edmonds, L. A. (2008). Attentive Reading and Constrained Summarization (ARCS) treatment in primary progressive aphasia: A case study. *Aphasiology, 22*(7–8), 763–775.

Rogalski, Y., Edmonds, L., Daly, V., & Gardner, M. (2013). Attentive Reading and Constrained Summarisation (ARCS) discourse treatment for chronic Wernicke's aphasia. *Aphasiology, 27*(10), 1232–1251.

Rose, M. (2006). The utility of arm and hand gestures in the treatment of aphasia. *Advances in Speech Language Pathology, 8*(2), 92–109.

Rose, M. L., Raymer, A. M., Lanyon, L. E., & Attard, M. C. (2013). A systematic review of gesture treatments for post-stroke aphasia. *Aphasiology, 27*(9), 1090–1127.

Sacchett, C., Byng, S., Marshall, J., & Pound, C. (1999). Drawing together: Evaluation of a therapy programme for severe aphasia. *The International Journal of Language and Communication Disorders, 34,* 265–289.

Sampson, M., & Faroqi-Shah, Y. (2011). Investigation of self-monitoring in fluent aphasia with jargon. *Aphasiology, 25*(4), 505–528.

Schonauer, K., & Denes, G. (1994). Graphemic jargon: A case report. *Brain and Language, 47,* 279–299.

Shuren, J., Smith Hammond, C., Maher, L., Rothi, L., & Heilman, K. (1995). Attention and anosognosia: The case of a jargonaphasic patient with unawareness of language deficit. *Neurology, 45,* 376–378.

Simmons, N., & Buckingham, H. (1992). Recovery in jargonaphasia. *Aphasiology, 6,* 397–401.

Simmons-Mackie, N., Raymer, A., Armstrong, E., Holland, A., & Cherney, L. (2010). Communication partner training in aphasia: A systematic review. *Archives of Physical Medicine and Rehabilitation, 91*(12), 1814–1837.

Stenneken, P., Hofmann, M. J., & Jacobs, A. M. (2008). Sublexical units in aphasic jargon and in the standard language. Comparative analyses of neologisms in connected speech. *Aphasiology, 22*(11), 1142–1156.

Strauss Hough, M. (1993). Treatment of Wernicke's aphasia with jargon: A case study. *Journal of Communication Disorders, 26,* 101–111.

Swinburn, K., Porter, G., & Howard, D. (2004). Comprehensive Aphasia Test. Hove, England: Psychology Press.

Turner, S., & Whitworth, A. (2006). Conversational partner training programmes in aphasia: A review of key themes and participants' roles. *Aphasiology, 20*(6), 483–510.

Weinstein, E. (1981). Behavioural aspects of jargonaphasia. In J. Brown (Ed.), *Jargonaphasia* (pp. 139–149). New York: Academic Press.

Weinstein, E., & Lyerly, O. (1976). Personality factors in jargon aphasia. *Cortex, 12,* 122–133.

Whitworth, A., Webster, J., & Howard, D. (2014). *A cognitive neuropsychological approach to assessment and intervention in aphasia: A clinician's guide* (2nd ed.). Hove, England: Psychology Press.

World Health Organization (WHO). (2001). The International Classification of Functioning, Disability and Health (ICF). Geneva, Switzerland: WHO.

Woolf, C., Panton, A., Rosen, S., Best, W., & Marshall, J. (2014). Therapy for auditory processing impairment in aphasia: An evaluation of two approaches. *Aphasiology, 28,* 12, 1481–1505.

CHAPTER 4

Agrammatic Aphasia

Yasmeen Faroqi-Shah
Angela Lea Baker

INTRODUCTION

The term *agrammatism* was first used by Kussmaul in 1877, and early references to this term are found in Pick (1913) and Kleist (1916) (both cited in Bastiaanse & Thompson, 2012). The central feature of agrammatic aphasia is impoverished sentence production that is markedly more affected than the person's lexical or motoric limitations. Another, less consistently reported symptom is difficulty comprehending grammatically complex verbal material despite relatively preserved comprehension of conversational speech. Given that agrammatism is a cluster of symptoms, there are varying theoretical accounts. Some focus on a single symptom while other accounts are based on a specific linguistic theory or on the presumed function of Broca's area for syntactic computation. Consequently, a vast range of rehabilitation approaches for agrammatism has been proposed, many focusing on a single symptom. This chapter is organized into four sections. First, the clinical profile of agrammatism is discussed, followed by a brief overview of theoretical accounts and neurological findings. Next, evidence-based rehabilitation approaches and general guidelines for intervention are presented. Finally, we illustrate an intervention plan for a person with agrammatic aphasia.

CLINICAL PROFILE OF AGRAMMATIC APHASIA

The four central symptoms of agrammatism include the characteristic triad of sentence production symptoms: limitations in sentence structure, verb retrieval, and functional morphology, as well as asyntactic comprehension. This is illustrated in the three sample descriptions of the Cookie Theft Picture:

> **69-year-old male, 2 years post-onset**: *Um…uh…a young boy…eeking on top…on… uh…stair uh…school…the school is…fell over…um…um…water uh…um um…the sink is overflowing.*
>
> **49-year-old female, 3 years post-onset**: *The boy is…the school…is …cookie jar… giving. And that's not a sentence. She's doing the …cookie jar. And reaching. She's…the girl…the…a woman…is …plate…and…the sink.*
>
> **56-year-old female, 2 years post-onset**: *The mother…* [laughs] *is watching* [washing]… *tichen* [kitchen]*…but some reason the sink is going…on the floor… and some reason dan dan they didn't notice that… and they key is…the son and the nother daughter's trying to get into the cookie jar… and the son is on the step sool* [stool]*… and they almost looked like they's going to fall and…and uh the…you know looking for the cookie…but some reason they don't about him almost falling….and…uh that's it for me* [laughs].

Sentence Structure

These three speech samples show a variety of sentence structural abnormalities, including absence of sentence structure, word order errors, and overly simplified sentences. While some individuals with agrammatic aphasia manage to produce simple sentences (e.g., subject-verb-object in English), these are characterized by overuse of a single sentence frame, such as *Noun is Verbing* in English (Saffran, Schwartz, & Marin, 1980). Complex sentence structures such as negatives, passives, or "wh-" questions are rarely produced (Bastiaanse, Rispens, Ruigendijk, Rabadaán, & Thompson, 2002; Saffran, Berndt, & Schwartz, 1989). In elicited contexts, there appears a hierarchy of difficulty even within complex structures, for example, object cleft structures (e.g., *It was the artist who the thief chased*) may be more impaired than wh- questions with object movement (e.g., *Who did the thief chase?*; Thompson, Shapiro, Kiran, & Sobecks, 2003). There is also intraindividual variability in accuracy and diversity of sentences based on task demands (Kok, van Doorn, & Kolk, 2007). Not surprisingly, spontaneous speech produces more severe agrammatic symptoms than sentence completion or sentence anagram tasks (Kok et al., 2007).

Verb Retrieval

In most people with agrammatic aphasia, sentences or sentence fragments show lexical difficulties that are relatively more pronounced for verbs and functional morphology (both free and bound grammatical morphemes) than for nouns. These lexical deficits are evident not only in spontaneous speech but also in elicited tasks such as confrontation naming (e.g., Kim & Thompson, 2000, 2004; Miceli, Silveri, Villa, & Caramazza, 1984; Zingeser & Berndt, 1990) and sentence completion (Faroqi-Shah & Thompson, 2004, 2007; Kok et al., 2007). Verb production of people with agrammatic aphasia shows two characteristics. First, there is a preference for people with agrammatic aphasia to retrieve more specific, heavy verbs (e.g., scrub vs. clean, run vs. go, bake vs. make) in elicited tasks (Breedin, Saffran, & Schwartz, 1998; Kim & Thompson, 2004). Another characteristic of verb deficits is a hierarchy of verb difficulty based on argument structure and thematic roles: verbs with single arguments (intransitives) are more successfully produced than transitive and ditransitive verbs (De Bleser & Kauschke, 2003; Dragoy & Bastiaanse, 2010; Jonkers & Bastiaanse, 1996; Kegl, 1995; Kemmerer & Tranel, 2000; Kim & Thompson, 2000, 2004; Thompson, Lange, Schneider, & Shapiro, 1997). Among single-argument verbs, those with simpler thematic roles are better produced than verbs that represent the theme as the sentential subject (Lee & Thompson, 2004; Thompson, 2003). For example, unergative verbs (i.e., intransitive verbs that take an agent as their subject) such as *sleeping* are more successfully produced than unaccusative verbs (i.e., intransitive verbs in which the subject is not responsive for the action of the verb) such as *melt*, where the thing that is melting is not the agent of the action. These verb impairment patterns were captured by Thompson's (2003) *argument structure complexity hypothesis* (ASCH), which proposes that production difficulty in agrammatism increases whenever verbs become more complex, either in terms of the number of associated arguments or the lack of direct mapping between argument structure of the verb and its sentence-structure representation. For example, verbs that allow for three arguments (e.g., *give, He gave Mary the flowers*) would be more difficult to retrieve than verbs that require only one argument (e.g., *sleep, He will sleep*). It needs to be pointed out that argument structure complexity also influences language production in neurologically healthy speakers, those with fluent aphasia, and children (Bastiaanse, Edwards, & Kiss, 1996; Pizzioli & Schelstraete, 2008).

Verb production deficits influence sentence production ability because failure to access verbs and their associated argument specifications limits the lexical material available for sentence construction. Berndt, Mitchum, Haendiges, and Sandson (1997) found a significant correlation between verb retrieval deficits and sentence production deficits. Further, when verbs were provided, individuals with verb retrieval deficits were able to produce "better-formed" sentences. This association between verb retrieval and sentence construction has implications for intervention: verb retrieval deficits should be targeted prior to sentence construction.

Functional Morphology

Functional morphology also shows a variety of deficits in people with agrammatism (Friedmann & Grodzinsky, 1997; Goodglass & Berko, 1960; Goodglass, Christiansen & Gallagher, 1993). Functional morphology refers to elements of the sentence that observe grammatical well-formedness and/or convey contextual and relational information, such as mood, gender, number, tense, aspect, case, and negation. These morphological impairments are observed both in free-standing elements, for example in English auxiliaries "do, be, have" (e.g., I *have* a car, I *have been* reading a book), modals *"can, could, may, might, must, shall, should, will, and would"* (e.g., He *may* go to the store), and affixes (a prefix, suffix, or infix added to a word to create a new word), as well as across languages that have very little grammatical morphology (such as Chinese dialects) and in languages rich in inflections (e.g., Russian and Finnish) (Dragoy & Bastiaanse, 2010; Law & Cheng, 2002; Lee, Milman, & Thompson, 2008; Penke, 2003; Wenzlaff & Clahsen, 2004; Yiu & Worrall, 1996). A similar general pattern is observed across languages: Verbal morphology tends to be more impaired than nominal morphology and semantic elements such as tense marking tend to be more impaired than structural elements such as agreement (Burchert, Swoboda-Moll & De Bleser, 2005; Faroqi-Shah & Thompson, 2004, 2007; Friedman & Grodzinsky, 1997; Goodglass et al., 1993). The errors can be either substitutions by incorrect morphemes or, in languages that allow it, omissions of functional morphology (Menn, Obler, & Goodglass, 1990). Although it was proposed that morphological deficits (such as past tense production) in agrammatism are due to a difficulty in morphological affixation (Ullman, Corkin, Coppola, & Hickok, 1997), a large-scale meta-analysis of verb morphology found little support for this account (Faroqi-Shah, 2007).

Asyntactic Comprehension

In terms of comprehension, people with agrammatic speech production may present with *asyntactic comprehension*, defined as a difficulty interpreting non-canonical sentences, such as passives, object clefts, and object relatives (Caplan & Hildebrandt, 1988). The characteristic error in asyntactic comprehension is incorrect attribution of thematic roles (e.g., agent, theme) to sentence nouns, especially in semantically reversible contexts. This results in what are typically called *role reversal* errors, in which the agent and patient roles are misinterpreted. For example, *the artist* in *"The artist was honored by the doctor"* is interpreted as the agent of the action. Although asyntactic comprehension typically refers to complex sentence interpretation, people with agrammatic aphasia are also impaired in interpreting functional morphology (Burchert, De Bleser, & Sonntag, 2003; Dickey, Milman & Thompson, 2008; Faroqi-Shah & Dickey, 2009). It is important to note that verb retrieval deficits and asyntactic comprehension are not unique to agrammatic aphasia, and could occur in other aphasia profiles as well (Berndt, Haendiges, & Wozniak, 1997; Berndt, Mitchum, & Wayland, 1997; Caplan, 1995). For example, people with fluent and mixed aphasia have been noted to exhibit verb retrieval deficits, whereas noun deficits tend to be associated with fluent aphasia only (Matzig, Druks, Masterson, & Vigliocco, 2009).

In summary, there is individual variability in the exact manifestation of agrammatic aphasia. The severity of sentence structural deficits, verb production impairments, or deficits in grammatical morphology differs from person to person, although all three impairments occur to some extent. Similar heterogeneity has been observed for asyntactic comprehension, that is, some agrammatic speakers present with asyntactic comprehension whereas others do not (Bastiaanse, 1995; Berndt, 1987; Berndt, Mitchum, & Haendiges, 1996; Berndt et al., 1997; Kolk & Friederici, 1985). This heterogeneity among patients with agrammatism poses challenges for diagnosis and intervention. That is, there is no single diagnostic measure of agrammatism, per se. Likewise, there is no unitary intervention for agrammatism, instead each of the symptoms is addressed individually. This is discussed further in the following sections.

DIAGNOSIS OF AGRAMMATIC APHASIA

The previous section identified four central symptoms of agrammatism, namely, impaired production of sentence structure, morphosyntax, and verbs, along with asyntactic comprehension. Published studies of agrammatism have used a variety of measures to identify and evaluate grammatical impairment. Not surprisingly, the choice of tests was primarily driven by the goals of the study. Typical measures have included comprehension of syntactically simple versus complex (reversible) sentences, grammaticality judgment of morphosyntactic anomalies, production (or fragment completion) of sentences with different syntactic constructions with picture support, syntactic priming of sentences, and verb naming (Bastiaanse & Edwards, 2004; Caplan, Waters, DeDe, Michaud, & Reddy, 2007; Faroqi-Shah & Dickey, 2009; Faroqi-Shah & Thompson, 2004, 2007; Linebarger, Schwartz, & Saffran, 1983; Saffran et al., 1980; Thompson & Lee, 2009; Thompson, Shapiro, Ballard, Jacobs, & Tait, 1997).

Despite the diversity of assessments across studies, one (nearly) consistently reported task is narrative speech, which could be elicited through conversation, story telling (e.g., Cinderella story), or picture description (e.g., Cookie Theft picture from the Boston Diagnostic Aphasia Examination [BDAE]; Goodglass, Kalpan, & Barresi, 2001, or Nicholas & Brookshire picture stimuli, 1993). The presence of short, fragmented utterances with morphosyntactic errors (e.g., word order, functional morphology such as tense) and a paucity of verbs is the most frequently described operational definition of agrammatism. While some studies provide objective measures of morphosyntax in narrative speech (e.g., Faroqi-Shah & Dickey, 2009), others cite clinical judgment as the basis of identifying agrammatism (e.g., Sahraoui & Nespoulous, 2012). Objective morphosyntactic measures for narrative speech include, but are not limited to, proportions of grammatical utterances, utterances with embedded clauses, utterances with verbs, verbs with correct morphology, noun to verb ratio, and mean length of utterance. Detailed analysis measures of narrative speech were developed by Saffran and colleagues (1989) in a method called Quantitative Production Analysis (QPA). The QPA includes lexical measures, such as proportion of closed class elements and ratio of nouns to pronouns; morphological measures, such as proportion of auxiliaries and ratio of determiners to nouns; and syntactic measures, such as proportion of well-formed sentences and elaboration of sentences. Using the QPA, Rochon and colleagues (Rochon, Saffran, Berndt, & Schwartz,

2000) supported Saffran and colleagues' findings that people with agrammatic aphasia presented with more morphological deficits than individuals without agrammatism, but that people with nonagrammatic, nonfluent aphasia presented with lower scores of sentence complexity. Normative data and data from individuals with agrammatic aphasia are provided for comparison and are an objective resource for clinicians and researchers analyzing narratives for agrammatic symptoms.

In summary, the diagnosis of agrammatism is derived from an examination of narrative speech *and* tests that assess grammatical competence. Among the commercially available language tests for aphasia, the Boston Diagnostic Aphasia Examination, Third Edition (Goodglass et al., 2001) and the Verb and Sentence Test (Bastiaanse, Edwards, Maas, & Rispens, 2003) provide a variety of subtests to evaluate grammatical impairments. While evaluating agrammatism, it is important to bear in mind that grammatical impairments can be significantly impacted by task and computational demands. For instance, agrammatic productions are more severely manifested in narrative speech compared to tasks where a single sentence or a sentence fragment is elicited (Kok et al., 2007; Sahraoui & Nespoulous, 2012). The modality in which sentences are presented in a comprehension task will influence performance if the person with aphasia has a limited verbal memory span or reading difficulty. It is also important to note if the stimuli have been matched for psycholinguistic variables, such as sentence length, event plausibility, word frequency, and even visual clarity/ambiguity, as these are known to influence performance due to increased task demands.

NEUROANATOMICAL FINDINGS

Traditionally, agrammatism has been linked with lesions of Broca's area (posterior left inferior frontal gyrus; Grodzinsky, 2000). However, recent findings reveal a far more complex neuroanatomical lesion profile. Several lesion studies have found that syntactic comprehension is not associated with a specific lesion; rather, there are multiple potential regions, including left superior/middle temporal, left angular gyrus, and right hemisphere structures (Caplan, Waters, Kennedy, et al., 2007; Dronkers, Wilkins, Van Valin, Redfern, & Jaeger, 2004; Wilson & Saygin, 2004). It is notable that across lesion studies, Broca's area has not been implicated for asyntactic comprehension. Using probabilistic tractography, Griffiths and colleagues (2013) integrated data from functional neuroimaging of neurologically healthy participants and lesion mapping of asyntactic comprehension to conclude that structural disconnections in either the arcuate fasciculus or the extreme capsule, can result in syntactic impairment. Sentence production impairments (especially complex syntax) are associated with left anterior lesions, specifically pars opercularis/triangularis in the inferior frontal regions, anterior superior temporal gyrus, anterior portions of the supramarginal gyrus, basal ganglia, and insula (Faroqi-Shah et al., 2014). As for verb deficits, these are associated with lesions in brain regions that have been implicated for motor representations (left precentral gyrus) and lexical and conceptual knowledge of actions (left inferior frontal gyrus, supramarginal gyrus, and middle temporal gyrus; Kemmerer, Rudrauf, Manzel, & Tranel, 2012; see also Matzig et al., 2009, for a review). In summary, the individual symptoms of agrammatism have relatively distinct neuroanatomical correlates, which probably accounts for the individual variability in severity of these symptoms.

THEORETICAL ACCOUNTS OF AGRAMMATISM

The underlying source of agrammatism has been a much researched and debated question over the past three decades. Several accounts have been proposed and empirically examined, and a complete discussion is beyond the scope of this chapter. Broadly speaking, most theories attempt to explain a single agrammatic symptom, and approach the symptom from one of three perspectives: cognitive neuropsychological, resource allocation, or linguistic (admittedly, these perspectives are not always mutually exclusive).

In the cognitive neuropsychological approach, a breakdown in one or more processes identified in normal language production is used to explain agrammatic symptoms. The most commonly adopted models have been those of Garrett (1975, 1988), Levelt (1989, 1999), and Bock and Levelt (1994). All of these models propose a *functional processing* stage during which thematic roles are assigned to lexical items (e.g., "boy" is "agent/subject"), often determined by which verb is selected (e.g., buy vs. sell, give vs. take). These models also propose a subsequent stage of *positional processing*, during which sentence structure is retrieved and built. One account of agrammatism, the mapping theory, pinpoints an impairment in mapping of thematic roles during functional processing as the source of role reversal errors in agrammatic production and asyntactic comprehension (Linebarger et al., 1983; Saffran, Schwartz, & Linebarger, 1998). Others have attributed impaired sentence structure and functional morphology to a failure of positional processing (Mitchum, Haendiges, & Berndt, 1993). Another account, diacritical encoding and retrieval, attributes a failure to link elements of the message, such as tense/aspect to specific functional morphemes during positional processing as the source of verb morphology errors (Faroqi-Shah & Thompson, 2007).

Detailed linguistic theories of morphosyntax such as Chomsky's Government and Binding theory (Chomsky, 1981) and the Minimalist Program (Chomsky, 2000) have been used as a framework to explain word order errors, role reversals, and functional morphology errors in agrammatism. The central idea is that all languages have a base word order (deep structure or d-structure), and all other sentences are derived from this base word order by movement operations. Moved elements leave behind a trace of their original position, a mental link between the d-structure and the surface structure (s-structure). For instance, passive structures in English are derived by moving the theme/recipient of the action to the subject position of the sentence, hence a trace of the theme exists in its initial post-verbal position (e.g., "*The chef cooked* **the meal**" becomes "**The meal** was cooked **[trace]** by *the chef*"). Grodzinsky (1986) proposed that asyntactic comprehension occurred because these traces were deleted (Trace Deletion Hypothesis), causing a failure to derive the d-structure (which maps onto sentence meaning) from s-structures. This difficulty in movement operations has also been implicated for sentence formulation deficits (Bastiaanse & van Zonneveld, 2005). Other linguistic accounts of impaired morphosyntactic production propose that syntactic tree representations are compromised, such that a part of the tree (usually higher nodes in the syntactic tree) cannot be computed. In the Tree Pruning Hypothesis (Friedmann & Grodzinsky, 1997), complementizers and tense morphology are considered to be higher in the syntactic tree and hence more affected than agreement morphology (see also Ouhalla, 1993).

The second type of theoretical construct involves resource allocation (Kolk & van-Grunsven, 1985). Given that producing and comprehending sentences is an incredibly complex, multifaceted process that must be implemented at a rapid speed by the brain, immense computational resources need to be allocated for sentence-level processes. Proponents of resource limitation accounts point out that agrammatism could be the cumulative outcome of impaired subprocesses of language formulation and comprehension. Or, given the presence of brain damage, there could be an overall reduction in the computational resources that are available for language processes. For example, Kolk (1995) proposed that the "telegraphic" speech, which included content words and lacked functional morphemes, was an adaptation to nonfluency and grammatical impairment. Many authors have found greater agrammatic symptoms with increasing task demands (Kok et al., 2007). A similar argument has been made for asyntactic comprehension, based on the argument that individuals with aphasia and neurologically healthy participants show similar patterns of performance in terms of order of difficulty (Caplan, Waters, Kennedy, et al., 2007; Faroqi-Shah & Dickey, 2009).

Finally, the third account focuses on complexity of linguistic structures as a weak point for agrammatism. Accounts such as the Argument Structure hypothesis for verbs (Thompson, 2003) can also be construed as resource limitation accounts. To summarize, there are numerous theories of specific symptoms of agrammatic aphasia, all with some empirical support. However, a single comprehensive theory of the entire symptom complex of agrammatism has yet to be developed.

REHABILITATION STRATEGIES

The fragmented language of agrammatic aphasia significantly impacts communicative effectiveness and is therefore an important focus of intervention. A crucial question is whether agrammatic symptoms must be specifically targeted during the intervention, or whether conventional aphasia therapy administered in clinical settings and theoretically motivated word-retrieval interventions generalize to sentence structure. The answer to this question had been elusive because relatively few word-retrieval intervention studies have reported sentence structural outcomes, even when the intervention used a discourse context. However, in the past decade, there has been a significant increase in the variety of outcome measures reported (e.g., Kempler & Goral, 2011; Wambaugh & Ferguson, 2007), and the emerging picture strongly suggests that improvement in agrammatic symptoms is found only when they are directly targeted in treatment (Faroqi-Shah & Virion, 2009; Kempler & Goral, 2011). For example, Faroqi-Shah and Virion (2009) examined morpho-syntactic outcomes following Constraint-Induced Language Therapy (CILT; Pulvermuller et al., 2001). CILT uses a natural conversational format with constraints placed on non-verbal communication and is delivered with high intensity, typically 10 to 15 hours per week. Treatment typically specifies the use of carrier phrases and politeness to increase utterance length (e.g., Pass the salt → Mr. Arthur, please pass the salt). Faroqi-Shah and Virion compared conventional CILT with a modified CILT, which specifically included grammaticality constraints (following Faroqi-Shah, 2008). Results with four speakers with agrammatism showed improvement in morphosyntactic production only when gram-maticality was specifically targeted. In another study, Kempler and Goral (2011) compared verb retrieval, sentence structure, and discourse outcomes following two different inter-vention approaches: *Drill*, in which verb names were repetitively practiced, and *conversa-tion*, which is a pseudo-conversational format that used event pictures to foster exchange of new information. The latter intervention emphasized use of complete sentences that included at least one verb. Outcomes from two participants with agrammatism showed that improvements were specific to the intervention: sentence measures only improved with conversational intervention, while isolated verb naming improved with drill.

The existing data suggest that this specificity of treatment outcomes is more often seen for measures of functional morphology (e.g., verb tense) and complex syntax (e.g., wh- questions) than for simple canonical sentences (Faroqi-Shah, 2008, 2013; Jacobs & Thompson, 2000; Schwartz, Saffran, Fink, & Myers, 1994). For example, there are a num-ber of verb retrieval interventions that have reported improved production of grammati-cal sentences, and in many instances, this was defined as the presence of a verb and its arguments yielding a subject-verb-object construction, without reference to grammatical morphology (Edmonds, Nadeau & Kiran, 2009; McCann & Doleman, 2011; Schneider & Thompson, 2003).

Given the general finding of relatively little transfer of treatment effects across agram-matic symptoms coupled with the relative dissociation of agrammatic symptoms dis-cussed earlier, the best intervention strategy for agrammatism is to target sentences, functional morphology, and verbs individually. As per many language production models, computation of sentence structure and functional morphology require prior successful selection of the verb (Eberhard, Cutting, & Bock, 2005; Levelt, 1999). For example, the argument structure of the selected verb dictates assignment of the grammatical frame of the sentence. Hence it is a judicious strategy to target any significant verb deficit prior to introducing intervention for sentence structure and functional morphology deficits. There is evidence that sentence production abilities are enhanced when people with apha-sia are provided with an isolated verb (Berndt et al., 1997). In this chapter, treatments for agrammatism are grouped into three categories: those that (a) aim to improve verb and verb argument structure production, (b) focus on production and comprehension of various sentence structures, and (c) target functional morphology. This is followed by a section on general considerations for intervention. As with all language therapy, it is important to build a therapy plan based on the specific needs and profile of the patient.

Intervention for Verb Deficits

Verb production deficits have a significant impact on language production skills in people with agrammatic aphasia because verbs form the core of the sentence, and verb retrieval is an essential prerequisite for sentence production (Loverso, Prescott, & Selinger, 1988, 1992). While there have been numerous intervention studies for word retrieval in aphasia, most have focused on nouns. Not surprisingly, a majority of the earliest verb retrieval intervention approaches were modeled after techniques used to train noun naming (e.g., Drew & Thompson, 1999; Linebaugh, Baron, & Corcoran, 1998; Nickels, 2002) and these approaches focused mostly on verb naming in isolation. More recent interventions for verbs have emphasized the sentential complements of the verb, including argument structure. These two broad categories of intervention approaches are discussed separately in the following sections.

Verb Naming in Isolation

One primary theoretical framework of aphasia intervention is that word retrieval deficits arise from either semantic or phonological impairments (Nickels, 2002). Consequently, the approach of strengthening semantic networks or phonological representations, based on the individual patient's deficit pattern, has been quite successful for noun retrieval (Beeson & Robey, 2006) and has also been applied to verb naming intervention (Drew & Thompson, 1999; Linebaugh et al., 1998; Nickels, 2002).

Semantically based intervention is implemented either by providing semantic cues during elicited verb naming (see **TABLE 4.1**) or practicing contextual associations of the action (see **FIGURE 4.1**). Generally, semantic cues proceed in an increasing hierarchy in which a failure to name the verb is followed by the least specific semantic cue such as a general description of the action. This is followed by cues with stronger semantic or contextual associations such as a sentence to complete.

Wambaugh and colleagues have examined the efficacy of semantic cueing for verb retrieval in comparison to phonemic cueing (Wambaugh, 2003; Wambaugh, Cameron, Kalinyak-Fliszar, Nessler, & Wright, 2004). Although there were positive outcomes on trained verbs for both semantic and phonemic cueing, there were individual differences in response to treatment: only one of the six participants showed superior response to semantic compared to phonemic cueing treatment. Generalization to untrained verbs was not typically observed (see Chapter 7, this volume).

Semantic Feature Analysis (SFA) is another semantic approach borrowed from noun interventions. It aims to improve access to verb names by strengthening the associations between the verb and related concepts in the mental lexicon, such as tool use, resulting

TABLE 4.1 Semantic cueing hierarchy, adapted from Wambaugh et al. (2002).

Step	Objective	Details
1	Provide description of verb	Clinician provides verbal description of the target action. For example, for the target verb *dig*, the description "when you move dirt to make a hole" is provided.
2	Prompt semantically neutral sentence completion cue	For example, "dogs love to…"
3	Prompt semantically loaded sentence completion cue	For example, "you use a shovel to…"

Data from Wambaugh et al. (2002)

state, and typical nouns/persons associated with the verb (Boyle & Coehlo, 1995; Faroqi-Shah & Graham, 2010; Peach & Reuter, 2010; Wambaugh & Ferguson, 2007; Wambaugh, Mauszycki, & Wright, 2014). Intervention consists of guiding the participant to generate various semantic features of each target verb, using a template illustrated in Figure 4.1 (from Peach & Reuter, 2010). The outcomes of SFA have been generally positive for trained verbs, with little generalization to untrained verbs. In an attempt to enhance generalization to untrained verbs, Faroqi-Shah and Graham (2010) selected training and generalization verbs based on overlap in semantic features (Levin, 1993). For example, the class of *Cut* verbs such as mince and dice have five semantic features (action, motion, contact, tool use, and change of state), of which the first three features also characterize the class of *Contact* verbs (e.g., nudge, tickle, kiss, bump). They hypothesized that training

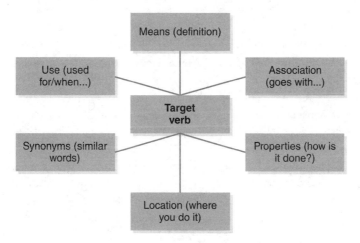

FIGURE 4.1 Semantic feature analysis for verb retrieval training

Data from Peach & Reuter, 2010

of the *Cut* class of verbs would generalize to the class of contact verbs because of overlap in trained semantic features. Their hypothesis was partially supported in a two-participant treatment study. This theoretically motivated treatment holds promise in terms of generalization to untrained exemplars, but needs further replication.

Errorless learning, which emphasizes the avoidance of errors during intervention, has also been used for verb retrieval (Abel, Schultz, Radermacher, Willmes, & Huber, 2005; Conroy, Sage, & Lambon Ralph, 2009a, 2009b, 2009c; Fillingham, Sage, & Lambon Ralph, 2005a, 2005b, 2006). Conroy and colleagues implemented errorless learning with decreasing phonological cues, that is, the verb label was provided soon after presentation of the action picture during the initial sessions. This was followed by partial phonological cues, such as the initial syllable in later sessions (see **TABLE 4.2**). In a series of studies that compared efficacy of errorless learning (with decreasing cues) and the more traditional intervention approach of increasing cues with each failed naming attempt, Conroy and colleagues found similar outcomes for both approaches. However, participants preferred decreasing cueing therapy because it ensured initial success and also challenged them as therapy progressed.

To summarize, semantic treatments generally have shown positive outcomes for verbs, as have phonological interventions (Raymer et al., 2007; Rodriguez, Raymer, & Gonzalez-Rothi, 2006; Wambaugh, Doyle, Martinez, & Kalinyak-Fliszar, 2002). A few points are worth noting: first, semantic treatments also engage phonological representations because word forms are used during treatment and are elicited to test confrontation

TABLE 4.2 Errorless learning approach with decreasing cues (Conroy et al., 2009).

Session	Word Cue	Sentence Cue for Transitive Verb
1–3	Whole word in spoken and written forms, e.g., "*driving*"	Sentence in spoken and written forms (pronoun always used for agent), e.g., "*She is bouncing the ball*"
4–5	CVC/CCVC phonemic and graphemic prompts, e.g., "*driv-*"	Sentence frame with C/CC phonemic and graphemic prompt for patient "ball," e.g., "*She is bouncing the b----*"
6	CV/CCV phonemic and graphemic prompts, e.g., "*dri-*"	Sentence frame with CV/CCV phonemic and graphemic prompt for verb, e.g., "*She is bou----* (await correct response) *the ----*"
7	C/CC phonemic and graphemic prompts, e.g., "*dr-*"	Sentence frame with C phonemic and graphemic prompt for verb, with action picture, e.g., "*She is b----* (await correct response) *the ----*"
8–10	Picture alone	Action picture with written prompt "*---- is ---- the ----*"

Data from Conroy et al., 2009

naming. Secondly, generalization to untrained verbs has been elusive. In many studies, verbs selected for treatment have been unrelated to one another or drawn from a list of unsuccessfully named items from test batteries (e.g., Kim, Adingono, & Revoir, 2007; Wambaugh & Ferguson, 2007). Therefore, during treatment, different semantic networks were likely stimulated, diminishing the potential for within-category generalization. Although it remains uncertain whether training verbs with semantic overlap leads to better generalization (Faroqi-Shah & Graham, 2010; Schneider & Thompson, 2003), more research is needed on the effects of semantically related verb stimuli.

Verb Naming with Sentential Complements

The intervention techniques described in this section integrate verb retrieval practice with related linguistic elements, such as the participant roles selected by the verb (i.e., argument structure and associated thematic roles), or a sentence frame (Bastiaanse, Hurkmans, & Links, 2006; Byng, Nickels, & Black, 1994; Edmonds & Kiran, 2006; Edmonds et al., 2009; Kim et al., 2007; Le Dorze, Jacob, & Coderre, 1991; Loverso et al., 1988, 1992; Schneider & Thompson, 2003; Thompson, Riley, den Ouden, Meltzer-Asscher, & Lukic, 2013; Webster, Morris, & Franklin, 2005). The theoretical justification for using verb arguments is that these are co-activated whenever a verb's representation is activated (e.g., measure/carpenter; Edmonds & Mizrahi, 2011; McRae, Hare, Elman, & Ferretti, 2005). The general procedure of argument structure-based interventions involves naming the verb, generating typical arguments for the verb using wh- questions (e.g., Who measures? What is measured?), and constructing a sentence that includes the verb and its typical arguments (see **TABLE 4.3**). Different argument combinations for a specific verb may also be elicited, such as chef/sugar, carpenter/lumber, and surveyor/land for the verb *measure* (Edmonds & Kiran, 2006; Edmonds et al., 2009). Verb Network Strengthening Treatment (VNeST) is an example of a treatment approach that focuses on generating agents and patients associated with a given verb (e.g., *chef/sugar* match with the verb *measure* because a chef can measure sugar; see Table 4.3). Following VNeST treatment, participants improved noun and verb retrieval and use of argument structure as measured by connected speech samples, and saw generalization to untrained verbs (Edmonds & Kiran, 2006; Edmonds et al., 2009). Another variation of sentential approach to verb retrieval includes a judgment of whether a given set of arguments matches the verb (Webster et al., 2005). Kim and colleagues' (2007) approach used theme-focused stories for verb training.

Another sentential approach used a fill-in-the-blank format by requiring participants to provide a verb for a sentence-picture pair (Bastiaanse et al., 2006). Infinitives and finite verbs were trained in separate steps, followed by a step requiring participants to form sentences without a cue. Schneider and Thompson (2003) provided auditory information about who did what to whom and then asked participants to produce target verbs. Overall, these approaches have reported improved verb retrieval outcomes and generally better generalization to sentence production than the isolated verb retrieval approaches described in the previous section (see Chapter 7, this volume).

TABLE 4.3 Verb network strengthening treatment (VNeST; Edmonds et al., 2009).

Step	Objective	Details
1	Generation of three agents or patients for verb	For example, clinician says, "Tell me who/what can *measure*." Clinician prompts as necessary with written response cards and foils (this same prompting approach is used in all successive steps).
2	Generation of corresponding agent or patient to complete agent–patient pairs	Say patients that correspond to the agents generated in Step 1. For example, chef/*sugar*, carpenter/*lumber*, and surveyor/*land*
3	Answer wh- questions about agent–patient pair	Client chooses one agent–patient pair to discuss in more detail. The clinician asks the client wh- questions (where, when, and why) about that pair. For example, "When does a chef measure sugar?" ... "*In the morning.*" "Why?" ... "*To get the correct amount.*" "Where?" ... "*In the kitchen.*"
4	Semantic judgment of sentences	Clinician reads 12 sentences containing the target verb (4 correct, 4 with inappropriate agent, 4 with inappropriate patient, 4 with agent and patient switched). Client then indicates whether the sentences make sense or not.
5	Generation of three agent–patient pairs (repeat steps 1–2)	Clinician asks the same question from Step 1, and the Client is then encouraged to produce up to three agents and their respective patients. General feedback is provided and no cue cards are used.

Data from Edmonds et al., 2009

Multimodal Approaches

Given that most frequently used verbs denote human actions, gestures have been used to augment language intervention. The theoretical rationale for using gestures is that actions (or gestures) and their corresponding verbal labels share a conceptual representation (de Ruiter, 2006). Further support for integrating gesture with verb retrieval intervention comes from neuroimaging and behavioral evidence that language representations are intertwined with sensorimotor representations, a view that is referred to as *embodied semantics* (Barsalou, 2008; some authors have questioned the embodiment of language, for example, Mahon & Caramazza, 2008). It has been argued that gestures facilitate and sustain access to the semantic features of a verb before the verb itself is retrieved (Morsella & Krauss, 2004; Rose, 2006). Investigators have compared various permutations of gesture and language therapy: gesture only, gesture plus semantic stimulation, repetition (phonological stimulation), and repetition plus orthographic treatments (Boo & Rose, 2011;

Raymer et al., 2006; Rodriguez et al., 2006; Rose & Sussmilch, 2008). In the gesture condition, participants are encouraged to imitate or produce hand/arm movements for the action verb. So far, outcomes have been generally positive if the person has a phonological locus of deficit; whereas no improvement in verb naming has been reported for people who have a semantic deficit that includes verb comprehension difficulties. Further, verb-naming outcomes are similar for semantic only and semantic plus gesture therapy, and so far, suggest no additional benefit of gestures. Generalization to untrained verbs did not occur in any of the studies. Possible reasons for the limited utility of gestures include overall severity of enrolled participants, and the combination of gesture with verbalization makes it a dual-task demand. Furthermore, some of the verb stimuli used in treatment were not hand/arm verbs (e.g., running; Boo & Rose, 2011), so the practiced gesture may not have activated the actual sensorimotor representations of the target verb. Further research is necessary to elucidate the value of gestures for verb naming. Interestingly, a treatment approach that utilized passive observation of action videos had a superior effect on verb naming compared to gestural treatment (Marangolo et al., 2010).

Intervention for Sentence Structural Deficits

This section describes approaches that target comprehension and/or production of sentences without explicitly addressing lexical difficulties. This is in contrast to the interventions described earlier (see section on *Verb retrieval with sentential complements*). There are relatively few replicated sentence-level treatment approaches, and existing treatments differ in their theoretical foundations. One early model relies on memorization and repetitive practice, referred to here as *script training* (Cherney, Halper, Holland, & Cole, 2008; Helm-Estabrooks, 1981). Other, more recent approaches, especially by Thompson and colleagues, have used a *reverse complexity* model, in which training is initiated with syntactically complex sentence structures and focuses on deriving the complex sentence from a simple canonical sentence in a stepwise progression (Treatment of Underlying Forms; Thompson, Ballard, & Shapiro, 1998; Thompson, Shapiro, Tait, Jacobs, & Schneider, 1996). A third approach focuses on strengthening the participant's ability to parse thematic roles in different sentence structures, referred to as *mapping* between form and meaning (Byng, 1988; Rochon, Laird, Bose, & Scofield, 2005; Schwartz et al., 1994). Mapping therapies emphasize comprehension, and some variations include production steps as well. Finally, there are approaches that broadly focus on the sentence level, but are less precise about the syntactic structures to include in training (Kempler & Goral, 2011; Linebarger, Romania, Fink, Bartlett, & Schwartz, 2008; Meinzer, Djundja, Barthel, Elbert, & Rockstroh, 2005; Pulvermuller et al., 2001). For example, in CILT, participants work towards producing progressively longer utterances (*Pass the salt* → *Mr. John, please pass the salt*), but there are no a priori hypotheses about underlying linguistic representations or patterns of transfer to untrained sentences (Pulvermuller et al., 2001). We will refer to these approaches as *general and conversational approaches*. In the following sections, selected interventions for sentence production are reviewed.

Script Training

The characteristic feature of script training methods is repeated practice and memorization of a fixed set of sentences. The earliest such program is the Helm-Estabrooks Language Program for Syntax Stimulation (HELPSS; Helm-Estabrooks, 1981; later commercially available as the Sentence Production Program for Aphasia; Helm-Estabrooks & Nicholas, 2000). This program involves progression from short phrase-like structures such as imperatives (e.g., Sit down, Watch out) to longer active sentences and wh- questions. It uses short picture scenarios and clinician modeling to train production of eight different sentence structures. Unlike the prespecified set of sentences used in HELPSS, other script training approaches train the use of personally relevant and individualized scripts, such as routines involved in small talk with strangers and ordering from a restaurant menu (Holland, Milman, Muñoz, & Bays, 2002). More recently, repeated practice of commonly used sentences and phrases has been implemented through a computer interface with a virtual therapist (AphasiaScripts; Cherney et al., 2008). In a pilot study, three participants who used AphasiaScripts showed improvements in the content, grammatical productivity, and rate of delivery of the scripts (Cherney et al., 2008). In general, while outcomes for trained scripts are generally positive, there is little generalization to untrained sentences and sentence structures (Doyle, Goldstein, & Bourgeois, 1987; Helm-Estabrooks & Ramsberger, 1986).

Treatment of Underlying Forms

Treatment of underlying forms (TUF, originally called Linguistic Specific Treatment) was developed by Thompson and colleagues for training complex sentences, such as object clefts and passives (Thompson, 2008; Thompson et al., 1997, 1998). In TUF, the training begins with reviewing an active sentence and identifying the verb and its arguments (or adjunct). Successive steps in the treatment focus on improving knowledge of the thematic roles of the verb in the sentence (who did what to whom), followed by changing the linear order of elements in the sentence, to derive the surface form of the target sentence. These steps are illustrated in **TABLE 4.4**. A computerized version of TUF with a virtual clinician is also available (Sentactics; Thompson, Choy, Holland, & Cole, 2010).

The theoretical rationale for this intervention is the Complexity Account of Treatment Efficacy (CATE), which proposes that training linguistically complex structures results in generalization to less complex structures, if the untrained structures encompass linguistic processes relevant to treated ones (Thompson et al., 2003). At the core of TUF are the syntactic tree structures of sentences, which provide a template for underlying linguistic representations (Chomsky, 1995). As an illustration, consider the sentences below, all of which refer to the same event.

1. The actress called the police. (active)

2. Who did the actress call? (object wh- question)

3. It was the police who the actress called. (object cleft)

4. The journalist saw the police who the actress called. (object relative)

5. The police was called by the actress. (passive)

6. The actress seems to have called the police. (subject raising)

7. When did the actress call the police? (adjunct wh- question)

8. Where did the actress call the police? (adjunct wh- question)

TABLE 4.4 Treatment of underlying forms illustrating training for wh- questions, from Thompson (2008).

Step	Objective	Details
1	Introduce the deep (d) structure	Clinician presents the underlying d-structure of the target question (e.g., The man is sending flowers.) and asks the client to read/repeat the sentence. Clinician instructs that the sentence will be changed to produce a new sentence.
2	Generation of target sentence/ question	Clinician presents the d-structure sentence elements on individual cards, and also *What, Who,* and *?* cards. Clinician instructs the Client to produce the target sentence/question (e.g., *What is the man sending?*)
3	Identify sentence elements	Clinician identifies the verb, subject NP (noun phrase) and object NP of the sentence. Clinician then explains (a) that the object NP is the "thing" (What questions) or "person" (Who questions) receiving the action and (b) that it is replaced by *What* or *Who*, respectively. Clinician then replaces the object NP with the *What/Who* card and places the *?* at the end, forming an echo question (e.g., *The man is sending What?*). The echo question is read/repeated by the Client.
4	Intermediate steps	In this step, any functional morphology changes are made, depending on the sentence being trained. For training wh- questions, it would be subject-auxiliary inversion (Is the man sending What?)
5	Generation of surface (s) structure	Clinician demonstrates movement of the wh- word to the sentence initial position (e.g., What is the man sending?). The key element of this training is demonstration of the movement of sentence elements from d-structure to s-structure position. The Client reads/repeats the target sentence.
6	Independent practice	Clinician rearranges the sentence cards to their d-structure order and places the What, Who and ? cards next to the sentence. Client is encouraged to generate the s-structure by replacing/moving the sentence cards. Assistance is provided. The client then reads/repeats the sentence.

Thompson (2008)

In transformational grammar of linguistics, the active sentence (1) can be used to derive the surface structure of sentences (2) through (6) using *movement* operations (Chomsky, 1995). Sentences differ in the element that is moved to generate the surface structure; object wh- questions (2), object clefts (3), and object relatives (4) are derived by moving the wh- element from the direct object position within the verb phrase (VP) to the Specifier of the complementizer phrase (Spec, CP). This is illustrated in **FIGURE 4.2** for an object wh- question. Passives (5) and subject raising (6) sentences are derived by moving the noun phrase (NP) from its direct object position in the VP to the Specifier of

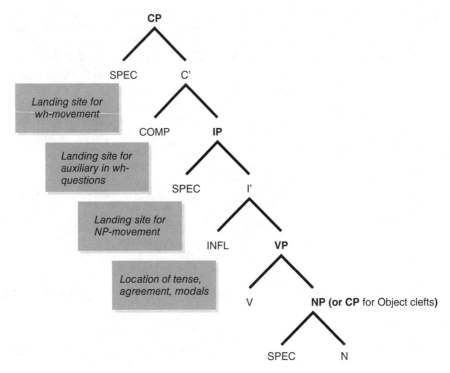

FIGURE 4.2A Tree structure of a sentence illustrating the hierarchical relationship between different functional elements, used as the basis for syntactic accounts and interventions of agrammatism (e.g., Treatment of Underlying Forms, Thompson, 2008; Tree Pruning Hypothesis, Friedmann & Grodzinksy, 1997). The heads of the different elements are CP (complementizer phrase), IP (inflectional phrase), and VP (verb phrase). The specifier of the CP (COMP=complementizer) can be filled either at d-structure or through wh-movement in the creation of wh-questions. The specifier of the IP can be filled either by the subject at d-structure or through NP-movement as in passive constructions. The local head, INFL, marks verb tense and agreement.

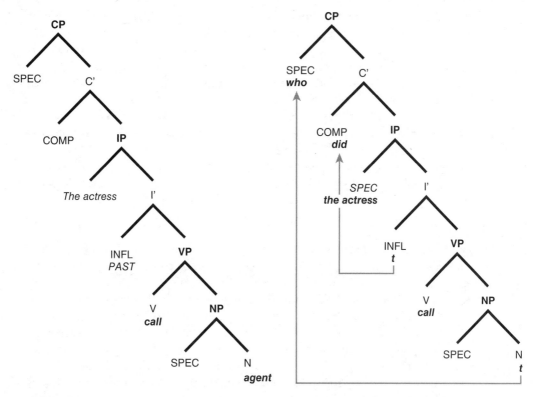

FIGURE 4.2B Example tree structure for an active sentence. (The actress called the agent.)

FIGURE 4.2C The object-extracted wh-question Who did the actress call? The object of the verb call moves to the SPEC of the CP, leaving a trace (t).

the inflectional phrase (Spec, IP). In other words, direct object elements move to different landing sites to derive object clefts and wh- questions (Spec, CP) compared to passives and subject raising sentences (Spec, IP). The *when* and *where* questions in (7) and (8) involve a different kind of movement, the wh- element is moved from the adjunct prepositional phrase to the Spec, IP.

Based on the distinct transformational operations involved in generating different surface structures, Thompson and colleagues tested and confirmed the hypothesis that training to produce one kind of sentence would generalize only to other sentences with the same movement operation. Thus training of object clefts generalized to object-extracted wh- questions (who and what), training of subject raising generalized to passives, and training of adjunct NP movement improved other adjunct NP structures (when and where) (Ballard & Thompson, 1999; Jacobs & Thompson, 2000; Thompson, 2008;

Thompson, Shapiro, & Roberts, 1993; Thompson et al., 1996, 1998, 2003). In addition, a complexity hierarchy predicted generalization patterns: training of more complex structures generalized to less complex structures with the same movement operation. Thus, training of object relatives improved production of object wh- questions and object clefts, but training of wh- questions did not improve the more complex object relative constructions (Thompson et al., 2003) (see Chapter 7, this volume). Active sentences, which are syntactically simplest, improved in all instances. TUF has been implemented in other languages, such as German (Stadie et al., 2008) and Kannada (Faroqi & Chengappa, 1997), and similar generalization patterns have been reported. In a single-case study of a multilingual person with agramamtic aphasia, Faroqi and Chengappa (1997) observed cross-language generalization of wh- and NP-training from the trained language (Kannada) to a linguistically similar language spoken by the individual (Telugu).

Mapping Therapies

Mapping therapies aim to improve production by improving comprehension of verbs and their thematic role assignments. The theoretical premise comes from psycholinguistic models of sentence production and comprehension, which propose three basic processing levels: the conceptual level, the functional (or lemma) level, and the positional level (e.g., Bock & Levelt, 1994; Levelt, 1999). The speakers' intentions from the conceptual level are lexicalized at the functional level. The functional level includes accessing words along with their grammatical specifications, such as word class, thematic roles, and combinatorial constraints. Finally, at the positional level, lexical elements are integrated into a grammatically well-formed sentence. Proponents of mapping therapy hypothesize a specific locus of impairment in agrammatism: difficulty in mapping information derived from the functional to the positional level and vice versa. In essence, the linking, or "mapping" between positional level and functional levels is faulty. Hence therapy aims to strengthen these connections (Berndt & Mitchum, 1997; Byng, 1988; Rochon et al., 2005; Schwartz et al., 1994).

There are several variations of mapping therapy, although they maintain the common theme of linking positional- and functional-level representations. This is achieved by identifying verbs and verb arguments of the target sentence. In lexical mapping therapy, which is recommended for people with a verb deficit, the emphasis is on treating verb and verb argument structure access (Schwartz et al., 1994). Hence the procedure is similar to approaches discussed earlier (see section on *Verb retrieval with sentential complements*). Procedural mapping therapy, on the other hand, is intended for people who show asyntactic comprehension and agrammatic production, specifically poorer performance on non-canonical compared to canonical sentences, with relative sparing of verb knowledge. The focus is on strengthening connections between meaning and structure, such as between thematic roles (agent, theme; who did what to whom) and subject and object positions of sentences. Connections between meaning and structure are trained by color-coding words and pictures in a matching task, enacting scenarios with figurines, and/or asking participants to respond to wh- probes. In the most frequently used version, participants identify verbs and their arguments by underlining the appropriate words in the sentence with a specific pen color for each element (e.g., blue for verb, red for agent; Schwartz et al., 1994). Sentence structure is not explicitly trained, which is unlike TUF where relationship between syntactic position and thematic roles is described by the clinician. Another difference with TUF is that training proceeds from structurally simple to complex structures, for example, from active forms to passive forms. Most mapping therapies focus on sentence comprehension, anticipating generalization to sentence production. However, Rochon and colleagues' (2005) mapping therapy directly trained sentence production of four sentence structures: active, subject cleft, passive, and object cleft sentences. Mapping therapy also has been adapted for computer delivery, using a computer-based microworld (Beveridge & Crerar, 2002; Crerar, Ellis, & Dean, 1996).

Outcomes of mapping therapies are generally positive, but somewhat diverse given the differences in procedures, participants, and language measures (Berndt & Mitchum, 1997; Beveridge & Crerar, 2002; Byng, 1988; Crerar et al., 1996; Rochon et al., 2005; Schwartz et al., 1994). Improved comprehension of trained and untrained canonical sentences has been found in studies that have trained and tested comprehension (Schwartz et al., 1994; Beveridge & Crerar, 2002), while outcomes for comprehension of non-canonical sentences have been mixed even with training. For example, Schwartz and colleagues' (1994) study did not find improvement of non-canonical sentences and Beveridge and Crerar (2002) found improvements in only a subset of participants. When mapping therapy was aimed at sentence production, improved production of trained canonical and non-canonical sentences and generalization to other tasks such as narrative speech have been found; however, there was no improvement in sentence comprehension (Rochon et al., 2005). To summarize, the evidence shows that mapping therapies result in improvements in trained structures and trained modalities (comprehension, production), with the possible exception of comprehension of complex sentences.

General and Conversational Approaches

Numerous approaches target overall conversational abilities for aphasia, but do not specifically focus on grammaticality. These interventions are nevertheless a valuable adjunct to other more impairment-focused interventions for agrammatism. One such approach is *Constraint-Induced Language Therapy* (CILT), more recently referred to as intensive language action therapy (ILAT; Pulvermuller & Berthier, 2008). CILT typically involves about 30 to 36 hours of weekly group interaction of aphasic participants in therapeutic language games (typically over 10 days; Breier, Maher, Novak, & Papanicolaou, 2006; Maher et al., 2006; Meinzer et al., 2005; Pulvermuller et al., 2001). Language and conversations are practiced in a group game format, typically with card games or board games. The therapist makes progressively increasing demands on verbal responses that need to be produced and provides general cues. Typically, the goals are to progressively increase utterance length by adding different parts of speech or politeness markers. The crucial manipulation (from which the approach gets its name) is that people must use the verbal modality for communication and not rely on gestures or writing. In some studies, visual barriers are placed between group members to preclude use of alternative nonverbal communication strategies. Most CILT efficacy studies have found reduction in overall aphasia severity, especially comprehension scores, an aspect that is not explicitly targeted in CILT (Pulvermuller et al., 2001; Szaflarski et al., 2008), but limited improvements in measures of grammatical production (Faroqi-Shah & Virion, 2009; Szaflarski et al., 2008, p. 250). As described earlier, one study examined the results of CILT on four individuals with agrammatism and tested the effect of adapting the CILT procedure to include morphosyntactic shaping (Faroqi-Shah & Virion, 2009). Two participants received CILT-O, that is, CILT as originally described in Pulvermüller and colleagues (2001), and two participants received CILT-G, or CILT with addition of grammatical constraints. Those constraints included a requirement to produce a temporal adverb (e.g., yesterday) and the appropriate verb tense morphology (e.g., held, not hold). Furthermore, for CILT-G participants, written cues for grammatical morphemes were available in the early sessions, and participants were required to make well-formedness judgments on their partner's requests. The two participants who received the modified CILT with grammaticality constraints (called grammatical-CILT by the authors) improved in overall sentence grammaticality compared to the two participants who received traditional CILT.

In contrast to CILT are approaches that do not place any constraints on the modality of communication. Instead, these approaches have emphasized the application of natural conversation rules for aphasia therapy with a focus on both conversational partners and their equal role in the interaction (Hopper, Holland, & Rewega, 2002; Marangolo et al., 2013; Cunningham & Ward, 2003). The rationale is, that if conversational partners, such as the clinician or spouse, have frequent cooperative communicative exchanges with the person with aphasia (PWA), the PWA will improve in his or her capacity to both convey and receive information during the conversations. Any communicative modality is allowed during the conversation (verbal, gestural, writing, drawing, mime) and there are no demands on lexical or syntactic accuracy, the main emphasis is on equal and active participation of both communication partners to exchange new information and ideas. Some approaches also include training for the conversational partners of PWAs, such as *Supported Conversation Analysis* (Kagan, Black, Duchan, Simmons-Mackie, & Square, 2001) and *Conversational Coaching* (Hopper et al., 2002; Cunningham & Ward, 2003; reviewed in Wilkinson & Wielaert, 2012). While some of the conversational approaches have been single-subject studies with individualized coaching and reported qualitative outcomes (Beeke, Wilkinson, & Maxim, 2007), others have been group studies with a more structured training program (e.g., Kagan et al., 2001). Although there is a wide variation in the experimental design and intervention approach, these studies have generally found modest improvements in the speaking behavior of both the PWA and conversational partner (Wilkinson & Wielaert, 2012).

Computer software applications have also been used to enhance and practice sentence production. One such system is Sentence Shaper, which allows the PWA to create, edit, and revise audio recordings of sentences (Linebarger, Schwartz, & Kohn, 2001). The rationale behind creating such off-line sentences is that agrammatism may be partially due to a processing limitation. People with agrammatic aphasia have the capacity to formulate sentences when given enough time, something that is not available during a real-time conversation (Linebarger et al., 2001). The Sentence Shaper program gives the PWA time to come up with utterances, record them, edit them by correcting or expanding them, and then play back the sentences. A more recent version also provides lexical support and pictures to practice sentence formulation. Given the time required to record and edit, the Sentence Shaper is most suitable for messages that can be anticipated (e.g., communications with store clerks and doctors, speeches, and toasts). In one study, home practice with the Sentence Shaper improved the sentence structural scores of two people with nonfluent aphasia, but not their production of grammatical morphemes (Linebarger, Schwartz, Romaina, Kohn, & Stephens, 2000), and these results were replicated in another study with five participants (Linebarger et al., 2001). As described earlier, AphasiaScripts is another computer software program that serves a similar function of practicing messages that are prepared in advance (Cherney et al., 2008).

Intervention for Functional Morphology

There are fewer theoretically motivated interventions for functional morphology compared to verb retrieval and sentence structure. Existing interventions are mostly designed to address tense/aspectual markings on verbs, and a few are designed to improve production of other functional categories such as complementizers (Boser & Weinrich, 1998; Faroqi-Shah, 2008, 2013; Harris, Olson, & Humphreys, 2012; Thompson, Kearns, & Edmonds, 2006; Weinrich, Boser, & McCall, 1999; Weinrich, Shelton, Cox, & McCall, 1997; Wieczorek, 2011). Two broad theoretical frameworks have been used to motivate interventions: psycholinguistic models of sentence production (Bock & Levelt, 1994; Garrett, 1975, 1988) and syntactic theories (Bobalijk & Thrainsson, 1998; Friedmann & Grodzinsky, 1997; Hagiwara, 1995). We first describe psycholinguistically based treatment approaches followed by syntactically based methods of intervention.

Interventions Guided by Sentence Production Models
While Garrett's (1988) model of sentence production considered functional morphology to be inherently bound to sentence frames, later frameworks recognized that functional morphology was influenced by conceptual, lexical, and syntactic constraints (e.g., Bock & Levelt, 1994). Therefore, there are different intervention approaches depending on the psycholinguistic framework adopted by the authors. Berndt and colleagues used Garrett's approach of the inseparability of functional morphology and sentence frames and targeted training of specific sentence frames (Mitchum & Berndt, 1994; Mitchum et al., 1993; Weinrich et al., 1997). For example, Mitchum et al. (1993) trained production of verb morphology referring to the future (will V), present (present progressive: is V-ing) and

past (present perfect: has V-ed) using written practice. All three verb clusters were trained using a *noun phrase + auxiliary + verb + noun phrase (The horse is jumping/has jumped over the fence)* sentence frame using a three-picture sequence to illustrate the future, present, and past. The first step of the treatment protocol was to chronologically sequence the pictures, followed by practice producing the corresponding sentences. Errors were corrected using a cueing hierarchy. In another study, the same procedure was used with the oral modality with a single client (Mitchum & Berndt, 1994). Both studies reported improvement in the production of sentence frames for all trained verbs. For example, following treatment, one patient produced the following sentences for the words *drill* and *dial*: *The mechanic will drill the tires* and *The lady has dialed the telephone* (pre-treatment sentences were *Take a drill* and *The dial is broken*; Mitchum & Berndt, 1994). However, no improvements were noted in morphosyntactic measures of narrative speech such as the proportion of grammatical sentences, use of trained verbs in narrative speech, the production of passive voice, or the variety of verbs used.

Intervention approaches that follow the multidimensional views of functional morphology include some sort of training on conceptual-semantic implications of morphemes. For example, Weinrich and colleagues developed a computer-based iconic system (called C-VIC) and trained verb tense in clients with severe nonfluent aphasia (Boser & Weinrich, 1998; Boser, Weinrich, & McCall, 2000, Weinrich et al., 1997, 1999). Weinrich and colleagues (1997) hypothesized that an improvement in the ability to link temporal information (past, present, etc.) with lexical representations of verbs would result in overall improvement in production of verb tense (based on LaPointe & Dell's model, 1989). The C-VIC training is nonverbal; participants describe pictures by arranging icons in *noun + verb + noun* sequences (Boser & Weinrich, 1998; Boser et al., 2000; Weinrich et al., 1997, 1999). Three participants were trained to place a clock-like icon indicating temporal reference (e.g., present, past) at the beginning of each C-VIC sentence, rather than to directly mark verbs with tense inflection. Following this, participants produced target sentences, either orally or in writing. Feedback and cues were provided as needed. After training, participants not only improved in the trained C-VIC iconic sentences, but also in verbal/written production of corresponding English sentences. There was also improved oral naming of verbs that were used in iconic training. Another step-by-step intervention approach that focuses on conceptual-semantic implications of tense is morphosemantic treatment (Faroqi-Shah, 2008), which is outlined in the next section.

Morphosemantic treatment.   The primary focus of this intervention is to associate the morphological shape that a verb could take with the meaning it conveys (e.g., *will + Verb* denotes an activity in the *future*). The theoretical rationale behind this approach is the Diacritical Encoding and Retrieval (DER) hypothesis proposed by Faroqi-Shah and Thompson (2007), which states that functional morphology errors in agrammatism result from impaired ability to select semantically appropriate diacritical features (e.g., tense, mood) and link those features to the correct verb form. The concept of diacritical encoding and retrieval was drawn from psycholinguistics models of language production (Bock & Levelt, 1994; Eberhard et al., 2005; Janssen, Roelofs, & Levelt, 2002; Levelt, 1999) The DER hypothesis was based on empirical findings that people with agrammatic aphasia perform relatively well when required to make decisions about the morphosyntactic constraints of verb morphology, such as grammaticality judgments (e.g., *will washed) or sentence completion (e.g., The boy will _____ his hands [washing, washed, wash, washes]; Faroqi-Shah & Dickey, 2009; Faroqi-Shah & Thompson, 2007). However, performance is severely affected when the semantic implications of verb morphology are considered, both in grammaticality judgment and sentence completion tasks (e.g., Yesterday the boy _____ his hands [is washing, washed, will wash, washes]). Moreover, this selectional difficulty was highly correlated with errors in production of verb morphology in a picture description task (Faroqi-Shah & Dickey, 2009).

The morphosemantic treatment explicitly focused on semantic features conveyed by verb inflections by training individuals with agrammatism on reference to the past (simple past), present (simple present), and future (*will* + *Infinitive*) using a series of steps, none of which required oral production of target forms (Faroqi-Shah, 2008, 2013). These steps are outlined in **TABLE 4.5**. The first step was grammaticality judgment (for example,

TABLE 4.5 Morphosemantic treatment for verb tense (Faroqi-Shah, 2013).

Step	Objective	Details
1	Verb naming	Clinician presents a three-picture sequence that represents the target action about to occur, in progress, and completed. Clinician asks the client to name the action.
2	Anomaly judgment—detect incorrect conceptual–verb morphology pairings	Clinician reads aloud a sentence for the client to judge correctness. Incorrect sentences contain mismatches between the temporal adverb and verb tense (e.g, Yesterday the boy will wash his hands). Feedback is provided and one more sentence is presented for judgment. Note that this step can be adapted for written presentation for clients with limited auditory memory span.
3	Auditory comprehension—learn temporal reference–verb morphology pairings	Clinician reads aloud a sentence without a temporal marker (e.g., The boy will wash his hands). The client is asked to match the sentence with one of three action pictures.
4	Sentence completion	Client writes (or selects from word cards) the correct completion for a sentence to match a picture (e.g, Yesterday, the boy _____ his hands).
5	Sentence construction	Client selects and arranges word cards (anagrams) to form a sentence that corresponds to a given picture.

Faroqi-Shah, 2013

Tomorrow the boy washed his hands). This was followed by a comprehension task where participants pointed to the picture that matched an auditorily presented sentence from a choice of three pictures (for example, *The boy will wash his hands*). The next two steps involved written sentence completion (fill in the blank, such as *The boy _____ his hands*) and an anagram arrangement task (e.g., arrange tiles, each with a sentence element, in grammatical order).

In efficacy studies of morphosemantic treatment, all participants successfully acquired trained morphology and carried over the trained morphological markings to untrained verbs (Faroqi-Shah, 2008, 2013). Across these two efficacy studies conducted by Faroqi-Shah, four (out of nine) participants were trained using verbs that had irregular past tenses only, either those that only involved a vowel change for the past tense (e.g., *ring-rang, drink-drank, wear-wore*), or those that required a vowel change along with a consonant addition (t/d; e.g., *sleep-slept, keep-kept, sell-sold*). The other five participants were trained using verbs with regular past tense forms. Generalization was tested to production of verbs with regular and irregular past tense forms. Participants trained with irregular verbs showed generalization to regular past, while the reverse pattern of improvement in irregular past for people trained on regular past was not found (except in one instance). Overall, improvements in untrained irregular past were limited, irrespective of whether regular or irregular verbs were trained. These outcomes are consistent with representational differences between regular and irregular verbs generally assumed by most authors (although differences exist between them; Bybee, 1995; Clahsen, 1999; Halle & Marantz, 1993; Pinker & Prince, 1991; Rumelhart & McClelland, 1986). Irregular verbs are assumed to represent the default affixation rule (add -ed), which is *blocked* when the lexically stored irregular (past tense) is accessed. This blocking principle prevents an over-regularized form from being produced (e.g., *singed* or *sanged*). Thus, the effects of irregular verb treatment, via activation of the affixation rule, could trickle down to the production of regular past tense forms. This predicts that practice of irregular verb inflections could potentially improve both irregular and regular verb production. However, practice with regular verb inflections is unlikely to benefit irregular verb production. These predictions were confirmed by the treatment outcomes observed in Faroqi-Shah (2008, 2013) and for C-VIC by Weinrich et al. (1999). The outcomes of both studies of morphosemantic treatment included improvements in a variety of verb-related and morphosyntactic measures such as the proportion of verbs, the proportion of affixed verbs, the accuracy of verb tense, diversity of verb tense (type-token ratio of tense), mean length of utterance, and the proportion of sentences produced.

The positive outcomes of morphosemantic treatment contrast with the outcomes of a *morphophonological* intervention approach tested by Faroqi-Shah (2008) in two individuals with agrammatic aphasia. The morphophonological approach was developed to address the proposal of a post-lexical affixation and phonological difficulty in agrammatic aphasia (Bird, Lambon Ralph, Seidenberg, McClelland, & Patterson, 2003; Braber, Patterson, Ellis, & Lambon Ralph, 2005; Kean, 1977; Ullman et al., 1997). Indeed, variables that increase phonological complexity, such as syllable stress, the number of syllables, and the presence of consonant clusters, negatively affect production of verb inflections in agrammatic aphasia (Bird et al., 2003; Kohn & Melvold, 2000; Lambon Ralph, Braber, McClelland, & Patterson, 2005; Meth, Obler, Harris, & Schwartz, 1995). The essential difference between the morphosemantic treatment described previously and the morphophonological treatment is that the latter technique targeted encoding and oral production of single words without semantic context. The treatment steps included auditory discrimination (e.g., *rob-robbed, rakes-raked*), followed by a lexical decision task where one half of the stimuli consisted of illegal morphological endings (e.g., *digged, rakely, robness*). This was followed by a morphology generation task, where participants were asked to generate all possible morphological variants of the verb being trained (free morphemes were included, such as *will rake, is raking, raked, rakes*). The last two steps included oral and written transformations based on a model (e.g., *ask-asked, rake-??*) and repetition of all morphological variants of the treatment verb. Both patients improved in production of the variety of morphological forms in narrative speech, as measured by the proportion of affixed verbs and the variety of verb forms to refer to past, present, and future. However, both remained unchanged in their ability to meaningfully and accurately use these morphological markings in sentence contexts. Thus, the morphophonological treatment produced selective improvements in the overall proportion of verbs produced and in the diversity and frequency with which verbs were affixed, but there were no changes in the accuracy of tense production in narrative speech.

Hierarchical Approaches to Treating Functional Categories

Hierarchical approaches to treatment for functional category deficits in agrammatic aphasia have been advanced to test the tree pruning hypothesis (TPH; Friedmann & Grodzinsky, 1997; Hagiwara, 1995). Briefly, the TPH posits that a breakdown at any level of the syntactic tree will impair not only that level but also all levels above it (see Figure 4.2). Thompson, Milman, et al. (2006) developed an intervention protocol for functional morphology to test the hierarchical breakdown claim of TPH. Twelve individuals with agrammatism were trained on complementizers (sentence (9) below), tense as in (10), and agreement as in (11). The order of treatment of the three forms was counterbalanced across participants. The treatment steps were modeled after TUF, and target forms were trained in simple active sentences (see Table 4.4).

(9) They wonder *if* the man is grabbing the woman. (complementizer)
(10) Yesterday the man grabb*ed* the woman. (tense)
(11) Nowadays the man grab*s* the woman. (agreement)

Treatment outcomes showed that all but one participant improved on production of trained sentences. However, the generalization patterns were not consistent with the predictions of TPH: training of complementizers did not generalize to tense/agreement or vice versa. The data pointed to the lack of a relationship between complementizer phrases and inflectional phrases, supporting syntactic theories that propose a distinction between the two (Chomsky, 1986; Cinque, 1999).

Two other case studies used syntactic hierarchies for intervention of agrammatism and tested the correspondence between sentence structure and functional morphology (Dickey & Thompson, 2007; Friedmann, Wenkert-Olenik, & Gil, 2000). Dickey and Thompson (2007) trained production of wh- movement structures using TUF in a person with agrammatic aphasia and, although his production of trained sentences improved, no changes in verb inflection were noted. In contrast, Friedmann et al. (2000) trained a Hebrew-speaking person with agrammatism to produce wh- questions using TUF and found improved production of verb tense. This latter finding is inconsistent with the general pattern of lack of generalization between sentence structure and functional morphology, and should be interpreted with caution because the study lacked experimental control in its design.

General Considerations for Intervention of Agrammatism

The previous section presented an overview of intervention approaches for verb retrieval, sentence structure, and functional morphology deficits in people with agrammatic aphasia. In this section, the current evidence on training and generalization effects will be used to propose general guidelines for intervention. Training effects refer to improvements in trained items and generalization refers to change in behaviors or stimuli that were not directly addressed in training. Given that generalization of treatment effects from trained to untrained material and conditions is the gold standard of successful treatment, we recommend that clinicians select treatment approaches for any domain after evaluating evidence for generalization effects.

In general, across all the three linguistic domains, intervention was found to be successful for improving the trained domain (verbs, sentence structure, functional morphology). Regardless of whether the goal of treatment is to improve sentence structure, verb production, or functional morphology, the evidence reviewed suggests that training in sentence contexts produced the greatest training effects. Training effects tend to be specific to the trained domain and, for verbs and verb morphology, also item specific. That is, training to name a set of verbs rarely generalized to other untrained verbs, although this needs to be more systematically investigated.

Generalization effects were mixed across approaches, but within-domain generalizations were consistently supported by the complexity account of treatment efficacy (Thompson et al., 2003), both in the domain of sentence structure and functional morphology. Specifically, training of NP- or wh- movement operations generalized to other sentences that were (1) syntactically simpler than the trained sentence, and (2) engaged the same movement operation (NP or wh-). For functional categories, training of the more complex irregular verbs generalized to past tense production of regular verbs. Generalization to grammatically accurate spontaneous speech occurs if the treatment approach includes practice with syntactically accurate sentences. Generalization across linguistic domains, for example from syntax to morphology, or from comprehension to production, appears not to derive from treatment; however, more research examining cross-domain generalization is warranted.

When planning interventions for people with agrammatic aphasia, a thorough evaluation of all three domains of agrammatism is a crucial first step in gleaning the relative severity of symptoms and prioritizing intervention goals. Given the central role of verbs in sentence production, any moderate to severe verb retrieval difficulty needs to be targeted as an early treatment goal. Furthermore, current evidence on limited across-verb generalization suggests that verb retrieval may be a long-term goal where different verb categories are targeted over time. For verb retrieval, both semantic and argument structure based interventions are effective, while there is little benefit from incorporating gesture in the intervention (at least as per the evidence to date). There is some evidence that people with a severe deficit in grammatical morphology fail to produce verbs because they lack the knowledge to inflect the verb (e.g., Druks, 2006). Although this has not been systematically tested yet, it is worth examining if training tense morphology prior to verb retrieval treatment is more efficient than the reverse sequence (as per CATE, Thompson et al., 2003). At present, there is little evidence to suggest whether there is a greater benefit from training sentence structure or verb morphology, one before the other. Irrespective of which domain is targeted, there is strong evidence that reverse complexity effects act in both domains: training complex sentences via movement rules and training irregular verbs using morphosemantic treatment, and both result in stronger generalization effects to untrained structures. Within complex sentence structures, both NP- and wh- movement need to be trained separately, as there is no generalization across these movement operations. In the domain of morphology, different irregular verbs need to be trained separately, as there is limited generalization from trained to untrained irregulars (but regular past consistently improves with training of irregular verbs). Morphosemantic treatment is more effective than morphophonological treatment unless the client shows specific difficulties with lexical morphology such as failure to affix any verb. Finally, while there is evidence that conversational practice per se does not improve grammatical accuracy in production, conversational approaches are an important supplement to intervention to enable generalization to daily speaking activities.

In conclusion, over the past two decades, there have been significant advances in our understanding of and intervention for agrammatism. However, there are also many gaps in our knowledge that need to be addressed, particularly with regard to developing a unified theoretical account of agrammatism, promoting generalization to untrained verbs, and to unconstrained sentence production.

CASE ILLUSTRATION

HM is a 56-year-old retired university professor of social work who continued to give lectures and volunteer in the local community after her retirement. Fourteen months prior to treatment, she sustained a left hemisphere ischemic stroke that spanned the inferior frontal, inferior parietal, and posterior temporal regions. HM received speech therapy during her 2-week hospital stay following the stroke, followed by outpatient rehabilitation once per week for the next 6 months. At the time of the current evaluation, HM's main concerns were finding words, speaking in complete sentences, and being able to ask questions. She noticed little difficulty in understanding conversational speech. She also expressed feeling socially isolated.

HM was strongly motivated to improve her speech so that she could better integrate into the community, particularly for service activities. The following battery of tests were administered as part of HM's evaluation: Western Aphasia Battery-Revised (WAB-R, Kertesz, 2006), Object and Action Naming Battery (OANB; Druks & Masterson, 2000), Verb Inflection Test (Faroqi-Shah & Thompson, 2004), and narrative speech tasks from the Aphasia Bank protocol (www.talkbank.org/aphasiabank). The evaluation revealed a profile of Broca's aphasia, with an Aphasia Quotient of 67.5 (WAB-R), and poorer naming of verbs (12/50) compared to nouns (42/50; OANB). HM scored 4/20 in the Verb inflection test, which uses pictures to elicit sentences in past, present, and future tenses. The low score on the Verb inflection test indicates impairment in using verb morphology to convey tense information. Narrative speech samples were transcribed and analyzed using CLAN (www.talkbank.org) for measures proposed in Saffran and colleagues' (1989) Quantitative Production Analysis (QPA). The perusal of HM's quantitative production analyses results revealed that the following indices fell within the range for people with agrammatic aphasia reported by Saffran and colleagues (1989): proportion of closed class words/narrative words, determiner/noun ratio, proportion of verbs, elaboration of auxiliary, proportion of well-formed sentences, structural elaboration of sentences, median length of utterance, and speech rate. Interestingly, in contrast to HM's low score on the Verb Inflection Test reported earlier, Saffran and colleagues' inflection index (verbs inflected/possible inflections) was higher than values reported for agrammatic aphasia. This was because HM overused the progressive verb ending (verb + ing) with every verb, yielding a high inflection index.

HM enrolled for three 60-minute individual sessions and one group speech therapy session per week. We developed a 4-month intervention plan for HM with the following goals: (1) improve verb retrieval in isolation and discourse during the first 3 months, (2) improve sentence production during months three and four, and (3) practice conversational speech in group situations during all four months. Verb retrieval intervention was the first and primary goal in order to build a core verb vocabulary that could later be used as the basis for sentence structure and tense morphology intervention. To target verb retrieval, the clinician largely followed the Verb Network Strengthening Treatment (VNeST) proposed by Edmonds et al. (2009; see Table 4.3) with a few modifications to personalize the intervention for HM. For example, the verbs to be targeted were based on HM's community involvement, interests, and daily habits and identified by consulting with HM's husband and adult daughter. Out of the 150 verbs identified, the clinician selected about 20 verbs for every 2-week period (this was increased to 30 verbs during the second month). To the extent possible, the 20-verb set consisted of semantically related verbs, to maximize strengthening of specific semantic networks. VNeST was further modified during the second month by using short animated video clips for additional practice with sentence construction.

During the third and fourth months of intervention, the clinician utilized Faroqi-Shah's (2008, 2013) morphosemantic treatment to address contextually accurate use of verb morphology. Given that irregular past verbs promoted generalization to regular past (but not vice versa), a set of 40 imageable irregular verbs were used to practice simple tenses (simple past, present, and future). The clinician continued to incorporate re-telling of animated video clips to promote generalization to discourse. After HM's production of simple tenses improved to nearly perfect accuracy, the clinician introduced verb aspect (progressive and perfect). During the fourth month, the computerized Sentactics program (Thompson et al., 2010) was initiated to train production of syntactically complex sentences.

During the 4-month period, HM also participated in one 60-minute group intervention session every week. There were four other group members, three with an agrammatic speech profile similar to HM, and one with Broca's aphasia with a severe verb impairment but no other agrammatic symptoms. During the first half of each group session, the clinician utilized Semantic Feature Analysis (SFA) modified for group settings (Antonucci, 2009; Falconer & Antonucci, 2012) and discourse (Peach & Reuter, 2010). The clinician used short nonfiction articles (read by participants as homework prior to the session) and commercially available picture sequences (such as Narrative Story Cards; Helm-Estabrooks & Nicholas, 2003) as materials to elicit discourse. The clinician followed the timeline of increasing stimulus difficulty used by Falconer and Antonucci (2012): participants described single-picture scenes during the first 2 weeks, followed by single-picture scenes that were anomalous in some way (e.g., a person with an upside down hat), story telling with picture sequences, fairy tales, re-telling a biography (week 7), and the plot of a favorite movie.

A complete evaluation (WAB-R, OANB, Verb Inflection Test, narratives) was readministered at the conclusion of the 4-month intervention period. HM showed significant gains in all of the production subtests of the WAB-R, aphasia quotient, accuracy of verb naming on OANB, accuracy of tense marking on Verb inflection test, and several indices of Quantitative Production Analysis, showing a less severe agrammatic profile, including higher proportion of grammatical utterances, lower open to closed class ratio (due to increase in number of function words), and higher verb morphology index (due to increased production of inflected verb phrases).

REFERENCES

Abel, S., Schultz, A., Radermacher, I., Willmes, K., & Huber, W. (2005). Decreasing and increasing cues in naming therapy for aphasia. *Aphasiology, 19*, 831–848.

Antonucci, S. M. (2009). Use of semantic feature analysis in group aphasia treatment. *Aphasiology, 23*, 854–866.

Ballard, K. J., & Thompson, C. K. (1999). Treatment and generalization of complex sentence production in agrammatism. *Journal of Speech, Language, & Hearing Research, 42*, 690–707.

Barsalou, L. W. (2008). Grounded cognition. *Annual Review of Psychology, 59*, 617–645. doi:10.1146/annurev.psych.59.103006.093639

Bastiaanse, R. (1995). Broca's aphasia: A syntactic and/or morphological disorder? A case study. *Brain and Language, 48*(1), 1–32.

Bastiaanse, R., & Edwards, S. (2004). Word order and finiteness in Dutch and English Broca's and Wernicke's aphasia. *Brain and Language, 89*, 91–107.

Bastiaanse, R., Edwards, S., & Kiss, K. (1996). Fluent aphasia in three languages: Aspects of spontaneous speech. *Aphasiology, 10*, 561–575.

Bastiaanse, R., Edwards, S., Maas, E., & Rispens, J. (2003). Assessing comprehension and production of verbs and sentences: The verb and sentence test (VAST). *Aphasiology, 17*, 49–73.

Bastiaanse, R., Hurkmans, J., & Links, P. (2006). The training of verb production in Broca's aphasia: A multiple-baseline across-behaviours study. *Aphasiology, 20*, 298–311.

Bastiaanse, R., Rispens, J., Ruigendijk, E., Rabadaán, O. J., & Thompson, C. K. (2002). Verbs: Some properties and their consequences for agrammatic Broca's aphasia. *Journal of Neurolinguistics, 15*, 239–264.

Bastiaanse, R., & Thompson, C. K. (2012). *Perspectives on Agrammatism*. East Sussex, UK: Psychology Press.

Bastiaanse, R., & van Zonneveld, R. (2005). Sentence production with verbs of alternating transitivity in agrammatic Broca's aphasia. *Journal of Neurolinguistics, 18*, 57–66.

Beeke, S., Wilkinson, R., & Maxim, J. (2007). Grammar without sentence structure: A conversation analytic investigation of agrammatism. *Aphasiology, 21*, 256–282.

Beeson, P. M., & Robey, R. (2006). Evaluating single-subject treatment research: Lessons learned from the aphasia literature. *Neuropsychological Review, 16*, 161–169.

Berndt, R. S. (1987). Symptom co-occurence and dissociation in the interpretation of agrammatism. In M. Coltheart, G. Sartori & R. Job (Eds.), *The cognitive neuropsychology of language* (pp. 221–232). Hillsdale, New Jersey: Erlbaum.

Berndt, R. S., Haendiges, A. N., & Wozniak, M. A. (1997). Verb retrieval and sentence processing: Dissociation of an established symptom association. *Cortex, 33,* 99–114.

Berndt, R., & Mitchum, C. (1997). An experimental treatment of sentence comprehension. In N. Helm-Estabrooks & A. Holland (Eds.), *Approaches to the treatment of aphasia* (pp. 91–111). San Diego, CA: Singular Publishing Group.

Berndt, R. S., Mitchum, C. C., & Haendiges, A. N. (1996). Comprehension of reversible sentences in "agrammatism": A meta-analysis. *Cognition, 58,* 289–308.

Berndt, R. S., Mitchum, C. C., Haendiges, A. N., & Sandson, J. (1997). Verb retrieval in aphasia-1. Characterizing single word impairments. *Brain and Language, 56,* 68–106.

Berndt, R. S., Mitchum, C. C., & Wayland, S. (1997). Patterns of sentence comprehension in aphasia: A consideration of three hypotheses. *Brain and Language, 60,* 197–221.

Beveridge, M. A., & Crerar, M. A. (2002). Remediation of asyntactic sentence comprehension using a multimedia microworld. *Brain and Language, 82,* 243–295.

Bird, H., Lambon Ralph, M. A., Seidenberg, M. S., McClelland, J. L., & Patterson, K. (2003). Deficits in phonology and past-tense morphology: What's the connection? *Journal of Memory and Language, 48,* 502–526.

Bobaljik, J., & Thrainsson, H. (1998). Two heads aren't always better than one. *Syntax, 1,* 37–71.

Bock, K., & Levelt, W. (1994). Language production: Grammatical encoding. *Handbook of psycholinguistics.* G. M. A. San Diego, Academic Press.

Boo, M., & Rose, M. L. (2011). The efficacy of repetition, semantic and gesture treatments for verb retrieval and use in Broca's aphasia. *Aphasiology, 25,* 154–175.

Boser, K. I., & Weinrich, M. (1998). Functional categories in agrammatic production: Evidence for access to tense projections. *Brain and Language, 65,* 207–210.

Boser, K. I., Weinrich, M., & McCall, D. (2000). Maintenance of oral production in agrammatic aphasia: Verb tense morphology training. *Neurorehabilitation and Neural Repair, 14,* 105–118.

Boyle, M., & Coelho, C. A. (1995). Application of semantic feature analysis as a treatment for aphasic dysnomia. *American Journal of Speech-Language Pathology, 4,* 94–98.

Braber, N., Patterson, K., Ellis, K., & Lambon Ralph, M. A. (2005). The relationship between phonological and morphological deficits in Broca's aphasia: Further evidence from errors in verb inflection. *Brain and Language, 92,* 278–287.

Breedin, S. D., Saffran, E. M., & Schwartz, M. F. (1998). Semantic factors in verb retrieval: An effect of complexity. *Brain and Language, 63,* 1–31.

Breier, J. I., Maher, L. M., Novak, B., & Papanicolaou, A. C. (2006). Functional imaging before and after Constraint-Induced Language Therapy for aphasia using magnetoencephalography. *Neurocase, 12,* 322–331.

Burchert, F., De Bleser, R., & Sonntag, K. (2003). Does morphology make the difference? Agrammatic sentence comprehension in German. *Brain and Language, 87,* 323–342.

Burchert, F., Swoboda-Moll, M., & De Bleser, R. (2005). Tense and agreement dissociations in German agrammatic speakers: Underspecification vs. hierarchy. *Brain and Language, 94,* 188–199.

Bybee, J. (1995). Diachronic and typological properties of morphology and their implications for representation. In L. B. Feldman (Ed.), *Morphological aspects of language processing* (pp. 225–246). Hillsdale, New Jersey: Lawrence Erlbaum Associates.

Byng, S. (1988). Sentence processing deficits: Theory and therapy. *Cognitive Neuropsychology, 5,* 629–676.

Byng, S., Nickels, L., & Black, M. (1994). Replicating therapy for mapping deficits in agrammatism: Remapping the deficit? *Aphasiology, 8,* 315–341.

Caplan, D. (1995). Issues arising in contemporary studies of disorders of syntactic processing in sentence comprehension in agrammatic patients. *Brain and Language, 50,* 325–338.

Caplan, D., & Hildebrandt, N. (1988). Specific deficits in syntactic comprehension. *Aphasiology, 2,* 255–258.

Caplan, D., Waters, G., DeDe, G., Michaud, J., & Reddy, A. (2007). A study of syntactic processing in aphasia I: Behavioral (psycholinguistic) aspects. *Brain and Language, 101*(2), 103–150.

Caplan, D., Waters, G., Kennedy, D., Alpert, N., Makris, N., DeDe, G., et al. (2007). A study of syntactic processing in aphasia II: Neurological aspects. *Brain and Language, 101*(2), 151–177.

Cherney, L. R., Halper, A. S., Holland, A. L., & Cole, R. (2008). Computerized script training for aphasia: Preliminary results. *American Journal of Speech-Language Pathology, 17,* 19–34.

Chomsky, N. (1981). *Lectures on government and binding.* Foris: Dordrecht.

Chomsky, N. (1986). *Barriers.* Cambridge, MA: MIT Press.

Chomsky, N. (1995). Categories and transformations. In N. Chomsky (Ed.), *The minimalist program* (pp. 219–394). Cambridge, MA: MIT Press.

Chomsky, N. (2000). Minimalist inquiries: The framework. In R. Martin, D. Michealis, & J. Uriagereka (Eds.), *Step by step* (pp. 89–155). Cambridge, MA: MIT Press.

Cinque, G. (1999). *Adverbs and functional heads.* New York: Oxford University Press.

Clahsen, H. (1999). Lexical entries and rules of language: A multidisciplinary study of German inflection. *Behavioral and Brain Sciences, 22,* 991–1060.

Conroy, P., Sage, K., & Lambon Ralph, M. A. (2009a). Errorless and errorful therapy for verb and noun naming in aphasia. *Aphasiology, 23,* 1311–1337.

Conroy, P., Sage, K., & Lambon Ralph, M. A. (2009b). A comparison of word versus sentence cues as therapy for verb naming in aphasia. *Aphasiology, 23,* 462–482.

Conroy, P., Sage, K., & Lambon Ralph, M. A. (2009c). The effects of decreasing and increasing cue therapy on improving naming speed and accuracy for verbs and nouns in aphasia. *Aphasiology, 23,* 707–730.

Crerar, M. A., Ellis, A. W., & Dean, E. C. (1996). Remediation of sentence processing deficits in aphasia using a computer-based microworld. *Brain and Language, 52,* 229–275.

Cunningham, R., & Ward, C. D. (2003). Evaluation of a training programme to facilitate conversation between people with aphasia and their partners. *Aphasiology, 17,* 687–710.

De Bleser, R., & Kauschke, C. (2003). Acquisition and loss of nouns and verbs: Parallel or divergent patterns? *Journal of Neurolinguistics, 16*(2–3), 213–229.

de Ruiter, J. P. (2006). Can gesticulation help aphasic people speak, or rather, communicate? Commentary on Rose, M. L. (2006). The utility of arm and hand gestures in the treatment of aphasia. *Advances in Speech-Language Pathology, 8,* 124–127.

Dickey, M. W., Milman, L. H., & Thompson, C. K. (2008). Judgement of functional morphology in agrammatic aphasia. *Journal of Neurolinguistics, 21,* 35–65.

Dickey, M. W., & Thompson, C. K. (2007). The relation between syntactic and morphological recovery in agrammatic aphasia: A case study. *Aphasiology, 21,* 604–616.

Doyle, P. J., Goldstein, H., & Bourgeois, M. S. (1987). Experimental analysis of syntax training in Broca's aphasia: A generalization and social validation study. *Journal of Speech and Hearing Disorders, 52,* 143–155.

Dragoy, O., & Bastiaanse, R. (2010). Verb production and word order in Russian agrammatic speakers. *Aphasiology, 24,* 28–55.

Drew, R. L., & Thompson, C. K. (1999). Model-based semantic treatment for naming deficits in aphasia. *Journal of Speech, Language, and Hearing Research, 42,* 972–989.

Dronkers, N. F., Wilkins, D. P., Van Valin, R. D., Redfern, B. B., & Jaeger, J. J. (2004). Lesion analysis of the brain areas involved in language comprehension. *Cognition, 92*, 145–177.

Druks, J. (2006). Morpho-syntactic and morpho-phonological deficits in the production of regularly and irregularly inflected verbs. *Aphasiology, 20*, 993–1017.

Druks, J., & Masterson, J. (2000). *An object and action naming battery*. Philadephia, PA: Taylor & Francis.

Eberhard, K. M., Cutting, J. C., & Bock, K. (2005). Making syntax of sense: Number agreement in sentence production. *Psychological Review, 112*(3), 531–559.

Edmonds, L. A., & Kiran, S. (2006, May). *The effects of verb network strengthening treatment (VNeST) on sentence production in individuals with aphasia*. Paper presented at the Clinical Aphasiology Conference, Ghent, Belgium.

Edmonds, L. A., & Mizrahi, S. (2011). Online priming of agent and patient thematic roles and related verbs in younger and older adults. *Aphasiology, 25*(12), 1488–1506. doi:10.1080/0268703 8.2011.599527

Edmonds, L. A., Nadeau, S. E., & Kiran, S. (2009). Effect of Verb Network Strengthening Treatment (VNeST) on lexical retrieval of content words in sentences in persons with aphasia. *Aphasiology, 23*, 402–424.

Falconer, C., & Antonucci, S. M. (2012). Use of semantic feature analysis in group discourse treatment for aphasia: Extension and expansion. *Aphasiology, 26*(1), 64–82. doi:10.1080/02687038.20 11.602390

Faroqi, Y., & Chengappa, S. (1997). Trace deletion and its implication for intervention in a multilingual agrammatic aphasic patient. *Osmania Papers in Linguistics, 22–23*, 79–106.

Faroqi-Shah, Y. (2007). Are regular and irregular verbs dissociated in non-fluent aphasia?: A meta-analysis. *Brain Research Bulletin, 74*, 1–13.

Faroqi-Shah, Y. (2008). A comparison of two theoretically driven treatments for verb inflection deficits in aphasia. *Neuropsychologia, 46*, 3088–3100.

Faroqi-Shah, Y. (2013). Selective treatment of regular versus irregular verbs in agrammatic aphasia: Efficacy data. *Aphasiology, 27*(6), 678–705.

Faroqi-Shah, Y., & Dickey, M. W. (2009). On-line processing of tense and temporality in agrammatic aphasia. *Brain and Language, 108*, 97–111.

Faroqi-Shah, Y., & Graham, L. E. (2010). Treatment of semantic verb classes in aphasia: acquisition and generalization effects. *Clinical Linguistics & Phonetics, 25*, 399–418.

Faroqi-Shah, Y., Kling, T., Solomon, J., Liu, S., Park, G., & Braun, A. (2014). Lesion analysis of language production deficits in aphasia. *Aphasiology, 28*, 258–277.

Faroqi-Shah, Y., & Thompson, C.K. (2004). Semantic, lexical, and phonological influences on the production of verb inflections in agrammatic aphasia. *Brain and Language, 89*, 484–498.

Faroqi-Shah, Y., & Thompson, C.K. (2007). Verb inflections in agrammatic aphasia: Encoding of tense features. *Journal of Memory and Language, 56*, 129–151.

Faroqi-Shah, Y., & Virion, C. (2009). Constraint-induced language therapy for agrammatism: Role of grammaticality constraints. *Aphasiology, 23*, 977–988.

Fillingham, J. K., Sage, K., & Lambon Ralph, M. A. (2005a). The treatment of anomia using errorless vs. errorful learning: Are frontal executive skills and feedback important? *International Journal of Language and Communication Disorders, 40*, 505–524.

Fillingham, J. K., Sage, K., & Lambon Ralph, M. A. (2005b). Further explorations and an overview of errorless and errorful therapy for anomia: The number of naming attempts during therapy effects outcome. *Aphasiology, 19*, 597–614.

Fillingham, J. K., Sage, K., & Lambon Ralph, M. A. (2006). The treatment of anomia using errorless learning. *Neuropsychological Rehabilitation, 16*, 129–154.

Friedmann, N., & Grodzinksy, Y. (1997). Tense and agreement in agrammatic production: Pruning the syntactic tree. *Brain and Language, 56*, 397–425.

Friedmann, N., Wenkert-Olenik, D., & Gil, M. (2000). From theory to practice: Treatment of aggrammatic production in Hebrew based on the tree pruning hypothesis. *Journal of Neurolinguistics, 13*, 250–254.

Garrett, M. F. (1975). The analysis of sentence production. In G.H. Bower (Ed.), *The psychology of learning and motivation* (vol. *9*; pp. 133–177). New York: Academic Press.

Garrett, M. F. (1988). Processes in language production. In N. Frederick (Ed.), *Linguistics: the Cambridge survey*. Cambridge: Cambridge University Press.

Goodglass, H., & Berko, J. (1960). Agrammatism and inflectional morphology in English. *Journal of Speech-Language and Hearing Research, 3*, 257–267.

Goodglass, H., Christiansen, J. A., & Gallagher, R. (1993). Comparison of morphology and syntax in free narrative and structured tests: Fluent vs. nonfluent aphasics. *Cortex, 29*, 377–407.

Goodglass, H., Kaplan, E., & Barresi, B. (2001). *Boston Diagnostic Aphasia Examination* (3rd ed.). Philadelphia: Lippincott Williams and Wilkins.

Griffiths, J. D., Marslen-Wilson, W. D., Stamatakis, E. A., & Tyler, L. K. (2013). Functional organization of the neural language system: Dorsal and ventral pathways are critical for syntax. *Cerebral Cortex, 23*, 139–147.

Grodzinsky, Y. (1986). Cognitive deficits, their proper description, and its theoretical relevance. *Brain and Language, 27*, 178–191.

Grodzinsky, Y. (2000). The neurology of syntax: Language use without Broca's area. *Behavioral and Brain Sciences, 23*, 1–71.

Hagiwara, H. (1995). The breakdown of functional categories and the economy of derivation. *Brain and Language, 50*, 92–116.

Halle, M., & Marantz, A. (1993). Distributed morphology and the pieces of inflection. In K. Halle & S. J. Keyser (Eds.), *The view from building 29: Essays in linguistics in honor of Sylvian Bromberger* (pp. 111–175). Cambridge, MA: MIT Press.

Harris, L., Olson, A., & Humphreys, G. (2012). Rehabilitation of past tense verb production and non-canonical sentence production in left inferior frontal non-fluent aphasia. *Aphasiology, 26*, 143–161.

Helm-Estabrooks, N. (1981). *Helm Elicited Language Program for Syntax Stimulation*. Austin, TX: Exceptional Resources Inc.

Helm-Estabrooks, N., & Nicholas, M. (2000). *Sentence Production Program for Aphasia*. Austin: TX: Pro-Ed Inc.

Helm-Estabrooks, N., & Nicholas, M. (2003). *Narrative Story Cards* (6th ed.). Austin, TX: Pro-Ed, Inc.

Helm-Estabrooks, N., & Ramsberger, G. (1986). Treatment of agrammatism in long-term Broca's aphasia. *British Journal of Disorders of Communication, 21*(1), 39–45.

Holland, A., Milman, L., Muñoz, M., & Bays, G. (2002, July). *Scripts in the management of aphasia*. Paper presented at the World Federation of Neurology, Aphasia and Cognitive Disorders Section Meeting, Villefranche, France.

Hopper, T., Holland, A., & Rewega, M. (2002). Conversational coaching: Treatment outcomes and future directions. *Aphasiology, 16*, 745–761.

Jacobs, B. J., & Thompson, C. K. (2000). Cross-modal generalization effects of training noncanonical sentence comprehension and production in agrammatic aphasia. *Journal of Speech, Language & Hearing Research, 43*, 5–20.

Janssen, D. P., Roelofs, A., & Levelt, W. J. M. (2002). Inflectional frames in language production. *Language and Cognitive Processes, 17,* 209–236.

Jonkers, R., & Bastiaanse, R. (1996). The influence of instrumentality and transitivity on action naming in Broca'a and anomic aphasia. *Brain and Language, 55,* 37–39.

Kagan, A., Black, S. E., Duchan, J. F., Simmons-Mackie, N., & Square, P. (2001). Training volunteers as conversation partners using "Supported Conversation for Adults with Aphasia" (SCA): A controlled trial. *Journal of Speech Language and Hearing Research, 44,* 624–638.

Kean, M.-L. (1977). The linguistic interpretation of aphasic syndromes: Agrammatism in Broca's aphasia, an example. *Cognition, 5,* 9–46.

Kegl, J. (1995). Levels of representation and units of access relevant to agrammatism. *Brain and Language, 50,* 151–200.

Kemmerer, D., Rudrauf, D., Manzel, K., & Tranel, D. (2012). Behavioral patterns and lesion sites associated with impaired processing of lexical and conceptual knowledge of actions. *Cortex, 48*(7), 826–848.

Kemmerer, D., & Tranel, D. (2000). Verb retrieval in brain-damaged subjects: 1. Analysis of stimulus, lexical, and conceptual factors. *Brain and Language, 73,* 347–392.

Kempler, D., & Goral, M. (2011). A comparison of drill- and communication-based treatment for aphasia. *Aphasiology, 25,* 1327–1346.

Kertesz, A. (2006). *Western Aphasia Battery-Revised.* New York: Grune Stratton.

Kim, M., & Thompson, C. K. (2000). Patterns of comprehension and production of nouns and verbs in agrammatism: Implications for lexical organization. *Brain and Language, 74*(1), 1–25.

Kim, M., & Thompson, C. K. (2004). Verb deficits in Alzheimer's disease and agrammatism: Implications for lexical organization. *Brain and Language, 88,* 1–20.

Kim, M., Adingono, M. F., & Revoir, J. S. (2007). Argument structure enhanced verb naming treatment: Two case studies. *Contemporary Issues in Communication Science and Disorders, 34,* 24–36.

Kohn, S., & Melvold, J. (2000). Effects of morphological complexity on phonological output deficits in fluent and nonfluent aphasia. *Brain and Language, 73,* 323–346.

Kok, P., van Doorn, A., & Kolk, H. (2007). Inflection and computational load in agrammatic speech. *Brain and Language, 102*(3), 273–283.

Kolk, H. (1995). A time-based approach to agrammatic production. *Brain and Language, 50,* 282–303.

Kolk, H., & Friederici, A. (1985). Strategy and impairment in sentence understanding by Broca's and Wernicke's aphasics. *Cortex, 21,* 47–67.

Kolk, H., & vanGrunsven, M. (1985). Agrammatism as a variable phenomenon. *Cognitive Neuropsychology, 2*(4), 347–384.

Lambon Ralph, M. A., Braber, N., McClelland, J., & Patterson, K. (2005). What underlies the neuropsychological pattern of irregular > regular past tense production. *Brain and Language, 93,* 106–119.

LaPointe, S. G., & Dell, G. S. (1989). A synthesis of some recent work in sentence production. In G. N. Carlson & M. K. Tanenhaus (Eds.), *Linguistic Structure in Language Processing* (pp. 107–156). Dordrecht: Kluwer Academic Publishers.

Law, S.-P., & Cheng, M.-Y. (2002). Production of grammatical morphemes in Cantonese aphasia. *Aphasiology, 16,* 693–714.

Le Dorze, G., Jacob, A., & Coderre, L. (1991). Aphasia rehabilitation with a case of agrammatism: A partial replication. *Aphasiology, 5,* 63–85.

Lee, J., Milman, L., & Thompson, C. K. (2008). Functional category production in English agrammatism. *Aphasiology, 22*(7–8), 893–905.

Lee, M., & Thompson, C. K. (2004). Agrammatic aphasic production and comprehension of unaccusative verbs in sentence contexts. *Journal of Neurolinguistics, 17*, 315–330.

Levelt, W. J. M. (1989). *Speaking: From intention to articulation*. Cambridge, MA: MIT Press.

Levelt, W. J. M. (1999). Producing spoken language: A blueprint of the speaker. In C. M. Brown & P. Hagoort (Eds.), *The neurocognition of language*. New York: Oxford University Press.

Levin, B. (1993). *English verb classes and alternations: A preliminary investigation*. Chicago, IL, University of Chicago Press.

Linebarger, M. C., Romania, J. R., Fink, R. B., Bartlett, M., & Schwartz, M. F. (2008). Building on residual speech: A portable processing prosthesis for aphasia. *Journal of Rehabilitation Research and Development, 45*(9), 1401–1414.

Linebarger, M. C., Schwartz, M. F., & Kohn, S. E. (2001). Computer-based training of language production: An exploratory study. *Neuropsychological Rehabilitation, 11*(1), 57–96.

Linebarger, M. C., Schwartz, M. F., Romania, J. R., Kohn, S., & Stephens, D. (2000). Grammatical encoding in aphasia: Evidence from a "processing prosthesis". *Brain and Language, 75*, 416–427.

Linebarger, M. C., Schwartz, M. F., & Saffran, E. M. (1983). Sensitivity to grammatical structure in so-called agrammatic aphasics. *Cognition, 13*, 361–392.

Linebaugh, C. W., Baron, C. R., & Corcoran, K. J. (1998). Assessing treatment efficacy in acute aphasia: Paradoxes, presumptions, problems, and principles. *Aphasiology, 12*, 519–536.

Loverso, F. L., Prescott, T. E., & Selinger, M. (1988). Cueing verbs: A treatment strategy for aphasic adults. *Journal of Rehabilitation Research and Development, 25*, 47–60.

Loverso, F. L., Prescott, T. E., & Selinger, M. (1992). Microcomputer treatment applications in aphasiology. *Aphasiology, 6*, 155–163.

Maher, L., Kendall, D. L., Swearengin, J., Rodriguez, A. D., Leon, S., Pingel, K., ... Gonzalez Rothi, L. J. (2006). A pilot study of use-dependent learning in the context of constraint-induced language therapy. *Journal of the International Neuropsychological Society, 12*, 843–852.

Mahon, B. Z., & Caramazza, A. (2008). A critical look at the embodied cognition hypothesis and a new proposal for grounding conceptual content. *Journal of Physiology - Paris, 102*, 59–70.

Marangolo P., Bonifazi S., Tomaiuolo F., Craighero L., Coccia M., Altoe, G., et al. (2010). Improving language without words: First evidence from aphasia. *Neuropsychologia, 48*, 3824–3833.

Matzig, S., Druks, J., Masterson, J., & Vigliocco, G. (2009). Noun and verb differences in picture naming: Past studies and new evidence. *Cortex, 45*, 738–758.

McCann, C., & Doleman, J. (2011). Verb retrieval in nonfluent aphasia: A replication of Edwards & Tucker, 2006. *Journal of Neurolinguistics, 24*, 237–248.

McRae, K., Hare, M., Elman, J. L., & Ferretti, T. R. (2005). A basis for generating expectancies for verbs from nouns. *Memory and Cognition, 33*, 1174–1184.

Meinzer, M., Djundja, D., Barthel, G., Elbert, T., & Rockstroh, B. (2005). Long-term stability of improved language functions in chronic aphasia after constraint-induced aphasia therapy. *Stroke, 36*(7 [electronic]), 1462–1466.

Menn, L., Obler, L. K., & Goodglass, H. (1990). *A cross-language study of agrammatism*. Philadelphia: John Benjamins.

Meth, M., Obler, L. K., Harris, K., & Schwartz, R. (1995, October). *A preliminary investigation of the role of verb stem features on agrammatic aphasics' affix production*. Paper presented at the Academy of Aphasia, San Diego, CA.

Miceli, G., Silveri, M. C., Villa, G., & Caramazza, A. (1984). On the basis for the agrammatic's difficulty in producing main verbs. *Cortex, 20*, 207–220.

Mitchum, C., & Berndt, R. (1994). Verb retrieval and sentence construction: Effects of targeted intervention. In M. J. Riddoch & G. Humphreys (Eds.), *Cognitive neuropsychology and cognitive rehabilitation*. Hove, England: Erlbaum.

Mitchum, C. C., Heandiges, A. N., & Berndt, R. S. (1993). Model guided treatment to improve written sentence production. *Aphasiology, 7,* 71–109.

Morsella, E., & Krauss, R. M. (2004). The role of gestures in spatial working memory and speech. *American Journal of Psychology, 117,* 411–424.

Nicholas, M., & Brookshire, R. (1993). A system for quantifying the informativeness and efficiency of the connected speech of adults with aphasia. *Journal of Speech Language and Hearing Research, 36,* 338–350.

Nickels, L. (2002). Therapy for naming disorders: Revisiting, revising and reviewing. *Aphasiology, 16,* 935–979.

Ouhalla, J. (1993). Subject-extraction, negation and the antiagreement effect. *Natural Language & Linguistic Theory, 11*(3), 477–518.

Peach, R. K., & Reuter, K. A. (2010). A discourse-based approach to semantic feature analysis treatment for the treatment of aphasic word retrieval failures. *Aphasiology, 24,* 971–990.

Penke, M. (2003). On the morphological basis of syntactic deficits. *Brain and Language, 87,* 50–51.

Pinker, S., & Prince, A. (1991). Regular and irregular morphology and the psychological status of rules of grammar. *Berkeley Linguistics Society, 17,* 230–251.

Pizzioli, F., & Schelstraete, M.-A. (2008). The argument-structure complexity effect in children with specific language impairment: Evidence from the use of grammatical morphemes in French. *Journal of Speech, Language, and Hearing Research, 51,* 706–721.

Pulvermuller, F., & Berthier, M. L. (2008). Aphasia therapy on a neuroscience basis. *Aphasiology, 22,* 563–599.

Pulvermuller, F., Neininger, B., Elbert, T., Mohr, B., Rockstroh, B., Koebbel, P., & Taub, E. (2001). Constraint-induced therapy of chronic aphasia after stroke. *Stroke, 32,* 1621–1626.

Raymer, A. M., Ciampitti, M., Holliway, B., Singletary, F., Blonder, L. X., Ketterson, T., ... Rothi, L. J. (2007). Semantic-phonologic treatment for noun and verb retrieval impairments in aphasia. *Neuropsychological Rehabilitation, 17,* 244–270.

Raymer, A. M., Singletary, F., Rodriguez, A., Ciampitti, M., Heilman, K. M., & Gonzalez Rothi, L. J. (2006). Effects of gesture+verbal treatment for noun and verb retrieval in aphasia. *Journal of the International Neuropsychological Society, 12*(6), 867–882.

Rochon, E., Laird, L., Bose, A., & Scofield, J. (2005). Mapping therapy for sentence production impairments in nonfluent aphasia. *Neuropsychological Rehabilitation, 15,* 1–36.

Rochon, E., Saffran, E. M., Berndt, R. S., & Schwartz, M. F. (2000). Quantitative analysis on aphasic sentence production: Further development and new data. *Brain and Language, 72,* 193–218.

Rodriguez, A., Raymer, A. M., & Gonzalez Rothi, L. J. (2006). Effects of gesture+verbal and semantic-phonologic treatments for verb retrieval in aphasia. *Aphasiology, 20,* 286–297.

Rose, M. (2006). The utility of gesture treatments in aphasia. *International Journal of Speech-Language Pathology, 8*(2), 92–109.

Rose, M., & Sussmilch, G. (2008). The effects of semantic and gesture treatments on verb retrieval and verb use in aphasia. *Aphasiology, 22,* 691–706.

Rumelhart, D., & McClelland, J. (1986). On learning the past tenses of English verbs: Implicit rules or parallel distributed processing. In D. Rumelhart & J. McClelland (Eds.), *Parallel distribute processing: Explorations in the microstructure of cognition* (pp. 216–271). Cambridge, MA: MIT Press.

Saffran, E. M., Berndt, R. S., & Schwartz, M. F. (1989). The quantitative analysis of agrammatic production: Procedure and data. *Brain and Language, 37,* 440–479.

Saffran, E. M., Schwartz, M. F., & Linebarger, M. C. (1998). Semantic influences on thematic role assignment: Evidence from normals and aphasics. *Brain and Language, 62*(2), 255–297.

Saffran, E. M., Schwartz, M. F., & Marin, O. S. M. (1980). The word order problem in agrammatism: II. Production. *Brain and Language, 10,* 263–282.

Sahraoui, H., & Nespoulous, J.-L. (2012). Across-task variability in agrammatic performance. *Aphasiology, 26,* 785–810.

Schneider, S. L., & Thompson, C. K. (2003). Verb production in agrammatic aphasia: The influence of semantic class and argument structure properties on generalization. *Aphasiology, 17,* 213–241.

Schwartz, M. F., Saffran, E. M., Fink, R. B., & Myers, J. L. (1994). Mapping therapy: A treatment programme for agrammatism. *Aphasiology, 8,* 19–54.

Stadie, N., Schroder, A., Postler, J., Lorenz, A., Swoboda-Moll, M., Burchert, F., & De Bleser, R. (2008). Unambiguous generalization effects after treatment of non-canonical sentence production in German agrammatism. *Brain and Language, 104,* 211–229.

Szaflarski, J. P., Ball, A. L., Grether, S., Al-fwaress, F., Griffith, N., Nells-Strunjas, J., ... Relchhardt, R. (2008). Constraint-induced aphasia therapy stimulates language recovery in patients with chronic aphasia after ischemic stroke. *Medical Science Monitor, 14,* 243–250.

Thompson, C. K. (2003). Unaccusative verb production in agrammatic aphasia: A syntactic account of verb production deficits. *Journal of Neurolinguistics, 16,* 151–167.

Thompson, C. K. (2008). Treatment of syntactic and morphological deficits in agrammatic aphasia: Treatment of underlying forms. In R. Chapey (Ed.), *Language intervention strategies in aphasia and related neurogenic communication disorders* (5th ed.; pp. 735–753). Baltimore: Williams & Wilkins.

Thompson, C. K., Ballard, K. J., & Shapiro, L. P. (1998). The role of syntactic complexity in training wh-movement structures in agrammatic aphasia: Optimal order for promoting generalization. *Journal of the International Neuropsychological Society, 4,* 661–674.

Thompson, C. K., Choy, J. J., Holland, A., & Cole, R. (2010). Sentactics®: Computer-automated treatment of underlying forms. *Aphasiology, 24,* 1242–1266.

Thompson, C. K., Kearns, K. P., & Edmonds, L. A. (2006). An experimental analysis of acquisition, generalisation, and maintenance of naming behaviour in a patient with anomia. *Aphasiology, 20,* 1226–1244.

Thompson, C. K., Lange, K. L., Schneider, S. L., & Shapiro, L. P. (1997). Agrammatic and non-brain-damaged subjects' verb and verb argument structure production. *Aphasiology, 11,* 473–490.

Thompson, C. K., & Lee, M. (2009). Psych verb production and comprehension in agrammatic Broca's aphasia. *Journal of Neurolinguistics, 22,* 354–369.

Thompson, C. K., Milman, L. H., Dickey, M. W., O'Connor, J. E., Bonakdarpour, B., Fix, S. C., ... Arcuri, D. F. (2006). Functional category production in agrammatism: Treatment and generalization effects. *Brain and Language, 99,* 79–81.

Thompson, C. K., Riley, E., den Ouden, D. B., Meltzer-Asscher, A., & Lukic, S. (2013). Training verb argument structure production in agrammatic aphasia: behavioral and neural recovery patterns. *Cortex, 49*(9), 2358–2376.

Thompson, C. K., Shapiro, L. P., Ballard, K. J., Jacobs, B. J., & Tait, M. E. (1997). Training and generalized production of wh- and NP-movement structures in agrammatic aphasia. *Journal of Speech, Language and Hearing Research, 40,* 228–244.

Thompson, C. K., Shapiro, L. P., Kiran, S., & Sobecks, J. (2003). The role of syntactic complexity in treatment of sentence deficits in agrammatic aphasia: The complexity account of treatment efficacy (CATE). *Journal of Speech, Language & Hearing Research, 46*, 591–607.

Thompson, C. K., Shapiro, L. P., & Roberts, M. M. (1993). Treatment of sentence production deficits in aphasia: A linguistic-specific approach to wh-interrogative training and generalization. *Aphasiology, 7*, 111–133.

Thompson, C. K., Shapiro, L. P., Tait, M., Jacobs, B. J., & Schneider, S. L. (1996). Training wh-question production in agrammatic aphasia: Analysis of argument and adjunct movement. *Brain and Language, 52*, 175–228.

Ullman, M. T., Corkin, S., Coppola, M., & Hickok, G. (1997). A neural dissociation within language: Evidence that the mental dictionary is part of declarative memory, and that grammatical rules are processed by the procedural system. *Journal of Cognitive Neuroscience, 9*, 266–276.

Wambaugh, J. L. (2003). A comparison of the relative effects of phonologic and semantic cueing treatments. *Aphasiology, 17*, 433–441.

Wambaugh, J. L., Cameron, R., Kalinyak-Fliszar, M., Nessler, C., & Wright, S. (2004). Retrieval of action names in aphasia: Effects of two cueing treatments in aphasia. *Aphasiology, 18*, 979–1004.

Wambaugh, J. L., Doyle, P. J., Martinez, A. L., & Kalinyak-Fliszar, M. (2002). Effects of two lexical retrieval cueing treatments on action naming in aphasia. *Journal of Rehabilitation Research and Development, 39*, 455–466.

Wambaugh, J. L., & Ferguson, M. (2007). Application of semantic feature analysis to retrieval of action names in aphasia. *Journal of Rehabilitation Research & Development, 44*(3), 381–394.

Wambaugh, J. L., Mauszycki, S., & Wright, S. (2014). Semantic feature analysis: Application to confrontation naming of actions in aphasia. *Aphasiology, 28*, 1–24.

Webster, J., Morris, J., & Franklin, S. (2005). Effects of therapy targeted at verb retrieval and the realization of the predicate argument structure: A case study. *Aphasiology, 19*, 748–764.

Weinrich, M., Boser, K. I., & McCall, D. (1999). Representation of linguistic rules in the brain: Evidence from training an aphasic patient to produce past tense verb morphology. *Brain and Language, 70*, 144–158.

Weinrich, M., Shelton, J. R., Cox, D. M., & McCall, D. (1997). Remediating production of tense morphology improves verb retrieval in chronic aphasia. *Brain and Language, 58*, 23–45.

Wenzlaff, M., & Clahsen, H. (2004). Tense and agreement in German agrammatism. *Brain and Language, 89*, 57–68.

Wieczorek, R. (2011). Tense/aspect category in fluent and nonfluent German aphasia: An experimental training programme for verb production. *Aphasiology, 25*, 851–871.

Wilkinson, R., & Wielaert, S. (2012). Rehabilitation targeted at everyday communication: Can we change the talk of people with aphasia and their significant others within conversation? *Archives of Physical Medicine and Rehabilitation, 93*(1 Suppl.), S70–S76.

Wilson, S. M., & Saygin, A. P. (2004). Grammaticality judgment in aphasia: Deficits are not specific to syntactic structures, aphasic syndromes or lesion sites. *Journal of Cognitive Neuroscience, 16*, 238–252.

Yiu, E. M. L., & Worrall, L. E. (1996). Agrammatic production: A cross-linguistic comparison of English and Cantonese. *Aphasiology, 10*, 623–647.

Zingeser, L. B., & Berndt, R. S. (1990). Retrieval of nouns and verbs in agrammatism and anomia. *Brain and Language, 39*, 14–32.

CHAPTER 5

Echophenomena in Aphasia: Causal Mechanisms and Clues for Intervention

Marcelo L. Berthier
Guadalupe Dávila
María José Torres-Prioris

INTRODUCTION

The word "echo" has different meanings depending upon the context. Its simplest definition is "a sound that is repeating after the original sound ended" (Echo, n.d.), yet the meaning that seems most popular makes reference to the repetition of a sound, typically heard in big, empty spaces (mountains, caves). In living creatures, such as bats, the term "echo" (or echolocator) refers to self-generated sounds that permit the animals to orient through labyrinthic environments in complete darkness (Wenstrup & Portfors, 2011). The noun "echolocator" is also used to designate individuals who are blind, who make clicking noises with their mouths, and use the reflected echoes to estimate the size and distance of perceived objects and surfaces (Milne, Anello, Gooddale, & Thaler, 2015). Also in humans, the definition of echo is "one who closely imitates or repeats another's words, ideas, or acts" (*Merriam-Webster's Dictionary of English Usage*, 1994). Moreover, imitation of different verbal and motor behaviors is a crucial component of "cultural learning" (Heyes, 2012).

In this chapter we review the production of echoes in the abnormal conditions of echophenomena (EP), paying more attention to those types that are integral constituents of aphasia syndromes (e.g., echolalia). We analyze the functional and neural mechanisms responsible for EP and the theoretical rationale for implementing interventions to reduce echolalia. Furthermore, we examine the use of repetition training as a strategy for improving speech production and related language and memory deficits. Also, we outline some implications for clinical practice and future research. Finally, we briefly describe a case study that exemplifies how theory-based interventions may improve echolalia.

ECHOPHENOMENA

The term EP, also known as *imitation behavior* (De Renzi, Cavalleri, & Facchini, 1996) or *resonance behavior* (Rizzolatti, Fadiga, Fogassi, & Gallese, 1999), refers to an act of social dependence (person-based activation) characterized by a strong tendency to imitate the gestures and utterances that the examiner makes in front of the patient even when no specific instruction has been given to do so (Ford, 1989; Stengel, 1947). EP includes a wide array of syndromes such as echolalia (imitation of heard words), echographia (involuntary copy of written material), and echopraxia (involuntary imitation of gestures) (Ganos, Ogrzal, Schnitzler, & Münchau, 2012; Hoffmann, 2014). EP is also described in terms of the time in which the different types of language and motor imitation occur relative to exposure to the trigger stimulus. Imitation which occurs directly after exposure is known as *immediate* EP. This behavior is in contradistinction to *delayed* EP in which the repetition/imitation of the trigger stimuli (verbal messages, gestures) that were previously heard or seen occurs after a time delay (minutes, hours, days) (Kanner, 1943). Delayed EP is a key symptom in individuals with autism spectrum disorders, but is only rarely reported in aphasia (Geschwind, Quadfasel, & Segarra, 1968).

Before advancing in the description of the different forms of EP, it should be noted that immediate EP rarely occurs in isolation. Affected individuals have been described as "captured" or "attracted" by ambient stimuli, which compel them to impulsively call out objects and persons (hypernomia) (Fujii, Yamadori, Fukatsu, Ogawa, & Suzuki, 1997) and to describe the gestures and actions of people nearby (forced hyperphasia) (Tanaka, Albert, Hara, Miyashita, & Kotani, 2000). Disinhibition during oral spelling (Ragno Paquier, & Assal, 2007), oral reading (hyperlexia, loss of silent reading) (Susuki et al., 2000; Vercuil & Klinger, 2001), and writing (hypergraphia) (Berthier, 1999; Cambier, Masson, Benammou, & Robine, 1988; Van Vugt, Paquier, Kees, & Cras, 1996) has also been reported. These disorders do not conform to the typical pattern of echo-reactions; rather, disinhibition of language functions in different output modalities (naming, reading, writing) induces behaviors that are considered fragments of the so-called "utilization behavior" (Berthier, Pulvermüller, Green, & Higueras, 2006; Lhermitte, Pillon, & Serdaru, 1986; Tanaka et al., 2000). The term *utilization behavior* makes reference to the execution of an instrumentally correct, yet exaggerated, motor response triggered by external stimuli that occurs in the absence of any specific instruction (Lhermitte et al., 1986). These disorders can also be classified as modality-specific utilization behavior because they imply the execution of an act of physical dependence (object-based activation) but are limited to a single modality. A full-blown utilization behavior and its modality-specific subtypes, as well as the more complex syndrome called "environmental dependency syndrome"[1] can coexist with EP (Della Salla & Spinnler, 1998). These conditions and EP share the same underlying mechanism. They result from an altered equilibrium between the activity of the frontal lobes and other cortical areas (temporo-parietal junction, occipital). Data from groups, single cases, and case series suggest that lesions in the anterior-medial frontal lobe (supplementary motor area [SMA], pre-SMA, anterior cingulate gyrus, orbitofrontal cortex) and fronto-striatal networks can reduce their normal inhibitory tone over related cortical areas (parietal, temporal, occipital) (De Renzi et al., 1996; Lhermitte et al., 1986). This faulty inhibition precipitates inappropriate motor acts and impulsive communication when the patient is confronted with visual and auditory stimuli (objects, written material, verbal questions) (Berthier et al., 2006; Denny-Brown & Chambers, 1958; Tanaka et al., 2000). These "exploratory" behaviors are actually the opposite of the so-called "rejection behavior" (patients with strong withdrawal or refusal to be touched and fed) in which large, symmetrical parieto-temporal lesions release the activity of intact medial frontal lobe areas implicated in tactile avoiding reactions (Denny-Brown & Chambers, 1958; Mori & Yamadori, 1989). All of these syndromes can be associated with EP and the astute clinician should be on the lookout for these clinical signs.

ECHOLALIA

Echolalia is generally defined as the automatic and noncommunicative repetition of words and/or utterances spoken by another person in the absence of the understanding of their meaning (Brain, 1965, p. 105). Several types have been described (Berthier, 1999; Wallesch, 1990). The more complex and socially embarrassing forms of echolalia (ambient, echoing approval) may or may not coexist with aphasia, but nearly always are associated with inappropriate behavioral and emotional changes. On the contrary, other forms of echolalia (automatic, mitigated, effortful) are integral constituents of aphasic syndromes (especially transcortical aphasias) and are not associated with grossly inappropriate behavioral changes, although they may coexist with psychological symptoms such as depression, anxiety, and apathy. In this section, we describe the different types of echolalia beginning with the most severe form.

---

1   The *environmental dependency syndrome* is a more complex form of utilization behavior, which occurs in environments that are more complex than typical patient/examiner interactions (Lhermitte, 1986). In complex and social situations (e.g., doctor's office) patients interact with the environment as if they actually are in charge of the situation by using purposefully available tools (e.g., reflex tester). The patients lose their personal autonomy and are "captured" by environmental cues that force them to perform complex tasks, which oftentimes exceed their expertise (Lhermitte, 1986).

Ambient Echolalia

The term ambient echolalia (Fisher, 1988) is applied when patients repeat words and sentences coming from unrelated conversations around them even when people are talking in a nearby room (Suzuki et al., 2012). Patients also repeat verbal information coming from other sources such as TV and CDs, but echolalic emissions do not appear when conversations and questions are directed to them (Della Salla & Spinnler, 1998; Suzuki, Itoh, Hayashi, Kouno, & Takeda, 2009). Ambient echolalia is a rare condition that mostly occurs in patients with dementia (Fisher, 1988) and nonfluent transcortical aphasias (Della Salla & Spinnler, 1998) although a case study not associated with these disorders has been reported (Suzuki et al., 2012). Ambient echolalia has been correlated with unilateral and bilateral lesions in the medial frontal and anterior cingulate regions (Suzuki et al., 2009, 2012) which play a role in inhibiting imitation (Brass, Ruby, & Spengler, 2009) as well as in "theory of mind" (Frith & Frith, 2006) and evaluation of outcomes (e.g., reflection on one's own performance) (Passingham, Bengtsson, & Lau, 2010).

In his original formulation of ambient echolalia, Fisher (1988) parsimoniously explained that incoming words automatically ignite the speech apparatus in patients with dementia, thus causing echolalia. This speculation aligns well with the findings of structural magnetic resonance imaging (MRI) in modern single-case studies (Suzuki et al., 2009, 2012). In these cases, the perisylvian language core responsible for speech perception and production was largely spared and presumably released from inhibition by the lesions in the SMA and anterior cingulate cortex which are implicated in the inhibition of inappropriate responses. Studies in healthy subjects using repetitive transcranial magnetic stimulation (rTMS) (Murakami, Restle, & Ziemann, 2012; Watkins, Strafella, & Paus, 2003) and event-related functional MRI (fMRI) (Pulvermüller et al., 2006) show that the perception of auditory speech reinforces the connectivity between areas of the auditory dorsal stream (arcuate fasciculus) and motor cortex responsible for verbal repetition, as well as the excitability of the left motor cortex underlying speech production. Also, stimulation of the left posterior inferior frontal gyrus with intermittent TMS (iTMS) in healthy subjects facilitates the repetition of foreign sentences (Restle, Murakami, & Ziemann, 2012). This neurophysiologic evidence highlights the causal role of heightened left perisylvian activity in the mediation of verbal repetition/imitation.

The mechanism championed by Fisher (1988) to account for ambient echolalia is probably accurate, but it is unlikely that it provides the whole story, insofar as it is necessary to explain the role of social context-dependent abnormal behaviors indicative of poor insight, foresight, and abstraction (Ibañez & Manes, 2012; Mesulam, 1986). Therefore, a complementary elucidation has been proposed (Suzuki et al., 2012). Suzuki and coworkers (2012) interpreted ambient echolalia as an "engagement of irrelevant codes in the decision-making process" (p. 335). Additionally, it is possible that key elements in ambient echolalia are the breakdown in self-other distinction (overlooking that the person is not addressing the patient but other people) and higher order social-cognition capacities like "theory of mind" or mentalizing (unconcern of the consequences of our own verbal behavior in others, reflection on one's own performance) (Brass et al., 2009; Frith & Frith, 2006; Hobson, 1993; Passingham et al., 2010; Santiestaban et al., 2012) together with a disinhibition of the mirror neurons (Berthier et al., 2006). In any case, further studies exploring the relative contribution of these interactive cognitive domains to the emergence of ambient echolalia are warranted.

Echoing Approval

Another astonishing form of echolalia has been termed *echoing approval* to distinguish it from typical echolalia (Ghika, Bogousslavsky, Ghika-Schmid, & Regli, 1996). Echoing approval is regularly elicited during a short dialogue or in replying to questions. In this type of echolalia, the words themselves are not repeated. Rather, affected individuals imitate the affirmative or negative syntactical construction of questions or the intonational patterns, even when questions are directed to other people (environmental-dependency syndrome) (Lhermitte, 1986). This unusual behavior was originally described by Karl Leonhard (1957) under the name *"speech-prompt catatonia"* in patients with catatonic schizophrenia and organic psychosis (Koehler & Jakumeit, 1976; Ungvari & Rankin, 1990). At that time the neural basis of echoing approval was not firmly established, but neuroimaging in modern cases discloses extensive bilateral involvement of fronto-subcortical regions (Ghika et al., 1996). In the following example, we transcribe a fragment of a discussion on the details of a neurological exam between the attending physician and a colleague in the presence of a patient (a 62-year-old woman). It is of note that although the physicians spoke using medical terms that were unknown to the patient, she made statements of agreement or disagreement about these scientific labels which wholly depended on the syntactical structure of the sentences or on their intonation patterns. For example, when the attending physicians commented on: *"We were impressed by the peculiar type of aphasia,"* the patient said: *Yes, yes ... yes, exactly, yes, yes."* And, when attending physicians added *"... with no phonemic or semantic paraphasia ..."* the patient reassured, *"No, no, absolutely not."*

Automatic Echolalia

This is the best-known type of echolalia. It is called "automatic" because echoes are generated in an impulsive, "parrot-like" manner. Patients do not appear inhibited by any type of verbal information including nonwords or foreign languages, and they repeat this information verbatim immediately after stimulus presentation. Automatic echolalia is nearly always elicited when patients are directly addressed, and not when comments and questions are directed to other people. This form of echolalia has recently been designated as *induced*[2] to distinguish it from the forms mentioned earlier (ambient echolalia and echoing approval) which are termed *incidental* (Grossi, Marcone, Cinquegrana, & Galluci, 2013). Although automatic echolalia does not entail any apparent communication purpose, and in fact some patients tend to inhibit it, the influence of deficits in other cognitive domains (self-other distinction, "theory of mind") on its emergence has not been examined.

Automatic echolalia nearly always occurs in transcortical motor aphasias with preserved comprehension (transcortical motor) or markedly impaired auditory comprehension (mixed transcortical), but it is rarely observed in transcortical sensory aphasia. In general, echolalic utterances in transcortical motor aphasia cases are easily enunciated but devoid of emotional coloring (flat intonation) (Berthier, Fernández, Martínez-Celdrán, & Kulisevsky, 1996; Speedie, Coslett, & Heilman, 1984). Individuals with impaired auditory comprehension are usually unconcerned about their irrepressible echolalic behavior, making the formal evaluation of other language domains impossible. By contrast, patients with preserved auditory comprehension have clear awareness of the echolalia but are unable to suppress unwanted emissions.

Traditional accounts (Brown, 1982; Wallesch, 1990) suggest that automatic echolalia results from both residual capacity of the left hemisphere (intact perisylvian cortex) and compensatory release of the right hemisphere. Modern models of echolalia maintain that lesions in the left medial frontal cortex may simultaneously cause a marked reduction of vocalization and self-initiated speech (mutism or adynamic speech) and automatic echolalia presumably due to overactivity of the mirror neurons in the inferior frontal cortex and temporo-parietal junction (Berthier et al., 2006). Anecdotal evidence suggests that automatic echolalia mostly occurs in *acute* aphasias. This may be interpreted as reflecting a rapid release of the repetition "reflex arc" (Wernicke, 1977) represented in the left perisylvian area (or less probably in homologous areas of the right hemisphere) soon after an acute brain injury (Berthier et al., 1991). Acute automatic echolalia should be distinguished from late-onset forms occurring in *chronic* aphasias associated with massive lesions of the left hemisphere which gradually evolve due to the takeover of repetition by the right hemisphere (Pulvermüller & Schönle, 1993). While acute echolalia is irrepressible, usually embracing the repetition of entire sentences, echolalia emerging in chronic stages is less severe and echoes can be limited to words or short phrases.

---

2   The use of the terms *induced* and *incidental* for classifying echolalia comes from an attempted fractionation of utilization behavior performed by Shallice, Burgess, Schon, and Baxter (1989). Based on the context and manner of elicitation of object use, Shallice and colleagues termed *induced* utilization behavior when the placement of objects in front of the patient immediately elicits their use. They also described a related subtype, which was termed *incidental,* because object utilization occurs when the patient is performing auditory-verbal cognitive tasks (Shallice et al., 1989).

Mitigated Echolalia and Its Variants

Mitigated echolalia is a minor form of EP, which refers to any language change in the echoed emission for communicative purposes (Pick, 1924). In some cases, it is not easy to determine whether and to what extent normal repetition can be separated from mitigated echoing. In mitigated echolalia entire sentences may be echoed, but more commonly only words or phrase fragments that sound ambiguous, equivocal, or are poorly understood are echoed (Berthier, 1999). Also, exact or approximate replicas may be heard including pronoun reversals (Question: "Where do you sleep?" Response: "I sleep."), grammatical conversions, and syntactical supplements (Question: "Is it a boy or a girl?" Response: "Huh? Boy or girl") (Fay & Butler, 1968).

Because patients with mitigated echolalia do not understand the meaning of certain words, they may either reproduce the linguistic intonational pattern of questions verbatim (Question: "Have you got any children?" Response: "Children? I am not married." in Stengel, 1947, p. 603) or change it (Question: "What is your name?" Response: "My name! Charles Frederick Leale" in Symonds, 1953, p. 4). The number of times that patients with mitigated echolalia verbally repeat a heard stimulus is variable and may be related to semantic deficits in auditory comprehension. Indeed, in a case of word meaning deafness[3] the patient (Dr. O) repeated several times a hard-to-define word, whereas he only repeated a word once when he was able to understand and define it correctly (Franklin, Turner, Lambon Ralph, Morris, & Bailey, 1996). For example, the word "slow" was incorrectly defined as: "*slow, slow, slow, slow, I know what it is but I can't get it, slow, slow,*" whereas the word "spare" was incorporated in the response and elicited the correct response "*a spare is something more than you actually need*" (see Table 4 in Franklin et al., 1996 and similar examples in Kohn & Friedman, 1986).

Mitigated echolalia has been described after focal brain lesions in patients with transcortical sensory aphasia, mild Wernicke's aphasia, conduction aphasia, anomic aphasia, and word-meaning deafness (Berthier, 1999), as well as in degenerative conditions such as Alzheimer's disease (Da Cruz, 2010) and semantic dementia (Snowden, Goulding, & Neary, 1989). Consider, for example, the case of semantic dementia. Language in this degenerative dementia is fluent but empty and characterized by preserved repetition and phonology in the face of impaired single-word comprehension (Hodges, Patterson, Oxbury, & Funnell, 1992). The dissociation between preserved repetition and impaired semantic comprehension of the same words justifies the frequent questioning of word meaning

---

3   Word meaning deafness (WMD) is a rare condition in which the patient "can repeat the words he heard without understanding their meaning" (Symonds, 1953, p. 3). The deficit in auditory comprehension is secondary to dissociation between accurate phonological and semantic information (Bormann & Weiller, 2012; Kohn & Friedman, 1986). While auditory comprehension is abnormal, comprehension of written and picture stimuli are normal. In general, word meaning deafness occurs in the context of transcortical sensory aphasia, Wernicke's aphasia, and conduction aphasia of mild severity. WMD should be distinguished from "pure word deafness," which is characterized by a dramatic deficit in auditory perception affecting phoneme identification and discrimination (Poeppel, 2001).

("Gorilla? ... gorilla ... what is gorilla?") (Kertesz, Jesso, Harciarek, Blair, & McMonagle, 2010). Thus, repetitive questioning of word meaning during conversation and language testing may represent instances of mitigated echolalia related to impoverished semantic comprehension associated to focal atrophy of the left temporal pole.

Another phenomenon akin to mitigated echolalia has been termed *echo-answer* (Lebrun, 1987; Lebrun, Rubio, Jongen, & Demol, 1971). Echo-answer refers to the superfluous inclusion of words from the question into the response. For example, when a patient with transcortical motor aphasia was asked "Are you in the hospital?" she replied "I am in the hospital" instead of using the more concise response: "Yes" (Brust, Plank, Burke, Guobadia, & Healton, 1982). According to Lebrun and colleagues (1971) this behavior results from an inability to grasp the meaning of auditory information and this would explain why instances of echo-answer and mitigated echolalia may co-occur in the same utterance, presumably to increase auditory comprehension. This repetitive behavior, usually termed *subvocalizing, rehearsal* and sometimes *reauditorization*, is used in rehabilitation as an augmentative strategy, although overreliance on auditory feedback may not always be beneficial (Civier, Tasko, & Guenther, 2010). The following example illustrates the blend between mitigated echolalia and echo-answer. When Byrom Bramwell asked a patient with word-meaning deafness (Case 11, 1897, in Ellis, 1984, p. 254) "Are you better?" she automatically repeated the word "better" and then voluntarily added, "Yes, better."

The last variant of mitigated echolalia reported up to now is named *effortful echolalia* and occurs in patients with transcortical motor aphasia (Hadano, Nakamura, & Hamanaka, 1998). Typically, echolalic emissions are extremely literal, precise, and automatic (Grossi et al., 2013). The speech act is fully preserved and devoid of effort, articulation errors, and abnormal linguistic prosody because the responsible lesions in the left medial frontal lobe spare the perisylvian area, which is responsible for the smooth generation of speech. In contrast, the term effortful echolalia has been coined to indicate the contamination of echolalic emissions by articulatory struggling, distorted prosody, and increased effort to produce and repeat sentences displayed by some patients with atypical transcortical motor aphasia (Goldstein, 1915; Hadano et al., 1998). Neuroimaging in the three cases of effortful echolalia reported so far (Hadano et al., 1998) disclosed the expected left medial frontal lobe involvement that accounted for the reduction of self-initiated speech, but the lesions were large enough to encompass the anterior perisylvian regions (Broca's area, anterior insula, basal ganglia), thus explaining why echolalia coexisted with disordered speech production. Importantly, effortful echolalia is not associated with completion phenomenon, another sign of release of the perisylvian areas. From a behavioral standpoint, effortful echolalia represents a form of mitigated echolalia because patients involuntarily repeat some words of the examiner's questions and subsequently produce their own responses. While typical echoing of words and utterances is nonintentional and associated with a variable awareness of its presence, patients with effortful echolalia are fully aware and embarrassed by their uncontrollable echoes (Hadano et al., 1998).

ECHOPRAXIA

Echopraxia is the automatic repetition of actions previously observed in other people without regard for the context and the meaning of this action. Echopraxia can occur in a variety of conditions including Tourette's syndrome (Ganos et al., 2012), autism (Kanner, 1943; Rutter, 1974), catatonia (Abrams & Taylor, 1976), schizophrenia (Pridmore, Brüne, Ahmadi, & Dale, 2008), left frontal lobe epilepsy (Cho, Han, Song, Lee, & Heo, 2009), and culture-bound syndromes (e.g., Latah or Indonesian startle response) (Bakker, van Dijk, Pramono, Sutarni, & Tijssen, 2013).

The association of echopraxia with aphasia is infrequent, and the description of automatic imitation of motor actions has been reported almost exclusively in patients with transcortical aphasias (motor and mixed types). The coexistence of echopraxia with transcortical aphasias has been associated with left parietal subcortical hemorrhage (Pirozzolo et al., 1981), bilateral damage to fronto-subcortical networks (Assal, 1985; Ghika et al., 1996; Gold et al., 1997), anterior cortical-subcortical atrophy/dysfunction in progressive supranuclear palsy (Ghika, Tennis, Growdon, Hoffman, & Johnson, 1995), and fronto-temporal dementia (patient NLE in Berthier, 1999, pp. 165–166) predominantly affecting the SMA, basal ganglia, and connected regions.

As mentioned previously, the association of echopraxia and aphasia is rare and limited to transcortical cases. One possible explanation for the lack of descriptions of echopraxia in aphasias with abnormal repetition (e.g., conduction, Wernicke's) would be that left hemisphere lesions causing these aphasic syndromes involve cortical areas (supramarginal and angular gyri) and neural networks (superior longitudinal fasciculus) that are also critical for the programming and execution (imitation) of skilled movements (Kertesz & Ferro, 1984; Mengotti et al., 2013). However, it is more difficult to explain why dysfunction of the SMA leads to either echopraxia or apraxia in different patients. On the one hand, focal vascular lesions and degenerative changes affecting the SMA have been associated with ideomotor apraxia (Leiguarda, Lees, Merello, Starkstein, & Marsden, 1994; Watson, Fleet, Gonzalez-Rothi, & Heilman, 1986). On the other hand, imitation behavior (echopraxia) has been described in patients with lesions in the pre-SMA and SMA (De Renzi et al., 1996). One possible explanation could be that different patients showing echopraxia or apraxia have overlapping but not identical involvement of the SMA. Although further neuroimaging studies are necessary, the role of the SMA and/or pre-SMA and anterior cingulate areas in suppressing automatic responses to environmental stimulation is undisputed (Finis et al., 2013).

ECHOGRAPHIA

Echographia is an unusual disorder characterized by the automatic translation of visual (and sometimes also auditory) stimuli into writing (Berthier et al., 2006; Pick, 1924). Echographia as described by Pick (1924; i.e., impulsive writing only elicited by visual stimuli with reluctance to copy foreign words, jargon aphasia, and frustration) is unique, since no similar cases have been reported so far. In modern cases, echographia occurred in patients with transcortical aphasias (two transcortical motor aphasias, one mixed transcortical aphasia) and it was triggered by both written and auditory stimuli. It coexisted with incessant writing activity (hypergraphia) and other environmentally induced behaviors such as utilization behavior, imitation, impulsive reading, and echolalia (Berthier, 1999; Cambier et al., 1988; Van Vugt et al., 1996). General behavior varied among patients, but it was always abnormal, ranging from apathy and slowness to disinhibition (distractibility, loss of decorum, or incomplete Klüver-Bucy syndrome). Structural neuroimaging revealed unilateral or bilateral lesions involving the medial frontal region in all cases and the temporal lobes in one (Berthier et al., 2006) with sparing of the perisylvian areas. It has been suggested that the involvement of the perisylvian language cortex in Pick's original case precluded the constellation of symptoms reported in modern cases (Berthier et al., 2006). Modern cases of echographia have been interpreted as forms of imitation and utilization behaviors selective for writing. It has been suggested that damage to the medial frontal lobe cortex (SMA), which plays a leading role in suppressing movements represented in premotor and motor cortices, triggers echographia by disinhibiting audio-visual mirror neurons that control writing actions (Berthier et al., 2006; Corballis, 2010; Longcamp, Hlushchuk, & Hari, 2011).

MECHANISMS UNDERLYING ECHOPHENOMENA

Breakdown of Inhibitory Control

A growing body of evidence indicates that the mere observation of an action triggers its corresponding motor representation in the observer (Brass et al., 2009; Gallese, Fadiga, Fogassi, & Rizzolatti, 1996). The neural mechanisms underpinning this active perception have been heightened by the discovery of the mirror neuron system (MNS) (Rizzolatti & Craighero, 2004). Mirror neurons are a specific class of cells that are activated and discharge both during observation of the same or similar motor act performed by another individual and during the execution of a motor act by oneself. The MNS is located in the inferior frontal gyrus (Brodmann's area [BA] 44), superior temporal gyrus (BA22), and inferior parietal lobule (BA40), a set of cortical areas connected by white matter tracts (dorsal stream) responsible for repetition/imitation (Arbib, 2010; Corballis, 2010). Imitation, action understanding, learning, and language may depend on the activity of the MNS and other sensorimotor neurons (Iacoboni et al., 1999; Keysers et al., 2003; Kohler et al., 2002; Pulvermüller, Moseley, Egorova, Shebani, & Boulenger, 2014). Seeing and hearing language signals facilitates the excitability of the motor system involved in speech and written production even in the absence of overt motor activity (Fadiga, Craighero, Buccino, & Rizzolatti, 2002; Papathanasiou, Filipovic, Whurr, Rothwell, & Jahanshahi, 2004; Tokimura, Tokimura, Oliviero, Asakura, & Rothwell, 1996; Watkins et al., 2003). Speech perception further enhances the connectivity between cortical areas (left temporo-parietal junction and primary motor cortex "lip area") linked by the auditory dorsal stream (Murakami et al., 2012).

The existence of the MNS confirms that action and perception share the same neural system and are mutually interdependent (Massen & Prinz, 2009; Pulvermüller & Fadiga, 2010). The activity of this neural system is controlled by inhibitory mechanisms that assure that imitative behavior is goal directed rather than impulsive, thus impeding the execution of strong but contextually inappropriate responses (Brass et al., 2009). The inhibition of unwanted actions depends on the activity of a bilateral large-scale network comprising premotor, posterior parietal, and frontal-parietal opercular cortices; right inferior frontal and superior temporal cortices, and basal ganglia (Aron, Robbins, & Poldrack, 2014; Bien, Roebroeck, Goebel, & Sack, 2009). Lesions disrupting the concerted action of this network can precipitate impulsive imitation when the subject perceives motor or verbal actions. These stimulus-bound behaviors result from unbalanced weighting between *decreased* inhibitory modulation of the frontal lobes (medial frontal cortex) and *increased* activity of connected regions (temporo-parietal junction), which enables the easy elicitation of motor and verbal plans (echolalia, echographia) by specific environmental stimuli (oral words, written material) (Berthier et al., 2006; Brass et al., 2009; Lhermitte et al., 1986; Pick, 1924). The presence of EP does not simply reflect disinhibition of brain areas involved in imitation but also the dysfunction of higher-level cognitive processes that are more susceptible to disruption than stimulus-based behaviors (Toates, 2006). In this regard, a hypothesis that still needs to be tested would suggest that lesions in the anterior fronto-median cortex responsible for dramatic imitative behaviors (ambient echolalia and echoing approval) could also alter the control of shared representations and complex social-cognitive processes (mental state attribution) (Brass et al., 2009; Frith & Frith, 2006). This being the case, treatment strategies acting on improving mental state attribution (e.g., increasing awareness of social interaction) might facilitate a better monitoring of echolalia. Other potential contributing factors to EP pending evaluation are awareness of abnormal imitation as well as the status of auditory comprehension and verbal/motor self-monitoring. These are briefly discussed in the next section.

Reduced Awareness, Auditory Comprehension, and Auditory Feedback

Denial (anosognosia) and reduced awareness of illness (anosodiaphoria) can affect motor, emotional, and cognitive domains, including language (Maher, Rothi, & Heilman, 1994; Shuren, Hammond, Maher, Rothi, & Heilman, 1995; Starkstein, Sabe, Chemerinski, Jason, & Leiguarda, 1996). The potential relationship between awareness deficits and EP has not been examined so far and little is known about the cognitive mechanisms underlying anosognosia/anosodiaphoria for aphasia. Interaction of impaired lexical-semantic comprehension, disturbed feedback, reduced attentional capacity, and psychological denial associated or not with depression has been entertained (Cocchini, Crosta, Allen, Zaro, & Beschin, 2013; Lebrun, 1987; Maher et al., 1994; Marshall, Robson, Pring, & Chiat,

1998; Shuren et al., 1995), but none of these hypotheses has been identified as the unique causative factor. Recent accounts prefer to define awareness deficits as "multifactorial" (Prigatano, 2009) or "multi-componential" (Vocat & Vuilleumier, 2010).

Clinical observation reveals that most patients with EP may have reduced awareness of their imitative behavior. For instance, automatic echolalia in transcortical aphasias with impaired auditory comprehension (mixed and sensory variants) is produced without conscious awareness and with no attempt to suppress it. By contrast, partial or complete awareness of stimulus repetition can be inferred in cases of mitigated echolalia. It has been argued that patients develop mitigated echolalia to improve semantic access for difficult words and utterances while they are engaged in auditory comprehension tasks (Berthier, 1999), an argument implying some cognitive control over the voluntary action of word repetition until its meaning is understood. This would explain why patients with mitigated echolalia tend to produce more repetitions when they have trouble understanding difficult words than when they access word meaning with ease (Brown, 1975; Franklin et al., 1996). Finally, reduced auditory feedback and error monitoring are probably implicated in severe forms of echolalia (echoing approval, and ambient and automatic forms). Healthy speakers use auditory feedback of their own voices to detect and correct errors (Postma & Noordanus, 1996) and also to improve high-level semantic monitoring (Lind, Hall, Breidegard, Balkenius, & Johansson, 2014). Verbal self-monitoring contributes to the conscious awareness of thought and to distinguish self from others. Conscious error perception has been attributed to the activity of a few brain areas (anterior insula, pre-SMA, anterior cingulate gyrus, and thalamus) (Klein, Ullsperger, & Danielmeier, 2013) whose damage can induce EP. Moreover, some of these areas (insula, frontal cortex) are integral components of the social context network (Ibañez & Manes, 2012), which may be dysfunctional in frontal patients with EP.

INTERVENTION STRATEGIES

At present, there is little empirical evidence on treatment strategies to attenuate echolalia in persons with aphasia (PWA). The paucity of reports on this issue is probably the consequence of viewing automatic echolalia in acute aphasia as a short-lived phenomenon. Additionally, echolalia is frequent in conditions for which aphasia therapy is not routinely indicated. In general, patients with echolalic aphasias associated to extensive, bilateral frontal lobe damage (Lhermitte et al., 1986), end-stage fronto-temporal dementia (Whitaker, 1976) and Alzheimer's disease (Cummings, Benson, Hill, & Read, 1985), and rapidly progressive dementias (Creutzfeldt-Jakob's disease) (McPherson et al., 1994; Shuttleworth, Yates, & Paltan-Ortiz, 1985) are rarely referred to language rehabilitation centers. These powerful arguments, however, should not undermine the need to look for potential therapeutic strategies to inhibit echolalia in severe cases. It should be noted, however, that echolalic repetition is not always a negative sign in PWA, because it can be used to stimulate speech production when other verbal functions are unavailable. Hence, the planning of therapies for echolalia needs to consider its *negative* or *positive* consequences on aphasia outcome. In other words, echolalia interfering with communication should be inhibited, whereas echolalic emissions in the presence of severely nonfluent speech could be redirected to gradually convert such automatic speech into a meaningful communicative function (Pulvermüller & Schönle, 1993).

To identify the best approach to control echolalia, it is important to realize that different mechanisms may underlie echolalic behavior. Some differences in echolalic behavior depend upon the type of transcortical aphasia and on the amount of time post-onset (acute vs. chronic). In acute transcortical motor aphasia (i.e., less than 2 months of evolution) the relative preservation of auditory comprehension and awareness may imply a better prognosis of echolalia than in acute transcortical sensory aphasia, in which impaired comprehension and anosognosia for aphasia are commonly observed.

Inhibiting Echolalia

Inhibiting automatic echolalia in PWA is an essential target in rehabilitation, because echolalia hampers communication by interfering with speech production and comprehension (Berthier, 1999; Della Salla & Spinnler, 1998). This also holds true for less severe mitigated echolalia, because reiterative repetition of auditory stimuli slows down functional communication (Franklin et al., 1996). Most of our knowledge about the clinical management of echolalic behavior in PWA comes from strategies used to reduce echolalia in individuals with autism spectrum disorders (Dobbinson, Perkins, & Boucher, 2003; Saad & Goldfeld, 2009; Stribling, Rae, & Dickerson, 2007). In some cases, increasing awareness and refocusing attention may help to reduce echolalia. Delay, rehearsal, and self-monitoring strategies (McMorrow & Foxx, 1986) have been successfully employed with two females with severe autism and developmental delay who also displayed echolalic behavior (McMorrow, Foxx, Faw, & Bittle, 1987). These two patients were successfully treated (i.e., reduction of echolalia) with an intervention called *"cues-pause-point language training."* This intervention encourages patients to remain silent before, during, and briefly after the auditory presentation of questions ("What do you wear on your feet?"). They are then allowed to verbalize the response on the basis of presentation of a visual cue (i.e., a picture or the actual object: shoes) (McMorrow et al., 1987). In other cases, introducing a nonverbal discriminative stimulus, such as a gesture (silence gesture), an iconic symbol (☺), or an auditory stimulus ("no," "shh") may serve to inhibit the echolalic response. Also, preventing the visual support of mouth movement and facial gestures that accompany speech (i.e., by using audiotapes instead of face-to-face interviews) may be a useful technique to manage echolalic behavior. However, the last strategy (i.e., hiding the speaker's face) could interfere with comprehension, and as a consequence, echolalic responses could increase.

Recent studies on imitation, action understanding, and social cognition in healthy subjects also suggest that imitative tendencies can be inhibited after extensive practice (Bardi, Bundt, Notebaert, & Brass, 2015). Thus, intensive therapies such as Constraint-Induced Aphasia Therapy (CIAT; also known as Constraint-Induced Language Therapy [CILT] and Intensive Language Action Therapy; Pulvermüller et al., 2001; Pulvermüller & Berthier, 2008) aimed to improve functional communication in everyday situations by discouraging the use of incorrect verbal strategies (echolalia, perseveration) and compensatory gestures unrelated to verbal communication may be useful to reduce echolalia in aphasia (see *Case Illustration* later in this chapter).

Echolalic Repetition as a Therapeutic Tool

Echolalic and perseverative speech is regarded as a meaningless and inappropriate communication strategy. Nevertheless, recent studies in autism spectrum disorders (Dobbinson et al., 2003; Saad & Goldfeld, 2009; Stribling et al., 2007) and dementing conditions (Alzheimer's disease, Huntington's disease; Da Cruz, 2010; Saldert & Hartelius, 2011) reveal that echolalia sometimes does entail a communicative function. In some patients with severe aphasia, echolalia is the only available overt language function. In this circumstance, the question that arises is whether there is any way to take advantage of echolalia to promote recovery of other language deficits (speech production, comprehension). Assuming that recovery relies on a dynamic interplay between abnormal and normal language processes that reflect the combined effects of brain damage and compensatory reorganization of neural networks (Berthier et al., 2011; Lambon Ralph, 2010), late-onset echolalia in aphasia may reflect brain reorganization (Berthier, 1999). This being the case, echolalia should not be viewed as a disinhibition deficit resulting from maladaptive plasticity. Rather, echolalia may be a hint of slow restorative plasticity, probably generated in right fronto-temporal networks or right basal ganglia, in cases with large lesions in the left perisylvian region (Berthier, 1999; Smania et al., 2010). In support of this argument, Pulvermüller and Schönle (1993) successfully took advantage of echolalic repetition to enhance speech production and comprehension skills in a formerly globally aphasic client (KS) who otherwise had no efficient communication. He was treated in a dyadic setting using repetitive card games (early version of CIAT) (Pulvermüller et al., 2001). Because KS was not able to use requests spontaneously (he could only repeat words and phrases), the paradigm used to elicit speech acts was termed "requesting by selective repetition." For example in the speech production paradigm—if KS had selected a card with a spoon depicted on it, the clinician asked questions such as "Do you want (a piece of) *cutlery* or *bread*?" and then KS could repeat the part of the sentence that matched his intention to ask for a *spoon* (that was the word "cutlery") (p. 145). In the comprehension paradigm, KS was requested to pass a particular card using sentences such as "Please give me the rabbit." or "Could I have the fork?" KS's speech production and comprehension improved significantly and these gains were attributed to strengthened synaptic connections of the auditory-motor networks in the right hemisphere. Using magnetoencephalography (MEG) in healthy subjects, Pulvermüller's group recently found that "requests" similar to the ones used with KS engaged mirror-neuron action-comprehension systems in both sensorimotor cortices but more strongly in the right hemisphere(Egorova, Pulvermüller, & Shtyrov, 2014).

Repetition/Imitation for Aphasia Treatment

Auditory repetition training forms part of the therapeutic catalogue for aphasia therapy mainly when the syndrome-specific standard approach is implemented. In this case, auditory repetition is applied in conjunction with other exercises, involving sentence completion, naming, spoken word–picture matching, reading, and writing to remediate aphasic deficits (Basso, Forbes, & Boller, 2013). However, the essential contribution of using auditory repetition as the key therapeutic tool in aphasia rehabilitation has not been appreciated until recently. Nowadays, rehabilitation focuses more readily on auditory repetition training, but only in certain types of aphasia. Although repetition/imitation training has successfully been used in transcortical motor aphasia (Salis, 2012) and mixed transcortical aphasia (Pulvermüller & Schönle, 1993), it may be anticipated that patients with severe echolalia are not good candidates for this type of intervention.

Auditory repetition is a complex function involving multiple domains (attention, phonological working memory, auditory-verbal short-term memory, and lexical-semantic, syntactic, phonemic, and motor production processes) that are supported by a large-scale neural network (Hope et al., 2014). Studies using functional magnetic resonance imaging (fMRI) (Saur et al., 2008) have revealed that auditory repetition is bilaterally (left > right) organized in the brain, so that not only is the left hemisphere mediating auditory repetition, but the right hemisphere can also contribute (Berthier, Lambon Ralph, Pujol, & Green, 2012). Complementary anatomical studies of the core language regions using diffusion tensor imaging (DTI) have mapped the architecture of the white matter pathways (e.g., arcuate fasciculus, ventral stream) underlying language repetition (Catani & Thiebaut de Schotten, 2012; Petrides, 2014). The neural basis of repetition is currently interpreted in a dual dorsal-ventral pathways framework (Hickok & Poeppel, 2007; Rauschecker & Scott, 2009). The ventral pathway is related to semantic function (comprehension) and is symmetrically represented, connecting the frontal and temporal cortices via the inferior fronto-occipital fasciculus, extreme capsule, and uncinate fasciculus (Saur et al., 2008; Petrides, 2014). By contrast, the arcuate fasciculus (dorsal stream) is related to auditory-motor transcoding (e.g., nonword repetition, auditory memory) and is more strongly developed in the left hemisphere than in the right one (Berthier et al., 2012; López-Barroso et al., 2013). Recent DTI (tractography) studies suggest that PWA with a fully developed right dorsal stream (long segment of the arcuate fasciculus) show better recovery from language deficits than those with undeveloped tracts (Forkel et al., 2014) because they also recruit the right arcuate fasciculus during word repetition (Berthier et al., 2013). Computational modelling investigations (Nozari & Dell, 2013; Nozari, Kittredge, Dell, & Schwartz, 2010; Ueno, Saito, Rogers, & Lambon Ralph, 2011;

Ueno & Lambon Ralph, 2013) and analysis of patients with brain damage (Berthier et al., 2012, 2013; Forkel et al., 2014) also increased our knowledge of the mechanisms under-pinning language repetition (Berthier & Lambon Ralph, 2014).

The advent of these technologies has motivated the study of brain reorganization promoted by intensive aphasia therapies. Intervention studies used repetition training in the presence of a picture (Heath et al., 2012) or embedded in Melodic Intonation Therapy (MIT; Schlaug, Marchina, & Norton, 2009; Sparks, Helm, & Albert, 1974; Zipse, Norton, Marchina, & Schlaug, 2012) and CIAT (Breier, Juranek, & Papanicolaou, 2011; Pulvermüller et al., 2001) to improve speech production. The main aim behind these therapies is to activate the remnants of left hemisphere white matter pathways (ventral stream) and/or to stimulate the compensatory activity of their homologues in the right hemisphere when the left ones are enduringly damaged. The improvements observed in picture naming (Heath et al., 2013) and speech production (Breier et al., 2011; Schlaug et al., 2009; Zipse et al., 2012) are attributed to therapy-promoted strengthening of auditory-motor assemblies or semantic-phonological connections in the right hemi-sphere (Heath et al., 2012; Zipse et al., 2012). Changes in white matter tracts promoted by intensive aphasia therapy can be identified with DTI.

Studies on PWA in whom repetition, though impaired, was more fluent than spon-taneous speech stimulated the selective use of repetition exercises as a therapeutic tool (Kohn, Smith, & Arsenault, 1990). The intention was to translate the gains obtained in auditory repetition performance after repetition practice to speech production (fluency), comprehension, and phonological working memory. Thus, patients with either moder-ately *impaired* or relatively *preserved* repetition performance at the word level underwent intensive auditory repetition of different stimuli (word, nonwords, sentences, digits, and idiomatic phrases) under immediate and/or delayed conditions. Significant benefits have been described for patients with conduction aphasia (Heath et al., 2013; Kalinyak-Fliszar, Kohen, & Martin, 2011; Koenig-Bruhin & Studer-Eichenberger, 2007; Kohn et al., 1990; Majerus, van der Kaa, Renard, Van der Linden, & Poncelet, 2005), Wernicke's aphasia (Francis, Clark, & Humphreys, 2003; Heath et al., 2013), mixed transcortical aphasia (Pulvermüller & Schönle, 1993), and anomic aphasia (Heath et al., 2013). Collectively, these studies revealed that training auditory repetition improved performance on repeti-tion tasks, and also that these gains generalized to speech production, naming, phono-logical short-term memory, and executive-attentional processes.

Nevertheless, most speech pathologists recognize that auditory repetition practice alone is not enough to promote manifest benefits in everyday language activities and functional communication. Therefore, in recent studies auditory and visual stimuli have been used simultaneously (Fridriksson et al., 2012; Heath et al., 2012, 2013; Lee, Fowler, Rodney, Cherney, & Small, 2010; Small, Buccino, & Solodkin, 2010). For example, a new computer-assisted intervention for aphasia (Intensive Mouth Imitation and Talking for Aphasia Therapeutic Effects [IMITATE]) has been devised (Lee et al., 2010; Mashal,

Solodkin, Dick, Chen, & Small, 2012; Small et al., 2010). The rationale behind this method is to use action observation and imitation of visual and auditory stimuli to enhance the activity of bilateral parietal-frontal pathways (audiovisual mirror neurons) (Iacoboni et al., 1999; Keysers et al., 2003; Kohler et al., 2002; Small et al., 2010). During an IMITATE session, patients silently observe audio-visually presented words and phrases spoken aloud by different speakers followed by a 20-second period during which they orally repeat the stimuli (Lee et al., 2010; Sarasso et al., 2014). Practice with this imitation-based therapy for 3.5 hours during a single day was correlated with improvement in the repetition subtest of the Western Aphasia Battery (WAB) (Kertesz, 1982) and electroencephalogram changes over the left central and frontal regions. Prominent functional changes were also found in the unaffected right hemisphere (Sarasso et al., 2014).

CONCLUSIONS AND DIRECTIONS FOR FUTURE RESEARCH

In this chapter we have described EP mainly highlighting those conditions (echolalia) which are inextricably linked with aphasia. Two forms of echolalia (ambient and echoing approval) are the most severe because their occurrence implies a major breakdown of higher-order cognitive processes (self-other distinction) and mentalizing, in addition to the distinctive inefficient control of stimulus-triggered repetition. Automatic echolalia is also a severe disorder because it interferes with verbal communication and is commonly associated with reduced awareness, auditory comprehension, and self-monitoring. Nevertheless, the preservation of full awareness of its irrepressible character, in some cases with preserved auditory comprehension, might reflect some preservation of social cognition. These forms of echolalia nearly always are associated with transcortical aphasias and their presence may denote inefficient control of the inhibitory network over the perisylvian language areas with release of the mirror neuron system and other sensorimotor circuits. Milder forms of echolalia (mitigated and its variants) occur in atypical transcortical aphasias and in residual aphasias (e.g., Wernicke's aphasia, conduction aphasia, word meaning deafness) and reflect incomplete damage to the perisylvian cortex and impaired connectivity of white matter tracts (dorsal and ventral streams).

This chapter further addressed rehabilitation strategies for inhibiting echolalia, but since echolalia often coexists with preserved or mildly impaired repetition performance, innovative rehabilitation strategies are employed to exploit these residual functions to improve speech production (fluency, naming), short-term memory, and executive-attentional and comprehension processes. Further studies are strongly needed to confirm preliminary evidence suggesting that benefits promoted by auditory repetition training in aphasia can be augmented using adjuvant therapy approaches such as medications and noninvasive brain stimulation. A promising option that is currently being investigated is the use of drugs to improve language deficits in PWA beyond the therapy effects (Berthier & Pulvermüller, 2011; Small et al., 2010). The main clinical goal of using drugs in aphasia is to accelerate and augment the benefits provided by aphasia therapy. Several combination strategies have been used. These include giving the drug before each language therapy session (Seniów, Litwin, Litwin, Leśniak, & Członkowska, 2009; Walker-Batson et al., 2001), beginning drug treatment and aphasia therapy simultaneously (Berthier et al., 2006), or initiating speech-language therapy in patients who were already receiving a drug treatment for a prolonged period (Berthier et al., 2009; Rothi et al., 2009). Drug administration before or simultaneously with aphasia therapy boosts the activity of dysfunctional areas surrounding the lesion and also stimulates the compensatory activity of remote areas ipsilaterally and contralaterally. In other words, drugs are used to prime brain structures for the concomitant or subsequent action of the language therapy. This does not mean that drug treatment alone is insufficient to ameliorate language deficits (Chen et al., 2010; Hong, Shin, Lim, Lee, & Huh, 2012), but rather that the combination of aphasia therapy with a drug regimen is more beneficial than drug treatment alone because it boosts experience-dependent plasticity (Berthier & Pulvermüller, 2011). In this regard, intensive auditory repetition practice in patients with chronic conduction aphasia who were receiving a cholinergic drug (donepezil) significantly improved not only repetition deficits but also speech production (Berthier et al., 2014).

The second adjuvant therapy approach that has received some attention recently involves stimulating the activity of cortical areas and neural networks underpinning language repetition with modern brain stimulation techniques (i.e., repetitive transcranial magnetic stimulation [rTMS] and transcranial direct current stimulation [tDCS]). These techniques are also emerging as viable strategies to improve speech production and naming in PWA. Two modes of intervention have been suggested for improving cognitive processing. One entails enhancing cortical or network activity to improve the efficiency of cognitive processing, and the other mode improves cognitive processing by inhibiting competing activity that interferes with task performance (Luber & Lisanby, 2014). Recent studies combining aphasia therapy (e.g., MIT) with inhibiting rTMS applied to the right hemisphere Broca's area homologue improved verbal fluency and phrase repetition in patients with nonfluent aphasia and large left hemisphere lesions (Al-Janabi et al., 2014; Vines, Norton, & Schlaug, 2011). Based on the fact that rTMS and tDCS temporarily modify neural activity, these methods are increasingly being used as therapeutic interventions for patients showing difficulties with inhibitory control (Hsu et al., 2011) or reduced task performance (Al-Janabi et al., 2014). Although these preliminary results are encouraging, the combination of brain stimulation with neuroscience-based rehabilitation techniques is still in its infancy.

A final issue requiring additional research involves service delivery models. Training audiovisual repetition is easy to implement and could be administered and monitored via telepractice procedures (e.g., Hall, Boisvert, & Steele, 2013). In fact, we were able to evaluate via an Internet-based service (Skype) the evolution of language deficits after audiovisual imitation training in clients with chronic global aphasia (De-Torres & Berthier, 2016).

CASE ILLUSTRATION

John was a 43-year-old right-handed man who was referred to our unit for evaluation of chronic aphasia 15 months after suffering a left temporal-parietal hemorrhage that left him with a moderately severe fluent aphasia (Western Aphasia Battery-Aphasia Quotient [WAB-AQ] score: 56.2/100) (Kertesz, 1982) and mitigated echolalia. In a re-evaluation 2 years later, it was noted that the aphasia had improved although mitigated echolalia persisted. Analysis of mitigated echolalia revealed that it was heard in casual conversations and in auditory comprehension tasks (yes/no questions, sequential commands) and during the praxis subtests of the WAB. John echoed entire sentences (Examiner: "Are you a doctor?" John: *Are you a doctor?... I'm not a doctor!*) and he occasionally modified the content of the echoed sentence to make it more appropriate (Examiner: "Does it snow in July?" John: *Does it snow in winter?*). In most cases, however, echoes were heard in syntactically complex constructions (Examiner: "Does March come before June?" John: *Come before?*). At times, when he had trouble understanding the meaning of a word (e.g., "chest") he produced a short phrase which contained the target word and repeated it several times to facilitate comprehension (e.g., "my *chest* hurts, my *chest* hurts"). John was fully aware of his auditory comprehension deficit and concerned by his inability to inhibit echolalia. He explained that he needed to incorporate fragments or the complete question into his responses in order to grasp their meaning.

Three years post-onset John still had severe mitigated echolalia that disturbed his functional communication. Previous treatments with standard speech-language therapy improved the aphasia symptoms but did not help reduce mitigated echolalia. Thus, John was invited to participate in a drug study to improve aphasic deficits (Berthier et al., 2009). He was randomly assigned to the placebo group. Initially, he received the placebo alone during 16 weeks, followed by a combined therapy with placebo and Constraint-Induced Aphasia Therapy (CIAT) (Pulvermüller et al., 2001; Pulvermüller & Berthier, 2008) during 2 weeks (weeks 16–18, 30 hours of therapy), then a period of placebo alone (weeks 18–20), and finally a period of washout (weeks 20–24). Post-baseline changes in aphasia severity were evaluated with the WAB at different times (weeks 16, 18, 20, and 24). The number of echolalic responses was tested using the Yes/No Questions subtest of the WAB. This task contains 20 questions that the client should answer only saying "yes" or "no." In 50% of the questions the correct answer is "yes" (e.g., question 15: "Will paper burn in fire?) and in the remaining ones the expected response is "no" (e.g., question 17: "Do you eat a banana before you peel it?).

During CIAT John was encouraged to avoid using echolalic repetition as a compensatory strategy when other participants asked him for an object depicted on a card. The use of mental echoing was also discouraged. To facilitate comprehension and reduce echolalia during the initial therapy sessions, only short, simple questions were used and more complex questions were introduced across training sessions. John did not show a clinically significant improvement in aphasia severity (week 16: 1.8 points; week 18: 2.0 points; week 20: 2.4 points; and week 24: 3.4 points. Note that only subjects improving > 5 points on the WAB-AQ are considered responders to treatment) (Berthier et al., 2009; Cherney, Erickson, & Small, 2010). Moreover, treatment with placebo alone (not associated to aphasia therapy) (week 16) did not improve echolalia either. However, the number of instances of mitigated echolalia in the 20 yes/no questions at baseline (12/20, 60%) showed a reduction of 50% immediately after CIAT (6/20, 30%; $p = 0.031$, McNemar test, two-tailed) and of 63% (2/20, 10%) 2 weeks later (week 20; $p = 0.002$, McNemar test, two-tailed). Six weeks after ending CIAT, the number of echolalic repetitions increased, but still remained lower than at baseline. Changes in echolalic behavior were not accompanied by improvement on the Yes/No Questions subtest, most likely due to a high baseline score (85% correct), but auditory comprehension (as measured by the WAB) showed improvement with CIAT (baseline: 7/10; week 18: 7.7/10). No clinically relevant benefits were observed in spontaneous speech or repetition.

Previous studies provided evidence that CIAT modifies repetition performance in PWA. Different changes have been reported, thus implying different mechanisms subserving residual repetition in chronic aphasia. Treatment with CIAT has been reported to improve impaired repetition (Breier et al., 2011). Breier and colleagues (2011) reported improved ability to repeat spoken sentences in a patient with chronic Broca's aphasia treated with CIAT. Improvement of aphasia was associated with functional and structural changes in white matter tracts mediating repetition (Breier et al., 2011). Alternatively, when repetition is relatively preserved, it can be used to improve other language functions (Kurland, Pulvermüller, Silva, Burke, & Andrianopoulos, 2012). Kurland and colleagues (2012) found that CIAT improved object naming in a client (HBL) with chronic transcortical motor aphasia who repeated verbal stimuli several times in a "self-generated ritual," whereas the improvement was less noticeable in another client (ITY) with chronic Broca's aphasia and impaired repetition of single words. The case of John provides new information on the role of CIAT on reducing disinhibited language function (echolalia). We implemented a strategy (discouraging the use of echolalia during comprehension of naming and requesting) embedded in CIAT (Egorova et al., 2014). Although CIAT is a group therapy, the intervention can be individually adjusted to the patient's needs, Thus, strategies to stop echolalia embedded in an activity/participation therapy such as CIAT produced beneficial effects which generalized to auditory comprehension.

REFERENCES

Abrams, R., & Taylor, M. A. (1976). Catatonia. A prospective clinical study. *Archives of General Psychiatry, 33*, 579–581.

Al-Janabi, S., Nickels, L. A., Sowman, P. F., Burianová, H., Merrett, D. L., & Thompson, W. F. (2014, February 4). Augmenting melodic intonation therapy with non-invasive brain stimulation to treat impaired left-hemisphere function: Two case studies. *Frontiers in Psychology, 5*, 37. doi:10.3389/fpsyg.2014.00037.

Arbib, M. A. (2010). Mirror system activity for action and language is embedded in the integration of dorsal and ventral pathways. *Brain and Language, 112*, 12–24.

Aron, A. R., Robbins, T. W., & Poldrack, R. A. (2014). Inhibition and the right inferior frontal cortex: One decade on. *Trends in Cognitive Sciences, 18*, 177–185.

Assal, G. (1985). An aspect of utilization behavior: Dependence on written language. *Revue Neurologique, 141*, 493–495.

Bakker, M. J., van Dijk, J. G., Pramono, A., Sutarni, S., & Tijssen, M. A. (2013). Latah: An Indonesian startle syndrome. *Movement Disorders, 28*, 370–379.

Bardi, L., Bundt, C., Notebaert, W., & Brass, M. (2015). Eliminating mirror responses by instructions. *Cortex, 70*, 128–136. doi:10.1016/j.cortex.2015.04.018.

Basso, A., Forbes, M., & Boller, F. (2013). Rehabilitation of aphasia. *Handbook of Clinical Neurology, 110*, 325–334.

Berthier, M. L. (1999). *Transcortical aphasias*. Hove, England: Psychology Press.

Berthier, M. L., Dávila, G., Green-Heredia, C., Moreno Torres, I., Juárez y Ruiz de Mier, R., De-Torres, I., & Ruiz-Cruces, R. (2014). Massed sentence repetition training can augment and speed up recovery of speech production deficits in patients with chronic conduction aphasia receiving donepezil treatment. *Aphasiology, 28*, 188–218.

Berthier, M. L., Fernández, A. M., Martínez-Celdrán, E., & Kulisevsky, J. (1996). Perceptual and acoustic correlates of affective prosody repetition in transcortical aphasias. *Aphasiology, 10*, 711–721.

Berthier, M. L., Froudist Walsh, S., Dávila, G., Nabrozidis, A., Juárez y Ruiz de Mier, R., Gutiérrez, A., ... García-Casares, N. (2013, Dec. 19). Dissociated repetition deficits in aphasia can reflect flexible interactions between left dorsal and ventral streams and gender-dimorphic architecture of the right dorsal stream. *Frontiers in Human Neuroscience, 7*, 873. doi:10.3389/fnhum.2013.00873.

Berthier, M. L., García-Casares, N., Walsh, S. F., Nabrozidis, A., Ruíz de Mier, R. J., Green, C, ... Pulvermüller, F. (2011). Recovery from post-stroke aphasia: Lessons from brain imaging and implications for rehabilitation and biological treatments. *Discovery Medicine, 12*, 275–289.

Berthier, M. L., Green, C., Higueras, C., Fernández, I., Hinojosa, J., & Martín, M. C. (2006). A randomized, placebo-controlled study of donepezil in poststroke aphasia. *Neurology, 67*, 1687–1689.

Berthier, M. L., Green, C., Lara, J. P., Higueras, C., Barbancho, M. A., Dávila, G., & Pulvermüller, F. (2009). Memantine and constraint-induced aphasia therapy in chronic poststroke aphasia. *Annals of Neurology, 65*, 577–585.

Berthier, M. L., & Lambon Ralph, M. A. (2014, Oct. 2). Dissecting the function of networks underpinning language repetition. *Frontiers in Human Neuroscience, 8*, 727. doi:10.3389/fnhum.2014.00727.

Berthier, M. L., Lambon Ralph, M. A., Pujol, J., & Green, C. (2012). Arcuate fasciculus variability and repetition: The left sometimes can be right. *Cortex, 48*, 133–143.

Berthier, M. L., & Pulvermüller, F. (2011). Neuroscience insights improve neurorehabilitation of poststroke aphasia. *Nature Reviews Neurology, 7*, 86–97.

Berthier, M. L., Pulvermüller, F., Green, C., & Higueras, C. (2006). Are release phenomena explained by disinhibited mirror neuron circuits? Arnold Pick's remarks on echographia and their relevance for modern cognitive neuroscience. *Aphasiology, 20,* 462–480.

Berthier, M. L., Starkstein, S. E., Leiguarda, R., Ruiz, A., Mayberg, H. S., Wagner, H., ... Robinson, R. G. (1991). Transcortical aphasia. Importance of the nonspeech dominant hemisphere in language repetition. *Brain, 114,* 1409–1427.

Bien, N., Roebroeck, A., Goebel, R., & Sack, A. T. (2009). The brain's intention to imitate: The neurobiology of intentional versus automatic imitation. *Cerebral Cortex, 19,* 2338–2351.

Bormann, T., & Weiller, C. (2012). "Are there lexicons?" A study of lexical and semantic processing in word-meaning deafness suggests "yes". *Cortex, 48,* 294–307.

Brain, R. (1965). *Speech Disorders.* London: Butterworths.

Brass, M., Ruby, P., & Spengler, S. (2009). Inhibition of imitative behaviour and social cognition. *Philosophical Transactions of the Royal Society B, 364,* 2359–2367.

Breier, J. I., Juranek, J., & Papanicolaou, A. C. (2011). Changes in maps of language function and the integrity of the arcuate fasciculus after therapy for chronic aphasia. *Neurocase, 17,* 506–517.

Brown, J. W. (1975). The problem of repetition: A study of "conduction" aphasia and "isolation" syndrome. *Cortex, 11,* 37–52.

Brown, J. W. (1982). Hierarchy and evolution in neurolinguistics. In M. A. Arbid, D. Caplan, & J. C. Marshall (Eds.), *Neural models of language processes* (pp. 447–467). New York: Academic Press.

Brust, J. C. M., Plank, C., Burke, A., Guobadia, M. M. I., & Healton, E. B. (1982). Language disorder in a right-hander after occlusion of the right anterior cerebral artery. *Neurology, 32,* 492–497.

Cambier, J., Masson, C., Benammou, S., & Robine, B. (1988). La graphomanie. Activité graphique compulsive manifestation d'un gliome fronto-calleux. *Revue Neurologique, 144,* 158–164.

Catani, M., & Thiebaut de Schotten, M. (2012). *Atlas of human brain connections.* New York: Oxford University Press.

Chen, Y., Li, Y. S., Wang, Z. Y., Xu, Q., Shi, G. W., & Lin, Y. (2010). The efficacy of donepezil for post-stroke aphasia: A pilot case control study. *Zhonghua Nei Ke Za Zhi, 49,* 115–118.

Cherney, L. R., Erickson, R. K., & Small, S. L. (2010). Epidural cortical stimulation as adjunctive treatment for non-fluent aphasia: Preliminary findings. *Journal of Neurology Neurosurgery and Psychiatry, 81,* 1014–1421.

Cho, Y. J., Han, S. D., Song, S. K., Lee, B. I., & Heo, K. (2009). Palilalia, echolalia, and echopraxia-palipraxia as ictal manifestations in a patient with left frontal lobe epilepsy. *Epilepsy, 50,* 1616–1619.

Civier, O., Tasko, S. M., & Guenther, F. H. (2010). Overreliance on auditory feedback may lead to sound/syllable repetitions: Simulations of stuttering and fluency-inducing conditions with a neural model of speech production. *Journal of Fluency Disorders, 35,* 246–279.

Cocchini, G., Crosta, E., Allen, R., Zaro, F., & Beschin, N. (2013). Relationship between anosognosia and depression in aphasic patients. *Journal of Clinical and Experimental Neuropsychology, 35,* 337–347.

Corballis, M. C. (2010). Mirror neurons and the evolution of language. *Brain and Language, 112,* 25–35.

Cummings, J. L., Benson, D. F., Hill, M. A., & Read, S. (1985). Aphasia in dementia of the Alzheimer type. *Neurology, 35*(3), 394–394.

Da Cruz, F. M. (2010). Verbal repetitions and echolalia in Alzheimer's discourse. *Clinical Linguistics & Phonetics, 24,* 848–858.

Della Sala, S., & Spinnler, H. (1998). Echolalia in a case of progressive supranuclear palsy. *Neurocase, 4,* 155–165.

Denny-Brown, D., & Chambers, R. A. (1958). The parietal lobe and behaviour. Research Publications. *Association for Research in Nervous and Mental Disease, 36*, 35–117.

De Renzi, E., Cavalleri, F., & Facchini, S. (1996). Imitation and utilisation behaviour. *Journal of Neurology, Neurosurgery and Psychiatry, 61*, 396–400.

De-Torres, I. & Berthier, M. (2016). Teletherapy for aphasia. Unpublished data.

Dobbinson, S., Perkins, M., & Boucher, J. (2003). The interactional significance of formulas in autistic language. *Clinical Linguistics & Phonetics, 17*, 299–307.

Echo (n.d.). Definition. Retrieved August, 25, 2016, from http://www.yourdictionary.com/echo.

Egorova, N., Pulvermüller, F., & Shtyrov, Y. (2014). Neural dynamics of speech act comprehension: An MEG study of naming and requesting. *Brain Topography, 27*, 375–392.

Ellis, A. W. (1984). Introduction to Byrom Bramwell's (1897) case of word meaning deafness. *Cognitive Neuropsychology, 1*, 245–248.

Fadiga, L., Craighero, L., Buccino, G., & Rizzolatti, G. (2002). Speech listening specifically modulates the excitability of tongue muscles: A TMS study. *The European Journal of Neuroscience, 15*, 399–402.

Fay, W. H., & Butler, B. V. (1968). Echolalia, IQ, and the developmental dichotomy of speech and language systems. *Journal of Speech, Language and Hearing Research, 11*, 365–371.

Finis, J., Enticott, P. G., Pollok, B., Münchau, A., Schnitzler, A., & Fitzgerald, P. B. (2013). Repetitive transcranial magnetic stimulation of the supplementary motor area induces echophenomena. *Cortex, 49*, 1978–1982.

Fisher, C. M. (1988). Neurologic fragments. I. Clinical observations in demented patients. *Neurology, 38*, 1868–1873.

Ford, R. A. (1989). The psychopathology of echophenomena. *Psychological Medicine, 19*, 627–635.

Forkel, S. J., Thiebaut de Schotten, M., Dell'Acqua, F., Kalra, L., Murphy, D. G., Williams, S. C., & Catani, M. (2014). Anatomical predictors of aphasia recovery: A tractography study of bilateral perisylvian language networks. *Brain, 137*, 2027–2039.

Francis, D. R., Clark, N., & Humphreys, G. W. (2003). The treatment of an auditory working memory deficit and the implication for sentence comprehension abilities in mild "receptive" aphasia. *Aphasiology, 17*, 723–750.

Franklin, S., Turner, J., Lambon Ralph, M. A., Morris, J., & Bailey, P. J. (1996). A distinctive case of word meaning deafness? *Cognitive Neuropsychology, 13*, 1139–1162.

Fridriksson, J., Hubbard, H. I., Hudspeth, S. G., Holland, A. L., Bonilha, L., Fromm, D., et al. (2012). Speech entrainment enables patients with Broca's aphasia to produce fluent speech. *Brain, 135*, 3815–3829.

Frith, C. D., & Frith, U. (2006). The neural basis of mentalizing. *Neuron, 50*, 531–534.

Fujii, T., Yamadori, A., Fukatsu, R., Ogawa, T., & Suzuki, K. (1997). Crossed mixed transcortical aphasia with hypernomia. *European Neurology, 37*, 193–194.

Gallese, V., Fadiga, L., Fogassi, L., & Rizzolatti, G. (1996). Action recognition in the premotor cortex. *Brain, 119*, 593–609.

Ganos, C., Ogrzal, T., Schnitzler, A., & Münchau, A. (2012). The pathophysiology of echopraxia/echolalia: Relevance to Gilles de la Tourette syndrome. *Movement Disorders, 27*, 1222–1229.

Geschwind, N., Quadfasel, F. A., & Segarra, J. M. (1968). Isolation of speech area. *Neuropsychologia, 6*, 327–340.

Ghika, J., Bogousslavsky, J., Ghika-Schmid, F., & Regli, F. (1996). "Echoing approval": A new speech disorder. *Journal of Neurology, 243*, 633–637.

Ghika, J., Tennis, M., Growdon, J., Hoffman, E., & Johnson, K. (1995). Environment-driven responses in progressive supranuclear palsy. *Journal of the Neurological Sciences, 130*, 104–111.

Gold, M., Nadeau, S. E., Jacobs, D. H., Adair, J. C., Rothi, L. J., & Heilman, K. M. (1997). Adynamic aphasia: A transcortical motor aphasia with defective semantic strategy formation. *Brain and Language, 57,* 374–393.

Goldstein, K. (1915). Die transkorticalen Aphasien. *Ergebnisse der Neurologie und Psychiatrie, 2,* 349–629.

Grossi, D., Marcone, R., Cinquegrana, T., & Gallucci, M. (2013). On the differential nature of induced and incidental echolalia in autism. *Journal of Intellectual Disability Research, 57*(10), 903–912.

Hadano, K., Nakamura, H., & Hamanaka, T. (1998). Effortful echolalia. *Cortex, 34,* 67–82.

Hall, N., Boisvert, M., & Steele, R. (2013). Telepractice in the assessment and treatment of individuals with aphasia: A systematic review. *International Journal of Telerehabilitation, 5*(1), 27.

Heath, S., McMahon, K. L., Nickels, L., Angwin, A., MacDonald, A. D., van Hees, S., ... Copland D. A. (2012). The neural correlates of picture naming facilitated by auditory repetition. *BMC Neuroscience, 13,* 21.

Heath, S., McMahon, K. L., Nickels, L., Angwin, A., MacDonald, A. D., van Hees, S., ... Copland, D. A. (2013). Facilitation of naming in aphasia with auditory repetition: An investigation of neurocognitive mechanisms. *Neuropsychologia, 51,* 1534–1548.

Heyes, C. (2012). Grist and mills: On the cultural origins of cultural learning. *Philosophical Transactions of the Royal Society of London. Series B, Biological Sciences, 367,* 2181–2191.

Hickok, G., & Poeppel, D. (2007). The cortical organization of speech processing. *Nature Reviews. Neuroscience, 8,* 393–402.

Hobson, R. P. (1993). *Autism and the development of mind. Essays in developmental psychology.* Hove, England: Lawrence Erlbaum Associates.

Hodges, J. R., Patterson, K., Oxbury, S., & Funnell, E. (1992). Semantic dementia: Progressive fluent aphasia with temporal lobe atrophy. *Brain, 115,* 1783–1806.

Hoffmann, M. (2014). The panoply of field-dependent behavior in 1436 stroke patients. The mirror neuron system uncoupled and the consequences of loss of personal autonomy. *Neurocase, 20,* 556–568.

Hong, J. M., Shin, D. H., Lim, T. S., Lee, J. S., & Huh, K. (2012). Galantamine administration in chronic post-stroke aphasia. *Journal of Neurology, Neurosurgery, and Psychiatry, 83,* 675–680.

Hope, T. M., Prejawa, S., Parker Jones, O., Oberhuber, M., Seghier, M. L., Green, D. W., & Price, C. J. (2014, May 6). Dissecting the functional anatomy of auditory word repetition. *Frontiers in Human Neuroscience, 8,* 246. doi:10.3389/fnhum.2014.00246.

Hsu, T. Y., Tseng, L. Y., Yu, J. X., Kuo, W. J., Hung, D. L., Tzeng, O. J., ... Juan, C. H. (2011). Modulating inhibitory control with direct current stimulation of the superior medial frontal cortex. *Neuroimage, 56,* 2249–2257.

Iacoboni, M., Woods, R. P., Brass, M., Bekkering, H., Mazziotta, J. C., & Rizzolatti, G. (1999). Cortical mechanisms of human imitation. *Science, 286,* 2526–2528.

Ibañez, A., & Manes, F. (2012). Contextual social cognition and the behavioral variant of frontotemporal dementia. *Neurology, 78*(17), 1354–1362.

Kalinyak-Fliszar, M., Kohen, F., & Martin, N. (2011). Remediation of language processing in aphasia: Improving activation and maintenance of linguistic representations in (verbal) short-term memory. *Aphasiology, 25,* 1095–1131.

Kanner, L. (1943). Autistic disturbance of affective contact. *Nervous Children, 43,* 217–250.

Kertesz, A. (1982). *The Western Aphasia Battery.* New York: Grune and Stratton.

Kertesz, A., & Ferro, J. M. (1984). Lesion size and location in ideomotor apraxia. *Brain, 107,* 921–933.

Kertesz, A., Jesso, S., Harciarek, M., Blair, M., & McMonagle, P. (2010). What is semantic dementia? A cohort study of diagnostic features and clinical boundaries. *Archives of Neurology, 67,* 483–489.

Keysers, C., Kohler, E., Umiltà, M. A., Nanetti, L., Fogassi, L., & Gallese, V. (2003). Audiovisual mirror neurons and action recognition. *Experimental Brain Research, 153*, 628–636.

Klein, T. A., Ullsperger, M., & Danielmeier, C. (2013, Feb. 4). Error awareness and the insula: Links to neurological and psychiatric diseases. *Frontiers in Human Neurosciences, 7*, 14. doi:10.3389/fnhum.2013.00014

Koehler, K., & Jakumeit, U. (1976). Subacute sclerosing panencephalitis presenting as Leonhard's speech-prompt catatonia. *British Journal of Psychiatry, 129*, 29–31.

Koenig-Bruhin, M., & Studer-Eichenberger, F. (2007). Therapy of short-term memory disorders in fluent aphasia: A single case study. *Aphasiology, 21*, 448–458.

Kohler, E., Keysers, C., Umiltà, M. A., Fogassi, L., Gallesse, V., & Rizzolatti, G. (2002). Hearing sounds, understanding actions: Action representation in mirror neurons. *Science, 297*, 846–848.

Kohn, S. E., & Friedman, R. B. (1986). Word-meaning deafness: A phonological-semantic dissociation. *Cognitive Neuropsychology, 3*, 291–308.

Kohn, S. E., Smith, K. L., & Arsenault, J. K. (1990). The remediation of conduction aphasia via sentence repetition. *British Journal of Disorders of Communication, 25*, 45–60.

Kurland, J., Pulvermüller, F., Silva, N., Burke, K., & Andrianopoulos, M. (2012). Constrained versus unconstrained intensive language therapy in two individuals with chronic, moderate-to-severe aphasia and apraxia of speech: Behavioral and fMRI outcomes. *American Journal of Speech-Language Pathology, 21*, S65–87.

Lambon Ralph, M. A. (2010). Measuring language recovery in the underlying large-scale neural network: Pulling together in the face of adversity. *Annals of Neurology, 68*, 570–572.

Lebrun, Y. (1987). Anosognosia in aphasia. *Cortex, 23*, 251–263.

Lebrun, Y., Rubio, S., Jongen, E., & Demol, O. (1971). On echolalia, echo-answer, and contamination. *Acta Neurologica Belgica, 71*, 301–308

Lee, J., Fowler, R., Rodney, D., Cherney, L., & Small, S. L. (2010). IMITATE: An intensive computer based treatment for aphasia based on action observation and imitation. *Aphasiology, 24*, 449–465.

Leiguarda, R., Lees, A. J., Merello, M., Starkstein, S., & Marsden, C. D. (1994). The nature of apraxia in corticobasal degeneration. *Journal of Neurology, Neurosurgery & Psychiatry, 57*(4), 455–459.

Leonhard, K. (1957). *Aufteilung der endogenen Psychosen*. Berlin, Germany: Akademie.

Lhermitte, F. (1986). Human autonomy and the frontal lobes. Part II: Patient behavior in complex and social situations: The "environmental dependency syndrome". *Annals of Neurology, 19*, 335–343.

Lhermitte, F., Pillon, B., & Serdaru, M. (1986). Human autonomy and the frontal lobes. Part I: Imitation and utilization behavior: A neuropsychological study of 75 patients. *Annals of Neurology, 19*, 326–334.

Lind, A., Hall, L., Breidegard, B., Balkenius, C., & Johansson, P. (2014, March 28). Auditory feedback of one's own voice is used for high-level semantic monitoring: The "self-comprehension" hypothesis. *Frontiers in Human Neurosciences, 8*, 166. doi:10.3389/fnhum.2014.00166

Longcamp, M., Hlushchuk, Y., & Hari, R. (2011). What differs in visual recognition of handwritten vs. printed letters? An fMRI study. *Human Brain Mapping, 32*, 1250–1259.

López-Barroso, D., Catani, M., Ripollés, P., Dell'Acqua, F., Rodríguez-Fornells, A., & de Diego-Balaguer, R. (2013). Word learning is mediated by the left arcuate fasciculus. *Proceedings of the National Academy of Sciences of the United States of America, 110*, 13168–13173.

Luber, B., & Lisanby, S. H. (2014). Enhancement of human cognitive performance using transcranial magnetic stimulation (TMS). *Neuroimage, 85*, 961–970.

Maher, L. M., Rothi, L. J., & Heilman, K. M. (1994). Lack of error awareness in an aphasic patient with relatively preserved auditory comprehension. *Brain and Language, 46*, 402–418.

Majerus, S., van der Kaa, M.-A., Renard, C., Van der Linden, M., & Poncelet, M. (2005). Treating verbal short-term memory deficits by increasing the duration of temporary phonological representations: A case study. *Brain and Language, 95,* 174–175.

Marshall, J., Robson, J., Pring, T., & Chiat, S. (1998). Why does monitoring fail in jargon aphasia? Comprehension, judgment, and therapy evidence. *Brain and Language, 63*(1), 79–107.

Mashal, N., Solodkin, A., Dick, A. S., Chen, E. E., & Small, S. L. (2012). A network model of observation and imitation of speech. *Frontiers in Psychology, 3,* 84. doi:10.3389/fpsyg.2012.00084.

Massen, C., & Prinz, W. (2009). Movements, actions and tool-use actions: An ideomotor approach to imitation. *Philosophical Transactions of the Royal Society of London. Series B, Biological Sciences, 364,* 2349–2358.

McMorrow, M. J., & Foxx, R. M. (1986). Some direct and generalized effects of replacing an autistic man's echolalia with correct responses to questions. *Journal of Applied Behavior Analysis, 19,* 289–297.

McMorrow, M. J., Foxx, R. M., Faw, G. D., & Bittle, R. G. (1987). Cues-pause-point language training: Teaching echolalics functional use of their verbal labeling repertoires. *Journal of Applied Behavior Analysis, 20,* 11–22.

McPherson, S. E., Kuratani, J. D., Cummings, J. L., Shih, J., Mischel, P. S., & Vinters, H. V. (1994). Creutzfeldt-Jakob disease with mixed transcortical aphasia: Insights into echolalia. *Behavioural Neurology, 7,* 197–203.

Mengotti, P., Corradi-Dell'Acqua, C., Negri, G. A., Ukmar, M., Pesavento, V., & Rumiati, R. I. (2013). Selective imitation impairments differentially interact with language processing. *Brain, 136,* 2602–2618.

Merriam–Webster's Dictionary of English Usage. (1994). Springfield, MA: Merriam–Webster.

Mesulam, M. M. (1986). Frontal cortex and behavior. *Annals of Neurology, 19,* 320–325.

Milne, J. L., Anello, M., Goodale, M. A., & Thaler, L. (2015). A blind human expert echolocator shows size constancy for objects perceived by echoes. *Neurocase, 21*(4), 465–470. doi:10.1080/13554794.2014.922994.

Mori, E., & Yamadori, A. (1989). Rejection behaviour: A human homologue of the abnormal behaviour of Denny-Brown and Chambers' monkey with bilateral parietal ablation. *Journal of Neurology Neurosurgery and Psychiatry, 52,* 1260–1266.

Murakami, T., Restle, J., & Ziemann, U. (2012). Effective connectivity hierarchically links temporoparietal and frontal areas of the auditory dorsal stream with the motor cortex lip area during speech perception. *Brain and Language, 122,* 135–141.

Nozari, N., & Dell, G. S. (2013). How damaged brain repeats words: A computational approach. *Brain and Language, 126,* 327–337.

Nozari, N., Kittredge, A. K., Dell, G. S., & Schwartz, M. F. (2010). Naming and repetition in aphasia: Steps, routes, and frequency effects. *Journal of Memory and Language, 63,* 541–559.

Papathanasiou, I., Filipović, S. R., Whurr, R., Rothwell, J. C., & Jahanshahi, M. (2004). Changes in corticospinal motor excitability induced by non-motor linguistic tasks. *Experimental Brain Research, 154,* 218–225.

Passingham, R. E., Bengtsson, S. L., & Lau, H. C. (2010). Medial frontal cortex: From self-generated action to reflection on one's own performance. *Trends in Cognitive Sciences, 14,* 16–21.

Petrides, M. (2014). *Neuroanatomy of Language Regions of the Human Brain.* San Diego, CA: Academic Press.

Pick, A. (1924). On the pathology of echographia. *Brain, 47,* 417–429.

Pirozzolo, F. J., Kerr, K. L., Obrzut, J. E., Morley, G. K., Haxby, J. V., & Lundgren, S. (1981). Neurolinguistic analysis of the language abilities of a patient with a "double disconnection syndrome": A case of subangular alexia in the presence of mixed transcortical aphasia. *Journal of Neurology Neurosurgery and Psychiatry, 44,* 152–155.

Poeppel, D. (2001). Pure word deafness and the bilateral processing of the speech code. *Cognitive Science, 25*, 679–693.

Postma, A., & Noordanus, C. (1996). Production and detection of speech errors in silent, mouthed, noise-masked, and normal auditory feedback speech. *Language and Speech, 39*, 375–392.

Pridmore, S., Brüne, M., Ahmadi, J., & Dale, J. (2008). Echopraxia in schizophrenia: Possible mechanisms. *The Australian and New Zealand Journal of Psychiatry, 42*, 565–571.

Prigatano, G. P. (2009). Anosognosia: Clinical and ethical considerations. *Current Opinion in Neurology, 22*, 606–611.

Pulvermüller, F., & Berthier, M. L. (2008). Aphasia therapy on a neuroscience basis. *Aphasiology, 22*, 563–599.

Pulvermüller, F., & Fadiga, L. (2010). Active perception: Sensorimotor circuits as a cortical basis for language. *Nature Reviews Neuroscience, 11*, 351–360.

Pulvermüller, F., Huss, M., Kherif, F., Moscoso del Prado Martin, F., Hauk, O., & Shtyrov, Y. (2006). Motor cortex maps articulatory features of speech sounds. *Proceedings of the National Academy of Sciences of the United States of America, 103*, 7865–7870.

Pulvermüller, F., Moseley, R. L., Egorova, N., Shebani, Z., & Boulenger, V. (2014). Motor cognition-motor semantics: Action perception theory of cognition and communication. *Neuropsychologia, 55*, 71–84.

Pulvermüller, F., Neininger, B., Elbert, T., Mohr, B., Rockstroh, B., Koebbel, P., & Taub, E. (2001). Constraint-induced therapy of chronic aphasia after stroke. *Stroke, 32*, 1621–1626.

Pulvermüller, F., & Schönle, P. W. (1993). Behavioral and neuronal changes during treatment of mixed transcortical aphasia: A case study. *Cognition, 48*, 139–161.

Ragno Paquier, C., & Assal, F. (2007). A case of oral spelling behavior: Another environmental dependency syndrome. *Cognitive and Behavioral Neurology, 20*, 235–237.

Rauschecker, J. P., & Scott, S. K. (2009). Maps and streams in the auditory cortex: Nonhuman primates illuminate human speech processing. *Nature Neuroscience, 12*, 718–724.

Restle, J., Murakami, T., & Ziemann, U. (2012). Facilitation of speech repetition accuracy by theta burst stimulation of the left posterior inferior frontal gyrus. *Neuropsychologia, 50*, 2026–2031.

Rizzolatti, G., & Craighero, L. (2004). The mirror-neuron system. *Annual Review of Neuroscience, 27*, 169–192.

Rizzolatti, G., Fadiga, L., Fogassi, L., & Gallese, V. (1999). Resonance behaviors and mirror neurons. *Archives Italiennes de Biologie, 137*, 85–100.

Rothi, L. J., Fuller, R., Leon, S. A., Kendall, D., Moore, A., Wu, S. S., et al. (2009). Errorless practice as a possible adjuvant to donepezil in Alzheimer's disease. *Journal of the International Neuropsychological Society, 15*, 311–322.

Rutter, M. (1974). The development of infantile autism. *Psychological Medicine, 4*, 147–163.

Saad, A. G., & Goldfeld, M. (2009). Echolalia in the language development of autistic individuals: A bibliographical review. *Pró Fono, 21*, 255–260.

Saldert, C., & Hartelius, L. (2011). Echolalia or functional repetition in conversation—A case study of an individual with Huntington's disease. *Disability and Rehabilitation, 33*(3), 253–260.

Salis, C. (2012). Short-term memory treatment: Patterns of learning and generalisation to sentence comprehension in a person with aphasia. *Neuropsychological Rehabilitation, 22*, 428–448.

Santiesteban, I., White, S., Cook, J., Gilbert, S. J., Heyes, C., & Bird, G. (2012). Training social cognition: From imitation to theory of mind. *Cognition, 122*(2), 228–235.

Sarasso, S., Määttä, S., Ferrarelli, F., Poryazova, R., Tononi, G., & Small, S. L. (2014). Plastic changes following imitation-based speech and language therapy for aphasia: A high-density sleep EEG study. *Neurorehabililation and Neural Repair, 28*, 129–138.

Saur, D., Kreher, B. W., Schnell, S., Kümmerer, D., Kellmeyer, P., Vry, M. S., ... Weiller, C. (2008). Ventral and dorsal pathways for language. *Proceedings of the National Academy of Sciences of the United States of America, 105,* 18035–18040.

Schlaug, G., Marchina, S., & Norton, A. (2009). Evidence for plasticity in white-matter tracts of patients with chronic Broca's aphasia undergoing intense intonation-based speech therapy. *Annals of the New York Academy of Sciences, 1169,* 385–394.

Seniów, J., Litwin, M., Litwin, T., Leśniak, M., & Członkowska, A. (2009). New approach to the rehabilitation of post-stroke focal cognitive syndrome: Effect of levodopa combined with speech and language therapy on functional recovery from aphasia. *Journal of the Neurological Sciences, 283,* 214–218.

Shallice, T., Burgess, P. W., Schon, F., & Baxter, D. M. (1989). The origins of utilization behaviour. *Brain, 112,* 1587–1598.

Shuren, J. E., Hammond, C. S., Maher, L. M., Rothi, L. J. G., & Heilman, K. M. (1995). Attention and anosognosia: The case of a jargon aphasic patient with unawareness of language deficit. *Neurology, 45,* 376–378.

Shuttleworth, E. C., Yates, A. J., & Paltan-Ortiz, J. D. (1985). Creutzfeldt-Jakob disease presenting as progressive aphasia. *Journal of the National Medical Association, 77,* 649–656.

Small, S. L., Buccino, G., & Solodkin, A. (2010). The mirror neuron system and treatment of stroke. *Developmental Psychobiology, 54,* 293–310.

Smania, N., Gandolfi, M., Aglioti, S. M., Girardi, P., Fiaschi, A., & Girardi, F. (2010). How long is the recovery of global aphasia? Twenty-five years of follow-up in a patient with left hemisphere stroke. *Neurorehabilitation and Neural Repair, 24,* 871–875.

Snowden, J. S., Goulding, P. J., & Neary, D. (1989). Semantic dementia: A form of circumscribed cerebral atrophy. *Behavioural Neurology, 2,* 167–182.

Sparks, R., Helm, N., & Albert, M. (1974). Aphasia rehabilitation resulting from melodic intonation therapy. *Cortex, 10,* 303–316.

Speedie, L. J., Coslett, H. B., & Heilman, K. M. (1984). Repetition of affective prosody in mixed trans-cortical aphasia. *Archives of Neurology, 41,* 268–270.

Starkstein, S. E., Sabe, L., Chemerinski, E., Jason, L., & Leiguarda, R. (1996). Two domains of anosognosia in Alzheimer's disease. *Journal of Neurology Neurosurgery and Psychiatry, 61,* 485–490.

Stengel, E. (1947). A clinical and psychological study of echo-reactions. *Journal of Mental Science, 93,* 598–612.

Stribling, P., Rae, J., & Dickerson, P. (2007). Two forms of spoken repetition in a girl with autism. *International Journal of Language & Communication Disorders, 42,* 427–444.

Susuki, K., Yamadori, A., Kumabe, T., Endo, K., Fujii, T., & Yoshimoto, T. (2000). Hyperlexia in an adult patient with lesions in the left medial frontal lobe. *Rinsho Shinkeigaku, 40,* 393–397.

Suzuki, T., Itoh, S., Arai, N., Kouno M., Noguchi, M., Takatsu, M., & Takeda, K. (2012). Ambient echolalia in a patient with germinoma around the bilateral ventriculus lateralis: A case report. *Neurocase, 18,* 330–335.

Suzuki, T., Itoh, S., Hayashi, M., Kouno, M., & Takeda, K. (2009). Hyperlexia and ambient echolalia in a case of cerebral infarction of the left anterior cingulate cortex and corpus callosum. *Neurocase, 15,* 384–389.

Symonds, C. (1953). Aphasia. *Journal of Neurology Neurosurgery and Psychiatry, 16,* 1–16.

Tanaka, Y., Albert, M. L., Hara, H., Miyashita, T., & Kotani, N. (2000). Forced hyperphasia and environmental dependency syndrome. *Journal of Neurology Neurosurgery and Psychiatry, 68,* 224–226.

Toates, F. (2006). A model of the hierarchy of behaviour, cognition, and consciousness. *Consciousness and Cognition, 15,* 75–118.

Tokimura, H., Tokimura, Y., Oliviero, A., Asakura, T., & Rothwell, J. C. (1996). Speech-induced changes in corticospinal excitability. *Annals of Neurology, 40*, 628–634.

Ueno, T., & Lambon Ralph, M. A. (2013, Aug. 26). The roles of the "ventral" semantic and "dorsal" pathways in conduite d'approche: A neuroanatomically-constrained computational modeling investigation. *Frontiers in Human Neuroscience, 7*, 422. doi:10.3389/fnhum.2013.00422.

Ueno, T., Saito, S., Rogers, T. T., & Lambon Ralph, M. A. (2011). Lichtheim 2: Synthesizing aphasia and the neural basis of language in a neurocomputational model of the dual dorsal-ventral language pathways. *Neuron, 72*(2), 385–396.

Ungvari, G. S., & Rankin, J. A. (1990). Speech-prompt catatonia: A case report and review of the literature. *Comprehensive Psychiatry, 31*, 56–61.

Van Vugt, P., Paquier, P., Kees, L., & Cras, P. (1996). Increased writing activity in neurological conditions. A review and clinical study. *Journal of Neurology, Neurosurgery and Psychiatry, 61*, 510–514.

Vercuil, L., & Klinger, H. (2001). Loss of silent reading in frontotemporal dementia: Unmasking the inner speech. *Journal of Neurology, Neurosurgery and Psychiatry, 70*(5), 705–706.

Vines, B., Norton, A., & Schlaug, G. (2011). Non-invasive brain stimulation enhances the effects of melodic intonation therapy. *Frontiers in Psychology, 2*, 230. doi:10.3389/fpsyg.2011.00230.

Vocat, R., & Vuilleumier, P. (2010). Neuroanatomy of impaired body awareness in anosognosia and hysteria: A multicomponent account. In G. P. Prigatano (Ed.), *The study of anosognosia* (pp. 359–406). Oxford, England: Oxford University Press.

Walker-Batson, D., Curtis, S., Natarajan, R., Ford, J., Dronkers, N., Salmeron, E., ... & Unwin, D. H. (2001). A double-blind, placebo-controlled study of the use of amphetamine in the treatment of aphasia. *Stroke, 32*, 2093–2098.

Wallesch, C. W. (1990). Repetitive verbal behaviour: Functional and neurological considerations. *Aphasiology, 4*, 133–154.

Watkins, K. E., Strafella, A. P., & Paus, T. (2003). Seeing and hearing speech excites the motor system involved in speech production. *Neuropsychologia, 41*, 989–994.

Watson, R. T., Fleet, W. S., Gonzalez-Rothi, L., & Heilman, K. M. (1986). Apraxia and the supplementary motor area. *Archives of Neurology, 43*(8), 787–792.

Wenstrup, J. J., & Portfors, C. V. (2011). Neural processing of target distance by echolocating bats: Functional roles of the auditory midbrain. *Neuroscience and Biobehavioral Reviews, 35*, 2073–2083.

Wernicke, C. (1977). *Wernicke's works on aphasia: A sourcebook and review* (pp. 91–145). [Der aphasische Symptomencomplex. Eine psychologische Studie auf anatomischer Basis]. (G.H. Eggert, Trans). New York: Mouton. (Original work published 1874).

Whitaker, H. (1976). A case of the isolation of the speech area. In H. Whitaker & H. A. Whitaker (Eds.), *Studies in neurolinguistics* (Vol. *1*; pp. 1–58). New York: Academic Press.

Zipse, L., Norton, A., Marchina, S., & Schlaug, G. (2012). When right is all that is left: Plasticity of right-hemisphere tracts in a young aphasic patient. *Annals of the New York Academy of Sciences, 1252*, 237–245.

CHAPTER 6

Stroke-Related Acquired Neurogenic Stuttering

Luc F. De Nil
Catherine Theys
Regina Jokel

INTRODUCTION

Neurological conditions, such as stroke, may result in the sudden or gradual development of speech disfluencies in adults. Quite frequently, these disfluencies in neurogenic stuttering closely resemble, at least behaviorally, the sound and part-word repetitions, prolongations, and blocks that are considered to be the core fluency disruptions of developmental stuttering. Stuttering-like disfluencies associated with neurological conditions in adults commonly are referred to as neurogenic stuttering (De Nil, Rochon, & Jokel, 2008; Helm-Estabrooks, 2005), although several other terms have been proposed such as cortical stuttering (Rosenbek, Messert, Collins, & Wertz, 1978), Stuttering Associated with Acquired Neurological Disorders (SAAND; Helm-Estabrooks, 1999), and adult onset stuttering, among others.

The recognition that stuttering or stuttering-like speech fluency disruptions can occur in adults following brain disease is not new. Indeed, Kussmaul (1877) reported on a young adult who suffered a mild stroke and subsequently developed stuttering-like disfluencies, which he called "Aphatische Stottern." A few years later, Pick (1899) reported on a 63-year-old stroke patient who also developed acquired stuttering. As an interesting aside, Pick had previously alluded to the fact that the study of such acquired stuttering may lead to greater insight into the nature and etiology of developmental stuttering, a question that until today has generated some interesting discussions (Krishnan & Tiwari, 2013; Theys,

De Nil, Thijs, van Wieringen, & Sunaert, 2013; Van Borsel & Taillieu, 2001). Since those early case reports, many more published case studies have appeared describing stuttering in adults with various neurological disorders including stroke, Parkinson's disease, amyotrophic lateral sclerosis, traumatic brain injury, and tumor. Less frequently, some patients have been reported to develop stuttering-like speech disturbances secondary to medication exposure, encephalitis, and anorexia nervosa (for a review see De Nil, Jokel, & Rochon, 2007).

In this chapter we will focus on the characteristics of acquired neurogenic stuttering in patients who have experienced a stroke. The emphasis will be on behavioral and neural characteristics of the speech disfluencies in these patients, complemented by a detailed description of a preferred assessment protocol for neurogenic stuttering and a review of treatment approaches that have been described in the literature. First, however, a few words about terminology. We prefer the term *acquired neurogenic stuttering* (ANS) when referring to the stuttering-like speech disfluencies that result from damage to the nervous system. We believe that this term may help to better differentiate this speech fluency disorder from developmental stuttering, which increasingly has been shown to be associated with both functional and structural neural deficits (Beal, Gracco, Lafaille, & De Nil, 2007; Chang, 2014; De Nil, 2004; Smits-Bandstra & De Nil, 2007) and thus could also be argued to be "neurogenic." In addition, we also will use the term *stroke-related neurogenic stuttering*, where it is helpful to differentiate the disfluencies observed in stroke patients from those seen in patients with other nervous system disorders. Finally, it is important to point out that acquired stuttering may also result from psychogenic disorders (Baumgartner, 1999; Binder, Spector, & Youngjohn, 2012), in which case it is often labeled *acquired psychogenic stuttering*, or *psychogenic stuttering* for short. While psychological factors undoubtedly may influence the development and manifestation of speech fluency disorders, whether developmental or acquired, acquired psychogenic stuttering as a separate disorder will not be discussed in detail in this chapter.

CHARACTERISTICS OF ACQUIRED NEUROGENIC STUTTERING

Pick (1899), as discussed by Bijleveld (2001), was one of the first clinician-researchers to try to identify speech characteristics that he believed to be specific to ANS (Pick himself used the term "stuttering with aphasia"). According to Pick, ANS could be characterized by (1) stuttering at word-initial positions especially for difficult words, (2) repetitions of syllables and one-syllable words, (3) repetitions in the middle of the word, and (4) possible repetitions of final consonants. More recently, Canter (1971) proposed that ANS could be differentiated into three subgroups (dysarthric stuttering, apraxic stuttering, and dysnomic stuttering) and described a number of speech characteristics that he thought would be useful in differentiating among these three subgroups. These characteristics have been widely quoted and have significantly influenced how subsequent clinicians and researchers have described and understood ANS. According to Canter, the seven general characteristics of ANS are: (1) repetitions and prolongations of final consonants; (2) stuttering primarily on /r/, /l/, and /h/; (3) no systematic relationship to the grammatical class of the words; (4) an inverse relationship between the likelihood of disfluencies and the propositionality of the text (e.g., choral speech and word repetitions more disfluent than self-formulated speech); (5) no decrease in disfluency with repeated reading of a text (adaptation effect); (6) no marked anxiety; and (7) no secondary behaviors. Helm-Estabrooks (1999) echoed Canter's observations when discussing differential speech characteristics of neurogenic, developmental, and psychogenic stuttering, but selected only five (leaving out the sound-specific stuttering and the link to propositionality) and added one more, namely that the occurrence of stuttering remains relatively consistent across various types of speech tasks.

While these attempts to characterize ANS have been important and influential in stimulating careful observation and better understanding of this speech fluency disorder, the story is far from clear. Subsequent observations and case studies as well as group studies and systematic reviews of the literature, have clearly pointed to the presence of significant interindividual variability (De Nil et al., 2008; Helm-Estabrooks, 2005; Theys et al., 2013; Van Borsel, 1997). Furthermore, different neural diseases or traumas have been shown to be associated with varying speech disfluency characteristics (De Nil et al., 2008; Theys, van Wieringen, & De Nil, 2008; Van Borsel, 2014). Indeed, it is important to note that most of the supposedly defining characteristics of speech disfluencies in ANS, like those listed in clinical textbooks such as Manning (2009) and Guitar (2014), have been described with little or no differentiation of the underlying neuropathological condition. As we have discussed elsewhere (De Nil et al., 2007), it is unlikely that such a general characterization will be clinically useful in light of the fact that the nature and frequency of disfluency characteristics differ between various neurodegenerative and traumatic brain conditions. Even more so, Van Borsel and Taillieu (2001) concluded "the demarcation between neurogenic stuttering and developmental stuttering as far as symptomatology is concerned, is not always very clear" (p. 392). In this study the researchers asked professional judges, each with experience in the assessment and treatment of people who stutter, to diagnose either neurogenic or developmental stuttering based on videotaped speech samples of eight patients (four neurogenic and four developmental). Twenty-four percent were diagnosed incorrectly and several responders admitted to being uncertain about their diagnosis, with correct diagnoses for individual patients ranging from 44 to 100%. Correct diagnosis was more likely for patients with more severe stuttering. The results from this study support the observation, shared by many clinicians who work with these patients, that while it may be possible to differentiate between ANS and developmental stuttering at a population level, it can be very difficult or sometimes impossible to make the differentiation at an individual level, especially when relying solely on observable disfluency levels or clinical observation of behavioral symptoms.

The fact that ANS cannot be associated with a homogeneous behavioral manifestation casts doubt on the validity of previous attempts to describe differential speech fluency characteristics in these patients. This prompted Lundgren, Helm-Estabrooks, and Klein (2010) to state that "it would appear that sufficient level of uncertainty has been raised about the validity of the 'six features of neurogenic stuttering' that they should be collectively regarded as a 'rule of thumb' rather than pathognomonic indicators of neurogenic stuttering" (p. 2).

Given the scope of this book, and recognizing the significant variation with which ANS can manifest itself, the remainder of this chapter will focus specifically on stroke-related ANS. We will nevertheless from time to time refer to the broader literature on ANS when it will assist in understanding an issue faced by clinicians and researchers. The discussion will be based on our own observations on ANS, as well as an in-depth review of case studies and patient reports in the literature to date. Finally, while much of the research discussed in this chapter will focus on characteristics of stuttering-like disfluencies in these patients' speech, in particular the presence of sound and part-word repetitions, prolongations, and blocks, which are considered the core disfluency characteristics of developmental stuttering, it must be recognized that many of these patients also display as part of their speech patterns, disfluencies that differ from those typically labeled as stuttering. Such disfluencies may include phrase repetitions and revisions, sound groping, incomplete phrases, word-finding difficulties, etc. These latter disfluencies are often described as typical, nonstuttering disfluencies in the developmental stuttering literature, but in stroke patients, some of these may also be associated with concomitant neurogenic speech or language problems, such as apraxia or anomia in stroke patients. Without a doubt, these nonstuttering disfluencies are important in characterizing the overall speech patterns of patients but clinically differentiating them from stuttering disfluencies in individual patients may not always be very straightforward.

INCIDENCE OF ACQUIRED NEUROGENIC STUTTERING IN STROKE

The incidence and prevalence of ANS in general and stroke-related acquired stuttering in particular have been described as "rare" or "infrequent" (Ludlow, Rosenberg, Salazar, Grafman, & Smutok, 1987; Osawa, Maeshima, & Yoshimura, 2006). Few studies have tried to obtain an accurate estimate of the true incidence and prevalence of this acquired disfluency disorder. Most of the reports on incidence or prevalence were based on indirect data and clinical impressions, while systematic estimates usually were deduced from survey studies of practicing clinicians. For instance, Market, Montague, Buffalo, and Drummond (1990) contacted more than 150 clinicians in a variety of clinical facilities from across the United States. Of these, 100 clinicians indicated that they or one of their colleagues had seen at least one person with acquired stuttering. These clinicians were mailed a questionnaire and 81 completed questionnaires were returned. While it is not known exactly from the article how the contacted facilities were initially selected, the results suggest that it may not be unusual for clinician to assess and treat individuals with ANS. Of the 81 patients for whom completed data were available, 37% were stroke patients, while just over 38% were identified as having experienced head trauma, confirming other reports that these etiologies are most commonly associated with ANS.

To our knowledge, the only direct prospective study of the incidence and prevalence of stuttering in stroke patients has been reported by Theys, van Wieringen, Sunaert, Thijs, and De Nil (2011). In this study, all patients who were admitted to the stroke unit in a large university hospital in Belgium during a 1-year period (*N* = 582) were screened for the presence of acquired stuttering. Of all admitted patients, 319 received a final diagnosis of stroke. Each of these patients was screened for speech fluency difficulties four times during a 12-month period following the initial diagnosis of the stroke. The first screening was completed during the acute phase shortly after admission to the hospital and consisted of a bedside conversation with the patient, information on past and current speech fluency, as well as other case information from a close relative. Three more follow-up screenings took place for all patients that could be contacted. The first follow-up screening was done by the clinician 1 month after the initial hospital admission. The second follow-up screening took place during the 3-month routine follow up in the hospital. This screening was conducted using a speech and language questionnaire that was completed jointly by the patient and his or her neurologist. The final screening took place 1 year after the initial hospital admission and was conducted again by the clinician. These screenings identified 33 patients with potential ANS. Subsequently, each of these patients was administered an in-depth battery of speech, language, and cognitive ability tests. Using the common criterion of 3% or more stuttering-like disfluencies (sound and syllable repetitions, sound prolongations, and silent or audible blocks in speech) during conversation, monologue, or reading of a text, 17 of the 33 patients were identified with ANS. This finding suggests an incidence of stroke-related ANS of 5.3%. Of the 17 stroke patients (age range 51–87 years) diagnosed with ANS 10 were male. This directly observed incidence coincides with the generally accepted incidence of approximately 5% for developmental stuttering (Bloodstein & Bernstein-Ratner, 2008), although the precise implications of this finding are not yet clear.

Fourteen of the 17 patients were available for extensive follow-up testing. For eight patients the stuttering persisted for more than 6 months following stroke onset, resulting in an incidence of persistent stuttering in 2.5%, among the total number of stroke patients investigated. Those patients who recovered from their stuttering did not receive speech fluency therapy, possibly implying that for approximately half of the patients, spontaneous recovery can be expected in the first months following their stroke. Of course, it cannot be excluded that language recovery during this time period, as well as indirect benefits from speech therapy not directly targeting speech fluency, also may have contributed to recovery from stuttering. This raises a number of important and interesting questions that deserve further investigation.

BEHAVIORAL AND NEURAL CHARACTERISTICS OF ACQUIRED NEUROGENIC STUTTERING ASSOCIATED WITH STROKE

In an attempt to obtain a comprehensive picture of ANS in stroke patients, we searched the literature for published case observations, case studies, and larger-scale studies. This resulted in a review of 53 published papers on neurogenic stuttering in stroke patients, published between 1996 and 2013 (these papers are identified in the reference list). While studies varied in the amount of data provided for each patient, our analysis yielded relatively detailed information on 127 stroke patients with ANS. The age range of these patients was 2 to 85 years with a median age of 56 years. As expected, the majority of the patients were older than 50 years, although we found a number of case reports of children younger than age 10 years who had suffered a stroke and who were suspected of having developed a juvenile form of acquired stuttering (Meyers, Hall, & Aram, 1990; Nass, Schreter, & Heier, 1994; Perez, Gubser-Mercati, & Davidoff, 1996). In these young children, it is possible that the neurological event caused ANS or, alternatively, acted as a trigger event for the onset of developmental stuttering. Future detailed analyses on a larger sample of young stroke patients focusing on factors predictive of developmental stuttering, such as family history, sex, and the differential time course of stuttering-like disfluencies and other disfluencies, may help with developing criteria for differential diagnosis.

Most stroke patients seen in clinical practice do not present with a history of developmental stuttering. As a result, the onset of ANS in these patients can with reasonable confidence be linked directly to the stroke. For some, however, there is a reported history of developmental stuttering from which the patient either recovered completely or experienced a decrease in severity over time. The stroke, then, most likely resulted in a recurrence of stuttering or an increase in severity (Mouradian, Paslawski, & Shuaib, 2000).

The majority of the stroke patients with ANS who were included in our literature review were male (N =92), while 34 of the patients were female (gender for one patient was not reported). Interestingly, this resulted in a sex ratio of approximately 2.5–3:1 which, coincidentally or not, is similar to that reported for developmental stuttering (Bloodstein & Bernstein-Ratner, 2008), and conforms to the data reported by Theys and colleagues (Theys et al., 2011). Of the patients for whom handedness reports were available, 56 were right-handed, 19 were left-handed, and one patient was ambidextrous.

Site of Stroke Lesion and the Relationship to Onset of Acquired Neurogenic Stuttering

Whether the onset of ANS can be linked to lesions in particular brain areas is an important question. The insights gained from this will not only contribute to our understanding of ANS but may also inform the development of neural models of speech production in general (Guenther, Ghosh, & Tourville, 2006). When analyzing the literature on stroke-related

ANS, 73 papers provided sufficiently detailed information regarding the site of the lesion. Not unexpectedly, the majority of the patients (N = 50) were reported to have a left-hemisphere lesion, 12 had right-hemisphere lesions, while eight patients developed ANS following a bilateral lesion. All but two of the 12 patients with right-hemisphere lesions were right handed. The two who were not were reported as ambidextrous. Similarly, most patients were diagnosed with cortical lesions (43 patients), but a significant number had subcortical (21 patients) or mixed cortical-subcortical lesions (10 patients). Slightly more patients were reported with intrahemispheric lesions in a single site (37 out of 79) than patients who experienced lesions in multiple sites (30 out of 79). When analyzing the location of the reported lesions it became apparent that both temporal and parietal cortical areas were most often associated with stroke-related ANS, but lesions were also reported in the frontal and, for a few patients, the occipital lobe. Among the subcortical regions associated with the onset of ANS, most lesions were located in the basal ganglia (most frequently the putamen and the caudate), but lesions were also seen in the cerebellum, brainstem, thalamus, and a number of other subcortical regions such as the internal capsule and corpus callosum. Clearly, the analysis of the lesion sites associated with ANS reported in these studies results in a rather complex picture, which may not be all that surprising given the complex distributed nature of the neural network involved in language and speech production (Guenther & Vladusich, 2012; Houde & Nagarajan, 2011).

The data discussed so far were based primarily on case studies, which differ significantly in the level of detail provided on the nature and site of lesion. To obtain more precise information on the relationship between lesion site and the onset of stroke-related ANS, we completed a large-scale prospective study during which detailed brain imaging data were obtained on 20 stroke patients who developed ANS (Theys et al., 2013). These data were then compared to those obtained from 17 stroke patients without ANS. Using voxel-based lesion-symptom mapping (vBLSM), the relationship between ANS and localization of the stroke lesion was analyzed in detail. In addition, all the patients were tested using an extensive battery, including cognitive, language, and speech tasks, and were diagnosed with stuttering using a 3% stuttering-like disfluencies criterion, as described above. Only right-handed patients were included in the analysis.

The results of the lesion-symptom analysis yielded nine specific brain regions that were significantly associated with the presence of ANS in stroke patients. Generally, these regions are located in the inferior frontal cortex, superior temporal cortex, intraparietal cortex, basal ganglia, and their white matter interconnections through the superior longitudinal fasciculus and internal capsule. All of these areas were localized in the left hemisphere and were identified as being part of a cortico-basal ganglia-cortical network, which largely overlaps with the neural speech production network (Guenther et al., 2006; Guenther & Vladusich, 2012). These findings allowed us to conclude that the presence of stroke-related ANS is not limited to lesions in one particular brain area, but rather it likely reflects the disintegration of a complex and highly integrated neural network of cortical and subcortical regions that have a crucial role in speech production. An interesting question would be how this neural network, or the lesions to this network, differs from the lesions associated with other speech disorders characterized by speech disfluencies, such as apraxia of speech. While the answer to this question still eludes us today, it could lead to more sophisticated and accurate differential diagnostic and intervention approaches for stroke-related ANS.

Disfluency Characteristics of Acquired Neurogenic Stuttering

Whether patients with ANS show differences in the nature and patterns of stuttering disfluencies is a question that has gained significant attention since the first systematic reviews on the topic were published (Canter, 1971). This interest has been fueled further by the belief that the type and pattern of disfluencies observed in ANS are useful indicators for differentiating neurogenic from developmental stuttering, or for identifying subgroups within the population of patients with ANS.

Subgroups
Despite considerable efforts, no clear subgroups have yet been identified based on observable disfluencies. Canter (1971), for instance, stated "since different foci of neural damage have systematically different effects on behavior, we should expect that there would be different types of neurogenic stuttering syndromes" (p. 140). As mentioned before, Canter suggested three types of ANS, which he identified as "dysarthric stuttering," "apraxic stuttering," and "dysnomic stuttering," based on the specific pattern of disfluency characteristics that is manifested. Few other authors have attempted to identify specific subgroups within ANS, but most recently, Van Borsel (2014) proposed a differentiation between "generally acquired" and "neurogenic" stuttering. He proposed that the first category could include subtypes such as psychogenic stuttering associated with acquired neurological disorders, and drug-induced stuttering, while the latter category could include subtypes such as thalamic stuttering and palilalia.

Core Characteristics
As part of our literature review on ANS in stroke patients, we analyzed the reported disfluency characteristics to assess if these would reflect an overall pattern different from that typically seen in developmental stuttering or other patients with ANS. In doing so, we focused primarily on the three types of disfluencies that are generally recognized to be core characteristics of developmental stuttering: sound or part-word repetitions, prolongations, and blocks (Bloodstein & Bernstein-Ratner, 2008).

   Of the 127 stroke patients for whom sufficient disfluency information was available, 22 were reported to show only sound, syllable, or single-word repetitions, and none exclusively demonstrated sound prolongations or articulation blocks. This finding confirms previous reports that repetitions are the most common stuttering disfluencies in stroke patients (De Nil et al., 2007). While many patients were observed to have repetitions accompanied by either prolongations or blocks, more (42 out of 127) experienced some combination of the three core stuttering disfluencies (repetitions, prolongations, and blocks).

It has often been stated that patients with ANS are more likely to demonstrate disfluencies in all positions within a word, especially final-word disfluencies, in contradistinction with developmental stuttering in which most disfluencies typically occur in the beginning of words (Canter, 1971; Helm-Estabrooks, 2005). We have argued earlier (De Nil et al., 2007) that this often-reported finding may not be accurate and, indeed, this seems borne out by our data obtained from the systematic case study review. Of the 72 patients for whom we had sufficient data to evaluate the location of disfluencies, 53 patients were reported with disfluencies that occurred exclusively or "mostly" in the initial word position. Only six of the 72 patients were observed to have some final sound disfluencies, while for 12 patients disfluencies were reported in the initial and/or medial (but not final) position of words. Among the patients who showed medial or final disfluencies, none was reported without demonstrating initial position disfluencies.

Frequency

The data from our longitudinal study of stroke patients in Belgium confirmed the heterogeneity in this population and demonstrated significant variability in their stuttering characteristics (Theys et al., 2011). In this study, 17 patients who were diagnosed with ANS showed significant variability in their overall frequency of stuttering. During conversation, the mean frequency of stuttering (as measured by percent syllables stuttered) was 6.0% (ranging from 0.6–19.4%), during monologue it was 4.1% (range: 1.0–10.9%), and during reading 2.6% (range: 0.0–10.3%). While stuttering frequencies during conversation and monologue were significantly correlated, no significant relationship was observed between reading and conversation or reading and monologue. Furthermore, and in agreement with other observations (Lundgren et al., 2010), a survey of clinicians who were experienced with assessing and treating stroke patients with ANS confirmed that the majority of their patients stuttered during multiple speech tasks, including singing, automatic speech, and reading, although some of the patients were reported to stutter only during spontaneous speech (Theys et al., 2008). The presence of stuttering during tasks that are often found to be fluency-inducing in developmental stuttering, may become a useful differential diagnostic marker.

Adaptation

Stuttering adaptation is one way in which stuttering has been observed to vary across speech tasks. Adaptation has been studied intensively in the developmental stuttering literature (Bloodstein & Bernstein-Ratner, 2008). In a typical stuttering adaptation task, participants are asked to repeatedly read aloud a standardized reading passage (typically about five consecutive times). On average, the frequency of stuttering decreases by about 50% from the first to the fifth reading (Max & Baldwin, 2010). Early interest in the adaptation effect was driven in part because of the belief that interindividual differences in adaptation could be predictive of treatment outcome (Bloodstein & Bernstein-Ratner, 2008), but this was not supported by the data, at least for developmental stuttering. More recently, it has been proposed that stuttering adaptation may provide an interesting phenomenon to study stuttering from a motor learning perspective (Max & Baldwin, 2010).

Several authors have proposed that patients with ANS are much less likely than those with developmental stuttering to show an adaptation effect. The absence of such an effect has been suggested to be one of the differentiating characteristics between neurogenic and developmental stuttering (Helm-Estabrooks, 2005; Krishnan & Tiwari, 2013) and that it may reflect a different etiology for the disorder. In an earlier review of the literature on ANS (De Nil et al., 2007), we suggested that stuttering adaptation may be more common than previously thought among patients with ANS, and that the likelihood of adaptation actually may differ based on the underlying neurological conditions that led to the development of stuttering in the first place. Our review of the literature yielded 28 cases of stroke patients for whom analysis of reading adaptation was part of the patient's assessment. Of these, 15 patients (10 males and five females) did not show reading adaptation during repeated reading of the same paragraph, while 13 patients did. This confirms our earlier observation (De Nil et al., 2008) that adaptation can be observed in about 50% of stroke patients who develop ANS. Similarly, Theys and colleagues (2011) tested reading adaptation in 13 stroke patients and found that approximately half ($N = 7$) showed a significant decrease in fluency during successive readings of a standardized text. It does not appear that the presence or absence of reading adaptation is linked to the lateralization of the stroke lesion. In our analysis, just under half of the patients who did not show adaptation ($N = 15$) had a lesion primarily located in the left hemisphere (seven patients), with four patients showing a right hemisphere lesion, and two patients demonstrating a bilateral lesion. Similarly, of the 13 patients (10 males and three females) who did show adaptation, just over half were reported to have lesions in the left hemisphere (7/13) with three patients having right hemisphere lesions, two had bilateral lesions and one had a lesion in the corpus callosum. In addition, no obvious differences were found in the site of the lesion within each hemisphere between the patients who showed adaptation versus those who did not.

While reading adaptation does not appear to be predictive of treatment outcome in developmental stuttering, we cannot say with certainty that this is also true for patients with ANS. Because stuttering disfluencies in these patients appear to be more consistent and less affected by temporal, situational, or task changes, it would not seem to be unreasonable to predict that if acquired stuttering in a given patient shows less consistency and decreased severity during repeated readings, this may point to greater sensitivity to the fluency-enhancing effects of treatment. However, for now, it is an empirical question that awaits further research. Unfortunately, while much of the research has focused on defining characteristics of ANS, far fewer investigators and clinicians have attempted to systematically document treatment outcomes, and such research is critically needed. The lack of strong evidence notwithstanding, we believe that assessing reading adaptation should be an integral part of assessment of stroke-related ANS because it may help identify elements of speech (e.g., specific sounds or words) that are consistently difficult for a given patient and, thus, should be specific targets for intervention.

CONCOMITANT BEHAVIORS AND SPEECH-RELATED ATTITUDES

Individuals who experience chronic speech fluency disorders often develop struggle and coping behaviors that over time may become habitual and form an integral part of their speech behavior, or in some cases, even be the predominant feature of their communication difficulties. Such behaviors are typically referred to as secondary or concomitant behaviors (Bloodstein & Bernstein-Ratner, 2008). In developmental stuttering, concomitant behaviors have been observed very early during the initial development of the disorder, but it is often thought that these behaviors are less likely to be seen in patients with ANS. In our review of the published studies on stroke-related ANS, sufficient detailed reports on concomitant behaviors were available for 40 stroke patients. Of these patients, half (20/40) displayed secondary behaviors. Most typically, the observed behaviors consisted of eye blinks, facial grimacing, and general signs of increased effort and tension. These behaviors can best be described as general indications of struggle behavior resulting from the efforts the patient is making during the attempt to produce a sound or word. Similarly, in a survey of clinicians (Theys et al., 2008), secondary behaviors were reported in approximately half of the 29 stroke patients with ANS (N = 16). The reported behaviors again consisted primarily of facial grimaces and associated movements of the limbs, although clinicians also reported postponement and avoidance behaviors used by patients to attempt to avoid saying the word on which stuttering was anticipated. Of special interest was the observation that most patients who reportedly did not display concomitant behaviors had lesions in the left hemisphere, while in the patients with such behaviors, the site of the lesion was more equally distributed between left and right hemispheres. In addition, a larger proportion of the 20 patients with secondary behaviors experienced lesions in cortical regions (10/20) than did patients without secondary behaviors (4/20). The reason for this difference, if indeed it is a real difference, is not clear. One possibility may be that the presence of concomitant behaviors is related to the severity and nature of additional speech and/or language deficits. Alternatively, the presence or absence of concomitant behaviors could be correlated with the severity of stuttering, or maybe with the length of time stuttering has been present. Our analysis did not allow us to answer these questions reliably and further research is needed. We believe that this is especially important because the presence of such behaviors may be of critical importance for mapping out the focus of intervention. For instance, the presence of avoidance or postponement behavior is often linked to a well-developed sense of anticipation of disfluencies in patients. The presence and accuracy of such anticipation may affect what strategies will be most effective during intervention. While anticipation of stuttering often results in increased tension and preparatory struggle in patients as they are preparing to utter the sound or word, typically resulting in even more severe stuttering, such anticipation also could be used with great effect to help a patient prepare to produce speech efficiently and more fluently or with less severe stuttering using strategies such as gentle onset or a slower, more stretched, production of the initial syllable or word (Guitar, 2013).

Similarly, the presence of speech-related attitudes and anxiety are important to assess, but unfortunately they are not commonly reported in studies on ANS, and even when they are, they often consist of subjective statements based on general clinical observations. The traditional view considers that ANS is not typically associated with negative speech attitudes or generalized communication anxiety (Canter, 1971). In our review of the literature, we were able to find sufficiently detailed descriptive data for 26 stroke patients. Of these patients, only eight were reported without signs of speech-related anxiety, while 15 of the 26 patients were reported to have anxiety, struggle, avoidance, or general negative attitudes toward their disfluencies, and three were said to be aware but not anxious. Similarly, in a recent survey study (Theys et al., 2008), 18 of the 29 stroke patients were reported by their clinicians to react emotionally to their stuttering, with reports of frustration, fear, anger, irritation, and crying in reaction to their stuttering. Clearly, these findings suggest that patients with stroke-related ANS often develop the same awareness and anxiety or frustration as is typically seen in adults with developmental stuttering. This observation was confirmed more systematically in a study by Jokel and colleagues (Jokel & De Nil, 2003; Jokel, De Nil, & Sharpe, 2007). These researchers administered the S-24 (Erickson, 1969), a questionnaire used to assess speech-related attitudes in individuals who stutter, the Locus of Control, version B (Craig, Franklin, & Andrews, 1984), and the Speech Situation Checklist (Vanryckeghem & Brutten, 2006), a self-assessment instrument for stuttering severity, to a group of stroke patients with ANS. The patients had an average score of 18 (out of 24) on the S-24 indicating a strong negative perception of their speech competency, although it is important to note that the items on this test mostly refer to speech in general and not specifically to speech fluency. Their score on the S-24 compares to an average score of 19 for adults with developmental stuttering. The results from the Locus of Control scale indicated a somewhat more external locus of control perception among stroke patients compared to individuals who stutter suggesting that they perceived their speech behaviors to be less under their personal control. The self-assessment of their severity across different situations yielded an average score of 3 on a 5-point scale, again suggesting that they perceive clear difficulties with speech fluency across a wide variety of situations in which communication is important.

Unfortunately, most reports on stroke-related ANS do not include detailed information on when the patient's speech fluency problems started. As such, it is possible that the absence of negative perceptions of speech, anxiety, or frustration in a number of patients may result from the fact that their lifetime experience with stuttering disfluencies has been relatively short. If this is true, one would expect a positive correlation between the duration of the speech fluency problems and the presence of such negative attitudes or reactions as the patient is repeatedly exposed to speech situations and tasks made difficult by the disfluencies. This limitation notwithstanding, it seems reasonable to assume that, at least in the case of stroke, while there may be some speech-related frustration and anxiety, the absence of extensive avoidance behaviors suggests that the experience of patients with their stuttering is sufficiently moderate as to be often overshadowed by the associated speech, language, or cognitive symptoms. Ironically, this may be one of the reasons why ANS is often underreported and may go unnoticed in clinical settings, precluding the initiation of appropriate intervention. Nevertheless, some patients with whom we worked did identify stuttering as their main problem, sometimes despite the presence of significant other cognitive and language problems, calling for greater attention to this disorder and more concerted efforts to find appropriate and effective treatment strategies.

COMORBID SPEECH, LANGUAGE, AND COGNITIVE IMPAIRMENTS

In the presence of comorbid speech and language impairments, it may be difficult or sometimes impossible to differentiate between certain types of speech (e.g., apraxia) or language (e.g., word finding) difficulties and stuttering.

Of the 95 stroke patients in our review for whom data on comorbid speech and language difficulties were reported, 27 patients (28%) were reported to have ANS as their only communication deficit. Given that approximately 30 to 40% of stroke patients experience dysarthria and/or aphasia (Flowers, Silver, Fang, Rochon, & Martino, 2013), this is not insignificant and points not only to the incidence of ANS in the clinical setting but also to the fact that ANS can and should be differentiated from other communication deficits. Of the 68 patients with reported comorbid disorders, the majority had either aphasia (20/95) or dysarthria without aphasia (15/95). Six patients had a combination of aphasia and dysarthria. Eight patients were reported to have comorbid anomia. Interestingly, only one of the 61 patients was reported with apraxia (in isolation) which provides further support that ANS is indeed different from the type of disfluencies often associated with apraxia of speech (Ballard, Granier, & Robin, 2000). Clinician reports, obtained as part of an earlier survey of ANS (Theys et al., 2008), revealed that the large majority of the reported patients with stroke-induced stuttering had other speech and language problems co-occurring with their stuttering. These included aphasia, specific word-finding problems, dysarthria, apraxia of speech, and dysphonia.

There did not appear to be a clear association between the lesion site and the comorbid occurrence of speech and language disorders in stroke patients with ANS. Maybe not surprisingly, most lesions in patients with such comorbid disorders were observed in the frontal, parietal, and temporal cortex, as well as the basal ganglia. An interesting observation was that while four times as many stroke patients with ANS had lesions primarily in the left hemisphere (50 patients) compared to right lateralized lesions (12 patients), the reverse was observed for patients with no comorbid speech and language disorders where 13 patients had primarily right lateralized lesions and lesions were left lateralized in six patients. This observation may lead one to conclude that while speech and language difficulties are primarily caused by lesions in left cortical and subcortical regions, the occurrence of stuttering may imply a greater involvement of disruptions of right hemisphere functions. This conclusion does find some support in the developmental stuttering literature (De Nil, Kroll, Lafaille, & Houle, 2003; Neef et al., 2011; Neumann et al., 2005) but deserves further investigation.

Some studies also report on comorbid cognitive deficits in stroke patients with ANS. Such reports are most often based on testing using the WAIS or Wechsler intelligence tests (Wechsler, 1997), or the Mini Mental State Examination (Folstein, Folstein, & McHugh, 1975). Of the 86 patients for whom such data were available, 37 were reported with cognitive deficits, primarily memory related, while 49 did not appear to have such deficits.

Direct testing of stroke patients (Theys et al., 2011) confirmed the findings from our literature review. When tested for the co-occurrence of ANS and aphasia, dysarthria, apraxia of speech, or cognitive problems, 14 of the 17 patients who were identified with ANS were diagnosed with one or more of these co-occurring disorders. Probably not surprisingly, aphasia was the most prevalent co-occurring disorder, with 11 of the 17 patients having aphasia. Dysarthria co-occurred with ANS in nine of the 17 stroke patients and cognitive problems were diagnosed in five patients. Apraxia of speech was only diagnosed in a minority ($N = 2$) of the patients. Interestingly, patients with co-occurring aphasia presented with a significantly higher frequency of stuttering compared to the group without aphasia, while such a relationship was not observed for the groups with co-occurring dysarthria or cognitive problems. Whether this implies a link between language deficits and ANS, as suggested for developmental stuttering (DiDonato, Brumbach, & Goffman, 2014; MacPerson & Smith, 2013), remains to be seen. Alternatively, it may be that concomitant language deficits place higher demands on motor planning and execution processes. For instance, research has demonstrated increased articulatory variability during syntactically more complex sentences, at least in children (MacPerson & Smith, 2013). It was also observed that the two patients with co-occurring apraxia of speech had relatively high frequencies of stuttering compared to the other patients (i.e., 6.5% and 19.4% stuttered syllables). This confirms that ANS is frequently part of a more complex picture of communication problems following stroke. Nevertheless, ANS was the only observed speech-language problem in three of the patients, confirming that this acquired speech fluency disorder can exist by itself.

CONCLUSIONS ON ACQUIRED NEUROGENIC STUTTERING

Our review of the existing literature on stroke-related ANS, combined with observations from our clinical experience and research, confirmed that while ANS is not present in all or even most patients who experience a stroke, it is not a rare component of these patients' overall communication difficulties. Indeed, most clinicians who work with stroke patients are likely to come across patients with ANS. Our review of the literature has shown that stroke-related ANS should indeed be seen as a communication disorder that deserves specific attention in terms of its identification and management (discussed later). In general, while differences may exist between the typical speech pattern seen in stroke-related stuttering compared to developmental stuttering, by and large these differences appear more quantitative than qualitative. This leads one to conclude that ANS in stroke patients appears to have more similarities than dissimilarities to developmental stuttering. This, in turn, points to a potentially common underlying neural signature for both types of atypical disfluencies. However, differential diagnosis of stuttering from other types of disfluencies in stroke patients can pose significant challenges and, as we will see next, an integrated assessment and treatment approach is often the best strategy to use.

ASSESSMENT OF ACQUIRED NEUROGENIC STUTTERING

As we have discussed, stroke-related ANS, similar to other forms of ANS, can manifest itself in many different ways depending on a number of factors, including nature and extent of the stroke lesion, the age of the patient, the time since onset, the presence of concomitant behaviors, and comorbid speech and language disorders. Patients also may exhibit motor or cognitive problems or have other related medical issues, which can affect their fluency performance. It is not surprising then that the assessment of ANS needs to be comprehensive, going beyond quantitative and qualitative speech fluency measures, and must be a highly individualized process. This will allow the clinician to consider the speech fluency difficulties in a patient from a broad and comprehensive perspective, form a coherent clinical picture, and design an individualized, well-grounded, and integrated intervention plan. Such a comprehensive assessment and treatment plan often will need to involve the expertise of a number of different health professionals. In this section, we will discuss some general strategies that we have found to be clinically useful for assessment.

One of the first questions to answer when assessing a patient is whether the observed stuttering is developmental or acquired. The answer to this question is not simply academic; it may lead one to contemplate what intervention strategies to use. For instance, if the patient has a history of developmental stuttering, the type of treatment received in the past may affect the decision about which intervention strategies are most promising in future treatment. In many cases, the answer to this differential diagnosis question is relatively clear, especially if the case history suggests that there is no reported or documented evidence of prior developmental stuttering, and there is a reasonable link between the onset or development of the neurological condition and the speech fluency difficulties. It is important to keep in mind, however, that even if there is evidence of pre-existing developmental stuttering, the neurological condition may have triggered a re-occurrence or aggravation of a pre-existing stuttering disorder (De Nil et al., 2007; Grant, Biousse, Cook, & Newman, 1999; Helm-Estabrooks, 2005; Marshall & Neuburger, 1987). In that case, the question may be raised whether the disfluencies can truly be called ANS, or rather should be considered developmental stuttering, or some combination of developmental and acquired stuttering. A definitive differential diagnosis may not be possible in all cases, and the speech and behavioral characteristics discussed in this chapter may provide some guidance in those cases where the differential diagnosis is unclear.

Another question that deserves some attention during the diagnostic process is whether the stuttering that is present is of neurogenic or psychogenic origin. Adults who experience a stroke may have significant psychological reactions, especially when the stroke has important implications for their daily activities, their quality of life, and their interactions with others in their environment. Stuttering itself, as we have seen, may result in strong negative attitudes toward one's ability to communicate.

Acquired neurogenic stuttering should also be clinically distinguished from psychogenic stuttering. According to Mahr and Leith (1992), psychogenic stuttering can best be identified by the following criteria: (1) a change in speech pattern suggesting stuttering; (2) a relationship to psychological factors as evidenced by an onset associated with emotional conflict and/or secondary gain; (3) the lack of evidence of an organic etiology; (4) a past history of mental health problems; (5) atypical disfluency features (stereotypical repetitions, no islands of fluency within conversational speech, and no secondary behaviors); (6) a perception of "la belle indifférence" in which the patient shows a lack of emotional responses to the disfluencies; and (7) interpersonal interactions of a somewhat unusual or bizarre quality. Duffy (2005) also includes the fact that intervention often has rapid (1–2 sessions) and dramatic fluency-improving effects in these patients, and there may be a lack of fluency reduction under choral reading, delayed auditory feedback, masking, singing, or even mimed speech. These criteria may be useful guidelines for assessing the presence or impact of psychogenic factors on stuttering. It is critical for diagnosis, however, to keep in mind that the apparent absence of a clearly identified neurological event preceding the onset of stuttering is not always a good indicator of the absence of ANS. The latter point is illustrated clearly by cases where the onset of stuttering effectively was the first observable symptom of a gradually developing medical condition (Lebrun, Leleux, Rousseau, & Devreux, 1983; Lebrun, Rétif, & Kaiser, 1983; Leder, 1996). Equally important is the fact that the presence of a neurological condition, such as stroke, does not preclude the diagnosis of psychogenic stuttering or the importance of psychological reactions in the development of stuttering severity. Indeed, people who experience a potentially devastating neurological disease, such as a stroke, may also develop psychological reactions that could manifest as psychogenic stuttering (Duffy & Baumgartner, 1997; Van Borsel, Van Lierde, Oostra, & Eeckhaut, 1997). It would indeed be very unusual for many stroke patients if they did not react with some degree of psychosocial concern to the often distressing neurological condition that they experience.

A Proposed Assessment Battery for Acquired Neurogenic Stuttering in Adults

In order to obtain a more detailed understanding of ANS, we have described a battery of tasks and tests known as the Assessment Battery for Acquired Stuttering in Adults

A. Case History
  a. Medical history, including neuroimaging data (structural and functional), if available
  b. Information on social and occupational history
  c. Information on personal and family speech and language history, including treatment history
  d. Detailed history and current status of disfluencies (onset and development) as well as previous treatment if applicable.
  e. Self-reported awareness of stuttering severity and secondary behaviors
B. Testing of General Functions
  a. Language functions (suggested tests: BDAE, BNT, PALPA, GORT, TROG, PPVT, PPTT)
  b. Speech production (suggested tests: ABA, Motor speech examination)
  c. Cognition (suggested test: MMSE)
C. Speech Fluency Assessment
  a. Reading: single words, short sentences, paragraph
  b. Spontaneous speech: monologue, conversation (minimum 200–600 syllables)
  c. More automatized speech such as counting, days, months, and singing
  d. Fluency enhancing techniques (suggested tasks: slowed speech, delayed auditory feedback, pacing)
  e. Speech situation checklist or self-reported stuttering severity in a variety of common communication situations
  f. Stuttering severity (SSI)
D. Self-Assessment of Attitudes (S-24, LCB)

FIGURE 6.1 Assessment Battery for Acquired Stuttering in Adults (ABASA), adapted from De Nil, Jokel, & Rochon (2007).

Abbreviations. MMSE = Mini-Mental State Examination (Folstein et al., 1975), BNT = Boston Naming Test (Goodglass et al., 2001), BDAE = Boston Diagnostic Aphasia Examination (Goodglass et al., 2001), TROG = Test for Reception of Grammar (Bishop, 1989), GORT = Gray Oral Reading Test (Wiederholt, 1992), PPVT-III = Peabody Picture Vocabulary Test (Dunn, 1997), PPTT = Pyramids and Palm Trees Test (Howard & Patterson, 1992), PALPA = Psycholinguistic Assessments of Language Processing in Aphasia (Kay, 1992), S-24 (Andrews & Cutler, 1974), SSI = Stuttering Severity Instrument (Riley, 1994), LCB – Locus of Control for Behavior (Craig et al., 1984).

(ABASA; see **FIGURE 6.1**) and described in greater detail later, that provides the clinician with a more complete picture of the nature and extent of the patient's stuttering difficulties (De Nil et al., 2007). Obviously not all of these tests and tasks need to be or can be administered for all patients. For instance, some reading or questionnaire tasks may be too difficult for some patients with aphasia. A clinician can and should use her or his discretion and clinical expertise to modify this battery depending on the patient, his or her needs, and the clinical setting in which the assessment takes place, by removing or adding additional speech, language, or cognitive tasks. This way, the information obtained as part of a clinical assessment is specific to each individual patient and will allow a clinician to form a well-informed and patient-specific clinical decision concerning the need for and the nature of further assessment and intervention.

Detailed Case History

Each assessment needs to include a detailed medical and developmental case history. In addition, medical stroke imaging information, if available, may provide important information to complement an assessment of the patient's stuttering. As outlined before, special attention should be given to the time since onset of the neurological problem in order to establish the connection between the stroke and the onset of stuttering. In addition, the presence of developmental stuttering as well as other speech and language problems and associated coping behaviors, should be thoroughly probed as it is not unusual for patients or their close relatives not to appreciate or recognize the presence of premorbid stuttering in light of the current communication difficulties.

If developmental stuttering was present prior to the stroke, special attention should be given to the early developmental years and changes in behavior as well as severity during the development of stuttering. The clinician should also probe the presence of secondary behaviors, and especially the nature and extent of any therapy that has been received, as well as the effectiveness of that treatment. Such information not only will be very useful in the planning of future intervention but also may help the patient to understand the nature of his or her fluency disorder and the rationale for the proposed intervention plan.

Speech Fluency Analysis

Any assessment of ANS should of course include a detailed analysis of the type, frequency, and severity of speech disfluencies. This is important in order to differentiate between disfluencies that occur in normal speech (and should not necessarily be treated) and those associated with stuttering (Guitar, 2013). For instance, research on patients with Tourette syndrome has shown that an overall higher frequency of typical disfluencies in the presence of infrequent stuttering disfluencies may nevertheless give the impression of stuttering in some patients (De Nil, Sasisekaran, Van Lieshout, & Sandor, 2005). In addition, a thorough fluency assessment should include the evaluation of how stuttering severity changes across speech tasks differing in complexity (De Nil et al., 2007). Such information, through direct testing in combination with self-reports, can be very critical in determining not only what intervention strategy to use, but also how effective the intervention is. For instance, if stuttering severity is measured in the clinic room, one should be careful in comparing the severity ratings obtained in that situation with those obtained during activities of daily living when measuring the impact of one's treatment.

It is important to evaluate the frequency and type of disfluencies in a variety of reading and spontaneous speech conditions, including monologue and conversation. Speech material should include simple (e.g., single word) and more complex utterances (e.g., sentences and continuous text). Clinicians can create their own tasks or use published material available in a number of widely available neurogenic language tests (e.g., Boston Diagnostic Aphasia Examination-3 [BDAE-3]; Goodglass, Kaplan, & Barresi, 2001) or clinical stuttering textbooks (Conture, 2000; Guitar, 2013; Shapiro, 1998). If possible, and depending on the language abilities of the patient, speech samples should be sufficiently long (at least 200–600 syllables) in order to provide a representative speech sample and an overall impression of the variability in stuttering severity. It is important to compare propositional speech (e.g., story telling or conversation) to simpler (e.g., single words) and automatic speech (e.g., counting or naming the days of the week), because people with ANS are more likely than people with developmental stuttering to continue experiencing significant disfluencies in the latter speech tasks (Duffy, 2005; Helm-Estabrooks, 2005). Because such simpler or automatic speech tasks may be the starting point for some treatment approaches, such as those in which fluency skills are first practiced on single syllables or words (Theys et al., 2008) it is important to assess the speech and language abilities of the stroke patient at that level of complexity. Sometimes it may be useful to test the effect of fluency-enhancing techniques, such as delayed auditory feedback, rhythmic speech, slowed speech, on the frequency and severity of disfluencies, because such testing may also suggest useful starting points for treatment (Theys et al., 2008; Van Borsel, Drummond, & de Britto Pereira, 2010).

Other Speech, Language, Cognitive, or Sensorimotor Tests

If possible and tolerated by the patient, the clinician should attempt to use standardized questionnaires, such as the S-24 (Andrews & Cutler, 1974) and the Locus of Control for Behavior (Craig et al., 1984), to assess perceptions and attitudes of the patient toward his or her own speech. Such questionnaires provide a useful and more objective complement to the clinician's own subjective impressions. In addition, it is good practice to administer cognitive tests, such as the Mini-Mental State Examination (Folstein et al., 1975) to screen for overall cognitive functioning. In light of the possible presence of concomitant speech, language, or cognitive deficiencies, it is important to test for comorbid deficiencies that may affect or aggravate the presence of disfluencies, or sometimes may even be mistaken for stuttering disfluencies (e.g., apraxia or word-finding difficulties). Several standardized tests for language and speech are available, including the BDAE-3 (Goodglass et al., 2001), the Boston Naming Test (BNT; Kaplan, Goodglass, & Weintraub, 2001), the Gray Oral Reading Test (GORT; Wiederholt & Bryant, 1992), the Psycholinguistic Assessment of Language Processing in Aphasia (PALPA; Kay, Lesser, & Coltheart, 1992), and the Apraxia Battery for Adults (Dabul, 2000) among others. Which specific tests should be administered clearly will depend on the nature of the stroke, as well as the presenting symptoms.

TREATMENT OF STROKE-RELATED ACQUIRED NEUROGENIC STUTTERING

Currently, there are no systematic reports on the relative effectiveness of one treatment approach over another for stroke patients who develop ANS. Furthermore, the study by Theys et al. (2011) showed that not all patients need treatment. About half of those who develop ANS recover in the absence of intervention, which is consistent with clinical observations. However, some patients do develop a more persistent form of ANS and may require targeted treatment intervention. Indeed, as we have seen, for some it is even the predominant or only communication disorder that persists following recovery from the stroke. Unfortunately, we do not yet have predictor variables to distinguish the patients who will recover spontaneously from those who will not.

A review of the available case studies of patients with stroke-related ANS shows that a wide variety of treatment techniques have been attempted, mostly corresponding to the variety of treatment approaches available for developmental stuttering, although none of these approaches has been specifically designed or evaluated for use with ANS. Typically, the reported intervention strategies can be classified along a continuum of fluency treatment, ranging from teaching and shaping of the speech motor skills necessary for fluency to approaches geared more toward general relaxation, cognitive reframing of the speech disfluencies, and acceptance of stuttering (Blomgren, 2013; Blomgren, Roy, Callister, & Merrill, 2005).

A survey of practicing clinicians (Theys et al., 2008) revealed that therapy focused specifically on the stuttering problems in 18 out of 23 stroke patients with ANS. The types of therapy included decreasing speech rate, increasing loudness, cognitive restructuring therapy, fluency shaping therapy, and breathing exercises. Our analysis of published reports revealed that only 11 of the 53 studies reported on speech fluency intervention with their stroke patients. Most of these reports only provided cursory descriptions of the intervention approach used and outcome data. Among those papers that reported some detail on the intervention protocol, all used either behavioral approaches (e.g., gentle onset, breathing exercises, slowed speech) or a combination of speech techniques with relaxation and cognitive restructuring. For instance, Krishnan, Nair, and Tiwari (2010) described a 51-year-old male who received three inpatient therapy sessions focusing on reducing stuttering by slowing down speech rate. They reported a reduction in stuttering from approximately 8 to 0.5% over those three sessions. The same authors (Krishnan & Tiwari, 2011) reported on another patient (56-year-old female) who received seven sessions of pacing therapy that resulted in fluent speech with occasional involuntary mouth movements. However, no further data were provided on treatment outcome. Rubow, Rosenbek, and Schumaker (1986) used a combination of breathing, relaxation, and cognitive reframing with an adult patient (no further details given). After 60 sessions, they reported reduced muscle activity in response to stress and improved fluency during single words and conversation. Meyers and colleagues (1990) report on the use of a speech fluency focused approach (reducing syllable repetitions, gentle onset, and systematic desensitization) with a 7-year-old boy who suffered a stroke. The boy received both language and stuttering treatment and showed a marked improvement in fluency after 4 months of intervention (from approximately 17% stuttering to 2%). However, further analysis by the authors cast doubt on whether the fluency improvement could indeed be attributed to the stuttering treatment, as opposed to the effects of general language recovery, spontaneous fluency recovery; or a combination of both. In the survey by Theys and colleagues (2008), clinicians reported improvement in speech fluency following treatment for 19 patients, including one patient who fully recovered. The stuttering was reported to remain unchanged after therapy in three patients. The survey did not allow the researchers to link improvement—or lack thereof—to particular treatment approaches. Clearly, the information available on treatment outcome remains very limited. While some case reports refer to successful outcomes of the treatment, others do not and in many reports the outcome data are of a highly subjective nature and do not provide sufficient evidence to evaluate the validity and reliability of such reports, let alone the long term maintenance of the reported improvements in speech fluency. In addition, based on the current literature, it is very difficult to assess whether the effectiveness of specific treatment approaches with ANS patients varies with differences in the underlying neurological conditions. Given differences in how ANS manifests itself in different etiologies (De Nil et al., 2007) this could be a fruitful direction for future research.

An interesting question is whether changes in stuttering frequency in stroke patients are independent of parallel changes in language ability resulting from aphasia treatment. Again, very little research has been done to shed light on this issue, but two reports provide some hints as to what the direction of the answer could be. Rosenbek and colleagues (1978) report on seven adult patients. Only two of these patients showed recovery from stuttering, while five did not. One of these patients received aphasia and stuttering treatment in parallel and both conditions improved. Two other patients also received both types of treatment. While these latter patients showed language improvement, their stuttering did not change. Tani and Sakai (2010) described a patient with a right cerebellar infarct. This patient received aphasia therapy only during a period of 43 days and actually experienced a severe increase in stuttering, from approximately 47 to 77% during conversation, as well as a remarkable increase in secondary behaviors. These preliminary, and admittedly limited, reports suggest that changes in stuttering may be independent from improvements in language, and that in most patients treatment should focus on both language and fluency difficulties. While these findings appear to confirm our belief that ANS constitutes a speech disorder that is separate from other language disorders in stroke patients, it is clear that much more research is needed to confirm this.

CONCLUSION

Stroke-related ANS is a communication disorder that affects a significant number of stroke patients and should be part of a diagnostic checklist used by each and every clinician working with this population. The acquired fluency disorder may sometimes go unnoticed among the other deficits the patient is demonstrating, but for a significant number of patients, the speech fluency difficulties form a major obstacle in their ability to communicate. As we have seen, there is strong evidence that stroke patients show signs of speech-related negative attitudes and concerns that are not much different from people with developmental stuttering. In this chapter we have provided an overview of the major speech characteristics of these patients, outlined a comprehensive assessment battery, and described some commonly used intervention techniques. Much work still needs to be done with regard to differential diagnosis of stuttering from other speech and language deficits, but the most pressing issue is future research concerning best practices for fluency treatment intervention. A very important first step will be for all clinicians who work with stroke patients to recognize the existence of these fluency difficulties. We hope that this chapter will have contributed to this growing awareness.

CASE ILLUSTRATION

CS was a 62-year-old, right-handed woman with disfluencies following a left basal ganglia stroke who was assessed 2 years after the onset of stuttering. She was a native English speaker with 10 years of education, born and raised in a small town where she worked for many years as a salesperson. Ten years before her stroke she moved to the city where she lived with her husband and two grown-up children. Her medical history was positive for hypertension and hypercholesterolemia managed with Norvasc (amlodipine) and Crestor (rosuvastatin), respectively. Two years prior to her fluency assessment she experienced a left-sided stroke to the basal ganglia resulting in rigidity of movements, mild difficulty with swallowing, and stuttering. Her MRI showed ischemic changes in the left basal ganglia consistent with an infarct. She recovered relatively well, with the exception of speech disfluencies, which consisted of initial syllable repetitions and sound prolongations. She was disfluent on 24% of the words during reading, 21% during conversational speech, and her Stuttering Severity Index (Riley, 1994) score was 24, indicating mild stuttering. Her fluency increased markedly during more automatic speech tasks (11%) and during repeated reading of a text (reading adaptation). During assessment, CS responded well to a variety of fluency enhancing conditions (singing, slowed speech, and pacing), but no change in frequency of stuttering was observed during masking and choral speech. Although there were no generalized anxiety and no secondary behaviors, she expressed a significant negative attitude toward her stuttering as demonstrated by a score of 18 on the S-24, a speech attitude test (Andrews & Cutler, 1974). Her score on this test was similar to the average score found for adults with developmental stuttering. She also expressed self-described moderate to severe disfluencies in a wide variety of speech situations as evidenced by a score of 86 on the Speech Situation Checklist (Vanryckeghem & Brutten, 2006).

Language Testing

CS was assessed 2 years after her stroke with an extensive battery that, in addition to fluency measures (Jokel et al., 2007), included the BDAE-3 (selected subtests) (Goodglass et al., 2001), BNT (Kaplan et al., 2000), The Word Test (Jorgensen, Barrett, Huisingh, & Zachman, 1981), selected subtests from the PALPA (Kay et al., 1992), Token Test (De Renzi & Vignolo, 1962), verbal fluency, interpretation of proverbs, the Peabody Picture Vocabulary Test (PPVT; Dunn & Dunn, 1981), selected items from the Arlin Test of Formal Reasoning (ATFR; Arlin, 1984), word and digit span, the story retelling test from the Arizona Battery for Communication in Dementia (ABCD; Bayles & Tomoeda, 1993), nonverbal motor-speech examination, and other nonstandardized tests to assess reading and writing skills.

Her pragmatic skills were intact in both the verbal and nonverbal domain. In addition to a mild stutter, CS presented with somewhat hypophonic speech and a mild word-finding deficit. Her other language skills were relatively intact, including auditory and reading comprehension, oral reading, and spelling.

Cognitive Testing

CS was well oriented to time and place; she also appeared well versed in recent cultural and political events. Her verbal memory was assessed with a story retell and appeared preserved. Verbal fluency, problem solving, interpretation of proverbs, and semantics were all within the average range, though some psychomotor slowing was evident. Digit span was somewhat low at 4 digits forward and 3 backward.

Motor Speech Testing

No anatomical or functional abnormalities were observed. Facial and speech praxis were normal. Her voice was hypophonic but otherwise unremarkable in quality.

In summary, CS presented with relatively preserved language, cognition, and speech with the exception of stuttering. She had a positive outlook and was willing to engage in a modified fluency shaping therapy that was offered over the next 12 weeks. She was seen twice per week for 1 hour (excluding the pre- and post-therapy assessments) and was assigned home-based exercises to be carried out between sessions. Each clinician-supervised session began with relaxation exercises focused on breathing (10 min) and transitioned into an easy-onset phonation of vowels and sounds (10 min) that are associated with free air flow (m, n, s, z, f, v, l). This was followed by practicing gentle onset with monosyllabic and multisyllabic single words (10 min). For words with initial airflow-stopping sounds (b, p, t, d, k, g) CS was introduced to a light contact technique whereby she practiced production of those sounds with the least amount of articulatory pressure. The final part of each session was spent on slow speech with stretched vowel phonation, because this was one of the techniques that yielded improvements during initial assessment. Although pacing also proved helpful during diagnostic testing, CS was reluctant to use pacing (the idea of moving a body part to facilitate speech was unattractive to her), hence it was not included in her therapy program.

In the second half of the therapy program (weeks 6–12), CS was introduced to two stuttering modification techniques whereby she was taught how to deal with instances of stuttering that were still occurring in her speech. They included pullouts and cancellations. *Pullouts* are characterized by a change from a "hard" stutter to an "easy" stutter so the word can be completed with the least amount of tension possible. A *cancellation* technique involves saying the stuttered word again but fluently. CS learned to use both techniques and employed them simultaneously, that is, a pullout followed by cancellation during the sessions, with a progressively increasing degree of success.

Home-based exercises capitalized on relaxation and were based on material practiced in the preceding session. They frequently included sounds or words that were particularly challenging to CS during the session. She was also asked to have at least one conversation a day (this increased with the program progression) using easy onset, light contact, and slow speech. She recorded the approximate number of stuttered moments and reported on the overall success with fluency techniques at the next session.

Immediately following 24 sessions and home-based exercises, CS's disfluency scores improved on all tasks by 7 to 23%. Most importantly, she felt confident about her ability to carry on using fluency-shaping techniques on her own. Two phone calls were placed post-treatment 3 months apart to perceptually evaluate CS's maintenance of treatment gains. Aside from occasional vowel prolongations on multisyllabic words she remained normally fluent.

REFERENCES

Abe, K., Yokoyama, R., & Yonifuki, S. (1993). Repetitive speech disorder resulting from infarcts in the paramedian thalami and midbrain. *Journal of Neurology, Neurosurgery and Psychiatry*, *56*(9), 1024–1026. [included in systematic review]

Ackermann, H., Hertrich, I., Ziegler, W., Bitzer, M., & Bien, S. (1996). Acquired dysflencies following infarction of left mesiofrontal cortex. *Aphasiology*, *10*, 409–417. [included in systematic review]

Andrews, G., & Cutler, J. (1974). Stuttering therapy: The relation between changes in symptom level and attitudes. *Journal of Speech and Hearing Disorders, 39*(3), 312–319.

Ardila, A., & Lopez, MV. (1986). Severe stuttering associated with right hemisphere lesion. *Brain and Language, 27*(2), 239–240. [included in systematic review]

Arlin, P. A. (1984). *Arlin Test of Formal Reasoning Test Manual.* East Aurora, NY: Slosson Educational Publications.

Bakheit, A. M. O., Frost, J., & Ackroyd, E. (2011). Remission of life-long stammering after posterior circulation stroke. *Neurocase, 17*(1), 41–45. [included in systematic review]

Balasubramanian, V. (1996). Phonological encoding deficits in a case of acquired neurogenic stuttering. *Brain and Language, 55*(1), 153–155. [included in systematic review]

Balasubramanian, V., Cronin, K. L., & Max, L. (2010). Dysfluency levels during repeated readings, choral readings, and readings with altered auditory feedback in two cases of acquired neurogenic stuttering. *Journal of Neurolinguistics, 23*(5), 488–500. [included in systematic review]

Balasubramanian, V., Max, L., Van Borsel, J., Rayca, K. O., & Richardson, D. (2003). Acquired stuttering following right frontal and bilateral pontine lesion: A case study. *Brain and Cognition, 53*(2), 185–189. [included in systematic review]

Ballard, K. J., Granier, J. P., & Robin, D. A. (2000). Understanding the nature of apraxia of speech: Theory, analysis, and treatment. *Aphasiology, 14*(10), 969–995.

Baumgartner, J. M. (1999). Acquired psychogenic stuttering. In R. F. Curlee (Ed.), *Stuttering and related disorders of fluency* (pp. 269–288). New York, NY: Thieme Medical Publishers, Inc.

Bayles, K. A., & Tomoeda, C. K. (1993). *The Arizona Battery for Communication Disorders of Dementia.* Tucson, AZ: Canyonlands Publishing.

Beal, D. S., Gracco, V. L., Lafaille, S. J., & De Nil, L. F. (2007). Voxel-based morphometry of auditory and speech-related cortex in stutterers. *NeuroReport, 18*(12), 1257–1260.

Behm, S. C., & Frohman, E. M. (2012). WEBINO and the return of the king's speech. *Journal of the Neurological Sciences, 315*(12), 153–155. [included in systematic review]

Bijleveld, H. (2001). Acquired stuttering. Retrieved from https://www.mnsu.edu/comdis/isad4/papers/bijleveld.html.

Bijleveld, H. A., Lebrun, Y., & van Dongen, H. (1994). A case of acquired stuttering. *Folia Phoniatrica et Logopaedica, 46*(5), 250–253. [included in systematic review]

Binder, L. M., Spector, J., & Youngjohn, J. R. (2012). Psychogenic stuttering and other acquired nonorganic speech and language abnormalities. *Archives of Clinical Neuropsychology, 27*(5), 557–568.

Bishop, D. V. M. (1989). *Test for reception of grammar.* London, UK: Harcourt Assessment.

Blomgren, M. (2013). Behavioral treatments for children and adults who stutter: A review. *Psychology Research and Behavior Management, 6*(1), 9–19.

Blomgren, M., Roy, N., Callister, T., & Merrill, R. M. (2005). Intensive stuttering modification therapy: A multidimensional assessment of treatment outcomes. *Journal of Speech Language and Hearing Research, 48*(3), 509–523.

Bloodstein, O., & Bernstein-Ratner, N. (2008). *A handbook on stuttering* (6th ed.). Clifton Park, NY: Delmar.

Burch, J. M., Kieman, T. E. J., & Demaerschalk, B. M. (2013). Neurogenic stuttering with right hemisphere stroke: A case presentation. *Journal of Neurolinguistics, 26*(1), 207–213. [included in systematic review]

Canter, G. J. (1971). Observations on neurogenic stuttering: A contribution to differential diagnosis. *British Journal of Disorders of Communication, 6*(2), 139–143.

Carluer, L., Marie, R. M., Lambert, J., Defer, G. L., Coskun, O., & Rossa, Y. (2000). Acquired and persistent stuttering as the main symptom of striatal infarction. *Movement Disorders, 15*(2), 343–346. [included in systematic review]

Chang, S. E. (2014). Research updates in neuroimaging studies of children who stutter. *Seminars in Speech and Language, 35*(2), 67–79.

Ciabarra, A. M., Elkind, M. S., Roberts, J. K., & Marshall, R. S. (2000). Subcortical infarction resulting in acquired stuttering. *Journal of Neurology, Neurosurgery and Psychiatry, 69*(4), 546–549. [included in systematic review]

Conture, E. (2000). *Stuttering: Its nature, diagnosis, and treatment.* Needham Heights, MA: Allyn & Bacon.

Craig, A. R., Franklin, J. A., & Andrews, G. (1984). A scale to measure locus of control of behaviour. *British Journal of Medical Psychology, 57*(2), 173–180.

Dabul, B. L. (2000). *Apraxia Battery for Adults* (2nd ed.). Austin, TX: Pro-Ed.

De Nil, L. F. (2004). Recent developments in brain imaging research in stuttering. In B. Maassen, H. F. M. Peters, & R. Kent (Eds.), *Speech motor control in normal and disordered speech. proceedings of the fourth international speech motor conference* (pp. 150–155). Oxford, England: Oxford.

De Nil, L. F., Jokel, R., & Rochon, E. (2007). Etiology, symptomatology, and treatment of neurogenic stuttering. In E. G. Conture & R. F. Curlee (Eds.), *Stuttering and related disorders of fluency* (3rd ed., pp. 326–343). New York, NY: Thieme.

De Nil, L. F., Kroll, R. M., Lafaille, S. J., & Houle, S. (2003). A positron emission tomography study of short- and long-term treatment effects on functional brain activation in adults who stutter. *Journal of Fluency Disorders, 28*(4), 357–380.

De Nil, L. F., Rochon, E., & Jokel, R. (2008). Adult-onset neurogenic stuttering. In M. R. McNeil (Ed.), *Clinical management of sensorimotor speech disorders* (2nd ed., pp. 235–248). New York, NY: Thieme.

De Nil, L. F., Sasisekaran, J., Van Lieshout, P. H. H. M., & Sandor, P. (2005). Speech disfluencies in individuals with Tourette's syndrome. *Journal of Psychosomatic Research, 58*(1), 97–102.

De Renzi, E., & Vignolo, L. A. (1962). The Token Test: A sensitive test to detect receptive disturbances in aphasics. *Brain, 85*(4), 665–678.

DiDonato Brumbach, A. C., & Goffman, L. (2014). Interaction of language processing and motor skill in children with specific language impairment. *Journal of Speech, Language, and Hearing Research, 57*(1), 158–171.

Doi, M., Nakayasu, H., Soda, T., Shimoda, K., Ito, A., & Nakashima, K. (2003). Brainstem infarction presenting with neurogenic stuttering. *Internal Medicine, 42*(9), 884–887. [included in systematic review]

Donnan, G. A. (1979). Stuttering as a manifestation of stroke. *Medical Journal of Australia, 1*(2), 44–45. [included in systematic review]

Duffy, J. R. (2005). *Motor speech disorders: Substrates, differential diagnosis, and management* (2nd ed.). St Louis, MO: Elsevier Mosby.

Duffy, J. R., & Baumgartner, J. (1997). Psychogenic stuttering in adults with and without neurologic disease. *Journal of Medical Speech-Language Pathology, 5*(2), 75–95.

Dunn, L., & Dunn, L. (1997). *Peabody Picture Vocabulary Test.* Circle Pines, MN: American Guidance Service.

Erickson, R. (1969). Assessing communication attitudes among stutterers. *Journal of Speech and Hearing Research, 12*(4), 711–724.

Fawcett, R. G. (2005). Stroke-associated acquired stuttering. *CNS Spectrums, 10*(2), 94–95. [included in systematic review]

Fleet, W. S., & Heilman, K. M. (1985). Acquired stuttering from a right hemisphere lesion in a right hander. *Neurology, 35*(9), 1343–1346. [included in systematic review]

Flowers, H. L., Silver, F. L., Fang, J., Rochon, E., & Martino, R. (2013). The incidence, co-occurrence, and predictors of dysphagia, dysarthria, and aphasia after first-ever acute ischemic stroke. *Journal of Communication Disorders, 46*(3), 238–248.

Folstein, M. F., Folstein, S. E., & McHugh, P. R. (1975). Mini-mental state: A practical method for grading the state of patients for the clinician. *Journal of Psychiatric Research, 12*(3), 189–198.

Franco, E., Casado, J. L., Lopez Dominquez, J. M., Diaz Espejo, C., Blanco, A., & Robledo, A. (2000). Stuttering as the only manifestation of brain infarct. *Neurologia, 15*(9), 414–416. [included in systematic review]

Gerratt, B. R. (1989). Effects of phonatory mode on fluency in a neurogenic stutterer. Unpublished paper. [included in systematic review]

Goodglass, H., Kaplan, E., & Barresi, B. (2001). *Boston Diagnostic Aphasia Examination.* Baltimore, MD: Lippincott, Williams & Wilkins.

Grant, A. C., Biousse, V., Cook, A. A., & Newman, N. J. (1999). Stroke-associated stuttering. *Archives of Neurology, 56*(5), 624–627. [included in systematic review]

Guenther, F. H., Ghosh, S. S., & Tourville, J. A. (2006). Neural modeling and imaging of the cortical interactions underlying syllable production. *Brain and Language, 96*(3), 280–301.

Guenther, F. H., & Vladusich, T. (2012). A neural theory of speech acquisition and production. *Journal of Neurolinguistics, 25*(5), 408–422.

Guitar, B. (2014). *Stuttering: An integrated approach to its nature and treatment* (4th ed.). Baltimore, MD: Lippincott, Williams & Wilkins.

Hagiwara, H., Takeda, K., Saito, F., Shimizu, T., & Bando, M. (2000). A case of callosal apraxia without agraphia and acquired stuttering associated with collosal infarction. *Clinical Neurology, 40*(6), 605–610. [included in systematic review]

Hajnšek, S., Basic, S., Sporis, D., Rados, M., Filipcic, I., Kovacevic, I., & Posavec, A. (2006). Acquired stuttering resulting from right parietal subcortical infarction. *Neurologia Croatia, 55*(3–4), 51–56. [included in systematic review]

Hamano, T., Hiraki, S., Kawamura, Y., Hirayama, M., Mutoh, T., & Kuriyama, M. (2005). Acquired stuttering secondary to callosal infarction. *Neurology, 64*(6), 1092–1093. [included in systematic review]

Helm-Estabrooks, N. (1987). Stuttering assessment and acquired brain lesions [reply]. *Neurology, 37*, 1434–1435.

Helm-Estabrooks, N. (1999). Stuttering associated with acquired neurological disorders. In R. F. Curlee (Ed.), *Stuttering and related disorders of fluency* (pp. 205–218). New York: Thieme.

Helm-Estabrooks, N. (2005). *Diagnosis and management of neurogenic stuttering in adults. The atypical stutterer: Principles and rehabilitation* (pp. 193–217). St. Louis, MO: Academic Press.

Helm-Estabrooks, N., Yeo, R., Geschwind, N., Freedman, M., & Weinstein, C. (1986). Stuttering: Disappearance and reappearance with acquired brain lesions. *Neurology, 36*(8), 1109–1112. [included in systematic review]

Heuer, R. J., Sataloff, R. T., Mandel, S., & Travers, N. (1996). Neurogenic stuttering: Further corroboration of site of lesion. *Ear, Nose & Throat Journal, 75*(3), 161–168. [included in systematic review]

Horner, J., & Massey, E. W. (1983). Progressive dysfluency associated with right hemisphere disease. *Brain and Language, 18*(1), 71–85. [included in systematic review]

Houde, J. F., & Nagarajan, S. S. (2011). Speech production as state feedback control. *Frontiers in Human Neuroscience, 5*, 82.

Howard, D., & Patterson, K. E. (1992). *The Pyramids and Palm Tree Test.* Bury St. Edmunds, England: Thames Valley Test Company.

Jokel, R., & De Nil, L. F. (2003). A comprehensive study of acquired stuttering in adults. In K. L. Baker & D. T. Rowley (Eds.), *Proceedings of the sixth oxford dysfluency conference* (pp. 59–64), Leicester, UK: KLB Publications.

Jokel, R., De Nil, L., & Sharpe, K. (2007). Speech disfluencies in adults with neurogenic stuttering associated with stroke and traumatic brain injury. *Journal of Medical Speech-Language Pathology*, *15*(3), 243–261. [included in systematic review]

Jones, R. K. (1966). Observations on stammering after localized cerebral injury. *Journal of Neurology, Neurosurgery and Psychiatry*, *29*(3), 192–195. [included in systematic review]

Jorgensen, C., Barrett, M., Huisingh, R., & Zachman, L. (1981). *The Word Test*. Moline, IL: LinguiSystems.

Kakishita, K., Sekiguchi, E., Maeshima, S., Okada, H., Okita, R., Ozaki, F., & Moriwaki, H. (2004). Stuttering without callosal apraxia resulting from infarction in the anterior corpus callosum: A case report. *Journal of Neurology*, *251*(9), 1140–1141. [included in systematic review]

Kaplan, E., Goodglass, H., & Weintraub, S. (2001). *Boston Naming Test* (2nd ed.). Philadelphia: Lippincott, Williams & Wilkins.

Kay, J., Lesser, R., & Coltheart, M. (1992). *PALPA: Psycholinguistic Assessments of Language Processing in Aphasia*. Hove, England: Lawrence Erlbaum Associates Ltd.

Kirk, A. (1993). The heterogeneity of acquired stuttering. *Journal of Clinical and Experimental Neuropsychology*, *15*(1), 45–46. [included in systematic review]

Kono, I., Hirano, T., Ueda, Y., & Nakajima, K. (1998). A case of acquired stuttering resulting from striatocapsular infarction. *Clinical Neurology*, *38*(8), 758–761. [included in systematic review]

Krishnan, G., Nair, R. P., & Tiwari, S. (2010). Clinical evidence for the compensatory role of the right frontal love and a novel neural substrate in developmental stuttering: A single case study. *Journal of Neurolinguistics*, *23*(5), 501–510. [included in systematic review]

Krishnan, G., & Tiwari, S. (2011). Revisiting the acquired neurogenic stuttering in the light of developmental stuttering. *Journal of Neurolinguistics*, *24*(3), 383–396. [included in systematic review]

Krishnan, G., & Tiwari, S. (2013). Differential diagnosis in developmental and acquired neurogenic stuttering: Do fluency-enhancing conditions dissociate the two? *Journal of Neurolinguistics*, *26*(2), 252–257.

Kussmaul, A. (1877). Monographie. In Pick, A. (1899). Ueber das sogenannte aphatische stottern als symptom verschiedenoertlich localisirter cerebraler herdaffectionen. *Archiv für Psychiatrie 32*(2), 447–469.

Lebrun, Y., Leleux, C., Rousseau, J. J., & Devreux, F. (1983). Acquired stuttering. *Journal of Fluency Disorders*, *8*(4), 323–330.

Lebrun, Y., Retif, J., & Kaiser, G. (1983). Acquired stuttering as a forerunner of motor-neuron disease. *Journal of Fluency Disorders*, *8*(4), 161–167.

Leder, S. B. (1996). Adult onset of stuttering as a presenting sign in a parkinsonian-like syndrome: A case report. *Journal of Communication Disorders*, *29*(6), 471–478.

Ludlow, C. L., Rosenberg, J., Salazar, A., Grafman, J., & Smutok, M. (1987). Site of penetrating brain lesions causing chronic acquired stuttering. *Annals of Neurology*, *22*(1), 60–66.

Lundgren, K., Helm-Estabrooks, N., & Klein, R. (2010). Stuttering following acquired brain damage: A review of the literature. *Journal of Neurolinguistics*, *23*(5), 447–454.

MacPherson, M. K., & Smith, A. (2013). Influences of sentence length and syntactic complexity on the speech motor control of children who stutter. *Journal of Speech, Language, and Hearing Research*, *56*(1), 89–102.

Mahr, G., & Leith, W. (1992). Psychogenic stuttering of adult onset. *Journal of Speech and Hearing Research*, *35*(2), 283–286.

Manning, W. H. (2009). *Clinical decision making in fluency disorders*. Clifton Park, NY: Delmar Cengage Learning.

Market, K. E., Montague, J. C., Buffalo, M. D., & Drummond, S. S. (1990). Acquired stuttering: Descriptive data and treatment outcome. *Journal of Fluency Disorders, 15*(1), 21–33.

Marshall, R. C., & Neuburger, S. I. (1987). Effects of delayed auditory feedback on acquired stuttering following head injury. *Journal of Fluency Disorders, 12*(5), 355–365.

Max, L., & Baldwin, C. J. (2010). The role of motor learning in stuttering adaptation: Repeated versus novel utterances in a practice-retention paradigm. *Journal of Fluency Disorders, 35*(1), 33–43.

Mazzucchi, A., Moretti, G., Carpeggiani, P., Parma, M., & Paini, P. (1981). Clinical observations on acquired stuttering. *British Journal of Disorders of Communication, 16*(1), 19–30. [included in systematic review]

Meyers, S. C., Hall, N. E., & Aram, D. M. (1990). Fluency and language recovery in a child with a left hemisphere lesion. *Journal of Fluency Disorders, 15*(3), 159–173. [included in systematic review]

Mouradian, M. S., Paslawski, T., & Shuaib, A. (2000). Return of stuttering after stroke. *Brain & Language, 73*(1), 120–123. [included in systematic review]

Nass, R., Schreter, B., & Heier, L. (1994). Acquired stuttering after a 2nd stroke in a 2-year-old. *Developmental Medicine and Child Neurology, 36*(1), 73–78. [included in systematic review]

Neef, N. E., Jung, K., Rothkegel, H., Pollok, B., von Gudenberg, A. W., Paulus, W., & Sommer, M. (2011). Right-shift for non-speech motor processing in adults who stutter. *Cortex, 47*(8), 945–954.

Neumann, K., Preibisch, C., Euler, H. A., Gudenberg, A. W. V., Lanfermann, H., Gall, V., & Giraud, A.-L. (2005). Cortical plasticity associated with stuttering therapy. *Journal of Fluency Disorders, 30*(1), 23–39.

Nowack, W. J., & Stone, R. E. (1987). Acquired stuttering and bilateral cerebral disease. *Journal of Fluency Disorders, 12*(2), 141–146. [included in systematic review]

Osawa, A., Maeshima, S., & Yoshimura, T. (2006). Acquired stuttering in a patient with Wernicke's aphasia. *Journal of Clinical Neuroscience, 13*(10), 1066–1069. [included in systematic review]

Perez, E. R., Gubser-Mercati, D., & Davidoff, V. (1996). Transient acquired stuttering in a child. *Neurocase, 2*(4), 347–352. [included in systematic review]

Pick, A. (1899). Ueber das sogenannte aphatische stottern als symptom verschiedenoertlich localisirter cerebraler herdaffectionen. *Archiv fur Psychiatrie, 32*(2), 447–469.

Riley, G. D. (1994). *Stuttering severity instrument for children and adults*. Austin, TX: Pro-Ed.

Rosenbek, J., Messert, B., Collins, M., & Wertz, R. T. (1978). Stuttering following brain damage. *Brain & Language, 6*(1), 82–96. [included in systematic review]

Rosenfield, D. B., Miller, S. D., & Feltovich, M. (1980). Brain damage causing stuttering. *Transactions of the American Neurological Association, 105*(1), 1–3. [included in systematic review]

Rubow, R. T., Rosenbek, J. C., & Schumaker, J. G. (1986). Stress management of stuttering following closed head injury. *Biofeedback and Self-Regulation, 11*(1), 77–78. [included in systematic review]

Sahin, H. A., Krespi, Y., Yilmaz, A., & Coban, O. (2005). Stuttering due to ischemic stroke. *Behavioral Neurology, 16*(1), 37–39. [included in systematic review]

Shapiro, D. (1998). *Stuttering intervention: A collaborative journey to fluency freedom*. Austin, TX: Pro-Ed.

Smits-Bandstra, S., & De Nil, L. F. (2007). Sequence skill learning in persons who stutter: Implications for cortico-striato-thalamo-cortical dysfunction. *Journal of Fluency Disorders, 32*(4), 251–278.

Soroker, N., Bar-Israel, Y., Schechter, I., & Solzi, P. (1990). Stuttering as a manifestation of a right-hemispheric subcortical stroke. *European Neurology, 30*(5), 268–270. [included in systematic review]

Tani, T., & Sakai, Y. (2010). Stuttering after right cerebellar infarction: A case study. *Journal of Fluency Disorders, 35*(2), 141–145. [included in systematic review]

Tani, T., & Sakai, Y. (2011). Analysis of five cases with neurogenic stuttering following brain injury in the basal ganglia. *Journal of Fluency Disorders, 36*(1), 1–16. [included in systematic review]

Theys, C., De Nil, L., Thijs, V., van Wieringen, A., & Sunaert, S. (2013). A crucial role for the cortico-striato-cortical loop in the pathogenesis of stroke-related neurogenic stuttering. *Human Brain Mapping, 34*(9), 2103–2112. [included in systematic review]

Theys, C., van Wieringen, A., & De Nil, L. F. (2008). A clinician survey of speech and non-speech characteristics of neurogenic stuttering. *Journal of Fluency Disorders, 33*(1), 1–23.

Theys, C., van Wieringen, A., Sunaert, S., Thijs, V., & De Nil, L. F. (2011). A one year prospective study of neurogenic stuttering following stroke: Incidence and co-occurring disorders. *Journal of Communication Disorders, 44*(6), 678–687. [included in systematic review]

Tsumoto, T., Nishioka, K., Nakakita, K., Hayashi, S., & Maeshima, S. (1999). Acquired stuttering associated with callosal infarction: A case report. *Neurological Surgery, 27*(1), 79–83. [included in systematic review]

Turgut, N., Utku, Y., & Balci, K. (2002). A case of acquired stuttering resulting from left parietal infarction. *Acta Neurologica Scandinavica, 105*(5), 408–410. [included in systematic review]

Van Borsel, J. (1997). Neurogenic stuttering: A review. *Journal of Clinical Speech and Language Studies, 7*(1), 17–33.

Van Borsel, J. (2014). Acquired stuttering: A note on terminology. *Journal of Neurolinguistics, 27*(1), 41–49.

Van Borsel, J., Drummond, D., & de Britto Pereira, M. M. (2010). Delayed auditory feedback and acquired neurogenic stuttering. *Journal of Neurolinguistics, 23*(5), 479–487.

Van Borsel, J., & Taillieu, C. (2001). Neurogenic stuttering versus developmental stuttering — an observer judgement study. *Journal of Communication Disorders, 34*(5), 385–395. [included in systematic review]

Van Borsel, J., Van der Made, S., & Santens, P. (2003). Thalamic stuttering: A distinct clinical entity? *Brain and Language, 85*(2), 185–189. [included in systematic review]

Van Borsel, J., Van Lierde, K., Oostra, K., & Eeckhaut, C. (1997). The differential diagnosis of late-onset stuttering. In Y. Lebrun (Ed.), *From the brain to the mouth. Acquired dysarthria and dysfluency in adults* (pp. 105–138). Dordrecht, The Netherlands: Kluwer Academic Publishers.

Van Borsel, J., Van Lierde, K., Van Cauwenberge, P., Guldemont, I., & Van Orshoven, M. (1998). Severe acquired stuttering following injury of the left supplementary motor region: A case report. *Journal of Fluency Disorders, 23*(1), 49–58. [included in systematic review]

Vanryckeghem, M., & Brutten, G. J. (2006). *Behavior assessment battery.* San Diego, CA: Plural Publishing.

Wechsler, D. (1997). *Manual for the Wechsler Adult Intelligence Scale* (3rd ed.). San Antonio, TX: Psychological Corporation.

Wiederholt, J. L., & Bryant, B. (1992). Gray Oral Reading Test. Austin, Tx: Pro-Ed.

Challenging Treatment Components

CHAPTER 7

Generalization in Aphasiology: What Are the Best Strategies?

Patrick Coppens
Janet Patterson

INTRODUCTION

The overarching goal of speech-language therapy is to establish or reestablish language behaviors that a patient with aphasia can apply when needed. When speech-language pathologists work with their clients on clinical goals, it is usually assumed that the therapy approach will not have to be practiced with all possible exemplars and in all possible settings. In other words, communication professionals expect that the successful establishment of a trained behavior will demonstrate generality and prove, "... durable over time ... environments ... and related behaviors." (Baer, Wolf, & Risley, 1968, p. 96). Such a change is viewed as the best possible outcome for a rehabilitation objective and represents "a meaningful change in processing ... rather than just the rote learning of specific responses" (Mitchum & Berndt, 1994, p. 319).

Even when generalization is optimal, historically it has appeared as a passive phenomenon in behavior change (i.e., rehabilitation) and a "natural" outcome rather than a planned and measured outcome (Stokes & Baer, 1977). To assess generalization, clinicians and researchers oftentimes measure patient success on untrained items to ascertain that the trained behavior has carried over to other exemplars or different environments. This rather passive approach to generalization has been referred to as "train and hope" (Stokes & Baer, 1977, p. 351) or as "fishing for evidence of change" (Webster, Whitworth, & Morris, 2015) which, in a way, represents a tacit acknowledgment that we do not really know how to plan for or maximize generalization and simply assume that our clinical interventions will result in generalization. Only a handful of studies in clinical aphasiology have reported generalization information and even fewer included any kind of training specifically designed for generalization purposes (Thompson, 1989). It has been demonstrated, though, that clients are better served when specific strategies are employed to facilitate generalization processes (e.g., Goldberg, Haley, & Jacks, 2012). If one considers aphasia rehabilitation to be a reactivation of inaccessible linguistic information as opposed to a loss of linguistic skills that have to be relearned, then generalization may be considered an automatic consequence of linguistic reactivation (Thompson, 1989). However, evidence from early experimental studies shows that generalization does not readily happen following anomia therapy (Thompson & Kearns, 1981) or syntax rehabilitation (Doyle, Goldstein, & Bourgeois, 1987).

In this chapter we examine what we know about the various types of generalization, and we suggest specific strategies that can be incorporated as active ingredients in a treatment protocol in order to plan for generalization and maximize the likelihood that behavior changes will generalize.

GENERALIZATION TYPES AND PRESUMED MECHANISMS

Generalization cannot be expected if the treatment itself is unsuccessful. Furthermore, if application of a treatment protocol yields significant improvement, the success of generalization is always of a lesser extent (quantitatively). This pattern is an indication that generalization is broadly dependent on overall therapy success and also that it is a more challenging process than stimulating direct therapeutic gain. For example, Wambaugh and Thompson (1989) noted that the level of generalization for their participants was related to the success rate of the acquisition of the target structure. That is, the more successful the training, the better the potential for generalization.

Alternatively, some experimental research suggests that improvements on trained stimuli and improvements on untrained stimuli (i.e., generalization) are subsumed by different neurological processes (Dickey & Yoo, 2010; Meinzer et al., 2010). For example, Dickey and Yoo (2013) reported that for their participants the extent of generalization to untrained items did not correlate with any of their predictor variables (i.e., aphasia severity, auditory comprehension, complex sentence comprehension). This important observation signifies that the potential for generalization may be difficult to predict within the confines of our current level of understanding of patient variables. Dickey and Yoo further stated that the rate of generalization is slower than that of acquisition (i.e., trained items). These observations led Dickey and Yoo to conclude that improvements on trained versus untrained items are based on different learning mechanisms that rely on different neurological processes. The implication for treatment planning is that successful generalization requires implementation of specific strategies that may be different than those underlying the success of direct therapy. Also, a longer or more intense treatment period may be needed.

We have used the term "generalization" as if it represents a unitary process. Although it is tempting, for ease of treatment planning, to maintain this view, in reality, generalization appears as several distinct types. The labels associated with the types of generalization have varied with time and authors, but from a behavioral standpoint, generalization can be classified as either *response generalization* or *stimulus generalization.* Response generalization refers to measurable improvements to similar untrained items, whereas stimulus generalization means that the learned, trained response was triggered in a different stimulus environment (e.g., a different linguistic situation, a different setting, a different conversation partner, etc.). Because of the major differences in generalization types, processes that have the potential in facilitating one type of generalization may not be useful in promoting another type. Therefore, developing specific strategies for overall generalization in therapy is probably meaningless; each individual type of generalization requires specific planning strategies. This conclusion is buttressed by the numerous research articles showing different results for stimulus versus response generalization (e.g., Milman, 2016).

Finally, it should be emphasized that generalization is also dependent upon the linguistic process underlying the target training items. Successful generalization following a treatment for a word-finding deficit is inherently different from that for syntactic/morphological production, as these linguistic elements are processed differently. Anomia may be viewed as a difficulty accessing semantic and/or lexical representations, whereas agrammatism is essentially the application of a rule-based syntactic system. An example of the latter is offered by Cannito and Vogel (1987). The authors trained their patient with Broca's aphasia on a program focusing on the regular plural morpheme. The patient improved significantly on trained exemplars. Generalization was present for untrained items as well as for conversational samples, but no change was noted for items requiring an irregular plural form. The client apparently re-learned and internalized the regular plural rule and was able to use it in all instances and settings, but that rule did not apply to irregular plural forms.

In the field of child language disorders, there are several reviews of generalization strategies that have been effectively used in the treatment of developmental language impairments in children (Baer, 1999; Hughes, 1985; Stokes & Baer, 1977; Wildman & Wildman, 1975). For example, Stokes and Baer (1977) recognized nine types of generalization techniques:

1. *Train and Hope:* the most prevalent approach in which generalization is not specifically trained;

2. *Sequential modification:* the active focus on generalization through systematic modification of target behavior in situations for which generalization was not noted;

3. *Introduce to natural maintaining contingencies:* the transfer of a learned behavior to a more naturally occurring environment;

4. *Train sufficient exemplars:* the number of practice items needed as well as their diversity to establish a behavior and trigger generalization;

5. *Train loosely:* the introduction of variations in the stimuli and the responses in preparation for the natural environment by exerting as little control over stimuli as possible;

6. *Use indiscriminable contingencies:* a progressively unpredictable reinforcement schedule;

7. *Program common stimuli:* the treatment stimuli are similar than in settings where generalization is expected;

8. *Mediate generalization:* the learned strategy shares common features with the generalization environment so as to be applicable to other situations; and

9. *Train to generalize:* the separate reinforcement of successful instances of behavior generalization.

Some of these techniques do not seem appropriate for a population of adults with aphasia (e.g., focusing on a reinforcement schedule), but most could be applicable. Indeed, inspired by Stokes and Baer's list, Thompson (1989) discussed techniques potentially useful in aphasia rehabilitation. She selected four strategies to stimulate response and stimulus generalization in patients with aphasia: *train enough exemplars, search for common stimuli, use sequential modification,* and *apply loose training.* She supported her selection and her conclusions with data from the aphasiology literature. Other examples of aphasia treatment based on techniques from Stokes and Baer's list are Response Elaboration Training (Kearns, 1985), which employs a loose training approach; Training Requesting Behavior (Doyle, Goldstein, Bourgeois, & Nakles, 1989), which focuses on introducing natural maintaining categories; and Computer Assisted Therapy for Anomia (Laganaro, Di Pietro, & Schnider, 2006), which emphasizes training sufficient exemplars.

In the remainder of this chapter, we have pursued an objective similar to Stokes and Baer's in an attempt to assist clinicians in identifying useful variables for planning generalization in their patients with aphasia.

RESPONSE GENERALIZATION

When patients with aphasia make significant improvements in their ability to name trained lexical items, is that improvement also observable to untrained exemplars? The answer to that question is: not likely. This disappointing answer seems to be valid regardless of the number of items actually trained (Laganaro et al., 2006; Snell, Sage, & Lambon Ralph, 2010), whether the training takes place through computer interface or in person (Laganaro, Di Pietro, & Schnider, 2003), whether nouns or verbs are targeted (Wambaugh, Mauszycki, & Wright, 2014), or whether errorless or errorful approaches are utilized (Fillingham, Sage, & Lambon Ralph, 2005a, 2005b). In other words, the direct training of lexical items does not automatically generalize to other exemplars. However, Thompson (1989) reported that generalization to untrained exemplars occurs more frequently when untrained exemplars are selected to be similar to the trained items. This effect progressively diminishes as the trained and untrained items become increasingly dissimilar. For example, one early attempt at probing response generalization was the matrix technique (Loverso & Millione, 1992; Thompson, 1989; Tonkovich & Loverso, 1982). The technique consisted of entering several exemplars of one type of stimulus on each axis of a matrix, for example nouns on the abscissa and verbs on the ordinate, creating different stimuli for each cell of the matrix (i.e., N + V). One diagonal of cells is directly trained (e.g., seven cells in Tonkovich & Loverso, 1982) and the remainder of the cells were used as within-task generalization probes. Training continued until generalization became significant, which typically did occur. Of course, in such a setup, all nouns and verbs *are* actually trained; the generalization applies to combinations that are novel.

In another example, Doyle and Goldstein (1985) used the Helm's Elicited Program for Syntax Stimulation (HELPSS) and reported response generalization within the same syntactic structures, but not to novel structures. Furthermore, several authors attempted to train subjects with nonfluent aphasia to produce "wh-" questions (Thompson & McReynolds, 1986; Wambaugh & Thompson, 1989). There was generalization within each type of question, but not across types. Kearns and Salmon (1984) trained two subjects with Broca's aphasia to produce *is* [auxiliary] (e.g., boy is drinking). They probed for generalization to spontaneous speech and the copula forms of the word: copula + noun (e.g., man is a sailor); copula + locative (e.g., doll is on bed); copula + adjective (e.g., man is tall). Generalization was evident to copula + adjective, minimal and variable to other copulas, and nonexistent to discourse. They interpreted the results in terms of response class differences. It could be argued that the progressive form of the verbs (e.g., drinking) can be used as adjectives (e.g., the drinking boy), thereby explaining generalization to copula + adjective. However, generalization cannot be expected to other structures using different grammatical elements.

What might be thought of as "typical generalization patterns" have exceptions, however. Although response generalization to untrained items may be observed when the stimuli are similar, it does not happen in all patients (Shewan, 1976; Thompson & Kearns, 1981). Alternatively, generalization across stimuli types is sometimes, but not always observed (e.g., Kearns & Salmon, 1984; Rose & Douglas, 2008). If individuals with aphasia are unable to generalize to untrained, yet similar items, it is necessary to posit that, in such cases, the patients are unable to internalize the underlying rule or process that may facilitate successful production of untrained responses. Many potential explanations come to mind, including severity of symptomatology (Carragher, Conroy, Sage, & Wilkinson, 2012; Leonard, Rochon, & Laird, 2008), associated linguistic or cognitive limitations (Carragher et al., 2012), personality, or motivation to treatment (see Chapter 12, this volume). In selected individuals, some of these issues may be surmounted by additional training (as suggested by Shewan, 1976). For example, if a patient is unexpectedly successful at generalizing responses across exemplar types, it is possible that the training stimulated associated rules (e.g., from one wh- question type to another); that the individual was particularly motivated, which may have prompted independent learning; or yet another possibility is that treatment stimulation facilitated broad access to lexical information (Rose & Douglas, 2008), thus promoting generalization in unanticipated areas. Current knowledge does not permit us to distinguish between these different hypotheses.

Two studies reported a direct comparison between exposure levels for untrained items and generalization measurements. Howard, Patterson, Franklin, Orchard-Lisle, and Morton (1985) directly compared response generalization between untrained items that were used as probes during the therapy period and exemplars that were never seen or named by the subjects until the post-treatment period. Interestingly, the generalization patterns were different. There was a clear advantage in favor of the untrained items used as probes, but the exemplars to which the subjects were never exposed showed some level of generalization as well, albeit to a lesser extent. However, the unexposed items consisted of different pictorial views of the trained items, which likely led to an overestimation of generalization. Pring, Hamilton, Harwood, and MacBride (1993) directly compared generalization to items that were used as foils during the therapy tasks versus items to which the patients were never exposed, all within the trained semantic categories. The authors observed that response generalization occurred for the items used as foils, but not for the totally new exemplars. They concluded that generalization does not extend automatically to an entire semantic category, but depends on item exposure during therapy, albeit a possibly more incidental semantic processing. This observation was confirmed in a subsequent meta-analysis. Wisenburn and Mahoney (2009) showed that measurable improvements on probe items can be explained by the repeated presentations. Still, related items showed greater improvement than unrelated items to which the subjects were exposed during generalization measurements. It is difficult to interpret this effect as a genuine generalization; however, the authors also reported that improvements were seen on exemplars that were never presented during the therapy phase. Although this effect was significantly smaller, it shows that a true response generalization is nevertheless possible.

Several strategies that have been shown to facilitate response generalization are reviewed in the next section. While evidence exists to support each strategy, none is guaranteed to facilitate generalization in any given individual, and selection of strategies must consider patient and environmental factors.

Internalize the Strategy

Regardless of the strategy used by the individual with aphasia to facilitate language production, it is evident that the reliance on cues must eventually be switched from clinician to patient. Moreover, the patient-generated facilitation strategies should be applicable to new exemplars if response generalization is to be expected. For example, Law, Yeung, and Chiu (2008) attempted to train Chinese individuals with aphasia to name pictures using a lexical (orthographic-phonetic) cueing mechanism. Although phonemic approaches are challenging in an ideographic language, the authors reported a strong treatment effect.

They further noted limited response generalization in two out of their four patients. They attributed that generalization to multiple exposures to untrained items (Howard et al., 1985); but also, in one patient, to the possible internalization of the strategy to rely on the Chinese equivalent of a grapheme-phoneme conversion strategy.

Hickin, Herbert, Best, Howard, and Osborne (2007) used a phonological-orthographic cueing approach with two individuals with aphasia who had naming deficits but minimal semantic impairment. The patient with nonfluent aphasia showed response generalization but the patient with fluent aphasia showed no generalization. The authors hypothesized that the two individuals processed the cues differently, and this accounted for the generalization difference. The patient evidencing response generalization seemed to process the cues as a combination of semantic and lexical information, whereas the other patient's strategy was to sound out the graphemes. This observation implies that the strategy itself (automatic or not) must be generalizable for an individual and that a challenge to clinicians is to find ways to specifically train the internal strategy.

Semantic Feature Analysis (SFA) is a therapy technique for anomia for which good treatment effects for trained stimuli have been demonstrated (Boyle, 2004; Boyle & Coelho, 1995) but response generalization remains a challenge (e.g., Kristensson, Behrns, & Saldert, 2015; Rider, Wright, Marshall, & Page, 2008). The mechanism of SFA, when successful, is to assist lexical retrieval by stimulating the target item with closely associated semantic features, following the precepts of the spreading activation theory, until the target item reaches activation threshold. If the approach is able to reestablish the semantic feature connections, response generalization to closely associated representations may be anticipated, although it is not expected to extend to concepts that share few or no features with the trained target. For the response generalization pattern to be possibly more widespread, SFA should be broadened as a strategy; that is, patients must be taught an SFA strategy that they can internalize and automatically apply to all word-finding attempts (Lowell, Beeson, & Holland, 1995; Wambaugh et al., 2014). At first glance this may seem an easy task, but implementing this process is challenging. For example, Wambaugh, Mauszycki, Cameron, Wright, and Nessler (2013) attempted to add a formal step to SFA to teach individuals with aphasia to internalize the technique, but observed weak to no response generalization. Internalizing the SFA strategy may be difficult (although not impossible, see Davis & Stanton, 2005) and may explain the spotty presence of positive generalization results. Furthermore, conceptually this strategy would be very difficult to apply to sentence- or discourse-level language (i.e., stimulus generalization, discussed later) as the SFA strategy is time-consuming to apply. What is more, the few positive response generalization results seen with SFA (e.g., Boyle, 2004; Boyle & Coelho, 1995; Davis & Stanton, 2005) have been challenged. It is possible that the observed generalization effect actually represents an improvement due to multiple exposures to the probed (i.e., untreated) stimuli, rather than a true generalization effect (Howard, 2000; Howard et al., 1985; Wambaugh et al., 2014; Weisenburn & Mahoney, 2009), although some more recent naming studies have attempted to minimize this threat (e.g., Greenwood, Grassly,

Hickin, & Best, 2010). The same arguments can be made for the Phonological Components Analysis (PCA, Leonard et al., 2008), which is the phonological equivalent of SFA.

In an attempt to maximize response generalization, Lowell et al. (1995) used a modified SFA approach. They asked three individuals with aphasia to select personalized cues that were then trained with SFA. In addition, the authors included two types of untrained items: those to which subjects were exposed as probes and those that were not used at all during the training. Two patients showed significant training effects and strong response generalization to all untrained exemplars, whether they were semantically related or not. The authors emphasized that the approach they developed was an attempt at maximizing the internalization of the semantic self-cueing strategy. Interestingly, the single subject who did not benefit from the therapy approach showed the lowest scores on cognitive measures and that variable could be a negative candidacy factor when attempting to teach patients to internalize a treatment strategy.

In sum, there is no doubt that any word-finding strategy needs to be internalized if any response generalization is to be expected. However, this process does not take place automatically, and can only become established if the strategy is generalizable and focuses on skills that the patient can rely on consistently. For SFA specifically, the generalization data are not encouraging, but it seems that the best results are demonstrated when semantic cues are client-specific rather than dictated by the approach.

Train Enough Exemplars

A universal numerical answer to this question is precluded by the many variables that influence treatment, from the characteristics of the therapy objective, to aphasia severity, to the specific therapy protocol selected. To further complicate the matter, the criterion typically used to answer this question is an example of circuitous logic: If you seek response generalization, train a variety of items until you measure response generalization on your untrained probes! Several specific implications emerge from this rationale, however. Firstly, clinicians must plan on measuring generalization probes. This is sensible, but needs to be planned cautiously, because of the observed therapy effect on generalization probes or response foils (Howard et al., 1985; Pring et al., 1993). It is thus recommended that each generalization probe contain previously unused items to avoid an exposure effect. Secondly, there are different mechanisms of generalization: Has the patient reactivated an underlying process, such as an overall improved access to the phonological output lexicon? Has the patient internalized a new strategy, such as evoking related semantic concepts to access a specific semantic representation? Has the patient internalized a learned rule, such as associating past tense with the -ed morpheme? Consider the case, as discussed earlier, where authors recognized that therapy approaches for anomia are successful but the improvement tends to be item-specific (e.g., Laganaro et al., 2006; Snell et al., 2010). When the therapy approach focuses on practicing the reactivation of specific lexical items, the underlying mechanism causing the improvement will be item-specific, and increasing the number of practiced items may increase the success of therapy, but it is unlikely to trigger response generalization. However, developing a process-oriented therapy approach (i.e., a therapy approach focusing on the underlying skill or on a replacement strategy) should lead to successful reactivation of untrained exemplars (e.g., Hinckley & Carr, 2001).

In conclusion, quantity alone is not an effective variable. That is, training more exemplars is not a de facto solution for generalization unless it is combined with an underlying process-oriented learning strategy. Also of note is the fact that patients with aphasia who obtained higher scores on cognitive tests (e.g., Raven's Progressive Matrices) are more likely to show generalization (Hinckley & Carr, 2001) than individuals who have lower scores.

Use Loose Training

Loose training is a concept long advocated for the purpose of stimulating both response and stimulus generalization (Stokes & Baer, 1977; Thompson, 1989). This concept requires that the stimulus variables as well as the response contingency be varied and not tightly scripted. Specifically for response generalization, the expectation is that there may be several acceptable target responses and the patient has some discretion regarding how to phrase the answer. Alternatively, a related interpretation of loose training involves the production of target responses that differ on a variety of features such as semantic relatedness, phonemic proximity, or syntactic environment. This latter interpretation is reminiscent of the issue of massed versus distributed practice in motor speech disorders. Distributed practice introduces variations in production that lengthened the learning period but facilitated generalization (Yorkston, Beukelman, Strand, & Hakel, 2010).

Response Elaboration Training (RET) is a therapy technique based on loose training that has shown positive response generalization (Kearns, 1985; Kearns & Scher, 1989). The patient is asked to comment on a picture stimulus and the clinician asks follow-up questions that lead the patient to comment further. The patient is then asked to repeat the longer target sentence. This loose training procedure leads the patient to produce more content words as answers to untrained stimuli. Other language symptoms, such as agrammatism, remained unchanged. However, when Husak and Marshall (2012) adapted RET to a different task and required their patients with Broca's aphasia to generate a sentence of their choice based on a picture representation of an action verb, the results showed an improvement in syntax production in addition to response generalization to untrained items. As an approach, RET may be more successful with people with nonfluent aphasia rather than fluent aphasia types (Wambaugh, Wright, & Nessler, 2012).

Because Semantic Feature Analysis (SFA) has shown weak response generalization, Conley and Coelho (2003) attempted to combine SFA with RET in an attempt to boost the generalization potential. In the spirit of the loose training approach, the patient led the SFA protocol, the clinician expanded on the patient's responses, and the patient repeated the expanded utterances. The results showed a significant increase in correct production of trained and untrained items. The authors attributed this generalization to the semantic activation triggered by SFA combined with the production of utterances containing the target item. This phrase-level step seems to be similar to a syntagmatic cueing mechanism that the patient appeared to use as a self-cue strategy. For example, one can imagine the client evoking *white* to find the target *car*, because of the utterance *my car is white*. The advantage of this process is that SFA may automatically get distilled to the most powerful personal cue, rather than to embark on the time-consuming process of visualizing and filling out the entire semantic feature diagram (see earlier discussion, Lowell et al., 1995).

In sum, loose training in aphasia therapy does not have the same level of experimental support that it has in rehabilitation of motor speech disorders, but overall, the response generalization results surpass those of single-word training. It seems that its main benefit resides in the flexibility given to the patients in terms of types of response and types of cues.

Consider the Client's Associated Symptoms and Characteristics

This variable groups a variety of candidacy issues based on patient characteristics and abilities for successful generalization that are still only minimally understood. Among the studies measuring response generalization, some patients always generalize significantly better or worse than others, even after controlling for patient characteristics and treatment procedures. Clearly, we are still unable to separate patient-specific candidacy variables. Only a few infrequent hypotheses have been mentioned in the literature, and they all involve *a posteriori* qualitative observations.

There is a significant body of literature devoted to understanding the relationship between aphasia and cognitive skills. Many researchers have reported that cognitive scores are depressed in individuals with aphasia. This observation holds, even when the linguistic demands of the cognitive tests are minimized. Helm-Estabrooks (2002) posited that, although cognitive test scores are poorly correlated with language test scores, therapy success may be partially dependent on patients' cognitive abilities. It is beyond the scope of this chapter to review this entire literature, but it behooves us to mention that some authors have relied on this hypothesis to explain the variability of treatment effects (Carragher et al., 2012; Dickey & Yoo, 2010; Fillingham et al., 2005a, 2005b; Hinckley & Carr, 2001; Lowell et al., 1995) and the variability of generalization results among their subjects with aphasia. For example, Hinckley and Carr (2001) found that individuals with aphasia with higher cognitive scores (as measured by the Wisconsin Card Sorting Test [Grant & Berg, 1981] and the Raven's Progressive Matrices [Raven, 1976]) took less time to achieve criterion and maintained their gains at follow up, whereas patients with lower cognitive scores took much longer to improve and lost their gains at follow up. Law et al. (2008) reported that two of their four patients with aphasia had very similar symptomatologies, yet one was able to show response generalization, whereas the other showed progress on trained items only. The only difference in measured ability between the two patients involved cognitive measures of problem-solving skills. The authors ventured to hypothesize that the patient with better executive skills was able to internalize the Chinese equivalent of a grapheme-phoneme conversion rule, whereas the patients with poorer problem-solving abilities was unable to do so. Kendall, Raymer, Rose, Gilbert, and Gonzalez Rothi (2014) described a therapy approach for anomia using a combination of multiple semantic and phonological cues. Treatment effects were present but limited response generalization was observed across their eight subjects (still generalization within semantic category was superior to across semantic category, as expected). Interestingly, the subject showing the best generalization had the highest score on the Raven's Progressive Matrices Test. The authors concluded that cognitive ability may be a predictor variable for generalization, just as it has been shown to be for treatment effects (Fillingham, Sage, & Lambon Ralph, 2006).

Another significant variable reported in the literature is the level of aphasia severity. For example, Wambaugh and Thompson (1989) concluded that generalization was worse if patients exhibited perseverative or stereotypic behaviors. Wiegel-Crump and Koenigsknecht (1973) used a stimulation approach with four subjects with anomic aphasia in an attempt to improve word-finding. They reported generalization to untrained exemplars in trained categories and also to exemplars in an untrained category (clothes). The positive response generalization results in this study may be explained by severity. Anomic aphasia is considered the least severe of the aphasia types (even if the anomia is severe) and severity may in turn be a limiting factor for the generalization process. Furthermore, level of anomia severity at onset has also been associated to success of response generalization (Raymer et al., 2007).

In conclusion, the observed variability in generalization between patients guarantees that there are candidacy variables at play. Among those, level of severity and associated cognitive skills have been identified as influencing generalization, but there are still too little data to draw precise quantitative conclusions. Many other variables are likely involved such as motivation (see Chapter 12, this volume) or level of comprehension. However, none of these has been reported systematically, and no variable has had its influence studied experimentally.

Include Semantic Processing

There is an argument in the literature about the type of cues to use when targeting word-finding difficulties: lexical (phonological and/or orthographic) versus semantic. Although the bulk of the discussion has focused on the strength of the treatment effect rather than the generalization effect, authors have generally concluded that semantic-based therapy facilitates response generalization more readily than phonologically-based approaches (Nickels & Best, 1996). In their meta-analysis of the effects of anomia treatments, Wisenburn and Mahoney (2009) argued that both phonological and semantic approaches were efficacious, but that semantic strategies were more successful at generalization to exemplars never used during therapy. Reinforcing this conclusion, several case studies using a lexical cueing protocol have shown poor response generalization (Best et al., 2011; Herbert, Best, Hickin, Howard, & Osborne, 2003; Herbert, Gregory, & Best, 2014). However, it has been argued that semantic and phonological (or lexical) processing are virtually impossible to isolate (Howard, 2000), and as a consequence, focusing on a phonological therapy approach does not preclude semantic processing on the subject's part. Thus, including a semantic processing task in the treatment protocol may serve to increase the likelihood of response generalization.

Focusing rehabilitation on semantic processing usually includes the manipulation of the semantic features associated with the target item. As discussed previously, SFA does not have a particularly good track record of response generalization, especially if the strategy is not internalized. An interesting and novel approach relies exclusively on asking the patient to evoke a mental picture of the object (i.e., mental imagery) in a passive way, without attempting to name the object. This technique can be interpreted as requiring the patient to manipulate a single semantic feature, namely the visual representation of an item. A case description with a patient with chronic anomic aphasia (Bhatnagar, Zmolek, DeGroot, Sheikh, & Buckingham, 2013) revealed a positive therapy effect for typical and atypical items as well as response generalization to untrained exemplars. The paucity of data in the literature on this technique makes it impossible to recommend this approach without more research, but the concept remains intriguing.

Treat More Complex Items

This hypothesis seeks to facilitate generalization by focusing on more difficult or complex therapy targets rather than simpler ones early in the treatment protocol, a concept in opposition to traditional thinking of establishing a behavior in simple context then expecting generalization to different targets. The idea of training complex items earlier in treatment traces its origins in motor learning theory and was first applied to phonological therapy with children (Dinnsen, Chin, Elbert, & Powell, 1990; Geirut, 2001; Tyler & Figurski, 1994). These authors showed that selecting phonological treatment targets based on linguistic complexity resulted in greater generalization without an increase in time to reach criterion. Thompson and Shapiro (2007) suggested applying this concept to aphasia treatment. In a series of experiments, Thompson and colleagues have shown that this logic holds for syntax training and that response generalization is possible within syntactic transformation types such as NP movements or wh- movements (Thompson, Ballard, & Shapiro, 1998; Thompson et al., 1997). Thompson et al. (1998) further noted that within the wh- movement structures, response generalization was better from object cleft training to who question than vice versa. It seemed that the difference lay in the level of intrinsic complexity between the two types of wh- movements. Indeed, object cleft is considered more complex because the wh- movement takes place in an embedded clause, whereas a who question does not require embedding. As predicted, the results showed response generalization from more complex structure (object cleft) to simpler syntactic structure (who question) but not the opposite. Predictably, neither training showed generalization to passive sentences, which require a different syntactic movement type altogether. This confirms that treating more complex elements of language facilitates response generalization within the confines of linguistically similar processes. These results were replicated using three types of wh- movements that differ in their linguistic complexity (Thompson, Shapiro, Kiran, & Sobecks, 2003). Interestingly, the same results were obtained using a computerized interface (Thompson, Choy, Holland, & Cole, 2010). Thompson and colleagues concluded that training the most complex form generalized to the simpler structures, but not the opposite. The authors coined this effect the Complexity Account of Treatment Efficacy (CATE). Thompson and Shapiro (2005) summarized the relevant studies providing the evidence for CATE and provided additional evidence that the CATE principle is further applicable to verb argument structure complexity. That is, verbs with fewer possible arguments (e.g., RUN: *the boy ran*) are easier to produce than verbs requiring more arguments (e.g., GIVE: *the boy gives the toy to the dog*). Stadie et al. (2008) attempted to replicate the results described by Thompson and colleagues. They trained (in German) seven patients with Broca's aphasia and agrammatism either on object clefts or who questions while using passives as probes. They confirmed that there was a tendency for the training to generalize from object clefts to who questions but not vice versa. However, they also noticed that some patients generalized to passive sentence structures as well, which is in conflict with the CATE principle that there should be no generalization to different syntactic structures. Stadie et al. (2008) argued that instead of analyzing complexity in terms of type of movements or number of transformations, complexity should be determined based on the number of nodes needed in the deep structure sentence analysis (following Chomsky). In this paradigm, passive structures have the same number of nodes as who questions and fewer than object clefts. Although this theoretical argument is ongoing, it is overall good news for clinicians. It shows that careful planning of a syntactic complexity hierarchy can facilitate response generalization.

CATE was further applied to anomia rehabilitation. Kiran (2007; Kiran & Thompson, 2003) argued that atypical exemplars of a category (e.g., ostrich–BIRD) are more complex than typical exemplars (e.g., robin–BIRD) based on their semantic feature structure. The semantic features associated with atypical exemplars within a semantic category (e.g., feature = has a long neck; exemplar = ostrich; category = BIRD) include both the features of the atypical exemplar and features of typical exemplars (e.g., feature = has wings; exemplar = robin). The reverse however, is not the case; that is, typical exemplars (e.g., exemplar = robin) do not include features of atypical exemplars. Consequently, training atypical items forces the patient to process prototypical features shared by most members of the category in addition to the distinctive features belonging to the atypical category exemplars and facilitates access to semantic and phonological levels of processing (Kiran, 2008), and thus increases the likelihood of generalization. Training prototypical category members will only activate prototypical semantic features. Kiran and Thompson (2003) investigated the typicality effect using a semantic therapy approach for anomia in four individuals with fluent aphasia. (Patients with fluent aphasia were selected because prior reaction time research demonstrated that patients with Wernicke's aphasia do not show a typicality effect, whereas individuals with Broca's aphasia do.) The authors selected three levels of typicality among two categories and the results clearly showed that when therapy focused on typical items (e.g., robin) there was no response generalization to less typical exemplars (e.g., ostrich), whereas when the therapy focused on atypical items (e.g., artichoke) generalization occurred to more typical exemplars (e.g., carrot). No generalization across categories was evidenced; hence, no significant improvement on formal naming tests was noted. These results were extended to inanimate categories in patients with nonfluent aphasia types (Kiran, 2008), and to goal-oriented categories, such as *things to take camping*, in patients with mild fluent aphasias (Kiran, Sandberg, & Sebastian, 2011). The complexity hypothesis was further examined using the abstract/concrete dimension (Kiran, Sandberg, & Abbott, 2009) in which training abstract exemplars (e.g., HOSPITAL: health) tended to show response generalization to concrete items in the same category (e.g., HOSPITAL: surgery) whereas training concrete exemplars (e.g., CHURCH: chapel) did not show generalization to abstract items (e.g., CHURCH: prayer). These subsequent examinations of the CATE hypothesis roughly confirmed the predictions of the theory, but several patients did not improve or did not generalize improvements (Kiran, 2008; Stanczak, Waters, & Caplan, 2006). It is possible that individuals with fluent aphasias are better candidates for this approach than patients with nonfluent types of aphasia. For example, Wambaugh and colleagues (2013) were unable to replicate the generalization effects with nonfluent aphasia patients. Furthermore, in Kiran (2008), the two patients with poor response to treatment had the lowest scores on cognitive assessments, and thus candidacy could also hinge on remaining cognitive skills (Helm-Estabrooks, 2002). Finally, this approach may be more appropriate for individuals with semantic-level rather than phonologically based naming difficulties (Stanczak et al., 2006).

Identifying categories and specific exemplars may not be straightforward, as pointed out by Rossiter and Best (2013). These authors reported that the typicality effect was intercorrelated with other word effects such as age of acquisition, frequency, and familiarity. When the influence of these effects on naming skills was measured independently, age of acquisition was the strongest predictor and typicality one of the weakest. Rossiter and Best (2013) did confirm that typical exemplars were easier to access than atypical ones, but that the typicality effect may actually be partially an artifact of confounding variables that may render the selection of items more challenging than expected.

In conclusion, the typicality effect has reasonably strong support in the literature, both for syntax and word-finding therapy goals, even if the underlying reason for the effect is still uncertain. However, this effect is only useful within narrow confines, either a specific set of syntactic structures or semantic categories; overall response generalization is not within the reach of this technique.

Train Verbs

Many authors have reported that patients with aphasia also have a significant impairment in verb naming in addition to the ubiquitous anomia for nouns. Jane Marshall (1999) developed a semantic approach for verb naming with her patient EM. The treated verbs improved significantly, whereas untreated items did not. The author reported that exemplars semantically close to the target verbs tended to improve, but she also noted that these synonyms had been presented as foils during therapy. Edwards and Tucker (2006) exposed three individuals with fluent aphasia to a program of verb elicitation. Only one subject showed response generalization to untrained verbs but the authors acknowledged that multiple exposures to the untrained probe exemplars may have caused the measured improvements. Similarly, Fink, Schwartz, Sobel, and Myers (1997) trained verb naming. The results showed that the treatment effect was strong for trained items and for the exemplars used as probes, but no response generalization was observed for untrained and unexposed exemplars. Some authors have attempted to use the SFA approach with verbs in the hope that response generalization may be better than for nouns (Faroqi-Shah & Graham, 2011; Raymer & Ellsworth, 2002; Wambaugh & Ferguson, 2007; Wambaugh et al., 2014). The results have been disappointing, as the activated semantic features seem to remain item specific. Taken together, these results suggest that when therapy is targeted at individual lexical items, be it nouns or verbs, response generalization remains problematic.

In an attempt to move beyond single-verb training, Conroy, Sage, and Lambon Ralph (2009) directly compared word- versus sentence-based cues for verb naming. The authors anticipated better results for sentence-level cues because sentences rely on explicitly stated verb arguments; however, both procedures led to significant increases of verb naming, whereas response generalization remained nonexistent.

In sum, it seems that training verbs as single lexical units does not facilitate response generalization better than training nouns (Boo & Rose, 2011; Michum & Berndt, 1994; Raymer et al., 2007; Webster & Whitworth, 2012).

Train Items in a Sentence Context

The process of word retrieval is different when the target is an isolated lexical item (as in confrontation naming) than when it is surrounded by linguistic context (as in spontaneous speech tasks). Mayer and Murray (2003) reported that their subjects tended to access lexical items somewhat more easily in connected speech compared to naming tasks, and they retrieved verbs better than nouns. Still, the authors acknowledged that the reverse patterns are certainly possible in some patients with anomia. Yet, because of the influence of linguistic context, focusing intervention at the sentence level may have a positive impact on therapy success as well as generalization patterns for some patients.

Prescott, Selinger, and Loverso (1982) developed a therapy intervention requiring their subjects to produce simple SV sentences. The results of the multiple baseline across word lists showed response generalization to untrained verbs. Links, Hurkmans, and Bastiaanse (2010) trained their subjects with Broca's aphasia to produce verbs within sentence contexts either in an infinitive (uninflected) or an inflected form. They found that training inflected forms triggered response generalization to untrained verbs, whereas training the uninflected form did not. They offered no hypothesis for that discrepancy (although the complexity effect may come to mind). They further noticed an improvement in confrontation naming for nouns, and concluded that this generalization was a side effect of working with sentences because nouns were included in the training, as each sentence was in SVO format. Edmonds, Nadeau, and Kiran (2009) went a step further and required their patient to produce a subject and an object, with the intent of practicing the verb within the context of its predicate structure, thereby strengthening the link between verbs and their thematic structures. Their Verb Network Strengthening Treatment (VNeST) focuses on verbs but also requires the processing of the verbs' thematic roles. For example, for the target verb "measure," the patients have to select "chef" and "sugar" or "carpenter" and "lumber" as appropriate agents and objects. The authors hypothesized that the relationship between a verb and its possible thematic roles could lead to co-activation between those elements and furthermore, that related verbs could also be co-activated, so that focusing on the verb "measure" could generalize to "weigh." Response generalization was clearly demonstrated, both for noun and verb naming. In a subsequent investigation of VNeST in patients with more severe aphasia (Edmonds & Babb, 2011), the authors reported that a longer therapy period was necessary to achieve response generalization. In this study, only one subject showed widespread response and stimulus generalization. The variable that the authors identified as responsible for the generalization discrepancy between their two patients was the production of the sequence agent-verb-patient in phase 2 of the treatment program. With the individual who showed scant generalization, this phase only required production of agent-patient, without the verb. This may indicate that processing a sentence format is necessary to maximize generalization. Interestingly, as an added bonus, this approach seems to benefit nouns as well as verbs.

In order to stimulate generalization using Semantic Feature Analysis (SFA), Papathanasiou, Mesolora, Michoy, and Papachristou (2007) combined SFA with the production of semantic features in sentences. Both subjects in their study showed response generalization to untrained words. This result suggests that embedding target lexical items within a sentence structure may provide additional processing power that may in turn facilitate word-finding in general.

Mitchum and Berndt (1994) reported the results of a therapy approach focusing on sentence structure with a patient with agrammatism. The authors trained the patient to produce SVO sentences with correct syntactic morphemes (e.g., prepositions, tense). Results showed clear response generalization, as the patient was able to correctly produce untrained sentences in various sentence production paradigms. The authors concluded that the patient was able to internalize the rules pertaining to the required morphological elements of the sentence structure. However, stimulus generalization to spontaneous discourse did not occur, once again showing that the two types of generalization patterns follow different rules.

Milman, Vega-Mendoza, and Clendenen (2014) developed integrated training for aphasia (ITA), a language rehabilitation program that trains isolated lexical items and short sentences simultaneously, based on part-whole learning principles. Their three patients with nonfluent aphasia showed strong treatment effects but no response generalization. However, some minimal stimulus generalization to connected speech (i.e., picture description) was noted for two out of three patients, mainly involving mean length of utterance (MLU).

In conclusion, treating anomia within a sentence context seems to trigger a much more consistent response generalization than focusing therapy on isolated lexical items, be it a noun or a verb. However, it also appears that focusing on verbs, as the central hinge of a sentence, may extend response generalization to nouns, but not vice versa.

Train the Underlying Mechanism

This variable is related to the type of rehabilitation objective targeted in therapy. Clinicians must decide (with patient and family input, of course) whether to use process-oriented or skill-oriented objectives to rehabilitate specific behaviors. The former targets an underlying skill (i.e., a process such as word-finding) and the latter focuses on specific items (e.g., naming 10 functional objects). Common sense, as well as cognitive theory, predicts that the therapy targeting the underlying skill has the potential for generalization, whereas a task-oriented approach does not (Hinckley & Carr, 2001). One interpretation ascribes the superior response generalization to treating a central process (e.g., semantic-based therapy) rather than a more peripheral process (e.g., phonologically based therapy). Thus within a language processing model, treating central processes has greater potential for generalization than treating peripheral processes (Nickels & Best, 1996). Naturally, the focus on central versus peripheral processes has to match the patient's locus of difficulty. Researchers, therefore, have attempted to target underlying processes in an attempt to facilitate generalization. Mitchum, Haendiges, and Berndt (1993) described a patient with nonfluent aphasia and agrammatism. The authors purposefully devised the rehabilitation protocol to target the early stages of sentence production, that is, before the process becomes modality-specific, and they trained writing output only. They observed some limited response generalization to the untrained oral output modality.

Another important variable in training an underlying mechanism seems to be time post-onset. As discussed earlier, the literature in general suggests that direct training on lexical items tends not to trigger response generalization. However, that body of literature is comprised of patients in chronic stages of recovery. It is likely that focusing on the underlying mechanism of a skill (e.g., naming) in therapy could be more successful in the earlier stages of recovery, and that later improvements reflect some internal compensatory processing that is likely to involve new learning (Papathanasiou, Coppens, Durand, & Ansaldo, 2017). The former process is likely to generalize readily, whereas the latter mechanism may do so only when the strategy is internalized. However, this distinction is far from clear cut, particularly at the level of an individual patient. For example, the chronic patient with fluent aphasia described by Robson, Marshall, Pring, and Chiat (1998) showed a specific impairment of accessing the phonological representations of words from the semantic system. The authors developed a therapy program focused on phonological processing, with the intent of teaching the patient a specific strategy that she could then generalize as a self-cueing mechanism. The results showed strong treatment effects as well as strong response generalization. However, it was clear that the patient was not using the strategy as a self-cue, but had rather improved the overall access to phonological representations. This "deblocking" of a skill when the patient is in the chronic stages may be unexpected, but clearly is not impossible. It can only happen, however, if the therapy approach is focused at the mechanism underlying the impairment. In turn, it emphasizes the importance of informal testing designed to identify the exact locus of impairment (see Chapter 13, this volume).

Kendall et al. (2008) developed a therapy program focusing on phonological knowledge. The rationale was that a stronger representation of phonemes should facilitate word-finding using a phonological route, and this facilitation should occur regardless of the specific word or language environment. The therapy tasks included associating individual sounds with depictions of their realization; verbal descriptions of features of sound and minimal pairs; general use of visual, auditory, and kinesthetic feedback for individual sounds; associating phonemes and graphemes; and phonological blending and parsing exercises at the syllable level. The authors reported evidence of response generalization (no words were actually trained in therapy) and stimulus generalization (i.e., picture description), as well as increases in various formal test results such as the Western Aphasia Battery (Kertesz, 2007). However, even such a seemingly broad-based approach cannot be universally successful. The authors mentioned that good results depended on good comprehension and residual phonological processing skills.

Response generalization across modalities is rarely observed, although possible (Hillis, 1989; Raymer, Thompson, Jacobs, & Le Grand, 1993; Rose & Douglas, 2008). In an early analysis of generalization performance following a cueing hierarchy protocol, Hillis (1989) compared two patients with aphasia and examined the difference in generalization patterns. The patient with a central semantic problem showed response and stimulus generalization, whereas the patient with a specific difficulty at the level of phonemic representation retrieval did not show any type of generalization. By relying on a cognitive model of language processing, Hillis (1989) postulated that if the naming difficulties arise from the lexicosemantic system common to oral and written modalities, generalization to both modalities should be expected, provided the therapy contains a semantic component. However, if the underlying problem involves specific phonological or orthographic representations, no cross-modal generalization should occur. Indeed, an additional logical requirement for generalization to occur is that the output modalities are intact, which is not always the case. Imagine a central linguistic process common to oral and written output modalities being impaired in a person with aphasia. Focusing therapy on that impaired underlying process can only generalize to both output processes if these are functioning properly. If, let us say, a specific element of the written output process is also damaged, there will be no generalization to writing.

Raymer et al. (1993) trained oral naming in four subjects with Broca's aphasia and reported cross-modal generalization to oral reading in three of the four subjects for the trained items but not for the untrained exemplars. Two of the four subjects also generalized performance in written naming for the trained items. The authors framed the results in terms of the cognitive-linguistic model and inferred that the direct stimulation of the phonological output lexicon also stimulated the orthographic output lexicon. Still, the generalization patterns were variable across subjects. The authors hypothesized that severity and a treatment period that is too short may hinder generalization in general. Rose and Douglas (2008) compared three types of semantic interventions in one patient with mild anomic aphasia: linguistic, gestural, and linguistic + gestural. Results revealed that all three types of interventions showed strong treatment effects as well as response generalization to untrained items. The patient was repeatedly presented with the control items, which could explain the improvement; however, the patient also improved on overall naming assessment tools and interestingly, cross-modally in written naming. The authors hypothesized that the generalization could be explained because "the treatments specifically addressed the underlying cause of her naming disorder" (p. 35).

Regarding treatment for syntactic deficit, an early criticism of these therapies was the focus of the rehabilitation protocols on surface structures of sentences rather than deep structures. Thompson, Shapiro, and Roberts (1993) stated that, "the lack of generalization could be attributed to the fact that the *underlying* deficit responsible for abnormal sentence production was not addressed" (p. 112). Since then, researchers have relied on linguistic theory in an attempt to facilitate response generalization across sentence types (mostly involving a complexity continuum [see earlier discussion of CATE]). For example, focusing therapy on the assignment of thematic roles (e.g., mapping therapy) should logically generalize to all exemplars of that syntactic structure as well as to other modalities because the targeted process is central to comprehension and production (Marshall, 1995). Jones (1986) designed a therapy approach centered on word order, ignoring the syntactic markers. The approach focused on the meaning of the various sentence components without requiring the patient to say the target sentences. Results showed that the patient improved not only in syntactic comprehension but also production. Interestingly, the use of functors also improved significantly. These results clearly showed that the mapping process is a mechanism that underlies output modalities and targeting this early mechanism triggers generalization (Marshall, 1995).

Thompson et al. (1997) trained two individuals with agrammatism on two different syntactic movements (according to Chomsky's theory). Wh- movements consisted of object clefts (e.g., it was the student who the biker lifted) and who questions (e.g., who has the biker lifted?) and NP movements included subject raising (the biker seems to have lifted the student) and passive (e.g., the student was lifted by the biker) structures.

By training the underlying (i.e., *deep*) structure, the authors predicted that all transformations relying on that underlying structure would benefit. The results showed that response generalization to untrained syntactic structures occurred within but not across movement types. For example, the subject who was trained on subject raising structures improved on untrained subject raising structures and on passives because both structures rely on the same underlying transformations, but no response generalization was observed on any of the wh- movement structures. These results were replicated with object-cleft and passive syntactic structures (Jacobs & Thompson, 2000). The success of this approach prompted Thompson and colleagues to formalize it as Treatment of Underlying Forms (TUF; Thompson & Shapiro, 2005). Based on their body of research with this technique, the authors concluded that TUF promotes response generalization to untrained but similar syntactic structures, and that the generalization patterns occur from more complex to less complex structures but not vice versa. A few remarks about TUF should be raised as they may have an impact on generalization. First, it should be noted that Ballard and Thompson (1999) limited candidacy for TUF to patients with an Aphasia Quotient (WAB, Kertesz, 2006) above 50. Second, some functors such as *who* and *that*, used for embedded sentences, will likely have to be trained directly (Ballard & Thompson, 1999).

In sum, these results suggest that focusing on a central process has better generalization potential than focusing on a modality-specific process or a task-specific objective. This includes response generalization as well as generalization to other modalities such as writing; and it holds for anomia and agrammatism. However, this result hinges on the clinician targeting the patient's underlying impairment in terms of specific language production processes. In this scheme, time post-onset may be a limiting factor in attempting to reestablish premorbid functioning of central language processes.

Combine Other Modalities

Using one modality to treat another is either a deblocking mechanism (e.g., using a gesture to access the representation of an object or a verb) or a compensatory strategy (e.g., writing the target). If effective and internalized, both approaches can be applied to all instances of anomia and possibly simple sentence structures. For example, Raymer et al. (2006) used a naming + gesture therapy paradigm with nine individuals with chronic aphasia. The results showed strong and comparable treatment effects for both nouns and verbs but no response generalization to untrained items for oral naming. On the other hand, a number of patients showed response generalization for untrained exemplars using gestures. The authors did not argue that the therapy increased some underlying ability to use gesture, but rather that the emphasis on gestures in the therapy approach taught the patients that the use of another modality could be a successful way to communicate.

Rose and Douglas (2008) compared three semantic treatments with a patient with anomia: linguistic, gestural, and linguistic + gestural. All three types of interventions showed strong treatment effects as well as response generalization. The authors concluded that the presence of meaningful gestures did not influence the results, and that the important treatment variable in this case was the emphasis on semantic processing. Hence, the addition of the gesture modality possibly enhanced the treatment effect by adding semantic information, and not by representing another modality per se. When non-meaningful gestures are added to an intensive word-finding treatment protocol (Altmann et al., 2014), the treatment effect and response generalization are still observed, but not attributable to the presence of the gesture, as the *no gesture* group showed the same results as the *gesture* group.

Fridriksson et al. (2009) investigated the effect of adding visual information when training naming in patients with nonfluent aphasia. The authors directly compared aural with aural-visual presentation of the stimuli and the respective effects on naming treatment and response generalization. Although there was a slight advantage in favor of the audiovisual condition for the treatment items, the response generalization observed was similar for the two conditions.

Overall, these results suggest that multimodality can be a useful tool for relearning trained items, but its impact on response generalization is doubtful. Of course, when multimodality is used as a compensatory strategy to augment communication, a person with aphasia may be able to use that strategy to communicate more effectively, provided that strategy is internalized (see Chapter 8, this volume).

STIMULUS GENERALIZATION

Stimulus generalization, the appearance of a learned behavior in a different set of circumstances, encompasses several different types. Generalization to spontaneous discourse is different from generalization to other linguistic environments. In fact, generalizing from the clinical setting to a more naturalistic environment may change several conditions at the same time: conversational partner, setting, and stimulus. Not surprisingly, not all patients are able to build this bridge, and it behooves the clinician to introduce these changes in conditions in a planned and controlled manner. In general, stimulus generalization to discourse has received less attention than response generalization to untrained exemplars. On the whole, therapeutic interventions focusing on single-word processing have shown spotty generalization to spontaneous speech.

Generalization to other settings and/or other conversation partners should occur in a shorter time frame than was required to establish the behavior in the first place (Baer, 1999), if the behavior has been well established in the therapy room. However, generalizing from smaller linguistic units (e.g., words or syntactic structure) to larger units (e.g., conversations) requires that a single process (e.g., finding a specific word) be embedded into a multiprocess event (e.g., finding that same word while at the same time processing pragmatics, suprasegmentals, syntax, and lexical and phonological information). This multiprocess event is further complicated by the fast pace at which it is occurring. Not surprisingly, this transition does not occur easily or spontaneously. Raymer and Ellsworth (2002), for example, trained verb naming in an individual with nonfluent aphasia and noticed an improvement in sentence production, but the improvement was limited to accessing trained verbs, not untrained verbs or syntax. Wambaugh and Thompson (1989) did not observe generalization to conversation unless directly trained. However, when training occurred in a conversational setting, progress was observed. The authors concluded predictably that therapy needs to take place within other environments and conditions to elicit stimulus generalization.

Carragher and colleagues (2012, 2015) reviewed the challenges facing stimulus generalization to conversations following therapy focusing on noun and/or verb retrieval. In general, there was a tendency for the subjects' conversations to have improved because the trained items provided more lexical variability. However, the authors highlighted three problems with this type of generalization pattern, suggesting that the success of stimulus generalization depends on how it is measured and on the type of conversation investigated. First, measuring vocabulary diversity or success of conversational turns may yield better results than measuring sentence correctness, as syntax is not addressed. For example, Rider and colleagues (2008) trained lexical items pertinent to the description of specific video clips. Using the Semantic Feature Analysis (SFA) therapy, the individuals with aphasia showed improvement in naming these items, as well as improvement in lexical measures during the clip descriptions. This shows that trained lexical items may be accessed speedily enough to be used in prescribed discourse exercises, such as during script training therapy. This approach, however, is not likely to affect unscripted functional conversational discourse on a wider scale. Second, training nouns may provide better stimulus generalization results than training verbs because syntactic structure (crucial to verbs) is not addressed in single-word verb retrieval treatment. Finally, conversations with examiners tend to be semi-structured rather than naturalistic, thus not offering maximum opportunity for stimulus generalization to conversation. The authors concluded that involving a variety of conversation partners within the therapy paradigm is likely critical to the success of stimulus generalization.

Recently, Milman (2016) reviewed the results of several reports focusing on *integrated discourse treatment for aphasia* (IDTA), a program she developed that focuses on promoting stimulus generalization. Essentially, in IDTA, a typical clinical session includes direct work on single-word retrieval, sentence production, and a functional discourse component reminiscent of RET. She reported that there was a strong therapy effect, an equally strong maintenance effect, a small response generalization effect, but a much stronger stimulus generalization effect, in which six out of eight patients improved significantly on at least one discourse measurement. These results confirm the observation that response and stimulus generalization respond to different types of training. Interestingly, Milman (2016) further reported that the patients who showed poorer stimulus generalization performed worse on cognitive tasks such as attention, memory, and reasoning.

In sum, it appears that stimulus generalization has several components and that each component needs to be actively addressed during the rehabilitation process. The next section reviews the strategies that may best help clinicians achieve these generalization objectives.

Use Loose Training

Thompson and Byrne (1984) recommended "loose training" to promote stimulus generalization by building intermediary steps between the therapy room and a more natural environment. In their study, question-asking was the most difficult to generalize among the sentence forms. The authors hypothesized that the reluctance of individuals with aphasia to initiate turns explained the results rather than an underlying difficulty with that sentence format per se. A similar hypothesis was advanced by Kearns and Scher (1989) regarding their loose training approach (RET) which they tested by probing target behavior (mean number of content words) in several generalization conditions. Their three individuals with aphasia improved equally well and showed stimulus generalization to untrained stimuli, different people (clinician and spouse), and new settings. Stimulus generalization to spontaneous conversation was demonstrated for two of their three subjects. The authors hypothesized that loose training, which emphasizes response flexibility, gave the patients more confidence in the communicative value of their productions. Wambaugh et al. (2012) examined a modified RET specifically for stimulus generalization to discourse. The authors described the results as "disappointing," as only one out of five individuals with aphasia showed increased information units in discourse (personal stories). This may indicate that direct intervention in a discourse context is necessary.

Script training is a therapy approach for patients with limited language output and mild to moderate comprehension difficulties. The patients select a small number of script topics that fulfill functional needs and they are trained to produce the utterances in the scripts holistically and automatically in a massed practice paradigm. In order to facilitate stimulus generalization, Youmans, Holland, Muñoz, and Bourgeois (2005) introduced an element of loose training subsequent to the script training. The therapist purposefully varied her answers and prompts to introduce a level of flexibility in the mastery of the scripts, thereby adding a phase of loose training after the massed practice period. The results showed that the patients were able to generalize the use of scripts with unfamiliar conversation partners. The authors underscored that the loose training phase was a crucial element to achieve stimulus generalization. These results have been replicated (Goldberg et al., 2012). Naturally, the generalization only applies to the specific scripts.

This approach is reminiscent of the *sequential modification* strategy advocated by Stokes and Baer (1977) and Thompson (1989), as well as *natural maintaining contingencies* (Stokes & Baer, 1977), the former because stimulus generalization may occur as an additional step subsequent to direct therapy and the latter because clinicians manipulate the contingencies to smooth the transition between therapy and functional applications. Indeed, the links between any given training and more naturalistic communication situations must be carefully planned and directly trained by developing and practicing appropriate intermediary steps. Adding a loose training phase can be one of these steps because it approximates the stimulus/response variability of functional communication and hence may facilitate stimulus generalization to discourse. However, it does not appear that this technique has the potential to generalize to all unscripted communicative situations.

Add Discourse/Conversational Training

This variable is, in part, a subset of the umbrella term of *sequential modification* (Stokes & Baer, 1977; Thompson, 1989). In essence, this principle requires that direct intervention be applied to conditions that are shown to be resistant to generalization after the implementation of a successful treatment. This implies that direct therapy for anomia or agrammatism should be accompanied by a treatment phase focusing on discourse or conversation. However, because stimulus generalization to conversation is challenging, this focus of therapy should be introduced early in the treatment program. This discussion is reminiscent of the traditional approach of group therapy for aphasia. Group therapy was originally advocated as a follow-up rehabilitation period targeting communication in more functional/naturalistic settings subsequent to dismissal from direct language intervention (Marshall, R. C., 1999, p. 61), whereas a more recent service delivery model would advocate the addition of group therapy from the inception of the rehabilitation period because of its value in promoting stimulus generalization (Kearns & Elman, 2008, p. 392).

Several authors have sought to promote stimulus generalization to spontaneous speech by modifying a therapy approach focusing on lexical (i.e., phonological/orthographic) cueing. These authors acknowledged that training isolated words is not conducive to stimulus generalization and hence have attempted to introduce a conversational discourse training phase in their treatment protocol. Herbert et al. (2003) used a lexical cueing protocol with six patients with aphasia. Stimulus items were line drawings representing functional items that were chosen by the patient and caregiver based on personal interests. In addition to lexical cueing, these personalized items were also trained as part of a more functional (i.e., PACE) conversational approach. Unfortunately, the participants showed poor response and poor stimulus generalization to discourse. Hickin et al. (2007) used a similar approach with two individuals with aphasia, in which the corpus of items was trained in a naming task and then in a more functional/conversational approach. They measured both response and stimulus generalization. One individual with nonfluent aphasia showed response generalization as well as some improvement in word-finding in spontaneous conversations. However, the patient with fluent aphasia showed neither type of generalization, which may be an indication that aphasia type could influence candidacy. Greenwood et al. (2010) employed the same therapy paradigm with a person with conduction aphasia. The patient showed response generalization and stimulus generalization to word-finding in unscripted conversations, which the authors ascribed to an improved link between lexical representations and phonemic realization. It should be emphasized that the patients described by Greenwood et al. (2010) and by Hickin et al. (2007) were selected because they were found to respond well to lexical cueing, which may have led to an overestimation of the results of therapy and generalization. Still, only two of the three patients showed some level of stimulus generalization, thereby suggesting that additional candidacy factors further influence generalization. Best et al. (2011) used a lexical cueing paradigm with their individuals with aphasia and measured generalization to functional conversation. In contrast to previous studies, Best et al. (2011) purposefully did not script the conversations to match the exemplars targeted in therapy and instead used an outcome measure designed to investigate the relationship between word retrieval in picture naming and functional conversation. They reported that, as a group, their subjects did not show generalization to conversation. However, when they analyzed the relationship between therapy effects and lexical retrieval scores in conversation, there was a significant correlation. This suggests that therapy effects are related to the presence and strength of stimulus generalization to discourse. The authors concluded that the therapy improved word-finding to a small extent—enough to show a correlation with conversation content—but not enough to show response generalization. In other words, if anomia therapy is successful, trained nouns may be accessed rapidly enough to be retrieved in conversation. However, in this case, stimulus generalization is only the extension of item-specific anomia training.

It is also possible that the nature of the therapy interaction can facilitate stimulus generalization to discourse. Kempler and Goral (2011) concluded that more functional, client-generated interaction showed better generalization than traditional drill exercises. The authors posited that the emphasis on oral discourse principles and client-generated functional stimuli facilitated generalization, although as mentioned earlier, Herbert and colleagues (2003) did not find stimulus generalization with the introduction of a PACE phase. Also, Kempler and Goral (2011) acknowledged that the breadth of stimuli was, by the nature of the interaction, less restrictive than that of the drill approach, which may also have facilitated generalization by introducing an element of loose training. Peach and Reuter (2010) adapted SFA for use in discourse contexts by using pictured scenes instead of object or verb depictions. They subsequently used the traditional SFA paradigm with the lexical items that the patient was unable to access (noun or verb) before finally reverting back to the original scene. It was anticipated that targeting discourse-level production would facilitate generalization to untrained discourse tasks, thus bypassing the stimulus generalization process which is a recognized challenge for the original SFA format. The results demonstrated only minimal improvement in productivity (in words per T-units) and informativeness (in correct information units). Finally, in her IDTA approach, Milman (2016) included an element of sentence production and discourse practice in all therapy sessions. The results showed good stimulus generalization to discourse and weaker response generalization. The author underscored the importance of using functional, patient-generated content and noted that the presence of cognitive functioning limitations impaired good stimulus generalization results.

Overall, many studies have reported that stimulus generalization is possible, albeit minimal (Best et al., 2011; Greenwood et al., 2010; Peach & Reuter, 2010). Merely exposing patients to a discourse environment is clearly not enough. However, better results are possible (Milman, 2016) provided the gap between restricted controlled practice in the therapy room and the required flexibility in a natural discourse context is carefully bridged by the selection of patient-specific conversational content. The transition to more unscripted functional discourse demands additional intermediary steps that have yet to be defined.

Train Items in a Sentence Context

The researchers who have trained lexical items in sentence contexts have also attempted to build logical intermediary steps between a lexical rehabilitation focus and spontaneous discourse. For example, Mitchum and Berndt (1994) trained their patient with agrammatism to produce SVO sentences correctly, including appropriate syntactic morphology. The patient generalized the successful intervention to untrained sentences (response generalization) but showed no stimulus generalization to discourse. Moreover, mapping still remained a problem, as the patient kept producing erroneous reversible sentences. This example, as well as others, suggests that training sentence structures yields overall disappointing results in terms of stimulus generalization. As discussed earlier, the explanation may lay in the type of transition used from smaller units of language to stimulate discourse-level communication. Therefore, a new approach was suggested by Herbert, Webster, and Dyson (2012). These authors developed a therapy approach designed to treat lexical items within syntactic contexts, rather than merely focusing on lexical retrieval tasks applied to discourse. This approach is not designed to train syntactic structure per se but to include the syntactic properties of single words, such as part of speech, gender, and number information in stimulus items. In theory, this approach is based on the concept of the lemma stage and should stimulate the production of complete noun phrases, thereby facilitating transfer to spontaneous speech. Herbert et al. (2012), using this "Noun Syntax Therapy," focused on the noun determiners "a" versus "some" followed by countable or uncountable nouns respectively. The results showed no response generalization to untrained items, but positive stimulus generalization to discourse, indicating that most patients had increased the use of trained determiners in their story telling (i.e., Cinderella). The authors stated that candidacy for this type of treatment includes residual use of determiners (i.e., no severe agrammatism) and good phonological processing. These results were replicated and extended in a subsequent case study (Herbert et al., 2014) in which the authors also measured significant improvements in spontaneous unscripted conversation in terms of noun and determiner use. These data clearly show that successful stimulus generalization "to narrative and to conversation requires intervention beyond single words" (Herbert et al., 2014, p. 171). Taken together, these results indeed indicate that stimulus generalization to discourse can be present but tends to be limited. At best, discourse measures may improve slightly if the patient with aphasia is able to retrieve the trained items fast enough in the demanding confines of a spontaneous speech situation. This conclusion holds for nouns in isolation and nouns with their syntactic environments.

Links et al. (2010) described a therapy approach for sentence production comprising several steps. The subjects are asked to insert an uninflected verb form into a sentence, then, to complete a sentence with the inflected verb, and finally, to produce the full sentence spontaneously. All sentences were nonreversible. The authors reported an increase in MLU, in proportion of finite verbs, and in number of different verbs in spontaneous discourse. However, comprehension scores did not change, thereby confirming that successful rehabilitation of language production does not automatically generalize to receptive language, and that the latter should be addressed separately.

As a therapy approach for anomia, the SFA approach has not yielded significant stimulus generalization. In an attempt to remedy this situation, some authors have combined SFA with a sentence-level paradigm. Papathanasiou et al. (2007) developed the Elaborated SFA (ESFA) which uses the traditional SFA approach but adds a sentence production step to the procedure, during which the patient is asked to generate sentences for each feature named. Two individuals with aphasia participated in this study: one patient with anomic aphasia and one with global aphasia. Both subjects showed stimulus generalization to picture description as measured by utterance length. In another attempt at combining sentences with SFA, Capilouto and Wright (2009) asked their patients with aphasia to generate utterances containing several information units based on an action picture. The action picture was placed in the target spot of a traditional SFA diagram, but the semantic features were replaced with mostly wh- words (why, who, where, when). Using these elements, the patient was expected to produce sentences such as: *A man helping a woman out of a car at a hotel entrance.* By measuring the number of these information components, the authors observed variable yet overall moderate generalization to untrained targets. A similar enhanced SFA method was used by Knoph, Lind, and Simonsen (2015) with a multilingual patient. The authors reported improvements in connected discourse (in treated and untreated languages) and ascribed the positive result to the focus on verbs and the use of sentence-level practice.

In sum, it appears that sentence-level practice, as opposed to single lexical item therapy objectives, does facilitate stimulus generalization to discourse. These results, albeit modest, seem to be more successful than introducing discourse-level practice as a subsequent step following the therapy phase. It is conceivable that inserting sentence-level practice in therapy represents one of the possible intermediary steps between restrictive drill work and discourse applications.

Train Verbs

Because of the lack of stimulus generalization when therapy focuses on nouns, some authors have turned their attention to the training of verbs. Within their semantic representation, verbs contain an argument structure, which determines the required syntactic structure surrounding the use of a particular verb. As such, successful verb retrieval may facilitate the production of sentence structures (Marshall, J., 1999; Marshall, Pring, & Chiat, 1998). However, as discussed earlier, training verb naming as an isolated lexical level may not be sufficient. Edwards and Tucker (2006) trained three individuals with fluent aphasia to name verbs and their stimulus generalization was limited. Mitchum and colleagues (1993) trained their patient with nonfluent aphasia to write trained verbs in isolation and in sentences. There was a strong item-specific training effect, and the patient was able to retrieve the trained verbs in constrained written discourse production, but not in unconstrained discourse tasks. Furthermore, there was no overall improvement in written discourse beyond the ability to produce the trained items. In their review, Webster and Whitworth (2012) concluded that therapy focusing on verbs as single lexical items showed poor stimulus generalization to discourse. In fact, that type of generalization may even be harder to achieve than for nouns because of the richer semantic representation of verbs. Verbs contain specific information about associated argument predicate structure, and direct training of that structure may be necessary (Whitworth, Webster, & Howard, 2015). In other words, "mapping meaning relations between semantics and syntax" (Jones, 1986, p. 63) may be required for more effective stimulus generalization. For verbs, an underlying semantic problem will give rise to more severe sentence generation difficulties, because the predicate argument structure (i.e., the number and type of propositions required by the verb) is an integral part of the semantic constructs of verbs (Marshall et al., 1998; Webster, Morris, & Franklin, 2005). On the other hand, an isolated difficulty in phonological access for verbs will not affect the predicate argument structure of the verb and sentence-level discourse may not be impaired. What is more, this lexical-level problem is distinct from a genuine syntax impairment, such as agrammatism. Finally, in a thorough review of verb-level therapies, Conroy, Sage, and Lambon Ralph (2006) report that using video samples for verb naming rather than static images may provide a facilitatory effect and a better verb naming performance (at least in patients with cognitive difficulties).

Jones (1986) developed a therapy program for an individual with chronic severe nonfluent aphasia. The program was based on a metalinguistic presentation of verb argument structures and was initially carried out without requests for verbal sentence production. The approach led to significant improvement in sentence-level discourse in picture description and spontaneous discourse. Interestingly, there was an associated improvement of functor use, which had not been targeted directly in the therapy program. Jones concluded that the patient's underlying impairment requiring remediation related to the predicate-argument structure of verbs, and that a "surface" approach focusing, for example, on prepositions could not achieve any success without the support of that core organizational structure. Webster et al. (2005) trained their individual with nonfluent aphasia to name verbs and to associate appropriate thematic roles to specific verbs. The results showed no response generalization to untrained verbs, which is in line with the lack of generalization in other studies when therapy focuses on lexical items in isolation, even verbs. However, there was stimulus generalization to sentence production, which the authors interpreted as improvement in the ability to "specify the arguments around verbs [the patient] could produce" (p. 761).

In sum, treating verbs as lexical items and limiting the therapy to naming without an accompanying sentence-context provides limited, if any, stimulus generalization (e.g., Mitchum & Berndt, 1994). Even when an individual with aphasia improves verb naming as a word-finding skill, it does not lead to improved sentence production (Boo & Rose, 2011; Mitchum & Berndt, 1994; Mitchum et al., 1993; Whitworth et al., 2015). In other words, the greater complexity of verbs, in terms of intrinsic morphological and syntactic characteristics, translates to better sentence production if these components are accessed during discourse, but not if the verb is merely accessed as a decontextualized lexical item. Generalization, then, can only be expected if the therapy focuses specifically on these internal features, such as thematic roles or argument structures (Whitworth et al., 2015). As expected, because stimulus and response generalization are independent processes, response generalization to untreated exemplars remained very limited (Conroy et al., 2006).

We have already discussed that the VNeST program (Edmonds et al., 2009) shows good response generalization. The data also demonstrate that there is positive stimulus generalization as well (Edmonds & Babb, 2011; Edmonds, Obermeyer, & Kernan, 2015). The training of verbs and thematic roles together led to improvements in sentence production in discourse, including for untrained verbs and for novel pictures. Interestingly, one of the important elements that the authors identified to explain the positive generalization results, was the "highly diverse modifications" (p. 419). That is, each verb can be associated with a wide variety of agents and objects, and this diversity of semantic links offers built-in exemplar variety, which we know contributes to response and stimulus generalization. Furthermore, the processing and production of the entire sentence format (agent-verb-patient) in the treatment protocol may be necessary to trigger generalization (Edmonds & Babb, 2011).

As we saw, focusing therapy on the verb agreement structure may improve sentence-level production in spontaneous discourse; however, true syntax impairments are often superimposed. Bazzini et al. (2012) describe a multiphase program that includes a dual focus of verb agreement structure and specific syntax deficits (e.g., subject-verb agreement, prepositions). The results showed that there was a strong therapy effect, response generalization to untrained nouns and verbs, and stimulus generalization (i.e., increased sentence length) to picture description and connected speech. The patients showed remaining syntactic difficulties, but the authors argued that these could be further remediated with a longer therapy period. Unfortunately, the authors have not ventured hypotheses regarding the specific cause of the generalization pattern. Still, these results indicate that the impairment inherent to thematic roles within verb representation and syntactic deficits are distinct, and that for best results, both difficulties must be directly addressed. Inclusion criteria for this program were adequate articulation and phonology, absence of severe lexical-level processing, and absence of severe comprehension problems.

As discussed earlier, the SFA approach is a type of intervention that focuses on lexical items in isolation. Several authors have reported that individuals with aphasia who are successful at SFA, are, in general, not successful at generalizing their results to spontaneous discourse (Boyle, 2004; Boyle & Coelho, 1995). To facilitate such generalization, some researchers have applied the SFA paradigm to verbs (Faroqi-Shah & Graham, 2011; Wambaugh & Ferguson, 2007; Wambaugh et al., 2014). Wambaugh and Ferguson (2007) not only used action verbs as targets, they also modified the SFA diagram to include three features specifically designed to evoke the thematic roles related to the target verb. This predicate-argument structure training had the additional benefit of adding noun retrieval practice. Results showed that spontaneous discourse improved in terms of efficiency (in words per minute) and content (in correct information units). The authors noted that the patient with aphasia did not seem to use the SFA approach consciously during spontaneous discourse tasks, thereby indicating that there was no internalization of the strategy. Instead, they attributed the observed stimulus generalization to easier verb access because of the facilitatory effect of the predicate-argument structure information. In other words, the sentence context contains additional information that facilitates lexical access. This hypothesis also explains why there was no response generalization. The patient was not able to access untrained action verbs, probably because their predicate information was not readily available.

In sum, it is clear that training verbs as isolated lexical items does not lead to stimulus generalization, as is the case for nouns. However, results are much more encouraging when verbs are treated in the context of their argument structure and reliance is made on thematic roles. This latter variable also has the added benefit of triggering learning and generalization of nouns. This approach is not a panacea, however, because additional syntactic difficulties may require specific intervention, for example, more complex syntax structures or specific functors.

Add Home Practice

Speech-language pathologists regularly rely on home practice in aphasia rehabilitation. At face value, additional time spent practicing the targeted tasks should lead to increased treatment effects. Although there are little data showing that home practice per se is improving outcome or facilitating generalization, there are a significant number of studies showing that treatment intensity is related to outcome (e.g., Bhogal, Teasell, Foley, & Speechley, 2003; Bhogal, Teasel, & Speechley, 2003; Cherney, Patterson, Raymer, Frymark, & Schooling, 2008; Lee, Kaye, & Cherney, 2009) (see Chapter 9, this volume). For example, Lee and colleagues (2009) report that patients using script training achieved better mastery the more they practiced at home. This is not surprising because script training is based on a massed practice paradigm (Youmans et al., 2005).

One program that has recently integrated a strict home practice requirement is Constraint-Induced Aphasia Therapy (CIAT). CIAT has been shown to be a successful therapy approach for individuals with aphasia (e.g., Pulvermüller et al., 2001). The approach attempts to counteract the learned nonuse phenomenon where the desired behavior (e.g., verbal speech) is suppressed. It is based on principles similar to Constraint-Induced Motor Therapy (CIMT) for hemiparesis: constraints on behavior (e.g., requiring verbal output), response shaping (e.g., providing increased levels of difficulty), context that focuses on real-life activity, and condensed practice (massed practice and intensity of treatment). CIAT requires the patient to use oral language only within an intensive treatment paradigm. Yet, the stimulus generalization results were not up to par with those of CIMT (Taub et al., 2012) which led Johnson et al. (2014) to expand the original CIAT program to model it more closely to CIMT, specifically the home program component. The strategies that were employed included the addition of functional and naturalistic role-playing exercises and the development of an intensive and required home practice program. The home practice program was rebranded as the "transfer package" and contained (a) daily language tasks, (b) a daily diary identifying communicative difficulties and strategies for overcoming them, and (c) a verbal activity log to report quality of communication. Adherence to the home program was closely monitored by the clinicians. The authors reported significant gains in communication participation as well as gains on the WAB-R. These results suggest that home practice programs are important for stimulus generalization; however, the home practice needs to be carefully designed and monitored for compliance.

In conclusion, although there is limited experimental data specifically for home practice, there is little doubt that it is a potentially useful addition to the rehabilitation program to facilitate stimulus generalization. However, the program cannot rely merely on repetitions (i.e., quantitative) but must contain well designed functional applications. In that sense, this procedure is similar to *natural maintaining contingencies* advocated by Stokes and Baer (1977). It is crucial that the home program be carefully monitored by the clinician to maximize stimulus generalization results.

Treat More Complex Items

This principle has received more attention regarding response generalization than stimulus generalization. However, in their review of the literature on the subject, Thompson and Shapiro (2007) reported that training more complex syntactic structures did facilitate stimulus generalization to discourse. Specific spontaneous discourse improvements have been noted for MLU, frequency of grammatically correct sentences, frequency of verbs, and number of correct informational units. Also, Reichman-Novak and Rochon (1997) developed a two-phase approach to improve sentence production in an individual with Broca's aphasia. The first phase consisted of a single verb naming paradigm. As expected, a strong treatment effect was observed and neither response nor stimulus generalization was evident. The second phase focused on passive voice training using verbs trained during the first phase as well as novel verbs. The results showed an increase in production of passive sentences, but also an improvement in syntactically simpler active sentences. This observation was much stronger for the verbs trained in the first phase of the program, which indicates that the specific training of verbs was a necessary component.

In conclusion, it appears that this variable yields good results when applied to syntax. No information is available for word-finding. However, we know from other investigations that therapy on individual lexical items is not conducive to either response or stimulus generalization.

Train the Underlying Mechanism

Rose and Douglas (2008) described a patient with mild anomic aphasia, which they believe stemmed from a difficulty in semantic-lexical processing, with predominately semantic error types. The authors developed a therapy approach focusing on semantic processing and the treatment effect was large. Furthermore, the patient showed response generalization to untreated items and stimulus generalization to discourse. Specifically, her ability to access lexical items in discourse improved significantly. Finally, she also improved in written naming, thereby showing that the interface between semantic and lexical processing was facilitated regardless of the output modality. There is little doubt that this patient had improved in the general ability of accessing lexical items thanks to the fact that therapy was targeted directly at the underlying problem. Unfortunately, not all patients show these positive results, and candidacy is still mostly a mystery. However, this individual patient's symptomatology was particularly mild.

Mitchum et al. (1993) focused a therapy protocol on the early stages of sentence production. They trained their patient with nonfluent aphasia and agrammatism to first write individual verbs and then to produce sentences focusing the training on verb morphology. They trained the written output modality only. The results showed limited generalization to other forms of sentence generation tasks and generalization to the spoken output modality. According to the authors, the successful cross-modal generalization pattern can be explained by the therapy targeting common nodes of language processing. Furthermore, stimulus generalization to other forms of discourse can be interpreted as the internalization of the strategy to construct verb tense morphology.

Mapping therapy purportedly focuses on syntactic processing stages that subsume modality specificity (Marshall, 1995). As such, this has the potential to show response generalization as well as stimulus generalization to discourse and other modalities. Thompson et al. (1997) focused their treatment approach on the underlying "deep" levels of syntactic structures. Specifically, they trained their two patients with agrammatism on two non-canonical syntactic structure transformations: wh- movements and NP movements. In addition to within-structure response generalization, the authors also reported stimulus generalization to discourse. Interestingly, there was no specific performance improvement for the non-canonical structures trained, but rather an increase in the proportion of grammatical and complex sentences, as well as the number of sentences with correct verb argument structure. The authors argued that this generalization was due to the use of reversible sentences, with emphasis on the thematic roles surrounding the verbs, as well as because "the treatment provided focused explicitly on the linguistic and psycholinguistic underpinnings that we hypothesized would influence sentence production" (p. 242). The same positive stimulus generalization results were later confirmed following training on types of wh- movements only (Ballard & Thompson, 1999; Thompson et al., 2003). Jacobs and Thompson (2000) used two non-canonical syntactic structures to investigate stimulus generalization to discourse and to other modalities. They trained four participants with agrammatism on one of the two sentence structures, either by focusing on comprehension or on production training. The results showed some generalization to discourse in most patients, as exemplified by increased MLU and sentence complexity. Also, comprehension training generalized to sentence production both orally and in writing, whereas production training generalized to written sentence production only. The fact that both therapy approaches improved writing production confirms that the targeted syntactic processes are central processes of language production and are thus independent of output modality. However, the authors acknowledged that written stimuli were used in both types of interventions and that this element may have triggered the cross-modal generalization. The authors further discussed why comprehension generalized to production but not vice versa. They hypothesized that comprehension engages a level of sentence analysis that is not required when only producing the same sentence. This somewhat contradicts later reports (Thompson et al., 2010) where generalization to comprehension was evidenced for the same complex structures trained. Overall, this approach, focusing on the deep syntactic structure, was labeled Treatment of Underlying Form (TUF; Thompson & Shapiro, 2005). In their review of supporting data, the authors concluded that TUF typically facilitates the following components of stimulus generalization to discourse: MLU, proportion of syntactically correct sentences, and frequency of verbs. However, in a later comparison, discourse improvements were limited to MLU, words per minute, and proportion of complex sentences. As stated previously, candidacy for TUF has been limited by severity level (patients with an AQ score < 50). Ballard and Thompson (1999) reported that the two individuals with aphasia who did not show stimulus generalization to discourse had a more severe level of Broca's aphasia.

In conclusion, treating the underlying mechanism seems to be as beneficial for stimulus generalization as it is for response generalization (see previous discussion). This may be one of the few strategies able to facilitate both types of generalization processes.

Internalize the Strategy

If the goal of anomia therapy is to provide the individual with aphasia with a word-finding strategy, that strategy must be patient-generated if stimulus generalization is to be successful. Moreover, the specific strategy must also be fairly rapid in its execution in order to take place within reasonable delays in a discourse environment. Wambaugh and colleagues (2014) used SFA to train verbs in four patients with aphasia. The significant treatment effect did not translate to discourse generalization, but the authors doubted that their patients internalized the strategy, because they did not appear to use SFA during discourse tasks. Antonucci (2009) trained two individuals with aphasia to use SFA in group therapy discourse environments and reported that her patients had clearly internalized the strategy, but overall stimulus generalization to discourse still remained minimal. The approach had clearly not improved word-finding as a skill. A slightly different approach was preferred by Olsen, Freed, and Marshall (2012), who trained individuals with aphasia to associate personalized cues to specific lexical items. The approach successfully increased word retrieval for trained items in discourse, but there was no change in untrained exemplars or any other discourse measures. So, the patients with aphasia were able to generalize trained exemplars to other settings and to discourse by internalizing the strategy, which remained item-specific by design.

In sum, an internalized strategy can be useful for discourse generalization if the mechanism itself can be automatized and fairly rapid in its execution. If the mechanism is compensatory, such as by making conscious use of a different modality or a multistep strategy (e.g., writing the first letter of the target word, generating the phoneme, saying the word), similar to the use of an external augmentative/alternative communication (AAC) device for example, stimulus generalization to discourse may take place, but the execution will remain cumbersome and unnaturalistic.

Combine Other Modalities

There is an extensive literature supporting the use of multimodal approaches as a cueing mechanism or as a compensation method (see Chapter 8, this volume). Using other modalities to communicate can generalize to functional settings if the strategy has been internalized. For example, if a patient is taught to write words rather than express them verbally, this strategy could generalize, provided the patient's writing skills are preserved. If the patient is trained to write a limited set of functional words, this strategy may generalize to other settings or conversation partners, but will not generalize to other exemplars. Similarly, the use of a communication book or an AAC device faces the same challenges.

In contrast, few data address the role of multimodality use for generalization of oral language skills. One approach that has received some attention in that respect is the use of gestures. Some authors have reported stimulus generalization to discourse when including meaningful gestures as part of the therapy approach, both when focusing on nouns (Rose & Douglas, 2008) or verbs (Rose & Sussmilch, 2008). However, the observed generalization was not attributed to the use of an additional modality, but rather to the fact that therapy focused on the underlying problem (Rose & Douglas, 2008) or on the use of nouns in addition to verbs (Rose & Sussmilch, 2008). Similarly, when using non-meaningful gestures (i.e., with no added semantic value) stimulus generalization to discourse was reportedly limited to an increase of propositions in responses to questions, but not in picture descriptions. These results remain unexplained (Altmann et al., 2014). Rose, Raymer, Lanyon, and Attard (2013) completed a systematic review of studies incorporating gesture into treatment protocols and reported that evidence for generalization is mixed. They suggested that treatment items should be carefully selected in order to plan for generalization, but also in the event generalization fails, to assure that the trained items are of functional use for the patient.

In conclusion, this variable is essentially limited to the generalization of trained exemplars to other settings or partners with the objective of improving functional communication, rather than facilitating oral language use.

Use Functional Items

To explain the lack of stimulus generalization in studies of patients with aphasia, Thompson (1989) suggests that there may be a disconnect between the trained stimuli and their functionality in the probed generalization task. For example, trained syntactic structures or wh- questions may not be functional in a picture description task. The more functional the target utterances are, the more successful the generalization to different conversation partners and environments will be. For example, Doyle, Goldstein, Bourgeois, and Nakles (1989) trained individuals with Broca's aphasia to request information on three distinct functional topics and noted that the target behavior generalized to unfamiliar conversational partners and settings.

In conclusion, this variable is a way to build a bridge between the therapy room and more functional communicative situations. Training items that the patient is most likely to need in everyday activities is bound to facilitate communication in these same situations. As was the case for the addition of multimodal strategies, the introduction of functional items primes generalization to predictable environments and different communication partners, but it is not designed to generalize more widely to the entire variety of possible contexts and communication needs.

CONCLUSION

First and foremost, response and stimulus generalization processes require planning and specific strategies to bear fruit. Clinicians must spend time devising these strategies equal to the dedication that they use to develop clinical rehabilitation goals (Kearns & Elman, 2008). Moreover, stimulus and response generalization are not the same processes, and they do not necessarily respond the same way to the same strategies. There is a double dissociation.

The literature provides some indication about some useful and some less effective strategies to facilitate generalization. Even approaches that have shown promise do not work for all patients. Every strategy to support generalization is likely to possess its own candidacy issues, yet these are not well understood. Some of the candidacy variables reported so far have included cognitive abilities, aphasia types, and aphasia severity. For example, TUF has some candidacy regarding aphasia severity: AQ > 50 (Ballard & Thompson, 1999). Furthermore, almost all of the studies published have involved chronic patients. We know very little about generalization patterns associated with acute rehabilitation and improvements. It is possible that the ideal set of beneficial generalization strategies varies with time post-onset.

Overall, it seems that targeting language processes common to all output modalities has the greatest potential for stimulus and response generalization. However, it is important that the clinician determine the exact underlying mechanism of impairment for each patient, in order to target the precise origin of the problem and thus maximize stimulus and response generalization (see Chapter 13, this volume). Time post-onset may represent an important candidacy limitation as over time process-oriented therapy objectives tend to be replaced with task-specific goals, thus potentially changing generalization expectations. Another strategy that may facilitate both types of generalization is the focus on sentences, particularly when patients are made aware of the central importance of verbs, their argument predicate structure, and the associated thematic roles.

Some of the other suggested generalization strategies may be more adequate for either stimulus generalization or response generalization but not both. However, some of these strategies are clearly related and can be combined. For example, loose training is related to number of exemplars trained, and its success probably depends on the internalization of a strategy. Therefore, it may be difficult to isolate the effects of each individual strategy experimentally.

CASE ILLUSTRATION

KC is a 57-year-old woman who suffered a CVA 2 months ago. Her language symptoms were severe at onset and she was diagnosed with global aphasia; however, she made some improvements and the current diagnosis is Broca's aphasia characterized by a nonfluent output, agrammatism, anomia, mild to moderate comprehension difficulties, and mild apraxia of speech. She can rely on a voice output AAC device for word-finding and basic functional sentences, but prefers to attempt oral communication and shuns the device most of the time. Her life participation was decreased in the acute stages of the disease, but thanks to the training that the clinician provided to caregivers, friends, and some local shop owners, KC does not shy away from social contacts. As a consequence, KC's attitude toward her aphasia is not negative (as measured by the ASHA FACS; Frattali, Holland, Thompson, Wohl, & Ferketic, 2003). KC's husband is very supportive and eager to try new methods for better communication with KC. They both wish that KC could make progress in her oral language, particularly word-finding and sentence length.

Our informal assessment revealed that KC has good semantic processing, as she is able to access concepts receptively. Her errors are mostly semantic paraphasias, no answers, and a few phonemic paraphasias. Her naming shows a frequency effect. Her writing skills are similar to her oral production; however, she is able to understand single written words. Consequently, her main problem seems to be the access to the graphemic and phonological lexicons from a preserved semantic system. In an attempt to identify the nature of KC's agrammatic difficulties, we first assessed her verb naming. She was able to name 80% of action pictures (although she rarely used verbs in discourse production.) In addition, she had no problem comprehending the verbs in isolation and she had no difficulty at the level of the event, as she was able to choose the appropriate picture to complete a story event (Marshall, 2017). We tested KC's processing of the verb argument structure by using a sentence to picture matching task involving reversible sentences. She made many mistakes in mapping roles onto the argument structure. She also showed poor comprehension of more complex syntactic structures such as passives and wh- movements.

In order to remediate the patient's anomia and at the same time promote response generalization, we decided to focus therapy on verbs within a sentence structure. The literature suggests that using an approach such as VNeST (Edmonds et al., 2009) can stimulate verb as well as noun retrieval. This strategy also focuses on the verbs' thematic structures, which can also have a facilitatory effect on sentence-level production.

To stimulate generalization to discourse, we decided to focus on developing KC's awareness of the verb argument structure and the mapping of thematic information onto that structure. The literature shows good stimulus generalization with such a strategy (Bazzini et al., 2012; Webster et al., 2005). If progress and generalization are realized, we are planning, as a subsequent therapy step, to focus on specific complex syntactic structures such as passives. The literature has suggested that these structures have to be specifically trained (Bazzini et al., 2012). Within the type of syntactic structures selected to therapy, we would focus on the most complex forms, because there tends to be generalization to less complex forms, according to CATE (Thompson & Shapiro, 2007).

Stimulus generalization to functional settings and other conversation partners will be addressed by including role playing, with a variety of interlocutors in the therapy setting and by developing a home practice program with the assistance of KC's spouse and possibly friends. The home program will include a wider variety of items than those covered in the clinic as well as slightly amended instructions and response targets, in order to introduce an element of loose training.

We believe that these therapy elements carry the highest potential for KC to maximize response and stimulus generalization. Still, attention must be paid to careful measurement of KC's progress. For example, the response generalization probes will include items never seen by KC in therapy. The stimulus generalization measures for discourse will include picture descriptions (i.e., scripted output fairly similar to therapy activities), storytelling (e.g., The Three Bears), and unscripted but functional conversations.

REFERENCES

Altmann, L. J. P., Hazamy, A. A., Carvajal, P. J., Benjamin, M., Rosenbek, J. C., & Crosson, B. (2014). Delayed stimulus-specific improvements in discourse following anomia treatment using an intentional gesture. *Journal of Speech, Language, and Hearing Research, 57*, 439–454.

Antonucci, S. M. (2009). Use of semantic feature analysis in group aphasia treatment. *Aphasiology, 23*(7–8), 854–866.

Baer, D. M. (1999). *How to plan for generalization.* Austin, TX: Pro-Ed.

Baer, D. M., Wolf, M. M., & Risley, T. R. (1968). Some current dimensions of applied behavior analysis. *Journal of Applied Behavioral Analysis, 1*(1), 91–97.

Ballard, K. J., & Thompson, C. K. (1999). Treatment and generalization of complex sentence production in agrammatism. *Journal of Speech, Language, and Hearing Research, 42,* 690–707.

Bazzini, A., Zonca, G., Craca, A., Cafforio, E., Cellamare, F., Guarnaschelli, C., ... Luzzatti, C. (2012). Rehabilitation of argument structure deficits in aphasia. *Aphasiology, 26*(12), 1440–1460.

Best, W., Grassly, J., Greenwood, A., Herbert, R., Hickin, J., & Howard, D. (2011). A controlled study of changes in conversation following aphasia therapy for anomia. *Disability and Rehabilitation, 33*(3), 229–242.

Bhatnagar, S., Zmolek, B., DeGroot, D., Sheikh, A., & Buckingham, H. (2013). Generalizing naming ability through mental imagery. *Procedia—Social and Behavioral Sciences, 94,* 24–25.

Bhogal, S. K., Teasell, R. W., Foley, N. C., & Speechley, M. R. (2003). Rehabilitation of aphasia: More is better. *Topics in Stroke Rehabilitation, 10*(2), 66–76.

Bhogal, S. K., Teasell, R. W., & Speechley, M. R. (2003). Intensity of aphasia therapy, impact on recovery. *Stroke, 34,* 987–993.

Boo, M., & Rose, M. L. (2011). The efficacy of repetition, semantic, and gesture treatments for verb retrieval and use in Broca's aphasia. *Aphasiology, 25*(2), 154–175.

Boyle, M. (2004). Semantic feature analysis treatment for anomia in two fluent aphasia syndromes. *American Journal of Speech-Language Pathology, 13,* 236–249.

Boyle, M., & Coelho, C. A. (1995). Application of semantic feature analysis as a treatment for aphasic dysnomia. *American Journal of Speech-Langauge Pathology, 4,* 94–98.

Cannito, M. P., & Vogel, D. (1987). Treatment can facilitate reacquisition of a morphological rule. In R. H. Brookshire (Ed.), *Clinical aphasiology conference proceedings* (pp. 23–28). Minneapolis, MN: BRK Publishers.

Capilouto, G., & Wright, H. H. (2009). Scripting information components to improve narrative discourse performance. *Journal of Medical Speech-Language Pathology, 17*(2), 99–110.

Carragher, M., Conroy, P., Sage, K., & Wilkinson, R. (2012). Can impairment-focused therapy change the everyday conversations of people with aphasia? A review of the literature and future directions. *Aphasiology, 26*(7), 895–916.

Carragher, M., Sage, K., & Conroy, P. (2015). Outcomes of treatment targeting syntax production in people with Broca's-type aphasia: Evidence from psycholinguistic assessment tasks and everyday conversation. *International Journal of Language and Communication Disorders, 50*(3), 322–336.

Cherney, L. R., Patterson, J. P., Raymer, A., Frymark, T., & Schooling, T. (2008). Evidence-based systematic review: Effects of intensity of treatment and constraint-induced language therapy for individuals with stroke-induced aphasia. *Journal of Speech, Language, and Hearing Research, 51*(5), 1282–1299.

Conley, A., & Coelho, C. A. (2003). Treatment of word retrieval impairment in chronic Broca's aphasia. *Aphasiology, 17*(3), 203–211.

Conroy, P., Sage, K., & Lambon Ralph, M. A. (2006). Towards theory-driven therapies for aphasic verb impairments: A review of current theory and practice. *Aphasiology, 20*(12), 1159–1185.

Conroy, P., Sage, K., & Lambon Ralph, M. A. (2009). A comparison of word versus sentence cues as therapy for verb naming in aphasia. *Aphasiology, 23*(4), 462–482.

Davis, L. A., & Stanton, S. T. (2005). Semantic feature analysis as a functional therapy tool. *Contemporary Issues in Communication Science and Disorders, 32,* 85–92.

Dickey, M. W., & Yoo, H. (2010). Predicting outcomes for linguistically specific sentence treatment protocols. *Aphasiology, 24*(6–8), 787–801.

Dickey, M. W., & Yoo, H. (2013). *Acquisition versus generalization in sentence production treatment in aphasia: Dose-response relationships.* Paper presented at the American Speech-Language-Hearing Association Convention, Chicago, IL.

Dinnsen, D. A., Chin, S. B., Elbert, M., & Powell, T. W. (1990). Some constraints on functionally disordered phonologies: Phonetic inventories and phonotactics. *Journal of Speech and Hearing Research, 33*, 28–37.

Doyle, P. J., & Goldstein, H. (1985). Experimental analysis of acquisition and generalization of syntax in Broca's aphasia. In R. H. Brookshire (Ed.), *Clinical aphasiology* (Vol. *15*, pp. 205–213). Minneapolis, MN: BRK Publishers.

Doyle, P. J., Goldstein, H., & Bourgeois, M. S. (1987). Experimental analysis of syntax training in Broca's aphasia: A generalization and social validation study. *Journal of Speech and Hearing Disorders, 52*, 143–155.

Doyle, P. J., Goldstein, H., Bourgeois, M. S., & Nakles, K. O. (1989). Facilitating generalized requesting behavior in Broca's aphasia: An experimental analysis of a generalization training procedure. *Journal of Applied Behavior Analysis, 22*(2), 157–170.

Edmonds, L. A., & Babb, M. (2011). Effect of verb network strengthening treatment in moderate-to-severe aphasia. *American Journal of Speech-Language Pathology, 20*, 131–145.

Edmonds, L. A., Nadeau, S. E., & Kiran, S. (2009). Effect of Verb Network Strengthening Treatment (VNeST) on lexical retrieval of content words in sentences in persons with aphasia. *Aphasiology, 23*(3), 402–424.

Edmonds, L. A., Obermeyer, J., & Kernan, B. (2015). Investigation of pretreatment sentence production impairments in individuals with aphasia: Towards understanding the linguistic variables that impact generalization in Verb Network Strengthening Treatment. *Aphasiology, 29*(11), 1312–1344.

Edwards, S., & Tucker, K. (2006). Verb retrieval in fluent aphasia: A clinical study. *Aphasiology, 20*(7), 644–675.

Faroqi-Shah, Y., & Graham, L. E. (2011). Treatment of semantic verb classes in aphasia: Acquisition and generalization effects. *Clinical Linguistics and Phonetics, 25*(5), 399–418.

Fillingham, J. K., Sage, K., & Lambon Ralph, M. A. (2005a). Treatment of anomia using errorless versus errorful learning: Are frontal executive skills and feedback important? *International Journal of Language and Communication Disorders, 40*(4), 505–523.

Fillingham, J. K., Sage, K., & Lambon Ralph, M. A. (2005b). Further explorations and an overview of errorless and errorful therapy for aphasic word-finding difficulties: The number of naming attempts during therapy affects outcome. *Aphasiology, 19*(7), 579–614.

Fillingham, J. K., Sage, K., & Lambon Ralph, M. A. (2006). The treatment of anomia using errorless learning. *Neuropsychological Rehabilitation, 16*(2), 129–154.

Fink, R. B., Schwartz, M. F., Sobel, P. R., & Myers, J. L. (1997). Effects of multilevel training on verb retrieval: Is more always better? *Brain and Language, 60*(1), 41–44.

Frattali, C.M., Holland, A.L., Thompson, C.K., Wohl, C. & Ferketic, M. (2003). *Functional Assessment of Communication Skills for Adults* (AHSA FACS). Rockville MD: American Speech-Language-Hearing Association.

Fridriksson, J., Baker, J. M., Whiteside, J., Eoute, D., Moser, D., Vesselinov, R., & Rorden, C. (2009). Treating visual speech perception to improve speech production in nonfluent aphasia. *Stroke, 40*, 853–858.

Gierut, J. A. (2001). Complexity in phonological treatment: Clinical factors. *Language, Speech, and Hearing Services in Schools, 32*, 229–241.

Goldberg, S., Haley, K. L., & Jacks, A. (2012). Script training and generalization for people with aphasia. *American Journal of Speech-Language Pathology, 21*, 222–238.

Grant, D. A. & Berg, E. A. (1981). Wisconsin Card Sorting Test. Torrance, CA: WPS.

Greenwood, A., Grassly, J., Hickin, J., & Best, W. (2010). Phonological and orthographic cueing therapy: A case of generalized improvement. *Aphasiology, 24*(9), 991–1016.

Helm-Estabrooks, N. (2002). Cognition and aphasia: A discussion and a study. *Journal of Communication Disorders, 35*, 171–186.

Herbert, R., Best, W., Hickin, J., Howard, H., & Osborne, F. (2003). Combining lexical and interactional approaches to therapy for word finding deficits in aphasia. *Aphasiology, 17*(12), 1163–1186.

Herbert, R., Gregory, E., & Best, W. (2014). Syntactic versus lexical therapy for anomia in acquired aphasia: Differential effects on narrative and conversation. *International Journal of Language and Communication Disorders, 49*(2), 162–173.

Herbert, R., Webster, D., & Dyson, L. (2012). Effects of syntactic cueing therapy on picture naming and connected speech in acquired aphasia. *Neuropsychological Rehabilitation, 22*(4), 609–633.

Hickin, J., Herbert, R., Best, W., Howard, D., & Osborne, F. (2007). Lexical and functionally based treatment: Effects on word retrieval and conversation. In S. Byng, J. Duchan, & C. Pound (Eds.), *Aphasia therapy files* (Vol. II, pp. 69–82). Hove, England: Psychology Press.

Hillis, A. E. (1989). Efficacy and generalization of treatment for aphasic naming errors. *Archives of Physical Medicine and Rehabilitation, 70*, 632–636.

Hinckley, J. J., & Carr, T. H. (2001). Differential contributions of cognitive abilities to success in skill-based versus context-based aphasia treatment. *Brain and Language, 79*, 3–6.

Howard, D. (2000). Cognitive neuropsychology and aphasia therapy: The case of word retrieval. In I. Papathanasiou (Ed.), *Acquired neurogenic communication disorders: A clinical perspective* (pp. 76–99). London, England: Whurr.

Howard, D., Patterson, K., Franklin, S., Orchard-Lisle, V., & Morton, J. (1985). Treatment of word retrieval deficits in aphasia. *Brain, 108*, 817–829.

Hughes, D. L. (1985). Language treatment and generalization. A clinician's handbook. San Diego, CA: College Hill.

Husak, R. S., & Marshall, R. C. (2012, May). *A new approach for quantifying the effects of response elaboration training*. Paper presented at the Clinical Aphasiology Conference, Lake Tahoe, CA.

Jacobs, B. J., & Thompson, C. K. (2000). Cross-modal generalization effects of training noncanonical sentence comprehension and production in agrammatic aphasia. *Journal of Speech, Language, and Hearing Research, 43*(1), 5–20.

Johnson, M. L., Taub, E., Harper, L. H., Wade, J. T., Bowman, M. H., Bishop-McKay, S., ... Uswatte, G. (2014). An enhanced protocol for Constrained-Induced Aphasia Therapy II: A case series. *American Journal of Speech-Language Pathology, 23*, 60–72.

Jones, E. V. (1986). Building the foundations for sentence production in a non-fluent aphasic. *British Journal of Disorders of Communication, 21*, 63–82.

Kearns, K. P. (1985). Response elaboration training for patient initiated utterances. In R. H. Brookshire (Ed.), *Clinical Aphasiology* (Vol. 15, pp. 196–204). Minneapolis, MN: BRK Publishers.

Kearns, K. P., & Elman, R. J. (2008). Group therapy for aphasia: Theoretic and practical considerations. In R. Chapey (Ed.), *Language intervention strategies in aphasia and related neurogenic communication disorders* (pp. 376–400). Baltimore, MD: Lippincott Williams & Wilkins.

Kearns, K. P., & Salmon, S. J. (1984). An experimental analysis of auxiliary and copula verb generalization in aphasia. *Journal of Speech and Hearing Disorders, 49*, 152–163.

Kearns, K. P., & Scher, G. P. (1989). The generalization of response elaboration training effects. In T. E. Prescott (Ed.), *Clinical Aphasiology* (Vol. 18, pp. 223–245). Boston, MA: College Hill Press.

Kempler, D., & Goral, M. (2011). A comparison of drill- and communication-based treatment for aphasia. *Aphasiology, 25*, 1327–1346.

Kendall, D., Raymer, A., Rose, M., Gilbert, J., & Gonzalez Rothi, L. J. (2014). Anomia treatment platform as a behavioral engine for use in research on physiological adjuvants to neurorehabilitation. *Journal of Rehabilitation Research and Development, 51*(3), 391–400.

Kendall, D. L., Rosenbek, J. C., Heilman, K. M., Conway, T., Klenberg, K., Gonzalez Rothi, L. J., & Nadeau, S. E. (2008). Phoneme-based rehabilitation of anomia in aphasia. *Brain and Language*, *105*, 1–17.

Kertesz, A. (2007). *Western Aphasia Battery Revised*. San Antonio, TX: PsychCorp.

Kiran, S. (2007). Complexity in the treatment of naming deficits. *American Journal of Speech-Language Pathology*, *16*, 18–29.

Kiran, S. (2008). Typicality of inanimate category exemplars in aphasia treatment: Further evidence for semantic complexity. *Journal of Speech, Language, and Hearing Research*, *51*, 1550–1568.

Kiran, S., Sandberg, C., & Abbott, K. (2009). Treatment for lexical retrieval using abstract and concrete words in persons with aphasia: Effect of complexity. *Aphasiology*, *23*(7–8), 835–853.

Kiran, S., Sandberg, C., & Sebastian, R. (2011). Treatment of category generation and retrieval in aphasia: Effect of typicality of category items. *Journal of Speech, Language, and Hearing Research*, *54*, 1101–1117.

Kiran, S., & Thompson, C. K. (2003). The role of semantic complexity in treatment of naming deficits: Training semantic categories in fluent aphasia by controlling exemplar typicality. *Journal of Speech, Language, and Hearing Research*, *46*, 773–787.

Knoph, M. I. N., Lind, M., & Simonsen, H. G. (2015). Semantic feature analysis targeting verbs in a quadrilingual speaker with aphasia. *Aphasiology*, *29*(12), 1473–1496.

Kristensson, J., Behrns, I., & Saldert, C. (2015). Effects on communication from intensive treatment with semantic feature analysis in aphasia. *Aphasiology*, *29*(4), 466–487.

Laganaro, M., Di Pietro, M., & Schnider, A. (2003). Computerised treatment of anomia in chronic and acute aphasia: An exploratory study. *Aphasiology*, *17*(8), 709–721.

Laganaro, M., Di Pietro, M., & Schnider, A. (2006). Computerised treatment of anomia in acute aphasia: Treatment intensity and training size. *Neuropsychological Rehabilitation*, *16*(6), 630–640.

Law, S.-P., Yeung, O., & Chiu, K. M. Y. (2008). Treatment for anomia in Chinese using an ortho-phonological cueing method. *Aphasiology*, *22*(2), 139–163.

Lee, J. B., Kaye, R. C., & Cherney, L. R. (2009). Conversational script performance in adults with nonfluent aphasia: Treatment intensity and aphasia severity. *Aphasiology*, *23*(7–8), 885–897.

Leonard, C., Rochon, E., & Laird, L. (2008). Treating naming impairments in aphasia: Findings from a phonological components analysis treatment. *Aphasiology*, *22*(9), 923–947.

Links, P., Hurkmans, J., & Bastiaanse, R. (2010). Training verb and sentence production in agrammatic Broca's aphasia. *Aphasiology*, *24*(11), 1303–1325.

Loverso, F. L., & Millione, J. (1992). Training and generalization of expressive syntax in nonfluent aphasia. *Clinics in Communication Disorders*, *2*(1), 43–53.

Lowell, S., Beeson, P. M., & Holland, A. L. (1995). The efficacy of a semantic cueing procedure on naming performance of adults with aphasia. *American Journal of Speech-Language Pathology*, *4*(4), 109–114.

Marshall, J. (1995). The mapping hypothesis and aphasia therapy. *Aphasiology*, *9*, 517–539.

Marshall, J. (1999). Doing something about a verb impairment: Two therapy approaches. In S. Byng, K. Swinburn, & C. Pound (Eds.), *The aphasia therapy file* (pp. 111–130). Hove, England: Psychology Press.

Marshall, J. (2017). Disorders in sentence processing in aphasia. In I. Papathanasiou & P. Coppens (Eds.), *Aphasia and related neurogenic communication disorders* (2nd ed., pp. 245–267). Burlington, MA: Jones & Bartlett Learning.

Marshall, J., Pring, T., & Chiat, S. (1998). Verb retrieval and sentence production in aphasia. *Brain and Language*, *63*, 159–183.

Marshall, R. C. (1999). *Introduction to group treatment for aphasia*. Boston, MA: Butterworth-Heimemann.

Mayer, J. F., & Murray, L. L. (2003). Functional measures of naming in aphasia: Word retrieval in confrontation naming versus connected speech. *Aphasiology, 17*(5), 481–497.

Meinzer, M., Mohammadi, S., Kugel, H., Schiffbauer, H., Floel, A., Albers, J., … Deppe, M. (2010). Integrity of the hippocampus and surrounding white matter is correlated with language training success in aphasia. *NeuroImage, 53*, 283–290.

Milman, L. (2016). An integrated approach for treating discourse in aphasia. Bridging the gap between language impairment and functional communication. *Topics in Language Disorders, 36*(1), 80–96.

Milman, L., Vega-Mendoza, M., & Clenderen, D. (2014). Integrated training for aphasia: An application of part-whole training to treat lexical retrieval, sentence production, and discourse-level communications in three cases of nonfluent aphasia. *American Journal of Speech-Language Pathology, 23*, 105–119.

Mitchum, C. C., & Berndt, R. S. (1994). Verb retrieval and sentence construction: Effects of targeted intervention. In M. J. Riddoch & G. W. Humphreys (Eds.), *Cognitive neuropsychology and cognitive rehabilitation* (pp. 317–348). Hove, England: Lawrence Erlbaum.

Mitchum, C. C., Haendiges, A. N., & Berndt, R. S. (1993). Model-guided treatment to improve written sentence production: A case study. *Aphasiology, 7*(1), 71–109.

Nickels, L., & Best, W. (1996). Therapy for naming disorders (part I): Principles, puzzles, and progress. *Aphasiology, 10*(1), 21–47.

Olsen, E., Freed, D. B., & Marshall, R. C. (2012). Generalization of personalized cueing to enhance word finding in natural settings. *Aphasiology, 26*, 618–631.

Papathanasiou, I., Coppens, P., Durand, E., & Ansaldo, A. I. (2017). Plasticity and recovery in aphasia. In I. Papathanasiou & P. Coppens (Eds.), *Aphasia and related neurogenic communication disorders* (pp. 63–80). Burlington, MA: Jones & Bartlett Learning.

Papathanasiou, I., Mesolora, A., Michoy, E., & Papachristou, G. (2007, November). Elaborated semantic feature analysis treatment: Lexicality and generalization effects. Poster presented at the meeting of the American Speech-Language-Hearing Association, Boston, MA.

Peach, R. K., & Reuter, K. A. (2010). A discourse-based approach to semantic feature analysis for the treatment of aphasic word retrieval failures. *Aphasiology, 24*(9), 971–990.

Prescott, T. E., Selinger, M., & Loverso, F. L. (1982). An analysis of learning, generalization and maintenance of verbs by an aphasic patient. In R. H. Brookshire (Ed.), *Clinical Aphasiology* (pp. 178–182). Minneapolis, MN: BRK Publishers.

Pring, T., Hamilton, A., Harwood, A., & MacBride, L. (1993). Generalization of naming after picture/word matching tasks: Only items appearing in therapy benefit. *Aphasiology, 7*(4), 383–394.

Pulvermüller, F., Neininger, B., Elbert, T., Mohr, B., Rockstroh, B., Koebbel, P., & Taub, E. (2001). Constraint-induced therapy of chronic aphasia after stroke. *Stroke, 32*, 1621–1626.

Raven, J. C. (1976). Raven's Progressive Matrices. Torrance, CA: WPS.

Raymer, A. M., Ciampitti, M., Holliway, B., Singletary, F., Blonder, L. X., Ketterson, T., … Rothi, L. J. G. (2007). Semantic-phonologic treatment for noun and verb retrieval impairments in aphasia. *Neuropsychological Rehabilitation, 17*, 244–270.

Raymer, A. M., & Ellsworth, T. A. (2002). Response to contrasting verb retrieval treatments: A case study. *Aphasiology, 16*(10/11), 1031–1045.

Raymer, A. M., Singletary, F., Rodriguez, A., Ciampitti, M., Heilman, K., & Rothi, L. J. G. (2006). Effects of gesture + verbal treatment for noun and verb retrieval in aphasia. *Journal of the International Neuropsychological Society, 12*, 867–882.

Raymer, A. M., Thompson, C. K., Jacobs, B., & Le Grand, H. R. (1993). Phonological treatment of naming deficits in aphasia: Model-based generalization analysis. *Aphasiology, 7*(1), 27–53.

Reichman-Novak, S., & Rochon, E. (1997). Treatment to improve sentence production: A case study. *Brain and Language, 60*(1), 102–105.

Rider, J. D., Wright, H. H., Marshall, R. C., & Page, J. L. (2008). Using semantic feature analysis to improve contextual discourse in adults with aphasia. *American Journal of Speech-Language Pathology, 17*, 161–172.

Robson, J., Marshall, J., Pring, T., & Chiat, S. (1998). Phonological naming therapy in jargon aphasia: Positive but paradoxical effects. *Journal of the International Neuropsychological Society, 4*, 675–686.

Rose, M., & Douglas, J. (2008). Treating a semantic word production deficit in aphasia with verbal and gesture methods. *Aphasiology, 22*(1), 20–41.

Rose, M. L., Raymer, A. M., Lanyon, L. E., & Attard, M. C. (2013). A systematic review of gesture treatments for post-stroke aphasia. *Aphasiology, 27*(9), 1090–1127.

Rose, M., & Sussmilch, G. (2008). The effects of semantic and gesture treatments on verb retrieval and verb use in aphasia. *Aphasiology, 22*(7–8), 691–706.

Rossiter, C., & Best, W. (2013). "Penguins don't fly": An investigation into the effect of typicality on picture naming in people with aphasia. *Aphasiology, 27*(7), 784–798.

Shewan, C. M. (1976). Facilitating sentence formulation: A case study. *Journal of Communication Disorders, 9*, 191–1979.

Snell, C., Sage, K., & Lambon Ralph, M. A. (2010). How many words should we provide in anomia therapy? A meta-analysis and a case series study. *Aphasiology, 24*(9), 1064–1094.

Stadie, N., Schröder, A., Postler, J., Lorenz, A., Swoboda-Moll, M., Burchert, F., & De Bleser, R. (2008). Unambiguous generalization effects after treatment of non-canonical sentence production in German agrammatism. *Brain and Language, 104*, 211–229.

Stanczak, L., Waters, G., & Caplan, D. (2006). Typicality-based learning and generalisation in aphasia: Two case studies of anomia treatment. *Aphasiology, 20*(2/3/4), 374–383.

Stokes, T. F., & Baer, D. M. (1977). An implicit technology of generalization. *Journal of Applied Behavioral Analysis, 10*(2), 349–367.

Taub, E., Johnson, M. L., Harper, L. H., Wade, L. H., Haddad, M. M., Mark, V. W., & Uswatte, G. (2012, November). *An enhanced version of CI aphasia therapy: CIAT II.* Paper presented at the meeting of the American Speech-Language-Hearing Association, Atlanta, GA.

Thompson, C. K. (1989). Generalization in the treatment of aphasia. In L. McReynolds & J. Spradlin (Eds.), *Generalization strategies in the treatment of communication disorders* (pp. 82–115). Toronto, Canada: B.C. Decker.

Thompson, C. K., Ballard, K. J., & Shapiro, L. P. (1998). The role of syntactic complexity in training wh-movement structures in agrammatic aphasia: Optimal order for promoting generalization. *Journal of the International Neuropsychological Society, 4*, 661–674.

Thompson, C. K., & Byrne, M. E. (1984). Across setting generalization of social conventions in aphasia: An experimental analysis of "loose training." In R. H. Brookshire (Ed.), *Clinical aphasiology conference proceedings* (pp. 132–144). Minneapolis, MN: BRK Publishers.

Thompson, C. K., Choy, J. J., Holland, A., & Cole, R. (2010). Sentactics®: Computer-automated treatment of underlying forms. *Aphasiology, 24*(10), 1242–1266.

Thompson, C. K., & Kearns, K. P. (1981). An experimental analysis of acquisition, generalization, and maintenance of naming behavior in a patient with anomia. In R. H. Brookshire (Ed.), *Clinical aphasiology conference proceedings* (pp. 35–45). Minneapolis, MN: BRK Publishers.

Thompson, C. K., & McReynolds, L. V. (1986). Wh interrogative production in agrammatic aphasia: An experimental analysis of auditory-visual stimulation and direct-production treatment. *Journal of Speech and Hearing Research, 29*, 193–206.

Thompson, C. K., & Shapiro, L. P. (2005). Treating agrammatic aphasia within a linguistic framework: Treatment of underlying forms. *Aphasiology, 19*(10/11), 1021–1036.

Thompson, C. K., & Shapiro, L. P. (2007). Complexity in treatment of syntactic deficits. *American Journal of Speech-Language Pathology, 16*, 30–42.

Thompson, C. K., Shapiro, L. P., Ballard, K. J., Jacobs, B. J., Schneider, S. S., & Tait, M. E. (1997). Training and generalized production of wh- and NP-movement structures in agrammatic aphasia. *Journal of Speech, Language, and Hearing Research, 40*, 228–244.

Thompson, C. K., Shapiro, L. P., Kiran, S., & Sobecks, J. (2003). The role of syntactic complexity in treatment of sentence deficits in agrammatic aphasia: The Complexity Account of Treatment Efficacy (CATE). *Journal of Speech and Hearing Research, 46*, 591–607.

Thompson, C. K., Shapiro, L. P., & Roberts, M. M. (1993). Treatment of sentence production deficits in aphasia: A linguistic-specific approach to wh-interrogative training and generalization. *Aphasiology, 7*(1), 111–133.

Tonkovich, J. D., & Loverso, F. L. (1982). A training matrix approach for gestural acquisition by the agrammatic patient. In R. H. Brookshire (Ed.), *Clinical aphasiology conference proceedings* (pp. 283–288). Minneapolis, MN: BRK Publishers.

Tyler, A. A., & Figurski, G. R. (1994). Phonetic inventory changes after treating distinctions along an implicational hierarchy. *Clinical Linguistics & Phonetics, 8*, 91–108.

Wambaugh, J. L., & Fergusson, M. (2007). Application of semantic feature analysis to retrieval of action names in aphasia. *Journal of Rehabilitation Research and Development, 44*(3), 381–394.

Wambaugh, J. L., Mauszycki, S., Cameron, R., Wright, S., & Nessler, C. (2013). Semantic feature analysis: Incorporating typicality treatment and mediating strategy training to promote generalization. *American Journal of Speech-Language Pathology, 22*, S334–S369.

Wambaugh, J. L., Mauszycki, S., & Wright, S. (2014). Semantic feature analysis: Application to confrontation naming of actions in aphasia. *Aphasiology, 28*(1), 1–24.

Wambaugh, J. L., & Thompson, C. K. (1989). Training and generalization of agrammatica aphasic adults' wh-interrogative productions. *Journal of Speech and Hearing Disorders, 54*, 509–525.

Wambaugh, J. L., Wright, S., & Nessler, C. (2012). Modified response elaborated training: A systematic extension with replications. *Aphasiology, 26*(12), 1407–1439.

Webster, J., Morris, J., & Franklin, S. (2005). Effects of therapy targeted at verb retrieval and the realization of the predicate argument structure: A case study. *Aphasiology, 19*(8), 748–764.

Webster, J., & Whitworth, A. (2012). Treating verbs in aphasia: Exploring the impact of therapy at the single word and sentence levels. *International Journal of Language and Communication Disorders, 47*(6), 619–636.

Webster, J., Whitworth, A., & Morris, J. (2015). Is it time to stop "fishing"? A review of generalization following aphasia intervention. *Aphasiology, 29*(11), 1240–1264.

Whitworth, A., Webster, J., & Howard, D. (2015). Argument structure deficit in aphasia: It's not all about verbs. *Aphasiology, 29*(12), 1426–1447.

Wiegel-Crump, C., & Koenigsknecht, R. A. (1973). Tapping the lexical store of the adult aphasic: Analysis of the improvement made in word retrieval skills. *Cortex, 9*(4), 411–418.

Wildman, R. W., & Wildman, R. W. (1975). The generalization of behavior modification procedures: A review—with special emphasis on classroom applications. *Psychology in the Schools, 12*, 432–448.

Wisenburn, B., & Mahoney, K. (2009). A meta-analysis of word-finding treatments for aphasia. *Aphasiology, 23*(11), 1338–1352.

Yorkston, K. M., Beukelman, D. R., Strand, E. A., & Hakel, M. (2010). *Management of motor speech disorders in children and adults* (3rd ed.). Austin, TX: Pro-Ed.

Youmans, G., Holland, A., Muñoz, M. L., & Bourgeois, M. (2005). Script training and automaticity in two individuals with aphasia. *Aphasiology, 19*(3/4/5), 435–450.

Complementing Therapy Using Multimodal Strategies

Sarah Wallace

INTRODUCTION

The purpose of this chapter is to provide current, evidence-based information regarding use of multimodal augmentative alternative communication (AAC) strategies by people with aphasia (PWA) and methods for integrating these strategies into traditional aphasia rehabilitation. The chapter begins with a description of the theoretical background and rationale for use of multimodal strategies by PWA. Although AAC is often thought of as a psychosocial approach, this chapter will emphasize the potential dual role of multimodal strategies that may simultaneously improve both communication (psychosocial approach) and linguistic skills (neuropsychological approach). Next, information about AAC assessment for PWA at various stages of recovery will be presented, followed by an overview of the evidence for individual multimodal strategies ranging from gestures to speech-generating devices. Finally, a review of clinical challenges related to AAC strategies for PWA and potential solutions are described.

What is AAC?

Augmentative and alternative communication (AAC) includes strategies and devices designed to supplement or replace, either permanently or temporarily, insufficient or ineffective communication skills (American Speech-Language-Hearing Association [ASHA],

2007–2014). AAC includes strategies that support spoken and written expression as well as auditory and reading comprehension (ASHA, 2002). AAC is a flexible system of strategies and devices designed to minimize barriers to communication. Most PWA do not use a single AAC strategy or device for all communication, but rather use a group of strategies and devices, or a *multimodal system of strategies*, that can be used flexibly to meet various communication needs. Even within a single conversational turn, PWA might use gesturing, drawing, and speaking to communicate their intent. Additionally, PWA may use multimodal strategies to repair communication breakdowns resulting from ineffective or inaccurate spoken communication. Finally, multimodal strategies may be requested from communication partners to support comprehension of PWA.

Why Is AAC Appropriate for People with Aphasia?

For PWA, the recovery of communication skills may occur over an extended period ranging from months to years. Although many PWA make considerable progress in language recovery through participation in speech-language therapy, most people continue to have communication needs that remain unmet (Holland & Beeson, 1993; LaPointe, 2011). AAC is one approach that can assist people with meeting these communication needs, thereby increasing their participation in daily activities. Traditionally, speech-language therapy for PWA during early phases of rehabilitation has focused solely on restoring linguistic function, and compensatory strategies were only considered when those deficits did not resolve and the period of treatment was coming to an end (Weissling & Prentice, 2010). However, as some evidence suggests (e.g., Boo & Rose, 2011; Raymer et al., 2007a), AAC strategies can have a comprehensive role in aphasia rehabilitation such that in addition to compensating for language impairments they may also facilitate restoration. The facilitation of restoration can occur as a self-cueing or a deblocking mechanism (e.g., Crosson et al., 2005; Dietz, Weissling, Griffith, McKelvey, & Macke, 2014; Ferguson, Evans, & Raymer, 2012; Lanyon & Rose, 2009; Luria, 1970; Raymer et al., 2006; Raymer et al., 2007a, 2007b; Rose, 2013; Rosenbek, Collins, & Wertz, 1976; Tompkins, Scharp, & Marshall, 2006).

Living with Aphasia: A Framework for Outcome Measurement (A-FROM) is one model that can guide clinical decision making during aphasia assessment and treatment through consideration of outcomes in various domains (Kagan et al., 2008). The four A-FROM domains are participation, language, personal, and environmental. Participation refers to a person's involvement in roles, responsibilities, activities, and relationships. Language includes the severity of the person's communication impairment across multiple modalities (speaking, reading, writing, and understanding). Personal aspects are those related to how the person feels about his or her communication impairment and how it affects his or her attitude and identity. Finally, the environmental domain refers to supports and barriers present in the multiple contexts in which the person needs to communicate. Consideration of a comprehensive role of AAC for PWA can help clinicians address all four domains. Descriptions of how AAC can target outcomes in the A-FROM domains are highlighted throughout the following sections.

When Do People with Aphasia Use AAC?

With an increased emphasis on life participation outcomes for PWA (Chapey et al., 2008; Kagan, 2011) and knowledge of potential facilitative effects on language abilities (e.g., Boo & Rose, 2011; Raymer et al., 2007a), AAC strategies will likely be incorporated into aphasia rehabilitation with greater frequency, especially during the early stages of rehabilitation. Importantly, AAC strategies are not intended to replace the implementation of restorative treatments, but rather may be integrated within or complement these traditional approaches.

Whether clinicians provide services to PWA during acute or chronic rehabilitation stages, early introduction of AAC can help address the A-FROM domains in an effective and efficient manner (**TABLE 8.1**). Related to the A-FROM participation domain, early implementation of AAC may allow PWA to actively partake in their rehabilitation and medical care. For example, PWA can ask questions about physical therapy exercises or state goals related to meal preparation if they have effective communication tools reliably available. Increased participation in medical care and rehabilitation resulting from improved communication may reduce the potential for adverse events (Downey & Hurtig, 2006) and enhance long-term rehabilitation outcomes (Denes, Perazzolo, Piani, & Piccione, 1996; Robey, 1998). Early introduction of AAC may also address the A-FROM personal domain through increasing the confidence and independence of PWA (Simmons-Mackie, King, & Beukelman, 2013). Just as failed communication attempts can leave some PWA with decreased feelings of self-worth, successful communication interactions, perhaps mediated by multimodal approaches, may increase self-worth and

TABLE 8.1 A-FROM domains addressed through early implementation of AAC during both acute and chronic stages.

A-FROM Domain	Early AAC Intervention
Participation	• Increased communication with healthcare providers and family members may increase participation in important medical and life decisions and improve health-related outcomes.
Language	• Multimodal strategies may increase linguistic abilities. • Multimodal strategies can be integrated into a restorative treatment approach.
Personal	• Increased confidence may result from successful communication interactions using multimodal strategies. • Greater acceptance of multimodal strategies may result from increased time to receive instruction in strategy use.
Environmental	• Family members and other communication partners can receive instruction on how best to support communication.

independence (see Chapter 12 this volume). Additionally, early introduction of AAC strategies can allow greater time for family members and other communication partners to be instructed in AAC strategy facilitation, thereby addressing the A-FROM environmental domain. Changes to the environment, such as partner training, may also improve the quality of the medical care and other services that PWA receive (Kagan, Black, Duchan, Simmons-Mackie, & Square, 2001). The A-FROM language domain is addressed through the potential facilitative effect of some AAC strategies and through recognition that despite introduction of AAC, restorative treatments can also be used. That is, restorative and compensatory strategies do not need to be mutually exclusive (Weissling & Prentice, 2010). See Chapter 10 for more information about combining restorative and compensatory approaches. Table 8.1 lists the A-FROM domains through early introduction of AAC during acute and chronic rehabilitation.

AAC can be implemented in the early stages of both acute and chronic rehabilitation. Ideally, clinicians begin during the first therapy session by evaluating and even trying a few multimodal strategies based on what is known about the person with aphasia (e.g., previous testing or reported use of multimodal strategies). The purpose of AAC approaches and the instruction provided to PWA will likely differ across the continuum of acute and chronic rehabilitation. For example, some AAC strategies and devices may be used temporarily during acute rehabilitation while others may be used long term if language abilities do not improve. Additionally, primary communication goals during acute care and inpatient rehabilitation may differ from those during chronic stages, thereby possibly changing the type of AAC used. For example, acute rehabilitation communication goals may relate to participating in ongoing medical care and decision making, as well as providing and receiving emotional support from family members. During chronic rehabilitation, major communication goals may focus on returning to previously enjoyed social roles. These differences may change the selection of AAC strategies or emphasize the flexible use of selected strategies. The following sections review appropriate assessment and intervention techniques, including some differences between AAC implementation in acute and chronic rehabilitation phases.

AAC-BASED ASSESSMENT FOR APHASIA

The primary goal of an AAC assessment for PWA is to develop a *capability profile* that highlights the strengths and limitations related to communication. A capability profile includes participation patterns and communication needs of PWA (Beukelman & Mirenda, 2013). Participation patterns can include the behaviors displayed by the person with aphasia as they relate to functional communication. The development of a capability profile dovetails with the goals of traditional, comprehensive aphasia assessment, and may differ with time post-onset.

During acute rehabilitation, frequent reevaluation is necessary because capability profiles may change often as PWA experience changes in medical status. Additionally, during acute rehabilitation impaired attention and fatigue are common in people with stroke or brain injury thus precluding a lengthy evaluation at any one point in time. Abbreviated versions of the tasks described below may be more appropriate. For example, formal assessment tools like the *Cognitive Linguistic Quick Test* (CLQT; Helm-Estabrooks, 2001) may be replaced by informal assessments of critical cognitive functions. Additionally, instead of a complete inventory of desired messages, clinicians may prioritize messages related to participation in medical decision making, counseling, medical procedures (e.g., describing pain), and rehabilitation services. Simple AAC systems like pain and body charts can assist with communicating about medical issues. Food and drink as well as assistance in the restroom are often provided for the person who is hospitalized thus they likely will not require complex AAC systems. In contrast, increased participation through implementation of AAC in communication interactions related to rehabilitation goals and medical decision making rather than in those related to basic needs may provide greater long-term benefit for PWA (i.e., for the participation domain of A-FROM). When PWA are not included in these discussions and are not provided tools to participate in important decisions, a type of learned non-use may occur, such that PWA begin to allow others to speak for them (Weissling & Prentice, 2010). Therefore, clinicians should prioritize strategies and devices that can assist with these communication needs.

What follows is a description of a comprehensive aphasia evaluation that is based on the A-FROM model and integrates aspects of traditional and multimodal assessment for aphasia. It may not be realistic for clinicians to complete all tasks in all settings; therefore, modified versions of tasks may be implemented as appropriate. Additionally, as part of a comprehensive assessment, PWA should have their visual perceptual, hearing, and motor skills assessed. Given the importance of these related abilities for AAC use and their potential effect on assessment and intervention tasks, it is optimal for speech-language pathologists to collaborate with other professionals such as an occupational therapist or physical therapist.

A comprehensive aphasia/AAC assessment should include five major components (**TABLE 8.2**). These may be completed over multiple sessions and may be modified depending on the service delivery site (e.g., outpatient versus inpatient).

TABLE 8.2 Components of an AAC/aphasia evaluation.

Pre-assessment: Interdisciplinary team evaluation of sensory and motor skills

1. Aphasia assessment
2. Perceived communicative effectiveness and functional language assessment
3. Cognitive assessment
4. Specific AAC/aphasia tools
5. Strategy and device trials

After gathering information about sensory and motor abilities from other professionals or a chart review as part of the pre-assessment, the clinician will either administer an aphasia battery or standardized test or review results from previously administered testing. In cases where the clinician does not already have that information available, he or she will conduct an assessment using a comprehensive aphasia battery. Although many aphasia tests are available, the Boston Assessment of Severe Aphasia (BASA; Helm-Estabrooks, Ramsberger, Morgan, & Nicholas, 1989) may be particularly appropriate for people with severe aphasia because it allows the clinician to score responses delivered using nonverbal modalities. Similarly, the Western Aphasia Battery – Revised (WAB-R; Kertesz, 2007) includes a supplemental section that evaluates the drawing of eight common objects. Although this type of task does not necessarily reflect the communicative use of drawing, it provides information about construction, visual perceptual, and motor skills, indicating the potential for functional use of this strategy. Another supplemental section within both assessment tools evaluates limb apraxia, which may affect the use of various multimodal strategies (e.g., gestures, drawing, pointing to a communication notebook, selecting a message on a speech-generating device). The use of an aphasia battery will provide clinicians will information about severity and type of aphasia. For example, PWA with characteristics associated with Broca's aphasia may benefit from different AAC strategies than people with characteristics associated with Wernicke's aphasia.

The second component of an AAC-based assessment of PWA is to evaluate the perceived communicative effectiveness and functional communication abilities. Some clinicians may develop their own informal interview questions to ask the person and his or her communication partners about perceived effectiveness and functional communication abilities (Kagan, 2011). Additionally, perceived communicative effectiveness can be measured through standardized interview tools such as the Burden of Stroke Scale (BOSS; Doyle, McNeil, Hula, & Mikolic, 2003), the CAT Disability Questionnaire (Swinburn, Porter, & Howard, 2005), the ASHA Quality of Communication Life (ASHA-QCL; Paul et al., 2004), the Communicative Effectiveness Index (CETI; Lomas et al., 1989), or the Stroke and Aphasia Quality of Life Scale (SAQOL-39; Hilari, Byng, Lamping, & Smith, 2003), which was designed specifically to measure quality of life in PWA. These scales differ in content and format such that some include scales with graphics (e.g., ASHA-QCL), while others include scales that use lines without numbers (e.g., CETI contains 10-millimeter divisions of a single 10-centimeter line), and still others use scales with linguistically complex end points (e.g., BOSS). Clinicians should be cautioned that these scales are not consistently sensitive to changes over time and response bias may appear when examinees have access to previous responses (Hirch, Beeson, & Holland, 2007).

Formal and informal assessments can also be used to determine functional use of verbal and nonverbal modalities. The Communication Activities of Daily Living-2 (CADL-2; Holland, Frattali, & Fromm, 1999) is one formal tool that is useful for measuring how PWA use various communication modalities (e.g., gestures, drawing, writing, speaking) across multiple role-play situations. Purdy and Koch (2006) describe an adapted method of measuring performance during the CADL-2 that captures the ability of PWA to switch to different modalities to repair communication breakdowns. This modified informal measure involves analysis of a subset of test items that require a verbal response or the use of nonverbal modalities (i.e., not items assessing auditory comprehension). Other informal assessments may allow clinicians to determine how PWA use modalities in personalized situations. For example, a clinician might show a video clip of a personally relevant topic and ask the person to retell the main ideas using whichever strategies he or she prefers. If cues are needed to prompt the person to use the available pen and paper, or to search through available photographs, clinicians should note this as part of the evaluation.

The third component is the administration of cognitive assessments, such as tests of memory, attention, and executive functions. Although cognitive evaluation in aphasia can be challenging because of the linguistic demands of many cognitive assessments (Helm-Estabrooks, 2002), cognition is increasingly being recognized as an important consideration for AAC selection and intervention (e.g., Nicholas, Sinotte, & Helm-Estabrooks, 2011; Wallace, 2010; Wallace, Hux, & Beukelman, 2010). The CLQT was designed to quickly assess multiple cognitive domains in people with acquired neurological disorders resulting from stroke, head injury, or dementia. In contrast to other popular cognitive assessments, the CLQT has norms for PWA. Further, the CLQT Design Memory and Trail Making Test subtests may provide clinicians with helpful information regarding the person's visual memory and cognitive flexibility—two skills that are important for AAC use. The Test of Everyday Attention (TEA; Robertson, Ward, Ridgeway, & Nimmo-Smith, 1994) Map Search subtest may also provide useful information about the person's visual attention and search patterns that may be particularly helpful for understanding navigation of high-technology devices or search through a communication notebook.

The fourth component involves clinician's selection of the appropriate assessment tools directly related to AAC use, some of which were designed for PWA. Clinicians may administer these assessments during initial sessions or as part of an ongoing evaluation of the person with aphasia. These often include informal assessment tools that are particularly important for PWA (see Chapter 13, this volume) because unlike many standardized assessments, during administration clinicians are permitted to use supportive communication strategies (e.g., written keywords, gestures, encouragement of multimodal responses), which may allow PWA to feel the "immediate experience of success" and perhaps help PWA see the value of multimodal communication strategies early on (Hersh et al., 2013; Kagan, 2011, p. 221).

Many of these AAC assessment tools will help clinicians identify participation patterns as well as barriers to successful communication. The most comprehensive of these tools is the Multimodal Communication Screening Task for Persons with Aphasia (http://cehs.unl.edu/documents/secd/aac/assessment/score.pdf; Garrett & Lasker, 2005), which examines various skills related to multimodal strategy use in PWA. The assessment, which makes use of a nonpersonalized communication notebook, guides clinicians to assess the person's ability to communicate using an external aid, search through pictures, categorize information, combine symbols, combine communication modalities (e.g., gesturing plus pointing to a photograph), and use pictures to tell a story and convey a message. One significant benefit of this evaluation tool is that it incorporates many multimodal strategies, and specifically evaluates a person's ability to integrate strategies within a single conversational exchange. Additionally, this assessment tool allows for spoken responses, thereby introducing PWA to the important concept that compensatory and restorative strategies are not mutually exclusive. One disadvantage of this assessment tool is the lack of personalization in that it does not include personally relevant photographs or topics. Research suggests that PWA perform best when content is personalized; therefore, clinicians may need to investigate personalization within other portions of the assessment (Dietz et al., 2014; McKelvey, Dietz, Hux, Weissling, & Beukelman, 2007).

In 1997 (revised 2006), Garrett and Beukelman developed another informal assessment tool, the Aphasia Needs Assessment (http://cehs.unl.edu/documents/secd/aac/assessment/aphasianeeds.pdf; Beukelman, Garrett, & Yorkston, 2007). This tool guides clinicians to ask questions relevant to how PWA currently communicate about difficult situations and topics of interest and explores communication skills that are challenging. Other questions can be used to gather information about facilitator behaviors and the strategies communication facilitators currently use. Finally, the Aphasia Needs Assessment guides clinicians to ask the person with aphasia questions about reading and writing preferences, topics of interest, and perceived communication abilities. Clinicians may need to provide written choices or augmented input during the interview when using this tool (Beukelman et al., 2007). It is important that PWA are involved in the identification of their needs and topics of interest, and that they have multiple opportunities for a successful communication exchange even during the assessment. Garrett and Lasker (2005) identified two major categories to describe PWA who use AAC: independent and partner-dependent communicators. Their tool, the AAC-Aphasia Categories of Communicators Checklist (http://cehs.unl.edu/documents/secd/aac/assessment/aphasiachecklist.pdf), assists clinicians with determining the communicator category of PWA by identifying skills and challenges that place PWA within one of six communicator types. The first two types pertain to *independent* communicators. These are people who initiate communication, are aware of communication breakdowns, locate messages within a stored system, and successfully switch among multiple communication modalities. PWA who are independent communicators are further identified as *stored message* or *generative message* communicators. In contrast, the next three types relate to *dependent* communicators. These individuals require assistance to successfully implement most AAC strategies except for some of the most routine, automatic social responses. Dependent communicators include *emerging*, *contextual choice*, and *transitional* communicators. A final communicator type, the *specific need* communicator, may be either dependent or independent and uses AAC for a specific communication task rather than relying on AAC strategies for all tasks. For example, the specific need communicator may use AAC to start a phone conversation, explaining that he or she has aphasia and needs extra time to communicate. After that message is produced, he or she may continue to use natural speech for the conversation.

During acute stages of rehabilitation, clinicians might determine broadly if the person with aphasia is a partner-dependent or an independent communicator to assist with developing appropriate multimodal strategies and interventions. During chronic stages of rehabilitation, clinicians may find it helpful to assign the person with aphasia to one of the six previously mentioned communicator types to develop a system of multimodal strategies within intervention programs. The AAC-Aphasia Category of Communicator Checklist may also be appropriate for developing rehabilitation goals and measuring progress.

A final AAC-specific tool is an informal assessment tool referred to as a topic inventory, which adds personalized information to the Aphasia Needs Assessment through the addition of photographs or drawings. Personalized photographs about topics of potential interest provided by the person with aphasia and his or her family might be appropriate for this task. Additionally, clinicians may use commercially available tools such as the Life Interest and Value Cards (Haley, Womack, Helm-Estabrooks, Caignon, & McCulloch, 2010; Haley, Womack, Helm-Estabrooks, Lovette, & Goff, 2013; Helm-Estabrooks & Whiteside, 2012). These 121 cards have black and white line drawings that depict activities that might be enjoyed by adults of all ages. Whether personalized or nonpersonalized images are used, the primary purpose is for the person with aphasia (with clinician assistance) to sort the potential topics into two groups: topics of interest and topics of no interest. The initial sorting of the topics can help the clinician identify some areas of vocabulary that will be relevant to the person with aphasia.

Strategy and Device Trials

Strategy and device trials are most appropriately conducted as the final step in the AAC assessment. However, some strategies may be trialed during an initial therapy session regardless of how much of the comprehensive evaluation has been completed. Strategies such as gestures, drawing, writing, pointing to readily available photographs, augmented input, and written choice (Garrett & Beukelman, 1995; Lasker, Hux, Garrett, Moncreif, & Eischeid, 1997) are inexpensive and can be suggested as temporary strategies to meet immediate communication needs. The clinician may recognize that additional instruction or evaluation is needed but may not want to leave the person with aphasia without some means of communication. Trials of electronic devices that might be incorporated into the person's multimodal system of strategies may be most appropriate only after a comprehensive evaluation. Additionally, formal trials may assist clinicians in determining the type and amount of intervention that is needed for strategies and devices. In this way, strategies may be trialed early to provide an immediate means of communication, and again following the completion of a comprehensive evaluation.

Based on the information collected from the comprehensive evaluation, the clinician will match the person with aphasia's communication needs and skills to the features of one or more strategies or devices. Feature matching is the process of determining the desired AAC features based on a person's current or predicted future skills and needs (Beukelman & Mirenda, 2013). For example, consideration of PWA's motor abilities is warranted for most strategies, including drawing, writing, and gesturing, as well as for access methods for electronic speech-generating devices. If communication needs include phone communication, PWA will likely require some type of speech-generating devices. Feature matching for speech-generating devices includes many aspects of the devices, as it is critical that clinicians consider the interface or software as well as the platform on which the interface runs. In terms of the interface, the clinician should consider the size and number of messages or buttons on the display, the dynamic or static nature of the display, the type of message representation (e.g., photographs or line drawings), and the use of text. These aspects will be influenced by factors such as vision, motor skills, and cognitive abilities. Regarding the platform, the clinician should consider the device size, weight, shape, and portability relative to PWA's physical and visual needs. Cost and third-party payer funding is an important consideration related to both the interface and the platform. Additional strategy and device considerations are highlighted in the following sections.

Once a few strategies and devices have been selected based on the best feature matching, PWA should practice using them in as many functional settings as possible. Sessions may begin in a therapy or hospital room, but quickly move to practicing the use of the strategy and device in a waiting room or at a nursing station. Then, PWA may practice using AAC to order food in the cafeteria or make an inquiry in the gift shop. If possible, PWA ideally should have the opportunity to practice using AAC at home, in the community or, at a minimum, with familiar communication partners such as family members or nurses. Clinicians can assign using AAC as home practice to be completed between therapy sessions. For example, a clinician might ask the person with aphasia to use gestures and a speech-generating device to retell an event from the last week to four familiar communication partners and then at the next therapy session ask people to discuss what worked and did not work. Group therapy sessions and support groups for people who experience some isolation may be appropriate places to trial AAC as well.

AAC DEVICES AND STRATEGIES

PWA most often use multiple AAC strategies as part of their multimodal communication system (Garrett & Lasker, 2013). Their system may include natural speech as well as non-verbal modalities, such as requesting augmented input, gesturing, drawing, writing and text messaging, pointing to written choices, and selecting messages within communication notebooks and speech-generating devices. Although these strategies are ideally used in an integrated manner, some PWA will find that various strategies are more appropriate for familiar versus unfamiliar partners. Additionally, some strategies will require the support of a communication partner and therefore may only be appropriate in certain situations or with specific communication partners. Although typically used as part of an integrated multimodal communication system, each strategy and device will be described individually in the following sections.

Augmented Input

Augmented input differs from some of the other strategies available for use by PWA because its purpose is to support auditory comprehension rather than spoken expression. Augmented input supplements spoken expression through focus on the communication partner's use of gestures, written keywords, photographs, drawings, or prosodic emphasis while simultaneously speaking (Garrett & Lasker, 2013). Although the communication partner is critical to the success of this strategy, PWA can learn to request its use during times of decreased comprehension or communication breakdown. To that end, the person with aphasia can carry a card or have a message programmed into a speech-generating device that indicates the need for the augmented input. The message might say "Please write keywords when talking because it helps me understand" or "Please gesture the main concepts when talking because it helps me understand." This approach allows PWA to affect their environment for improved communication success, thus addressing the A-FROM environmental domain.

Clinicians should carefully evaluate each person with aphasia to determine which types of augmented input are most appropriate. Although more research is needed, individual differences are evident in studies that have compared the use of photographs and line drawings in supporting auditory comprehension of narratives (Wallace et al., 2012). Additionally, although not well studied, it is likely that PWA need a degree of self-awareness to request this strategy as they have to recognize the communication breakdown resulting from impaired auditory comprehension and realize that picture, written, or gestural support may assist their comprehension. Finally, individual needs may differ across acute and chronic stages of aphasia. During acute stages, the clinician or other family members may provide communication partners with instruction in its use, whereas, during chronic stages, some PWA may learn to independently request its use.

Gestures

Gestures used by PWA to improve communicative interactions include pointing to desired objects, nodding one's head, using facial expressions to express feelings (e.g., raising eyebrows to indicate surprise), or using iconic (i.e., pantomime) gestures that typically represent an item or action. Iconic or pantomime gestures are described as having specific meanings that represent single words (Marshall, 2006). Examples include the use of a curved hand moving upward toward a person's mouth to communicate "drink," "cup," or "thirsty." Gestures may require the use of both hands (e.g., opening hands away from each other to indicate "book" or "reading") or a single hand (e.g., "cup" or "drink" example from above). Thus, it is important that clinicians examine the presence and effect of limb apraxia or hemiparesis on the production of gestures.

People without language impairments use gestures naturally; however, some PWA may require instruction in their use for effective and efficient communication. One review found positive outcomes from 18 studies focusing on teaching the use of gestures to compensate for aphasia-related language impairments (Rose, 2006). Instructional strategies include Visual Action Therapy (Helm-Estabrooks, Albert, & Nicholas, 2014), drill and practice, imitation, and practice in simulated role-play or real-life situations. Promoting Aphasics' Communicative Effectiveness (PACE; Davis & Wilcox, 1985) is a multimodal intervention strategy that promotes the use of verbal and nonverbal modalities through a communicative interaction. The person with aphasia and the clinician take turns sending and receiving novel information using any modality possible, including gestures.

Of note, gesture intervention research has mostly included people with chronic aphasia (e.g., Visual Action Therapy); however, a few studies (de Jong-Hagelstein et al., 2011; Wallace, Purdy, & Skidmore, 2014) have found that a multimodal approach to aphasia rehabilitation, which included gestures, was effective during acute stages of aphasia as well. Increased acceptance of gestures as an AAC strategy during acute and chronic stages may be seen if PWA are provided instruction in the use of gestures combined with natural speech whenever possible (e.g., Ferguson et al., 2012; Raymer et al., 2007a, 2007b). Furthermore, clinician, family, and client concerns about learned non-use may be alleviated by the fact that, even during acute rehabilitation, multimodal instruction that includes gestures does not reduce use of spoken expression (Wallace, Purdy, & Skidmore, 2014).

The facilitative effect of gestures to improve word retrieval is of great interest to researchers and clinicians, perhaps because of the possibility of increasing acceptance of multimodality approaches. That is, many PWA may be more likely to use AAC strategies if they are introduced to them informally, as a tool that might help them to produce a word rather than as a tool to replace their spoken expression. Gesture intervention programs may cue spoken expression, particularly when combined with semantic and phonological interventions (e.g., Boo & Rose, 2011; Raymer et al., 2007b; Rose, 2013; Rose, Raymer, Lanyon, & Attard, 2013). Additionally, if PWA do not experience improved word retrieval, instruction in the use of pantomime gestures will provide them with an alternative communication modality. Thus, gestures are one of many nonverbal modalities that may be easily integrated into traditional aphasia treatment approaches at any stage of the rehabilitation process.

Despite the many benefits and natural aspects of using communicative gestures, PWA may experience limitations related to limb apraxia and the lack of specificity of many communication gestures (e.g., gesturing petting a small animal could communicate any number of pets such as *cat, dog,* or *bunny*). Thus, it is important to consider a multimodal system that includes other strategies with greater specificity such as drawing and writing (Beeson & Ramage, 2000).

Drawing

Drawing has been examined as a strategy to compensate for language impairments (Beeson & Ramage, 2000; Lyon, 1995; Lyon & Helm-Estabrooks, 1987; Sacchett, Byng, Marshall, & Pound, 1999; Ward-Lonergan & Nicholas, 1995) and to facilitate word retrieval (Taylor, 2012). The use of communicative drawing may be particularly valuable because drawings create a permanent record of the interaction that PWA and their communication partners can refer back to at a later time. Although dry-erase boards may be used in some settings, drawings on paper that can be stored for future use are often preferred. Some PWA carry spiral-bound notebooks to keep previous drawings readily available. Additionally, because communicative drawings are displayed in a shared visual space, they can also be used with partner assistance to co-construct meaning (Lyon, 1995). Some communication partners may require instruction in how to co-construct messages using drawing and how to interpret the drawings of PWA (Lyon & Helm-Estabrooks, 1987).

Although previous artistic talents should not significantly affect the use of drawing to communicate, given motor, cognitive, and linguistic changes, most PWA will likely benefit from communicative drawing instruction. Without intervention, some PWA may omit or distort the general shape or form of an object even though they are able to construct the details of the object (Lyon & Helm-Estabrooks, 1987; Pons & Stark, 2013). Other PWA may not initiate communicative drawing without intervention (Ward-Lonergan & Nicholas, 1995).

Therefore, the purpose of drawing intervention programs is to increase initiation of communicative drawing, improve the quality of the drawings relative to a communicative function, and address limitations related to limb apraxia or other motor impairments. Additionally, some people with aphasia will need to learn how to draw with their nondominant hand due to significant motor impairments in their previously dominant hand. Instructional programs might include the following tasks to increase PWA's communicative drawing effectiveness and accuracy: copying; tracing; matching a drawing to a photograph or a real object; listening to instructions for drawing; and creating drawings that communicate items, actions, scenes, or short stories. One example of a drawing intervention protocol, The Communicative Drawing Program (Helm-Estabrooks et al., 2014), includes multiple steps with the purpose of using drawing to communicate complex information. The steps in this program include selecting the color for common objects with distinctive colors (e.g., stop sign), outlining common objects, copying geometric shapes, completing drawings with missing parts, drawing objects to command, and drawing cartooned scenes. The cartooned scenes used for this particular program are appropriate for developing the skills to communicate interactions and relationships between people, objects, and the environment. Clinicians may select personal photographs for the person with aphasia to use in a similar way as the cartooned scenes with the intention to promote generalization to real-life events. Drawing may also be practiced in an interactive, communicative manner through the use of PACE (Davis & Wilcox, 1985). Finally, drawing can be integrated into restorative word retrieval interventions such as semantic feature analysis (Taylor, 2012) as it is believed that the process of drawing target words is similar to generating semantic features of the words and therefore an integrated approach may result in improved word retrieval and communication effectiveness.

Despite the benefits of communicative drawing interventions, challenges to implementing this strategy exist. One such challenge relates to the hemiparesis and limb apraxia experienced by many PWA, making it necessary for them to draw with their nondominant hand. They may be concerned that the drawings won't be as accurate or detailed as desired due to poor motor control in their nondominant hand. Similarly, some PWA may hesitate to participate in drawing intervention because of poor premorbid artistic abilities. However, drawings that are somewhat simplistic can still communicate a great deal of information. Clinicians may counsel PWA about the use of their nondominant hand or poor artistic abilities. Perhaps the clinician can even show examples of simplistic or slightly imperfect drawings that still accurately communicate a message or model successful communicative drawing during PACE therapy sessions, for example. Additionally, many PWA may be most comfortable using air drawing rather than drawing on a piece of paper. This strategy is similar to gesturing, but includes more details about how an intended concept looks rather than the action with which it is associated. For example, to communicate the concept "hammer," instead of gesturing holding a hammer to pound a nail, the person would air draw the outline of the handle and then the head of hammer with his or her finger. Although this strategy has fewer benefits than drawing on paper, it might work as a transition strategy for people who are hesitant about drawing.

Other challenges to using communicative drawing relate to the limitations of the strategy in general rather than PWA's personal preferences. For example, abstract words are difficult to communicate via a drawing (e.g., "acceptable," "important," or "begin"). Additionally, the time it takes to draw may interrupt the flow of conversation more than other AAC strategies. These challenges highlight the importance of developing a robust multimodal system of communication strategies for PWA. Additionally, drawing might be combined with another strategy such as writing to increase its effectiveness as a communication strategy.

Writing and Texting

Many researchers have explored methods to improve writing in PWA—some with the goal of improving its use for communication when verbal expression alone cannot meet the person's communication needs. This strategy may be particularly appropriate for people whose hand motor control is more preserved than speech motor control, due to coexisting apraxia of speech or dysarthria. Additionally, people for whom orthographic representations are better preserved than phonologic representations may be ideal candidates for using written expression to supplement or replace verbal expression. Similar to drawing, writing provides a permanent record of communicative interactions that can be referred to later by PWA and their communication partners, thus emphasizing the importance of using pen and paper for communication rather than a dry-erase board.

Beeson and colleagues (Beeson, 1999; Beeson, Rising, & Volk, 2003; Clausen & Beeson, 2003) described two writing instructional programs: Anagram and Copy and Treatment (ACT) and Copy and Recall Treatment (CART). Aspects of these programs include anagramming, copying, and tracing target words, as well as using writing to communicate with unfamiliar and familiar partners. Typically CART includes the following three steps. First, the clinician presents the person with aphasia with a picture of the target word, models the spoken production of the target word, and then asks the person with aphasia to repeat the spoken production. Second, the clinician writes the target word and the person with aphasia copies it until he or she accurately produces three copies. Third, the written target words are covered and the person with aphasia writes the target word without support. If the person with aphasia makes an error during this last step, he or she will review the model and copy the word three times, until the target word is written without support. Often this treatment involves daily home practice such as writing and then copying the written target word eight times given a photograph prompt. For home practice, clinicians may provide correct answers for the person with aphasia to check his or her written productions. Overall, these writing treatments appear to improve the written communication skills of PWA for the dual purposes of creating written messages and using writing as an alternative to spoken expression.

Some PWA report interest in using text messages, much like written communication, to replace or supplement their spoken communication (Greig, Harper, Hirst, Howe, & Davidson, 2008). Text messaging sent via cellular phone can be helpful for PWA because it reduces some of the time pressure involved in formulating face-to-face messages. Additionally, preserved text messages can be shown later to a communication partner during face-to-face conversations much like a written message. Some features of text messaging that may be particularly supportive for PWA include word prediction and autocorrect, although people unfamiliar with technology may need instruction in the use of these features. Additionally, the shorter format commonly used for text messages, including partial sentences or grammatically incorrect messages, may be easier for PWA. Some AAC applications can be used to create messages using picture support and these messages can be entered into a text message screen and sent to a communication partner. In this way, PWA are supported to formulate text messages to communicate with others. Despite these supports, many PWA may require instruction in the use of text messaging and/or intervention for linguistic skills needed for texting.

The goal of a recently examined CART-texting intervention (Beeson, Higginson, & Rising, 2013) was to improve text messaging for the dual purposes of sending messages via cellular phone and showing the phone's screen to communication partners for face-to-face conversations. The steps for CART-texting were similar to traditional CART; however, both the person with aphasia's written productions and the clinician's models were produced using the keyboard on a cellular phone. CART-texting home practice was completed in a similar manner to CART home practice. The development of text-based interventions is in early stages; however, as technological advances continue to occur, treatments like CART-texting will likely serve an important function for PWA.

To successfully use text messaging to communicate, PWA also need to comprehend text messages sent to them by communication partners. In particular, PWA report challenges with word and sentence formulation and comprehension of phonetic abbreviations (Greig et al., 2008). Thus, clinicians may need to provide instruction to communication partners who will be texting PWA (e.g., simplifying syntax, avoiding abbreviations). PWA may also explore cellular phone features such as text to speech that may support their comprehension of communication partners' text messages.

Written Choice

Written choice strategy supports decision making, and thereby increases the independence of PWA (Garrett & Beukelman, 1995; Lasker et al., 1997). Traditionally, this strategy involves the communication partner asking a question and providing three to four answer choices. The choices will be selected by the partner based on the topic of conversation and his or her previous experiences communicating with the person with aphasia. The final choice is often a message that can be selected if the person does not select any of the offered choices (e.g., "something else"). The communication partner both speaks and writes keywords for the question and response choices. Once a selection is made, the communication partner says the selection aloud and circles or points to it to confirm the person's response. Part of a clinician's role is to instruct through modeling and role play the use of written choice strategy to family members and other communication partners (Arroyo, Goldfarb, & Sands, 2012) therefore addressing the A-FROM environmental domain. Written choice strategy (Garrett & Beukelman, 1995; Lasker et al., 1997) can provide a means for PWA to communicate about important medical decisions and rehabilitation preferences that may be particularly important during acute rehabilitation. Additionally, during hospitalization, clinicians may encourage family members to consistently use the same notebook for written choice communication so that previous conversations can be referenced easily. Because the choices are produced in the moment rather than preplanned, this strategy allows communication partners to flexibly adapt to different contexts and situations. An example of this strategy appears in **TABLE 8.3**.

Communication Boards and Notebooks

The purpose of communication notebooks or boards can vary based on the person with aphasia. However typically, these AAC strategies are used to convey basic wants and needs,

TABLE 8.3 Example of written choice strategy.

Clinician's Spoken Message	Clinician's Written Message
"Where did you grow up?" "In Michigan, Nebraska, Pennsylvania, or somewhere else?" [PWA points to Michigan]	Where? • Michigan • Nebraska • Pennsylvania • Somewhere else
"Michigan?" [PWA nods affirmatively] "That's great."	Where? • (Michigan) • Nebraska • Pennsylvania • Somewhere else

to assist in specific communication situations (e.g., ordering in a restaurant), or to establish social closeness. It is important that clinicians remember to provide instructions for communication partners and develop a plan for a facilitator to update the notebook or board as appropriate, thus addressing the A-FROM environmental domain. Communication notebooks might include a pocket or pages for artifacts such as maps, an alphabet card, and other artifacts such as concert tickets or vacation souvenirs (Garrett, Beukelman, & Low-Morrow, 1989). Research regarding communication notebooks suggests that shared used (i.e., the notebook viewed by both PWA and their communication partners) results in the greatest amount of information exchanged (Hux, Buechter, Wallace, & Weissling, 2010). Therefore, it may be appropriate for clinicians to instruct facilitators to engage in a shared approach for this communication strategy. Specifically, if the person with aphasia approves, a communication partner can be instructed to sit side by side and point to items within the communication notebook during a conversation, thereby co-constructing the message with the person with aphasia. Additional considerations, such as message representation and organization of the notebook, are addressed in the next section on speech-generating devices as the interface design needs are similar. Templates are available to create communication notebooks with personalized photographs (http://cehs.unl.edu/aac/visual-scene-resources/).

Speech-Generating Devices and Applications

Various speech-generating devices and mobile AAC applications with speech output capabilities may be appropriate for some PWA. Given the wide variety of language, cognitive, physical, and sensory impairments that may occur following a stroke, the process of selecting a speech-generating device or application is complex. Generally, successful use of speech-generating devices is influenced by cognitive abilities, linguistic skills, instructional approach, facilitator support, and interface features. Both traditional speech-generating devices and mobile AAC applications can have different degrees of complexity such that some produce single words or phrases on a specific topic while others are multilevel applications that allow for formulation of unique phrases or words. Less complex speech-generating devices might be appropriate for the acute care setting or early teaching of AAC strategies, for people who have difficulty with the dynamic displays, and for specific communication situations such as answering the phone. Additionally, less complex speech-generating devices may be used initially to increase comfort or skill levels prior to introducing a complex, multiscreen speech-generating device. High technology, complex speech-generating devices might be most appropriate for people who are fairly independent communicators, with high levels of cognitive flexibility and visual attention, and people who are already familiar with computerized devices.

In addition to applications designed for AAC purposes, existing mobile device applications may help support communication. For example, photographs may be organized, retrieved, and then shown to a communication partner to communicate a complex topic. Additionally, PWA may take screen shots of map, weather, clock, or calendar applications and show these to a communication partner to illustrate an important concept. Finally, the address book or list of contacts may be used to help communicate a message about a specific person during an interaction.

Despite significant potential, traditional and AAC mobile applications have been minimally investigated with PWA. However, the interface features required in mobile applications are likely similar to those in speech-generating devices designed for PWA (Steele & Woronoff, 2011). Given the growing market for mobile AAC applications and new speech-generating devices, continued examination of interface features that are appropriate for PWA is warranted. It is critical that clinicians and researchers explore ways to integrate the strengths of PWA into interfaces while still accounting for the individual differences due to cognitive and language skills as well as familiarity and comfort with technology. Some strengths that are consistent across many PWA include visual acuity, world knowledge, recognition memory, and intellectual functions (McNeil, Odell, & Tseng, 1991). Limitations for some PWA are the presence of limb apraxia and impaired executive functions, both of which may affect high technology AAC device use (e.g., Nicholas et al., 2005; Nicholas, Sinotte, & Helm-Estabrooks, 2011). Although sensory and cognitive abilities are not prerequisites for effective AAC use, clinicians should consider modified interfaces or specially designed instructional programs for PWA based on their strengths and limitations. At least four speech-generating device interface-design considerations warrant investigation by clinicians: message representation, phrase formulation, content organization, and navigation strategies.

Messages Representation

Many types of message representation have been examined in PWA including images (e.g., photographs, iconic line drawings) and text (e.g., Koul & Harding, 1998; McKelvey, Hux, Dietz, & Beukelman; 2010). Recent research has emphasized the use of high-context photographs because they capitalize on strengths of PWA (Dietz, Hux, McKelvey, & Beukelman, 2009; Dietz, McKelvey, & Beukelman, 2006; McKelvey et al., 2010; Wallace et al., 2012). These photographs represent situations, places, and experiences through depiction of people or objects in relation to one another in a natural environment. The four evaluation criteria for high-context photographs are: (1) environmental context; (2) interaction between animals, people, or objects, or with the environment; (3) personal relevancy; and (4) clarity. Research suggests that high-context personal photographs are preferred by PWA (Dietz et al., 2014; McKelvey et al., 2010) because they can be identified with greater accuracy than line drawings (McKelvey et al., 2010) and they can better support the reading and auditory comprehension of some PWA (Dietz et al., 2009; Wallace et al., 2012). Another consideration is placing text representing a key concept or phrase, such as keywords, below or next to a photograph. Some PWA appear to benefit from the presence of written keywords regardless of their reading comprehension abilities (Griffith, Dietz, & Weissling, 2014).

Phrase Formulation

A number of interfaces require formulation of phrases and sentences through selection of individual words (e.g., Hough & Johnson, 2009; Koul, Corwin, & Hayes, 2005; McCall, Shelton, Weinrich, & Cox, 2000). To use these interfaces, PWA need to select individual words in the correct order, perhaps from different screens or pages to communicate a multiword phrase such as *I am going on vacation*. Given the syntactic and navigation skills required, the process may be too difficult for some PWA. Although not studied extensively, clinical experience tends to indicate that phrase formulation is easiest for people with nonfluent aphasia whose communication is also impaired by apraxia of speech. That is, people with relatively good comprehension and perhaps better language formulation skills than suggested by their verbal output due to the apraxia of speech may be best suited for this interface design. If sentence formulation skills within the speech-generating device are appropriate to target during intervention, a step-by-step intervention that helps PWA create sentences of various levels of syntactic complexity should be implemented (Hough & Johnson, 2009; Koul et al., 2005).

In contrast, other speech-generating device interfaces emphasize information exchange through preconstructed phrases. For example, a single navigation and selection would be required to communicate the message *I am going on vacation*. The disadvantage of this type of interface is that novel messages that meet the specific needs of a communication interaction in real time are more difficult to create than they would be through phrase formulation strategies. However, the reduction in navigation and linguistic skills required may be well worth the effort for some PWA. Additionally, preconstructed phrases may allow PWA to respond quickly and therefore participate more fully in desired activities. Given these apparent differences, it is important that clinicians evaluate which approach is most appropriate for each person with aphasia.

Content Organization

Whether the phrases are preconstructed or need to be formulated, PWA will need to locate information within a dynamic or static display. Static displays usually make it easier to find information, but they hold less content. Therefore, most PWA will prefer to use a dynamic display or have multiple pages within a static display system. In either situation, a strategy for organizing the content is needed and this organization can play a large role in the ability of PWA to quickly and efficiently locate desired messages. During trials with these devices, clinicians can test various organizational approaches to determine which are most appropriate for that person with aphasia. Most frequently in published research studies, semantic or categorical organization is used with PWA (e.g., Hough & Johnson, 2009). However, because many PWA demonstrate at least minimal semantic deficits, researchers have begun to examine organizational approaches that capitalize on areas of relative strength for PWA such as procedural memory and world knowledge. One such approach, episodic organization, sorts messages based on events, and has been used in visual scene displays designed specifically for PWA (e.g., Dietz et al., 2006). These two organizations may be the most appropriate starting point for clinicians who seek to determine which is best for each person with aphasia and accomplished through role-play scenarios designed to elicit messages from multiple sections (i.e., pages) of an AAC interface or notebook.

Navigation Strategies

Similar to efforts to support message location through careful selection of organizational approaches, researchers have also investigated interface features that might help make PWA efficient communicators when using speech-generating devices. Navigation rings (Dietz et al., 2006; Wallace & Hux, 2014) were developed to assist people with communication impairments locate messages within high technology, dynamic display AAC devices. Navigation rings include electronic folders that might normally be included as the main or home page on an AAC system, and are the superordinate level of organization. Instead of only appearing on the main page, the navigation ring appears in the area around the buttons or text used for communication. The navigation ring remains unchanged on each page and is therefore visible even after a person selects a message. Navigation rings were used more efficiently and learned more quickly than main or home page systems (Wallace & Hux, 2014), although PWA learned to use both systems after a minimal number of instruction sessions (as few as five sessions). Clinicians may wish to include a navigation ring or static buttons that lead to frequently used messages for PWA who wish to use dynamic display AAC devices. Additionally, folder tabs can be used within a communication notebook to allow for easy navigation of the messages organized within the book.

Reading and Writing Supports

As the definition of AAC suggests, reading and writing supports are intended to enhance reading comprehension and written expression in addition to the supports for spoken expression and auditory comprehension described earlier. Reading comprehension supports include aphasia-friendly formatting of texts such as simplification of words and sentences, use of ample white space, large text, and inclusion of images (i.e., photographs, drawings) (Brennan, Worrall, & McKenna, 2005). Technology such as text-to-speech may also improve reading efficiency of some PWA (Dietz, Ball, & Griffith, 2011; Harvey & Hux, 2012). People with aphasia report using both types of supports to increase their participation in functional reading activities (Knollman-Porter, Wallace, Hux, Brown, & Long, 2015).

In addition to the compensatory use of writing to support PWA when spoken expression is not sufficient, some PWA may use AAC to support their written expression. Two types of technology may be particularly helpful for PWA relative to facilitating written expression: speech-to-text and word prediction. Initial reports of speech-to-text suggest that with intensive intervention using this technology, PWA demonstrated improved quantity and quality of their written expression (Ball, Grether, Garza, & Romich, 2009; Bruce, Edmundson, & Coleman, 2003). Word prediction software typically provides word choices following first or second letter selection such that it provides support similar to written choice strategy (Armstrong & MacDonald, 2000; Garrett & Beukelman, 1995; Murray & Karcher, 2000). Because these supports for written expression rely on technology, they would be most useful for PWA interested in using email communication.

BARRIERS TO IMPLEMENTATION

Despite multiple examples in the literature and anecdotal evidence of PWA successfully using AAC strategies, several barriers may limit or hinder their use in functional communication interactions. These barriers can be identified through the use of the informal and formal tools described previously and considering the A-FROM domains. Some of these barriers are specific to individual multimodal strategies and therefore were included in previous sections (e.g., drawing with the nondominant hand). The barriers described here relate to implementation of a multimodal approach in general rather than to specific strategies and include issues of AAC acceptance and generalization.

Acceptance

Acceptance on the part of PWA and their family members can play a large role in the success of multimodal AAC interventions. The need for clinicians to consider, evaluate, and provide intervention related to family members' acceptance in addition to acceptance by PWA is supported by the environmental A-FROM domain. Additionally, although AAC acceptance has not been directly studied in aphasia, examination of acceptance in people with traumatic brain injury highlights the importance of AAC facilitators. That is, clinicians reported high levels of acceptance of high and low technology AAC strategies in people with traumatic brain injury, and suggested that lack of facilitator support rather than dismissal of technology resulted in the greatest amount of AAC abandonment (Fager, Hux, Beukelman, & Karantounis, 2006). Therefore, it is critical that clinicians carefully consider acceptance by facilitators and PWA.

The involvement and responsibility of AAC facilitators may vary depending on the needs of PWA and the AAC strategies that compose their multimodal system. For example, the facilitator responsibilities for maintaining a high technology AAC device may include programming and adding new content. In contrast, facilitators for a person who primarily uses writing, drawing, and gesturing may be responsible for ensuring that pen and paper are always available and for teaching communication partners how best to communicate with the PWA using these strategies. Some people may have difficulty identifying a consistent facilitator thus clinicians may need to train multiple potential facilitators or assemble training materials that can be passed on to new facilitators as needed. Despite the varied roles and the individual differences of the facilitators and PWA, a few primary issues related to acceptance are evident. These issues of acceptance may overlap between PWA and their family members.

One reason PWA may be reluctant to use AAC strategies is that they want to feel "normal" and not appear different from people without communication impairments. This situation is frequently seen in people who recover physically from the stroke or brain injury, but whose communication skills are not sufficient to meet their everyday needs. Because they look otherwise "normal," they do not want any device or other nonverbal strategy to interfere with that image. Additionally, the extra time required to draw or write their message may slow communication interactions, contributing to their perception of differing from their peers. Similarly, family members may be concerned with their loved one looking "normal" or being accepted by nonimpaired peers. Although these feelings may change over time, it is important that clinicians are prepared to address both PWA and family members' apprehensions.

Clinicians' therapeutic approaches with PWA concerned about appearing "normal" may consider issues related to the personal A-FROM domain. That is, it might be appropriate to implement counseling to improve confidence and renegotiation of self-identity related to using a multimodal system of communication strategies (Shadden, 2005). Additionally, some PWA may feel more comfortable practicing AAC strategies in settings that are perceived as safe, such as group therapy or a support group. These settings also allow the PWA to have positive experiences using their strategies in a supportive environment. Then, with time, the PWA may feel empowered to try a strategy in a more public context. Similarly, multimodal strategies can be successfully integrated in functional communication within the therapy room and at home with familiar partners (trained by a speech-language pathologist). Conversation partners can either use the techniques themselves or suggest their use to the person with aphasia. For example, if a person with aphasia shows difficulty saying the word *ice cream,* the clinician or a family member could casually suggest that the person with aphasia use a gesture to communicate the message without emphasizing that the gesture is used to replace spoken expression. This technique, designed to encourage multimodal strategies, has the added benefit of emphasizing their use to repair communication breakdowns and may result in facilitation of spoken expression. Finally, if deemed appropriate, the person with aphasia may want to try an application on a mobile device because they are frequently used by people without communication impairments. Using a device that is used by the general population may result in the person feeling that he or she still appears "normal." However, clinicians should caution that mobile applications may not be appropriate for every person with aphasia.

A second reason for poor acceptance by PWA and facilitators is a lack of interest in using technology or other nonverbal methods of communication due to fear or inexperience. Because many PWA and their facilitators may be older adults, their fear may relate to unfamiliarity with the latest technology rather than a fear of technology in general. Many older adults take longer to adopt newer technologies and instead rely on familiar devices with which they have greater experience.

Although designed to explain behaviors related to technology use in general rather than AAC, the Technology Acceptance Model (TAM; Davis, 1989; Davis, Bagozzi, & Warshaw, 1989) may help unravel barriers related to acceptance of various multimodal strategies. This model suggests two important constructs related to increasing acceptance of technology: perceived usefulness and perceived ease of use. As these constructs suggest, acceptance is not necessarily directly related to the existence of benefits but rather the perception of benefits and ease of use of the technology (Mitzner et al., 2010). The technology acceptance model constructs can be integrated into the design of assessments and interventions to support AAC acceptance. For example, during trials of multimodal strategies clinicians may initially provide significant support to assist the person with aphasia and reduce frustration during new learning (i.e., implement errorless learning strategies) thereby facilitating perceived ease of use. The same type of support can be provided to facilitators as they are learning to encourage, manage, and support multimodal communication strategies. For example, backward or forward chaining can be used to teach the multiple steps needed to navigate to the desired message (Wallace & Hux, 2014). An errorless learning approach can also be used to teach the facilitator the steps for programming a message into a device while minimizing frustration and increasing success.

Group therapy sessions or other functional practice of multimodal strategies can illustrate the usefulness and value of these approaches. If possible, it is also appropriate for family members or other facilitators to observe or watch video recordings of the use of multimodal strategies to see their value in different situations. Finally, PWA who remain reluctant to try nonverbal modalities in these settings may benefit from mentoring. Clinicians may introduce PWA who successfully use AAC strategies to mentor or model these strategies to new clients and their families (e.g., Cole & Snow, 2011). If mentoring is unavailable, clinicians and communication partners may model the use of nonverbal modalities to augment their verbal communication, thereby demonstrating some of the benefits of these strategies (Beeson & Ramage, 2000).

Another reason for lack of acceptance is the fear of learned non-use. That is, some people believe that a multimodal approach to communication may result in changes in the motivation and ability of PWA to speak. The literature suggests that these fears are unfounded (e.g., Dietz et al., 2014; Griffith et al., 2014); rather, as described earlier in this chapter, evidence suggests that some nonverbal strategies (e.g., gestures) may actually facilitate improvements in spoken language. Above all, it is important for clinicians to remember that AAC strategies and traditional restorative approaches do not need to be mutually exclusive (Weissling & Prentice, 2010). That is, a comprehensive approach to aphasia rehabilitation should include restorative as well as compensatory strategies (see Chapter 10, this volume). Discussion of this evidence and highlighting the value of a comprehensive, multimodal (verbal and nonverbal) approach with PWA and family members may result in greater acceptance of AAC. Furthermore, it is critical that family members and PWA understand that use of AAC does not hinder recovery of speech and language. Additionally, multimodal approaches can be described as strategies that are used "for now" in hopes that restorative treatment will continue to improve linguistic abilities.

Generalization

An ongoing challenge for PWA relative to their successful use of multimodal strategies is limited evidence of generalization of these strategies to functional communication interactions. Factors limiting generalization include cognitive impairments and the lack of evidence-based interventions related to generalization (see Chapter 7, this volume). In particular, the interventions described in the literature are often designed to teach PWA to produce a single modality (e.g., gesture) rather than to use multiple modalities in a way that is closer to what communication interactions require. Without direct multimodal intervention, some PWA may fail to switch to nonverbal modalities when attempts at spoken communication result in a breakdown (Purdy & VanDyke, 2011).

One approach to addressing the use of AAC strategies to resolve communication breakdowns is the multimodal communication treatment (Carr & Wallace, 2013; Purdy & VanDyke, 2011; Wallace & Purdy, 2013; Wallace, Purdy, & Skidmore, 2014). This intervention was designed to emphasize the multimodal nature of communication and the benefits of integrated practice. Specifically, it aims to improve switching among verbal and nonverbal modalities through integrated instruction in multiple AAC strategies and devices. For example, the clinician provides instruction in the use of gestures, drawing, writing, and speaking to communicate a single concept before providing instruction in a second concept. The preliminary results from this series of studies suggest that some PWA benefit from this integrated approach during both acute (Wallace, Purdy, & Skidmore,

2014) and chronic (Carr & Wallace, 2013; Purdy & VanDyke, 2011; Wallace, Purdy, & Mesa, 2014) stages of rehabilitation. Because it emphasizes both verbal and nonverbal modalities, PWA and their family members who have concerns about nonverbal interventions may view this approach as most acceptable.

Findings related to the multimodal communication treatment indicate that PWA with significant semantic impairments appear to benefit from additional or combined semantic interventions (Carr & Wallace, 2013; Purdy & VanDyke, 2011). For example, in addition to practicing verbal and nonverbal productions of a target concept, the person with aphasia may also sort semantic features into categories or identify key semantic features of the target word. This combined approach is supported by a two-step process of lexical retrieval that aims to improve the lexical access step and circumvent the phonological access step (Dell, Lawler, Harris, & Gordon, 2004). An additional benefit of the combined approach is the potential to improve word retrieval and semantic processing. This multimodal communication intervention still warrants further examination; however, Wallace and Purdy (2013) provide a list of basic tenets for clinicians when developing an intervention program for a person with aphasia (Wallace & Purdy, 2013). **TABLE 8.4** displays five tenets; four from Wallace and Purdy (2013) and one related to communication partner instruction.

TABLE 8.4 Multimodal communication treatment tenets and examples.

Tenet	Examples

1. Assessment should guide intervention	• Select modalities based on evaluation of
	  ○ Limb apraxia and handedness
	  ○ Semantic processing skills
	  ○ Pre-stroke interests and abilities

2. Treatment should aid integration of verbal and nonverbal representations	• Practice nonverbal and verbal productions of a concept before moving on to the next concept
3. Treatment should support comprehension	• Use augmented input • Confirm comprehension of treatment instructions
4. Treatment should integrate existing evidence	• Use evidence-based treatments for each modality (e.g., Copy and Recall Treatment for writing)
5. Treatment should extend to communication partners	• Model techniques that encourage multiple modalities so that communication partners can assist with carry-over to everyday conversations • Give communication partners opportunities to practice encouraging multiple modalities and provide feedback as needed

Other multimodal interventions also integrate verbal and nonverbal modalities during instruction and have demonstrated some improvements in verbal expression following treatment (Ferguson et al., 2012; Lanyon & Rose, 2009; Raymer et al., 2006; Rose, 2013). Although these interventions are in early stages of development, their potential to improve functional use of AAC strategies is evident. Similar to the multimodal communication treatment, these strategies may be more acceptable to PWA and their family members because they combine verbal and nonverbal approaches.

CONCLUSION

In summary, many PWA benefit from the use of a flexible multimodal communication system that includes verbal and nonverbal strategies and devices. AAC strategies and devices can address all four domains of the A-FROM model if introduced early. Although differences are evident in assessment and intervention during acute and chronic strategies of aphasia rehabilitation, it is critical that a multimodal approach be included within a traditional aphasia rehabilitation program to assist PWA in meeting all communication needs in all stages of the rehabilitation process. Clinicians can overcome barriers related to AAC implementation through strategies that increase acceptance and use of evidence-based instruction for multimodal AAC approaches.

CASE ILLUSTRATION

John is a 45-year-old Caucasian man who is 2 years post left hemisphere cerebral vascular accident. Before his stroke, John worked as a security manager for the Pittsburgh Pirates Major League Baseball team. His responsibilities as manager included supervising security officers, completing payroll and scheduling, reviewing officer round logs and surveillance tapes, as well as developing and managing the yearly budget for the security office. He has a bachelor's degree in psychology and began his career as a security officer and eventually become the security manager.

John lives with his wife of 17 years, Jean, in Pittsburgh. His parents and five sisters and his brother live nearby. He is very close to his family and his in-laws and sees most of them at least once a week. He and his wife have three sons ages 14, 12, and 7 years. His wife works as a human resources manager for a local radio station.

John's stroke occurred during a family vacation to Lake Erie. His oldest son noticed that John was unable to speak or stand up from the table after lunch. He was immediately taken by ambulance to a small local hospital, was given tissue plasminogen activator (TPA) about 2 hours after onset of symptoms, and was air-lifted to a stroke center at a larger nearby hospital where he remained for 10 days until he was transferred to rehabilitation. At discharge from inpatient hospitalization he was mostly alert (although easily fatigued). He was unable to produce any intelligible speech beyond his first name, but did follow some simple, familiar commands. He had no voluntary movement on his right side and full movement on his left side. He was diagnosed with severe Broca's aphasia with severe apraxia of speech.

Acute Stages of Rehabilitation

Before meeting with the speech-language pathologist, John's hearing and vision were determined to be within normal limits and further testing of motor skills suggested hemiparesis on his right side. John's speech-language pathologist conducted an informal assessment of his language and cognitive skills because, based on her chart review, his fatigue would have interfered with the results of a formal assessment. The results of her informal evaluation indicated that John had significant difficulty with confrontation naming but could produce some highly familiar words given a model. Auditory comprehension was a relative strength as he followed some familiar commands in context and correctly identified single words during a listening task. His reading comprehension was fairly intact at the single-word level; however, he was only able to write his name after a model was provided. John completed a trail-making task (cognitive flexibility) and a letter scan task (visual attention) with a few errors that he self-corrected when given extra time. The clinician determined that John would need support in all areas to have his communication needs met.

The clinician used written choice strategy (Garrett & Beukelman, 1995) and card sorting (photographs with written text) to determine topics that were important to John and to interview him about communication needs. Like most PWA who are hospitalized, John had many messages he wanted to communicate to the medical professionals and his family members. He wanted to ask his doctors questions about his stroke and the stroke recovery, and he had specific questions for various clinicians related to the return of his pre-stroke abilities (e.g., asking the speech-language pathologist "Will I be able to speak again?"). The nurses and nurse assistants felt it was important that he be able to indicate his pain level, describe areas in which he felt discomfort, and request PRN (i.e., as needed) medications when appropriate.

During the interview, the clinician encouraged John's use of alternative modalities by casually suggesting he try to gesture or write his responses to her questions. This gave her the opportunity to observe his use of communication modalities

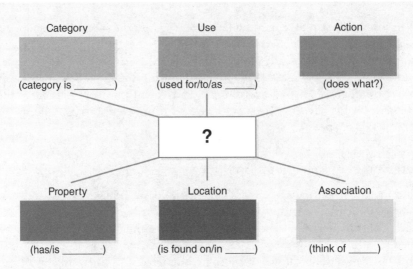

FIGURE 8.1 Example of a semantic feature analysis chart

during a functional task and allowed him to experience some initial success using a multimodal communication system. Based on these evaluations and trials of augmented input, gesture, drawing, and writing, the clinician determined that the best initial strategies for John would be augmented input, written choice (Garrett & Beukelman, 1995), gestures, and photographs on a small communication board.

During their limited number of sessions together, the speech-language patholo-gist integrated the use of AAC strategies into other restorative therapy approaches. For example, she asked John to say four features out of the six (e.g., category, use, action, location) related to personally relevant target concepts using a semantic feature analysis chart (see **FIGURE 8.1**). He was often unable to say the features so she encouraged him to first gesture the feature and then try to say it. She used a hierarchy of cues such as modeling with imitation to assist with John's nonverbal and verbal productions of features. She followed this same procedure to support his verbal and nonverbal production of the target concept before moving on to the next target concept and associated features. Toward the end of his inpatient reha-bilitation, John no longer needed the clinician's models for nonverbal productions relying instead of her verbal cue to "gesture it." John gravitated toward gesturing despite his right hemiparesis and with minimal counseling from the clinician he accepted the use of his left hand for mastering a number of one-handed gestures. As he began to master the use of gestures, the clinician also introduced a communi-cation board during the restorative treatment. Integration of verbal and nonverbal strategies appears to improve use of AAC strategies to resolve communication breakdowns and sometimes facilitate word retrieval (Carr & Wallace, 2013; Purdy & VanDyke, 2011; Wallace, Purdy, & Skidmore, 2014).

After trialing various line drawings and photographs, John's clinician determined that photographs best supported John's auditory comprehension. John indicated he preferred the high-context photographs so whenever possible, these photographs were selected as supports. His family members were provided with multiple examples of high-context photographs to ensure they could take or select the most appropriate photographs.

The speech-language pathologist provided photographs of key items in John's hospital room and of his medical team for a simple communication board. The back of the communication board had a drawing of the human body with written words and short phrases related to medical care. Although many PWA can simply point to body parts, John needed this extra support because his hemiparesis limited his ability to point to every body part. The speech-language pathologist's intention was for John to use the communication board to communicate messages related to his medical care (e.g., pain, discomfort); however, she determined that he would need support through modeling during role-play activities to achieve this goal. In addition to the communication board, his clinician sought to develop a communication notebook that would support social closeness and conversations related to family roles and family decisions. She asked John's family members to collect photographs of important people and places with written labels for each. **FIGURE 8.2** shows an example of a high-context photograph of John's in-laws for his communication notebook. Each page of the communication notebook had a tab that was labeled and color coded for easy navigation.

Finally, the clinician identified John's wife and his brother as his primary communication facilitators and trained them to use multiple approaches that would be useful for his many other communication partners. Specifically, she provided instruction in the use of written choice strategy (Garrett & Beukelman, 1995) and augmented input and encouraged communication partners to use the communication board and notebook to support comprehension as well as model use of nonverbal modalities. She emphasized that communication partners should cue John to encourage his gesturing and pointing to photographs to repair communication breakdowns or facilitate his word retrieval. She modeled this approach by showing his family how John could sometimes say the word *glasses* when he gestured with his left hand to indicate the two lenses of a pair of eyeglasses. The speech-language pathologist asked John's brother to create a photo dictionary of gestures that John frequently used that could be made available to medical team members and other visitors. Examples of therapy activities and the A-FROM domains addressed during acute rehabilitation are available in **TABLE 8.5**.

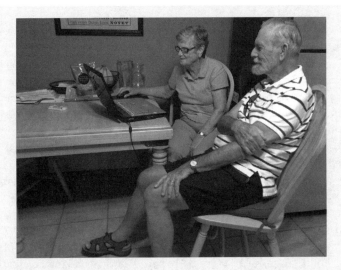

FIGURE 8.2 Example of high context photograph

© Sarah Wallace

At the time of discharge from acute rehabilitation, John had improved his communicative use of gesturing and pointing to a communication notebook and board with familiar communication partners. The speech-language pathologist was eager to implement other nonverbal modalities (e.g., writing, drawing) given his initial success, but she did not want to overwhelm him during the acute phase. When his communication partners remembered to use augmented input with gestures and drawings, John's participation in family discussions was increased. However, he required cues to use nonverbal modalities and to request the use of augmented input or written choice strategy (Garrett & Beukelman, 1995) from his communication partners. At this time, John was still a dependent communicator in that he relied on communication partner support to use his multimodal system of strategies (Garrett & Lasker, 2005). His verbal expression improved such that he was producing one to two word phrases that included familiar concrete nouns and verbs with some paraphasic errors.

Chronic Stages of Rehabilitation

John received speech-language, occupational, and physical therapies at his home following hospital discharge. After 3 weeks of home health services, he began outpatient therapy. He was initially approved for 8 weeks of outpatient speech-language

TABLE 8.5 A-FROM domains addressed during acute rehabilitation.

A-FROM Domain Addressed	Acute Therapy Activity

Participation	• Interventions to teach the following strategies to communicate with family members and medical team:
	  ○ Gestures
	  ○ Communication notebook
	  ○ Communication board with photographs
	  ○ Written choice strategy
	  ○ Augmented input

Language	• Restorative language approaches • Use of nonverbal modalities to facilitate verbal expression
Personal	• Use assessment strategies (e.g., written choice strategy) that facilitate successful communication therapy improving confidence • Continue to work on verbal communication goals
Environmental	• Facilitators identification and instruction provided • Facilitators instruction to encourage nonverbal modalities to repair breakdowns • Facilitators learn how to teach other communication partners • Create dictionary of gestures used

therapy; his clinician applied for and received 8 additional weeks before he was discharged from outpatient therapy. He joined a local stroke support group and began to attend the weekly group meetings with his wife.

After a short break in services due to lack of funding, John began attending individual and group speech-language therapy at a university clinic 1 day per week. As requested by the clinician, he brought the communication board and notebook from acute rehabilitation to this initial evaluation. His wife indicated that these tools were rarely used at home although he kept them in the bag on the back of his wheelchair so they were always available. The speech-language pathologist identified that perhaps the vocabulary within these tools was not currently relevant to John's current communication goals and needs. It became evident that John would benefit from a comprehensive AAC evaluation as part of his initial aphasia evaluation as he had unmet communication needs and AAC strategies and devices that were no longer helping him meet these needs.

During John's initial multisession evaluation he completed the WAB-R (Kertesz, 2007), the CADL-2 (Holland, et al., 1999), the CLQT (Helm-Estabrooks, 2001), an interview guided by the Aphasia Needs Assessment, and a topic inventory via card sort. Additionally, he and his wife completed the BOSS (Doyle et al., 2003). Based on his success during acute rehabilitation with a communication notebook and gestures, the clinician also completed sections from the Multimodal Communication Screening Task for Persons with Aphasia.

John's current communication abilities are described as follows. He has moderate-severe Broca's aphasia and moderate apraxia of speech. His auditory comprehension is better than his expressive language skills as he follows familiar multiple-step directions. He complains that he cannot follow family dinner conversations, however, because everyone "talks too fast." His WAB-R Aphasia Quotient Score (**TABLE 8.6**) confirms the challenges he describes related to auditory comprehension, although this is an area of relative strength for John. His verbal expression is not sufficient to meet his daily communication needs (e.g., 4.9/10

TABLE 8.6 John's results of the Western Aphasia Battery-Revised (WAB-R) and the Cognitive Linguistic Quick Test (CLQT).

WAB-R Subtests	Score
Spontaneous Speech	11/20
Auditory Verbal Comprehension	6.8/10
Repetition	3.4/10
Naming and Word Finding	4.9/10
Aphasia Quotient	52.2/100
CLQT Key Domains	Score (Description)
Attention	178/215 (Mild)
Memory	139/185 (Mild)
Executive Functions	20/40 (Mild)
Visual Spatial	89/105 (Within normal limits)
Key Subtests	Score
Symbol Trails	10/10
Design Memory	5/6

on the Naming and Word Finding Domain). His CADL-2 raw score was 62/100 placing him in the 24-40 percentile. Many of his errors on the CADL-2 reflect difficulty using nonverbal modalities without cueing. John's CLQT domain scores (Table 8.6) suggest a potential mild impairment in attention, memory, and executive function domains; however, subtests within these domains require significant language abilities likely resulting in a lower score given his poor spoken language skills (Helm-Estabrooks, 2002). He scored well on the Symbol Trails and Design Memory subtests indicating that his nonverbal cognitive flexibility and visual memory are fairly intact.

Information from the BOSS and an informal interview with John and his wife described the communication challenges he faces in his daily life. He used one-handed gestures to supplement his spoken expression and requested augmented input and written choice strategy (Garrett & Beukelman, 1995) from his communication partners. Additionally, he inconsistently showed communication partners photographs on his iPhone to express complex messages or set the context prior to requesting the written choice strategy (Garrett & Beukelman, 1995). John's family reported that his biggest challenge related to expression was using his communication strategies to resolve breakdowns (e.g., "He just doesn't seem to think to use other ways to communicate even though he can gesture"). Additionally, his brother and sisters would like him to communicate over the phone or via text. He is interested in communicating over the phone particularly as his sons get older and spend more time outside the home. John stated he would still prefer to use spoken expression whenever possible and hopes that his speech-language therapy sessions can improve his talking.

Further information was gathered from an interview guided by the Aphasia Needs Assessment. Now retired from his job at the ballpark, he has a new goal of returning as a volunteer for some of the team's charity activities. Volunteer roles might include helping to organize the volunteers who sell raffle tickets for various fundraising activities at the park or handing out water at the charity 5K walk/run and the annual golf outing. Additional goals include participating in family get-togethers, helping his sons with their homework, watching televised football games with his brother and sisters, and assisting his wife with household tasks. Finally, during medical appointments (which are now less frequent), John wants to communicate effectively with his physician and the nurse practitioners. His wife will often attend these appointments; however, it is important to both of them that all professionals address questions and comments to John rather than permitting his wife to speak for him. John continues to attend the weekly stroke support group meetings and uses the hospital gym facilities two times per week to work on his physical therapy exercises.

Given the changes in John's primary goals and his current frustrations related to lack of success with verbal expression, the speech-language pathologist decided to integrate AAC within sessions, with an emphasis on using nonverbal modalities to repair communication breakdowns. However, she wanted to also honor his interest in improving his verbal expression for functional settings. Therefore, she implemented an integrated multimodal approach within a treatment program designed to address verbal expression, motor planning, auditory comprehension, and reading comprehension, and she developed a plan to address all four A-FROM domains.

Related to the A-FROM environmental domain, the clinician held a brief meeting with John's wife and brother who serve as his primary communication facilitators. She reemphasized issues related to encouraging the use of nonverbal modalities to resolve breakdowns and training additional communication partners. She also invited them to attend therapy sessions so they could witness successful resolution of communication breakdowns when nonverbal modalities were implemented. Together John, his family, and the clinician created a cue card that John would keep with him to request augmented input and written choice strategy (Garrett & Beukelman, 1995) from communication partners thereby increasing his independence with unfamiliar partners. Related to the A-FROM language domain, his clinician provided restorative treatment such as response elaboration treatment, emphasizing the formation of short phrases and sentences. However, within this treatment she modeled gesture use and encouraged John to produce gestures combined with his natural speech as this was found to facilitate his word retrieval. The clinician addressed the A-FROM personal domain through a discussion with John related to his preference for verbal approaches and self-image as a verbal communicator. She provided examples of how people without communication impairments are often verbal and nonverbal communicators. She also encouraged him to discuss these issues at the next support group meeting as it was likely other group members shared his feelings on this issue. Finally, during group therapy sessions, she highlighted examples of other PWA successfully using nonverbal strategies to communicate.

The clinician addressed the A-FROM participation domain by first selecting vocabulary targets related to functional situations in which he was eager to participate. For example, vocabulary targets selected for the response elaboration treatment and multimodal communication treatment related to ballpark charity events, football, household tasks, and his son's homework. As part of the multimodal communication program, the clinician started with the modalities John was familiar with—gestures and speaking. Then, she added drawing and writing to the integrated multimodal practice of each target word. Once John was comfortable with these modes of communication, his clinician began to encourage him to also reference his cell phone photographs when the images matched a target message. As stated previously, these pictures helped to communicate complex topics and served as a topic setter when John initiated a conversation. His clinician frequently provided natural models of these strategies during their conversations within a treatment session. Given John's reported difficulty with initiating use of nonverbal strategies to repair breakdowns, the clinicians guided the multimodal communication treatment with a small cue card (**FIGURE 8.3**; Carr & Wallace, 2013). She frequently cued him by asking "How else could you tell me that?"

To address John's communication needs related to texting with his cell phone, his clinician implemented a CART-texting intervention using similar target words (Beeson et al., 2013). Texting provided another mode of communication that was aimed at increasing his communication with family members and friends who were not present. The clinician also provided training for his primary communication partners related to appropriate modifications to messages sent by communication partners. John also liked to send photographs via text messages to communicate and frequently combined a keyword with a photograph in the messages he sent.

When possible, role-play situations were constructed and practiced within therapy sessions to emphasize the multimodal communication strategies practiced. For example, John's wife participated in a therapy session during which she and John role played a communication interaction regarding a lawn service they use. His wife was instructed to encourage nonverbal modalities when John did not initiate their use on his own. Finally, the clinician asked John to practice use of the communication strategies in functional contexts and report back to her about what worked and did not work. John also sent text messages to his clinician during the week to give an update on his home practice of target words. In these ways, the clinician provided a progressive means for John to increase participation in contexts that are important to him. **TABLE 8.7** displays the A-FROM domains addressed through the therapy activities in the chronic rehabilitation stage.

Future Goals

The treatment program described in this case study details information about how John's most immediate communication needs across the A-FROM domains were

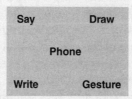

FIGURE 8.3 Multimodal communication treatment cue card

TABLE 8.7 A-FROM domains addressed in chronic rehabilitation.

A-FROM Domain Addressed	Therapy Activity
Participation	Progressive approach: • Introduction of functional vocabulary for desired activities • Role play with communication partners in therapy setting • Real life practice and reporting back
Language	• Restorative language approaches • Use of nonverbal modalities to facilitate verbal expression
Personal	• Counseling related to self-identity as a verbal communicator • Suggestion to discuss self-identity as verbal communicator at support group • Continue intervention aimed at verbal communication goals
Environmental	• Facilitator training • Facilitator observation of multimodal use

addressed using AAC. To develop clinical goals for the next phases of the rehabilitation plan, and given John's initial success using his communication notebook, the clinician administered the Multimodal Communication Screening Task for Persons with Aphasia. The test demonstrated John's inconsistent use of nonverbal modalities; however, he successfully located messages and combined symbols within the test administration notebook indicating that he may be candidate for continued use of a communication notebook. Additionally, this initial success and his use of the iPhone to communicate indicate that he may be a candidate for a high technology AAC device with speech output. A speech-generating device would increase John's independence in that a device would allow him to communicate better on the phone with his sons (and other family members). Gesturing, writing, and drawing are difficult to see even on video chat platforms. Unfamiliar listeners would be better able to understand John's communication attempts, enabling him to participate in a greater number of community activities. Additionally, John could use the speech-generating device to make doctor's appointments, to communicate with physicians and other medical professionals who may not be familiar with his nonverbal strategies or may pose complex medical questions not easily answered by these strategies. Thus, the clinician will begin to trial high technology AAC devices that are appropriate for John's skills and communication needs.

If John obtains a speech-generating device, the clinician will provide training for his primary communication partners and perhaps provide instruction for his oldest son, wife, and brother regarding the programming of the device. She will begin to integrate the speech-generating device into his multimodal treatment program with an integrative approach that includes other nonverbal and verbal modalities. To increase use of the speech-generating device outside of therapy sessions she will follow a similar procedure as she did for the other nonverbal modalities, including role playing and home practice.

REFERENCES

American Speech-Language-Hearing Association. (2002). Augmentative and alternative communication: Knowledge and skills for service delivery [Knowledge and Skills]. Retrieved from http://www.asha.org/policy/ks2002-00067.htm.

American Speech-Language-Hearing Association. (2007–2014). Augmentative and alternative communication. Retrieved from http://www.asha.org/public/speech/disorders/AAC/.

Armstrong, L., & MacDonald, A. (2000). Aiding chronic written language expression difficulties: A case study. *Aphasiology, 14*, 93–108.

Arroyo, C. G., Goldfarb, R., & Sands, E. (2012). Caregiver training in an AAC intervention for severe aphasia. *Journal of Speech-Language Pathology and Applied Behavior, 5*, 59–64.

Ball, A., Grether, S., Garz, K., & Romich, B. (2009, November). *A case with severe agraphia using word prediction technology.* Paper presented at the American Speech-Language-Hearing Association Annual Convention, New Orleans, LA.

Beeson, P. M. (1999). Treating acquired writing impairment: Strengthening graphemic representations. *Aphasiology, 13*(9–11), 767–785.

Beeson, P. M., Higginson, K., & Rising, K. (2013). Writing treatment for aphasia: A texting approach. *Journal of Speech, Language, and Hearing Research, 56*, 945–955.

Beeson, P. M., & Ramage, A. E. (2000). Drawing from experience: The development of alternative communication strategies. *Topics in Stroke Rehabilitation, 7*, 10–20.

Beeson, P., Rising, K., & Volk, J. (2003). Writing treatment for severe aphasia: Who benefits? *Journal of Speech, Language, and Hearing Research, 46*, 1038–1060.

Beukelman, D. R., Garrett, K. L., & Yorkston, K. M. (Eds.). (2007). *Augmentative communication strategies for adults with acute or chronic medical conditions.* Baltimore, MD: Paul H. Brookes Publishing Company.

Beukelman, D., & Mirenda, P. (2013). *Augmentative and alternative communication: Supporting children and adults with complex communication needs* (4th ed.). Baltimore, MD: Paul H. Brookes Publishing Company.

Boo, M., & Rose, M. (2011). The efficacy of repetition, semantic, and gesture treatments for verb retrieval and use in Broca's aphasia. *Aphasiology, 25,* 154–175.

Brennan, A. D., Worrall, L. E., & McKenna, K. T. (2005). The relationship between specific features of aphasia-friendly written material and comprehension of written material for people with aphasia. *Aphasiology, 19,* 693–711.

Bruce, C., Edmundson, A., & Coleman, M. (2003). Writing with voice: An investigation of the use of a voice recognition system as a writing aid for a man with aphasia. *Aphasiology, 38,* 131–148.

Carr, S., & Wallace, S. E. (2013, May). Effects of semantic + multimodal communication program for switching behavior in severe aphasia. Paper presented at the Clinical Aphasiology Conference, Tucson, AZ.

Chapey, R., Duchan, J., Elman, R., Garcia, L., Kagan, A., Lyon, J. G., & Simmons-Mackie, N. (2008). Life participation approach to aphasia: A statement of values for the future. In R. Chapey (Ed.), *Language intervention strategies in aphasia and related neurogenic communication disorders* (5th ed., pp. 279–289). Baltimore: Lippincott Williams & Wilkins.

Clausen, N. S., & Beeson, P. M. (2003). Conversational use of writing in severe aphasia: A group treatment approach. *Aphasiology, 17,* 625–644.

Cole, J., & Snow, B. (2011). Applying the principles of peer mentorship in persons with aphasia. *Topics in Stroke Rehabilitation, 18,* 106–111.

Crosson, B., Bacon Moore, A., Gopinath, K., White, K. D., Wierenga, C. E., Gaiefsky, M. E., ... Rothi, L. J. G. (2005). Role of the right and left hemispheres in recovery of function during treatment of intention in aphasia. *Journal of Cognitive Neuroscience, 17,* 392–406.

Davis, F. (1989). Perceived usefulness, perceived ease of use, and user acceptance of information technology. *MIS Quarterly, 13,* 318–340.

Davis, F., Bagozzi, R., & Warshaw, R. (1989). User acceptance of computer technology: A comparison of two theoretical models. *Management Science, 35,* 982–1003.

Davis, G. A., & Wilcox, M. J. (1985). *Adult aphasia rehabilitation: Applied pragmatics.* San Diego: College-Hill.

de Jong-Hagelstein, M., van de Sandt-Koenderman, W., Prins, N., Dippel, D., Koudstaal, P., & Visch-Brink, E. (2011). Efficacy of early cognitive–linguistic treatment and communicative treatment in aphasia after stroke: A randomised controlled trial (RATS-2). *Journal of Neurology, Neurosurgery, & Psychiatry, 4,* 399–404.

Dell, G. S., Lawler, E. N., Harris, H. D., & Gordon, J. K. (2004). Models of errors of omission in aphasic naming. *Cognitive Neuropsychology, 21,* 125–146.

Denes, G., Perazzolo, C., & Piccione, F. (1996). Intensive versus regular speech therapy in global aphasia: A controlled study. *Aphasiology, 10*(4), 385–394.

Dietz, A., Ball, A., & Griffith, J. (2011). Reading and writing in the 21st century: Technological applications of supported reading comprehension and written expression. *Topics in Stroke Rehabilitation, 18,* 758–769.

Dietz, A., Hux, K., McKelvey, M., & Beukelman, D. (2009). Reading comprehension by people with chronic aphasia: A comparison of three levels of visuographic contextual support. *Aphasiology, 23,* 1053–1064.

Dietz, A., McKelvey, M., & Beukelman, D. (2006). Visual scene display: New AAC interface for persons with aphasia, *Perspectives on Augmentative and Alternative Communication, 15,* 13–17.

Dietz, A., Weissling, K., Griffith, J., McKelvey, M., & Macke, D. (2014). The impact of interface design during an initial high-technology AAC experience: A collective case study of people with aphasia. *Augmentative and Alternative Communication, 30,* 314–328.

Downey, D., & Hurtig, R. (2006). Rethinking the use of AAC in acute care settings. *Perspectives on Augmentative and Alternative Communication, 15*, 3–8.

Doyle, P., McNeil, M., Hula, W., & Mikolic, J. (2003). The Burden of Stroke Scale (BOSS): Validating patient-reported communication difficulty and associated psychological distress in stroke survivors. *Aphasiology, 17*, 291–304.

Fager, S., Hux, K., Beukelman, D. R., & Karantounis, R. (2006). Augmentative and alternative communication use and acceptance by adults with traumatic brain injury. *Augmentative and Alternative Communication, 22*, 37–47.

Ferguson, N. F., Evans, K. J., & Raymer, A. M. (2012). A comparison of intention and pantomime gesture treatment for noun retrieval in people with aphasia. *American Journal of Speech Language Pathology, 21*, S126–S139.

Garrett, K. L., & Beukelman, D. R. (1995). Changes in the interaction patterns of an individual with severe aphasia given three types of partner support. *Clinical Aphasiology, 23*, 237–251.

Garrett, K. L., & Beukelman, D. R. (2006). Aphasia needs assessment. Retrieved from http://aac.unl.edu/screen/aphasianeeds.pdf

Garrett, K., Beukelman D., & Low-Morrow, D. (1989). A comprehensive augmentative communication system for an adult with Broca's aphasia. *Augmentative and Alternative Communication, 5*, 55–61.

Garrett, K. L., & Lasker, J. P. (2005). The multimodal communication screening test for persons with aphasia (MCST-A). Retrieved from http://cehs.unl.edu/documents/secd/aac/assessment/aphasiachecklist.pdf.

Garrett, K., & Lasker, J. P. (2013). Adults with severe aphasia. In D. Beukelman & P. Mirenda (Eds.), *Augmentative and alternative communication* (4th ed., pp. 405–446). Baltimore, MD: Paul H. Brookes Publishing Company.

Greig, C. A., Harper, R., Hirst, T., Howe, T., & Davidson, B. (2008). Barriers and facilitators to mobile phone use for people with aphasia. *Topics in Stroke Rehabilitation. 15*(4), 307–324.

Griffith, J., Dietz, A., & Weissling, K. (2014). Supporting narrative retells for people with aphasia using AAC: Photographs or line drawings? Text or no text? *American Journal of Speech Language Pathology, 23*, S213–S224.

Haley, K. L., Womack, J., Helm-Estabrooks, N., Caignon, D., & McCulloch, K. (2010). *The Life Interest and Values Cards*. Chapel Hill, NC: University of North Carolina Department of Allied Health Sciences.

Haley, K. L., Womack, J., Helm-Estabrooks, N., Lovette, B., & Goff, R. (2013). Supporting autonomy for people with aphasia: Use of the Life Interests and Values (LIV) cards. *Topics in Stroke Rehabilitation, 20*, 22–35.

Harvey, J., & Hux, K. (2012, November). Using text-to-speech technology to support reading: An aphasia case study. Paper presented at the American Speech-Language-Hearing Association Annual Convention, Atlanta, GA.

Helm-Estabrooks, N. (2001). *Cognitive Linguistic Quick Test*. San Antonio, TX: The Psychological Corporation.

Helm-Estabrooks, N. (2002). Cognition and aphasia: A discussion and a study. *Journal of Communication Disorders, 35*(2), 171–186.

Helm-Estabrooks, N., Albert, M. L., & Nicholas, M. (2014). *Manual of Aphasia and Aphasia Therapy* (3rd ed.). Austin, TX: Pro-Ed.

Helm-Estabrooks, N., Ramsberger, G., Morgan, A., & Nicholas, M. (1989). *Boston Assessment of Severe Aphasia*. Austin, TX: Pro-Ed.

Helm-Estabrooks, N., & Whiteside, J. (2012). Use of life interests and values (LIV) cards for self-determination of aphasia rehabilitation goals. *Perspectives on Neurophysiology and Neurogenic Speech and Language Disorders, 22*, 6–11.

Hersh, D., Worrall, L., O'Halloran, R., Brown, K., Grohn, B., & Rodriguez, A. (2013). Assess for success: Evidence for therapeutic assessment. In N. Simmons-Mackie, J. King, & D. Beukelman (Eds.), *Supporting communication for adults with acute and chronic aphasia* (Augmentative and alternative communication series) (pp. 145–164). Baltimore, MD: Paul H. Brookes Publishing.

Hilari, K., Byng, S., Lamping, D. L., & Smith, S. C. (2003). Stroke and Aphasia Quality of Life Scale (SAQOL-39): Evaluation of acceptability, reliability, and validity. *Stroke, 34*(8), 1944–1950.

Hirsch, F., Beeson, P., & Holland, A. (2007, May). Evaluating change in the communication abilities of aphasia group participants: An investigation of informed versus blind responses on the Communicative Effectiveness Index (CETI). Poster presentation at the Clinical Aphasiology Conference, Phoenix, AZ.

Holland, L., & Beeson, P. (1993). Finding a new sense of self: What the clinician can do to help. *Aphasiology, 7*, 581–584.

Holland, A., Frattali, C., & Fromm, D. (1999). *Communication Activities of Daily Living* (2nd ed.). Austin, TX: Pro-Ed.

Hough, M., & Johnson, R. K. (2009). Use of AAC to enhance linguistic communication skills in an adult with chronic severe aphasia. *Aphasiology, 23*(7), 965–976.

Hux, K., Buechter, M., Wallace, S., & Weissling, K. (2010). Using visual scene displays to create a shared communication space for a person with aphasia. *Aphasiology, 24*, 643–660.

Kagan, A. (2011). A-FROM in action at the Aphasia Institute. *Seminars in Speech and Language, 32*, 216–228.

Kagan, A., Black, S. E., Duchan, F. J., Simmons-Mackie N., & Square, P. (2001). Training volunteers as conversation partners using 'supported conversation for adults with aphasia' (SCA): A controlled trial. *Journal of Speech, Language, and Hearing Research, 44*(3), 624–638.

Kagan, A., Simmons-Mackie, N., Rowland, A., Huijbregts, M., Shumway, E., McEwen, S., Threats, T., & Sharp, S. (2008). Counting what counts: A framework for capturing real-life outcomes of aphasia intervention. *Aphasiology, 22*, 258–280.

Kertesz, A. (2007). *Western Aphasia Battery-Revised*. San Antonio, TX: PsychCorp.

Knollman-Porter, K., Wallace, S. E., Hux, K., Brown, J., & Long, C. (2015). Reading experiences and use of supports by people with chronic aphasia. *Aphasiology*, (Published online: 28 Apr 2015), 1–25.

Koul, R. K., Corwin, M., & Hayes, S. (2005). Production of graphic symbol sentences by individuals with aphasia: Efficacy of a computer-based augmentative and alternative communication intervention. *Brain and Language, 92*, 58–77.

Koul, R., & Harding, R. (1998). Identification and production of graphic symbols by individuals with aphasia: Efficacy of a software application. *Augmentative and Alternative Communication, 14*(1), 11–24.

Lanyon, L., & Rose, M. (2009). Do the hands have it? The facilitation effects of arm and hand gesture on word retrieval in aphasia. *Aphasiology, 23*, 809–822.

LaPointe, L. L. (2011). Humanistic basics: Adaptation, accommodation, and aristos. In L. L. LaPointe (Ed.), *Aphasia and related neurogenic language disorders* (4th ed., pp. 9–26). New York: Thieme.

Lasker, J., Hux, K., Garrett, K., Moncrief, E., & Eischeid, T. (1997). Variations on the written choice communication strategy for individuals with severe aphasia. *Augmentative and Alternative Communication, 13*, 108–116.

Lomas, J., Pickard, L., Bester, S., Elbard, H., Finlayson, A., & Zoghaib, C. (1989). Communicative Effectiveness Index (CETI). *Journal of Speech and Hearing Disorders, 54*, 113–124.

Luria, A. R. (1970). *Traumatic aphasia*. The Hague, The Netherlands: Mouton & Co.

Lyon, J. G. (1995). Drawing: Its value as a communication aid for adults with aphasia. *Aphasiology, 9*, 33–94.

Lyon, J. G., & Helm-Estabrooks, N. (1987). Drawing: Its communicative significance for expressively restricted aphasic adults. *Topics in Language Disorders, 8*, 61–71.

Marshall, J. (2006). The role of gesture in aphasia therapy. *International Journal of Speech-Language Pathology, 8*, 110–114.

McCall, D., Shelton, J. R., Weinrich, M., & Cox, D. (2000). The utility of computerized visual communication for improving natural language in chronic global aphasia: Implications for approaches to treatment in global aphasia. *Aphasiology, 14*, 795–826.

McKelvey, M., Dietz, A., Hux, K., Weissling, K., & Beukelman, D. (2007). Performance of a person with chronic aphasia using a visual scenes display prototype. *Journal of Medical Speech Language Pathology, 15*, 305–317.

McKelvey, M. L., Hux, K., Dietz, A., & Beukelman, D. R. (2010). Impact of personal relevance and contextualization on word-picture matching by people with aphasia. *American Journal of Speech-Language Pathology, 19*(1), 22–33.

McNeil, M. R., Odell, K., & Tseng, C. H. (1991). Toward the integration of resource allocation into a general theory of aphasia. *Clinical Aphasiology, 20*, 21–39.

Mitzner, T. L., Boron, J. B., Fausset, C. B., Adams, A. E., Charness, N., Czaja, S. J., ... Sharit, J. (2010). Older adults talk technology: Technology usage and attitudes. *Computers in Human Behavior, 26*, 1710–1721.

Murray, L., & Karcher, L. (2000). A treatment for written verb retrieval and sentence construction skills. *Aphasiology, 14*, 585–602.

Nicholas, M., Sinotte, M., & Helm-Estabrooks, N. (2005). Using a computer to communicate: Effect of executive function impairments in people with severe aphasia. *Aphasiology, 19*, 1052–1065.

Nicholas, M., Sinotte, M., & Helm-Estabrooks, N. (2011). C-Speak aphasia alternative communication program for people with severe aphasia: Importance of executive functioning and semantic knowledge. *Journal of Neuropsychological Rehabilitation, 21*, 322–366.

Paul, D., Frattali, C., Holland, A., Thompson, C., Caperton, C., & Slater, S. (2004). *Quality of Communication Life Scale*. Rockville, MD: American Speech-Language Hearing Association.

Pons, C., & Stark, J. (2013). Recovery of drawing ability in persons with aphasia. *Procedia-Social and Behavioral Sciences, 94*, 191–193.

Purdy, M., & Koch, A. (2006). Prediction of strategy usage by adults with aphasia. *Aphasiology, 20*, 337–348.

Purdy, M., & VanDyke, J. (2011). Multimodal communication training in aphasia: A pilot study. *Journal of Medical Speech-Language Pathology, 19*, 45–53.

Raymer, A. M., Ciampitti, M., Holliway, B., Singletary, F., Blonder, L. X., Ketterson, T., ... Gonzalez-Rothi, L. J. (2007a). Semantic-phonologic treatment for noun and verb retrieval impairments in aphasia. *Neuropsychological Rehabilitation, 17*(2), 244–270.

Raymer, A. M., Kohen, F., Blonder, L. X., Douglas, E., Sembrat, J. L., & Rothi, L. (2007b). Effects of gesture and semantic–phonologic treatments for noun retrieval in aphasia. *Brain and Language, 103*, 219–220.

Raymer, A., Singletary, F., Rodriguez, A., Ciampitti, M., Heilman, K., & Rothi, L. (2006). Effects of gesture + verb treatment for noun and verb retrieval in aphasia. *Journal of the International Neuropsychological Society, 12*, 867–882.

Robertson, I. H., Ward, A., Ridgeway, V., & Nimmo-Smith, I. (1994). *The Test of Everyday Attention*. Bury St. Edmunds, England: Thames Valley Test Company.

Robey, R. R. (1998). A meta-analysis of clinical outcomes in the treatment of aphasia. *Journal of Speech, Language, and Hearing Research, 41*(1), 172–187.

Rose, M. L. (2006). The utility of arm and hand gesture in the treatment of aphasia. *Advances in Speech-Language Pathology, 8,* 92–109.

Rose, M. L. (2013). Releasing the constraints on aphasia therapy: The positive impact of gesture and multimodality treatments. *American Journal of Speech-Language Pathology, 22,* S227–S239.

Rose, M. L., Raymer, A. M., Lanyon, L. E., & Attard, M. C. (2013). A systematic review of gesture treatments for post-stroke aphasia. *Aphasiology, 27,* 1090–1127.

Rosenbek, J. C., Collins, M., & Wertz, R. T. (1976). Intersystemic reorganization for apraxia of speech. In R. H. Brookshire (Ed.), *Clinical Aphasiology Conference Proceedings* (pp. 255–260). Minneapolis, MN: BRK Publishing.

Sacchett, C., Byng, S., Marshall, J., & Pound, C. (1999). Drawing together: An evaluation of a therapy programme for severe aphasia. *International Journal of Language and Communication Disorders, 34,* 265–289.

Shadden, B. B. (2005). Aphasia as identity theft. Theory and practice. *Aphasiology, 19,* 211–223.

Simmons-Mackie, N., King, J. M., & Beukelman, D. R. (Eds.). (2013). *Supporting communication for adults with acute and chronic aphasia.* Baltimore, MD: Paul H. Brookes Publishing Company.

Steele, R., & Woronoff, P. (2011). Design challenges of AAC apps, on wireless portable devices, for persons with aphasia. *Perspectives on Augmentative and Alternative Communication, 20,* 41–51.

Swinburn, K., Porter, G., & Howard, D. (2005). *The Comprehensive Aphasia Test.* Hove, England: Psychology Press.

Taylor, A. (2012). *The effect of drawing to enhance word retrieval in individuals with chronic severe aphasia.* (Unpublished Master's thesis). East Carolina University, Greenville, NC.

Tompkins, C. A., Scharp, V. L., & Marshall, R. C. (2006). Communicative value of self cues in aphasia: A re-evaluation. *Aphasiology, 20,* 684–704.

Wallace, S. E. (2010). AAC use by people with TBI: Effects of cognitive impairments. *Perspectives on Augmentative and Alternative Communication, 19,* 79–86.

Wallace, S. E., Dietz, A., Hux, K., & Weissling, K. (2012). Augmented input: The effect of visuographic supports on the auditory comprehension of people with chronic aphasia. *Aphasiology, 26,* 162–176.

Wallace, S. E., & Hux, K. (2014). Effect of two layouts on high technology AAC navigation and content location by people with aphasia. *Disability and Rehabilitation: Assistive Technology, 9,* 173–182.

Wallace, S. E., Hux, K., & Beukelman, D. R. (2010). Navigation of a dynamic screen AAC interface by survivors of severe traumatic brain injury. *Augmentative and Alternative Communication 26*(4), 242–254.

Wallace, S., & Purdy, M. (2013, September 01). *More than words.* The ASHA Leader.

Wallace, S. E., Purdy, M., & Mesa, A. (2014, June). Intensive multimodal communication intervention for people with chronic aphasia. Paper presented at the Clinical Aphasiology Conference, St. Simon's Island, GA.

Wallace, S. E., Purdy, M., & Skidmore, E. (2014). A multimodal communication program for aphasia during inpatient rehabilitation: A case study. *Neurorehabilitation, 35,* 615–625.

Ward-Lonergan, J., & Nicholas, M. (1995). Drawing to communicate: A case report of an adult with global aphasia. *European Journal of Disorders of Communication, 30,* 475–491.

Weissling, K., & Prentice, C. (2010). The timing of remediation and compensation rehabilitation programs for individuals with acquired brain injuries: Opening the conversation. *Perspectives on Augmentative and Alternative Communication, 19,* 87–96.

CHAPTER 9

Treatment Intensity in Aphasia Rehabilitation

Janet Patterson
Anastasia Raymer
Leora Cherney

INTRODUCTION

In 1972, Darley wrote that several parameters, including the intensity of the therapy, must be considered in designing treatment for people with aphasia. However scant attention was paid to defining the parameter of intensity until 1998 when Robey published an influential meta-analysis of outcomes in aphasia treatment. Reviewing 55 articles reporting aphasia treatment results, Robey coded patient characteristics, treatment type, and aphasia type. Amount of treatment, that is, what some may term *treatment intensity*, was coded as low (<1.5 hours of treatment per week), moderate (2 to 3 hours per week) or high (>5 hours per week). Despite the small number of studies for which the amount of treatment was available and the variability among them, Robey reported that a trend of greater change was observed with more intense treatment, and he advised a minimum of 2 hours of treatment per week, anticipating that treatment in excess of that would result in greater behavioral gains.

In this chapter we investigate the parameter of treatment intensity from several perspectives. We begin by defining intensity and examining how the study of intensive treatment for aphasia has evolved since Robey's publication (1998). Then we present methods of calculating treatment intensity to be used in clinical practice and to guide research comparing treatment outcomes at different levels of intensity. Next, we turn to contemporary clinical practice and a discussion of how clinicians might implement an intensive treatment program or deliver an intervention protocol in an intensive manner instead of or in addition to face-to-face treatment sessions. Two exemplars of delivering intensive treatment are highlighted, Constraint-Induced Language Therapy (CILT; Pulvermüller et al., 2001) and an Intensive Comprehensive Aphasia Program (ICAP; Rose, Cherney, & Worrall, 2013). We conclude with a case study demonstrating one plan to implement intensive treatment in a hybrid clinic-based and home-based program.

DEFINING TREATMENT INTENSITY

Intensity in behavioral treatment, such as speech-language therapy, is a multifaceted term. Treatment described as intensive may be concentrated on a single area or subject, compressed into a short time, or delivered in a very thorough or vigorous manner (Dignam, Rodriguez, & Copland, 2016; Intensive, Oxford English Dictionary, n.d.). Accordingly, aphasia treatment could be defined as intensive if a specific technique is delivered for several hours per week for a few weeks. Examples of studies following this definition are reported by Marcotte and colleagues (Marcotte et al., 2012; Marcotte, Perlbarg, Marrelec, Benali, & Ansaldo, 2013). These authors delivered semantic feature therapy for 1 hour per day, 3 days per week until participants reached criterion or 6 weeks passed. Alternatively, intensive treatment could be defined as a concentration of different treatments for several hours per day for a defined period, as in an ICAP (e.g., Babbitt, Worrall, & Cherney, 2015). It has become clear that the term "treatment intensity" is insufficient as a descriptor when attempting to capture the varied methods and amounts of treatment an individual may receive (Cherney, Patterson, & Raymer, 2011).

Bhogal, Teasell, and Speechley (2003) defined intensive treatment as at least 8 hours per week for 2 to 3 months. To arrive at this definition they correlated treatment intensity and a treatment outcome measure (Porch Index of Communicative Abilities; Porch, 2001, 1981; or Token Test; McNeil & Prescott, 1978) across eight studies, four of which showed a positive effect of treatment and four of which did not. The studies varied in treatment type (e.g., clinic-based or home-based treatment; conventional speech therapy; or emotional counseling), hours of treatment per week, number of weeks of treatment, and total hours of treatment. In the four studies that showed a positive treatment effect, the amount of treatment averaged 8.8 hours per week over 11.2 weeks for an average of 98.4 total hours. The four studies that showed a negative treatment effect averaged 2 hours of treatment per week over 22.9 weeks for an average of 43.6 total hours. Bhogal et al. (2003) concluded that more intensive therapies delivered over a shorter period of time resulted in a significant improvement in scores on these two outcome measures.

Five studies further illustrate the variable definitions of intensive treatment. Wertz et al. (1986) reported data for 94 participants who received 8 to 10 hours of treatment per week for 12 weeks (90–120 hours), either delivered by or directed by a speech-language pathologist. Mackenzie (1991) reported on five participants who received an average of 85 hours of individual and group treatment in a 4-week program (approximately 4 hours per day, 5 days per week for 4 weeks). The intensive treatment period in this study was preceded and followed by a period of no treatment. Hinckley and Craig (1998) retrospectively examined treatment schedules for 40 participants who were enrolled in three 6-week treatment periods; a period of no treatment that was preceded and followed by periods of intensive treatment. In the intensive periods each participant received 23 hours of treatment per week (individual, group, and computer) for about 130 total hours. Denes, Perazzolo, Piani, and Piccione (1996) compared 6 months of intensive treatment (6–7 sessions per week and 94–160 total hours) to regular treatment (3 sessions per week and 56–70 hours) for 17 individuals. Basso and Caporali (2001) reported data for participants enrolled in intensive treatment (5 hours clinic-based per week plus 2 to 3 hours home-based per day for as much as 20 hours per week) over those in less intensive treatment (5 hours per week). Participants in all these studies showed a positive effect following periods of treatment that were defined by the authors as intensive. This outcome occurred despite variations in participant factors (e.g., aphasia type and severity), treatment grouping (e.g., group, individual, or computer), therapy program (e.g., cueing treatment for anomia, Melodic Intonation Therapy), and schedule (e.g., hours per day, days per week, and length of treatment).

Robey (1998) and Bhogal et al. (2003) suggest that intensive treatment delivered in a short period of time (massed practice) can result in greater treatment gains when compared to less intensive treatment over a longer period of time (distributed practice). However, these authors offered different definitions of "intensive treatment," likely due to the different definitions of intensive treatment in the papers included for review. All five of the studies described here meet Robey's (1998) definition for a high amount of treatment (>5 hours per week); however, only two meet Bhogal and colleagues' definition (8.8 hours per week).

Two recent systematic reviews examined nine studies contrasting treatment intensity, grouping them by time post-onset (acute or chronic), outcome measure (impairment or activity/participation), and study phase (discovery, efficacy, or effectiveness) (Cherney, Patterson, Raymer, Frymark, & Schooling, 2008, 2010). Studies included in these systematic reviews were selected because the term *intensity* or *amount of treatment* appeared in the abstract. The amount of treatment per week ranged from 5 hours per week to 23 hours, and total duration of treatment, if reported, ranged from 2 weeks to 40 months. Cherney et al. (2008) reported positive outcomes on impairment-based measures associated with more intensive treatment for individuals with chronic aphasia, and mixed results on activity/ participation measures. Minimal data addressed behavior maintenance or individuals with acute aphasia. While recognizing the clinical value of the general statement that the "more intense the treatment, the greater the change" (Robey, 1998; p. 180), caution against oversimplifying the case is urged, considering the limited number of studies and the variability in the definitions of intensity (e.g., session frequency or duration, or cumulative amount of treatment) that exists among them (Cherney et al., 2008, 2011; Marshall, 2008; Robey, 1998).

The concept of intensive treatment was included in the influential paper published by Kleim and Jones (2008) who described the application of principles of neural plasticity gleaned from animal research to human learning and rehabilitation. The fifth principle, *intensity matters*, states that neural plasticity, which is essential for learning, is induced with training of a sufficient intensity (Kleim & Jones, 2008, p. S229). Not surprisingly, neither the criterion for a treatment to be labeled as "intense" nor the timing of treatment is clear. Kleim and Jones noted that it is also possible that overuse (too much intensive practice) could result in worsened function. Intensity (principle 5) is related to but should not be confused with the fourth principle, *repetition matters* (Kleim & Jones, 2008). Repetition of a newly learned behavior is required to drive neural plasticity and induce lasting neural and behavioral change; however, similar to intensity, the amount or schedule of repetition needed to achieve change is unknown. What is clear is that the parameters of intensity and repetition must be examined to understand how they influence aphasia intervention and outcome and how they relate to use-dependent learning (Kent, Rutherford, Breier, & Papanicoloau, 2009; Kerr, Cheng, & Jones, 2011; Maher et al., 2006; Raymer et al., 2008; Raymer, Maher, Patterson, & Cherney, 2007).

The review of these studies reveals three important points that require closer attention. First, authors have defined the concept of intensity in a variety of ways. As described by Warren, Fey, and Yoder (2007), several variables contribute to understanding treatment intensity: dose (i.e., the number of teaching episodes per intervention session); session length (i.e., the number of minutes of each session); dose frequency (i.e., the number of sessions per time period—per day or per week); and total intervention duration (i.e., the time period over which intervention occurs—weeks or months). Combining dose, dose frequency, and total intervention duration yields cumulative intervention intensity, which is a general indicator of treatment intensity. Second, the concepts of massed and distributed practice have been linked with intensity. In one view, the treatment protocol can remain constant but the length of the treatment period varies (i.e., high dose frequency in massed practice and low dose frequency in distributed practice). From another perspective, the content of the therapy can have a narrow focus—yielding concentrated practice on specific therapy target(s) (i.e., massed practice)—or it can include a wider scope of objectives, allowing for variety and variability in therapy targets and intervention schedule (i.e., distributed practice). Third, even when therapy delivery is constant, not all patients respond similarly to therapy. This suggests that patient characteristics, such as aphasia type, severity, or motivation also influence therapy outcomes. In sum, the impact of intensity on rehabilitation outcomes can only be understood when the independent influences of all these variables are known. In the next section we examine intensity according to delivery variables such as dose and duration.

QUANTIFYING TREATMENT INTENSITY

Traditionally, treatment intensity has been described in terms of frequency and duration; that is, how often a patient is seen each week and for how many weeks; however, there has been little empirical or theoretical support to determine these values. Furthermore, the varying definitions of intensive treatment pose obstacles in replicating a treatment or understanding its effectiveness.

As noted previously, Robey (1998) and Bhogal et al. (2003) reported that aphasia treatment studies that provided higher intensity treatments had considerably larger effect sizes (Robey, 1998) and better outcomes (Bhogal et al., 2003) than those that provided treatment on a low intensity schedule. Therefore, a number of aphasia treatment studies purport to provide intensive treatment for aphasia as part of the intervention protocol (e.g., Kendall, Oelke, Brookshire, & Nadeau, 2015; Wan, Zheng, Marchina, Norton, & Schlaug, 2014; Wilssens et al., 2015). However, not all studies of intensive aphasia treatment contrast different levels of treatment intensity as part of an experimental manipulation.

As part of systematic reviews of the aphasia treatment literature, Cherney et al. (2008, 2010, 2011) discussed the influence of intensity on treatment outcomes in aphasia. All 11 studies included in those reviews directly compared two levels of treatment intensity as an experimental manipulation, except for Lee, Kaye, and Cherney (2009) who explored intensity in a correlational analysis. Findings among the studies were mixed in favoring intensive over less intensive forms of treatment. At that time, however, we did not carefully distinguish the form of intensive treatment that was provided among the studies identified. As we described earlier, an intensity manipulation can concern different elements that contribute to a *cumulative intervention intensity*, including dose, intervention session duration, dose frequency, and intervention duration (Warren et al., 2007). Definitions of these terms and the formula for calculating *cumulative intervention intensity* appear in **TABLE 9.1**. Calculating cumulative intervention intensity requires that a clinician identify therapeutic acts (i.e., actions taken by the clinician) and client acts (i.e., responses to therapeutic acts) (Baker, 2012a), a task which is easier said than done. These clinician and client acts become the active ingredients of a teaching episode designed to induce behavioral change. Off, Griffin, Spencer, and Rogers (2015) provide an example of specifying dose, active ingredient, dose frequency, and total intervention duration in a study in order to calculate cumulative intervention intensity for two dose conditions: low dose and high dose.

In **TABLE 9.2**, we have refined our earlier reviews of aphasia treatment intensity and discuss aphasia treatment studies by the type of intensity comparison that was incorporated. For most studies on aphasia, the intensity comparison centered on dose frequency. Expanding upon our past work, we will add to the discussion studies that to some extent speak to issues of dosage in aphasia treatment, which we had not addressed in our earlier reviews.

Dose Frequency

When speaking of intensity comparisons, most aphasia treatment studies tend to refer to the treatment schedule or dose frequency in terms of number of sessions per week that treatment is provided. Table 9.2 lists several studies that varied dose frequency as an experimental manipulation. What is also important to note in those studies is what

TABLE 9.1 Terminology to measure intervention intensity.

Term	Definition
Teaching episode	Clinician behavior designed to induce behavior change and which can be identified and measured
Dose	Number of properly administered teaching episodes during a single intervention session
Dose form	Task or activity in which teaching episodes are delivered
Dose frequency	Number of times a dose of intervention is provided in a unit of time (e.g., per minute, in 60-minute session)
Total intervention duration	Time period over which intervention is presented
Cumulative Intervention Intensity (CII)	Dose × Dose frequency × Total intervention duration
Therapeutic Intensity Ratio (TIR)	Total number of therapy hours in a treatment program divided by the total number of potential treatment hours

Data from Babbitt et al.; 2013; Baker, 2012a; Warren, Fey, & Yoder, 2007.

happened to session duration and intervention duration to contribute to the overall cumulative intensity of treatment. For some studies cumulative intensity differed and for others cumulative intensity was the same across conditions. These studies are presented separately in Table 9.2.

*Dose Frequency Varied—Intervention Duration
Constant—Cumulative Intervention Intensity Different*
Some intensity studies, while systematically varying the dose frequency of treatment, held the intervention duration constant to control for the influence of time or spontaneous recovery in individuals with aphasia. In these studies, the combination of varied dose frequency and constant intervention duration led to large discrepancies in cumulative intervention intensity between high dose frequency and low dose frequency schedules. For example, in one of the first intensity comparisons by Denes et al. (1996), one group received six to seven sessions of treatment per week and the other received three sessions per week. Both groups took part in treatment for an average of 6 months. Therefore differences reported between groups at 6 months on a written language test may be a result of not only the dose frequency difference but also the greater cumulative amount

TABLE 9.2 Intensity comparisons of dose frequency across aphasia treatment studies; cumulative intensity different or same across studies.

Study	Design	Dose Frequency	Session Duration/ Day	Intervention Duration	Cumulative Intervention Intensity	Overall Result: High Versus Low Intensity Comparisons
Studies where cumulative intensity differs						
Denes et al., 1996	Two group controlled trial	Varied Not reported vs. 3 sessions/wk	Constant	Constant 6 months	Different Average 130 sessions vs. 60 sessions	High > Low—Written Language No difference in all other measures
Hinckley & Craig, 1998 Study 2	Retrospective within group	Varied 23 hr/wk vs. up to 3 hr/wk	Not reported	Constant 6 wk	Different 138 hr vs. up to 18 hr	High > Low—BNT Naming, Content Units
Bakheit et al., 2007	Three group controlled trial	Varied 5/wk vs. 2/wk	Constant	Constant 12 wk	Different 35.6 hr vs. 19.3 hr	No difference—Western Aphasia Battery; target cumulative frequencies not achieved (i.e., 60 hr vs. 24 hr)
Basso & Caporali, 2001	Paired case studies	Varied by case	Varied	Constant	Different in each pair	High > Low—AAT
Hinckley & Carr, 2005	Two group controlled trial	Varied 20 indiv. + 5 grp vs. 4 indiv.	Varied	Varied? Trained to criterion	Different?	Low > High—CADL-2 High > Low—PALPA Written naming No difference—Catalog ordering, PALPA Oral naming

(Continues)

TABLE 9.2 Intensity comparisons of dose frequency across aphasia treatment studies; cumulative intensity different or same across studies. (Continued)

Study	Design	Dose Frequency	Session Duration/Day	Intervention Duration	Cumulative Intervention Intensity	Overall Result: High Versus Low Intensity Comparisons
Lee et al., 2009	Correlational study	Varied 1.9–16.9 hr/wk	Varied	Constant 9 wk	Different 17.4–68.8 hr	Higher amount of treatment correlated with greater outcomes in content and rate of speech
Godecke et al., 2014	Two group cohort trial	5 hr/wk vs. 11 min/wk	Varied	Same 4–5 wk	Different avg. 18.65 sessions vs .3 sessions	High > Low*—WAB, Discourse analysis *85% in control/low group—no treatment
Godecke et al., 2013	Regression analysis of two prior cohorts combined (N = 70)	Varied	Varied 0–88.4 min/session	Varied 3–49 days	Different 0–1415 min. 0–21 sessions	Higher minutes/day (12.1 min) associated with greater improvement (7.6% greater)
Wenke et al., 2014	Two group cohort trial	Varied 4–5 days/wk 3–4 days/wk	Varied 2–2.5 hr/day 1 hr/day	Varied 11 weeks 8 weeks	Different 84–91 hr 25 hr	No difference between groups on CAT spoken language subtest or Disability Questionnaire
Studies where cumulative intensity is constant						
Pulvermüller et al., 2001	Two group controlled trial	Varied 5 day/wk 2–3 hr/wk	Varied 3–4 hr/day Not stated	Varied 2 wk vs. 3–5 wk	~Same 31.5 hr 33.9 hr	High CILT > Low Standard—AAT, AAT Oral naming, AAT Auditory comprehension, Communication activity log

Raymer et al., 2006	Single-subject design	Varied 3–4 day/wk 1–2 day/wd	Constant	Varied 3–4 wk 6–7 wk	Same 12 sessions	High > Low—Oral naming No difference—Auditory comprehension
Ramsberger & Marie, 2007	Single-subject design	Varied 5 sessions/wk 2 sessions/wk	Constant	Varied 3–4 wk 7–10 wk	Same 15–20 sessions	High > Low—Oral naming
Sage et al., 2011	Case series	Varied 5 sessions/wk 2 sessions/wk	Constant	Varied 2 wk 5 wk	Same 10 sessions	No difference—Oral naming acquisition Low > High—Oral naming follow up
Harnish et al., 2008	Case study	Varied 5 day/wk 2 day/wk	Varied 1.5 hr/day 1 hr/day	Varied 2 wk vs. 7.5 wk	Same 15 hr	High > Low—Naming, Auditory Comprehension, fMRI changes
Martins et al., 2013	Two group controlled trial	Varied 5/wk vs. 1/wk	Same 2 hr/day	Varied 10 wk vs. 50 wk	Same 100 hrs	No difference—Aphasia quotient, FCP
Dignam et al., 2015	Two group controlled trial	Varied	Varied 16 hours/week 6 hours/week	Varied 3 weeks Versus 8 weeks	Same 48 hours	High > Low for BNT No Difference for CETI, CCRSA, ALA

Data from Babbitt et al., 2013; Baker, 2012a; Warren, Fey, & Yoder, 2007

AAT = Aachen Aphasia Test (Huber et al. 1984); Assessment of Living with Aphasia (Kagan et al., 2010); BNT = Boston Naming Test; CADL-2 = Communication Activities of Daily Living (2nd ed.); CETI = Communicative Effectiveness Index; CCRSA = Communicative Confidence Rating Scale for Aphasia; CAT = Comprehensive Aphasia Test; FCP = Functional Communication Profile; PALPA = Psycholinguistic Assessment of Language Processing in Aphasia; WAB = Western Aphasia Battery of treatment delivered in a more intensive schedule in the high dose frequency group (average 130 sessions) compared to the low dose frequency group (average 60 sessions). Perhaps more surprising is that several other outcome measures showed no difference in outcomes despite the large differences in dose frequency and cumulative intensity.

Hinckley and Craig (1998) included a similar contrast in their retrospective within group study that compared intensive speech therapy (23 hours/week for 6 weeks) to nonintensive therapy (2 to 3 hours/week for 6 weeks or 3 to 5 hours/week for 6 weeks). Although the duration of the treatment interval remained constant at 6 weeks, the dose frequency per week varied dramatically, so the amount of treatment (cumulative intervention frequency) equaled, on average, 138 hours versus 18 to 30 hours in the high and low dose frequency conditions, respectively. Not surprisingly, therefore, the high cumulative intervention intensity group had very large effect sizes on a standardized picture naming test, whereas the less intensive group had small effect sizes.

Bakheit et al. (2007) also varied dose frequency while holding intervention duration constant at 12 weeks in their study of aphasia treatment intensity. While both groups improved performance on an aphasia battery following treatment, the high dose frequency group, which received treatment for 5 hours/week, had the same outcomes in a standard aphasia battery as their low dose frequency group, which received treatment 1 to 2 hours/week.

Another study that warrants mention was a small case series by Basso and Caporali (2001). In this study, not only was dose frequency varied, but also duration of treatment per day varied. The intensive treatment was delivered using volunteers to provide assistance at home in addition to daily clinical intervention, such that patients received 2 to 4 hours per day of treatment for 7 days each week. The lower intensity treatment was provided by a clinician for 1 hour per day for 5 days per week. This mostly descriptive comparison suggested that the higher intensity treatment had better recovery. Again, the cumulative frequency difference was considerable in the higher versus lower intensity participants, making it difficult to determine the influence of the dose frequency variable on the results.

In a correlational investigation with 17 individuals who used a computer to practice script production over 9 weeks, Lee et al. (2009) reported significant positive correlations between greater amount of time spent in the computer practice and better treatment outcomes.

The highest form of research investigation, a randomized controlled trial was conducted by Hinckley and Carr (2005) who compared two groups receiving aphasia treatment, one that received intensive treatment (20 hours/week individual + 5 hours/week group) and one with a "nonintensive" schedule (4 hours/week individual treatment). That is, the groups varied in both dose frequency and session duration per day. Further complicating the intensity story here is that intervention duration also varied. Whereas one would presume that the cumulative frequency of the intensive group was higher than the nonintensive group, it is not clear because treatment stopped when participants reached a preset criterion and the overall duration of treatment was not specified. The findings of this study were mixed—the intensive group was superior on the Psycholinguistic Assessments of Language Processing in Aphasia, Written Naming subtest (PALPA; Kay, Lesser, & Coltheart, 1992) and the nonintensive group was superior on the Communication Activities of Daily Living–2nd Edition (CADL-2; Holland, Frattali, & Fromm, 1999). Finally, no frequency difference was evident on a catalog-ordering task and on the PALPA Oral Naming subtest.

While all of the previous studies took place primarily with individuals who had chronic aphasia, some recent work examined treatment outcomes in individuals in the subacute and acute stages of aphasia recovery. A cohort investigation in a subacute setting by Wenke et al. (2014) compared treatment outcomes in two groups, an intensive group that received 9 hours/week of treatment for 11 weeks (1 hour/day of individual therapy + either computer, group, or speech pathology assistant for 1–1.5 hours/day), and a standard service group that received 3 hours per week for 8 weeks of individual therapy sessions. Although outcomes did not focus on functional language effects, it was noted that there was no difference between intensity groups on a standard aphasia assessment and on a disability measure.

Godecke and colleagues (2013, 2014) completed studies in the very early stage of aphasia recovery. They conducted large cohort trials that were used to complete a regression analysis on 70 patients to evaluate factors that influence aphasia recovery from early onset. In addition to initial aphasia severity and stroke disability, amount of aphasia treatment had an equally important impact on recovery. For every 12.1 minutes of treatment per day, patients could anticipate a 7.6% improvement in aphasia prognosis on a standardized aphasia battery.

Examining the findings of this set of studies in detail, where cumulative intervention intensity varied for high and low dose frequency conditions, demonstrated that there was no clear direct association between amount of treatment provided and resulting outcomes. Although correlation and regression analyses showed that more treatment was associated with better language outcomes, the results of at least three larger trials, including two controlled group trials (Bakheit et al., 2007; Denes et al., 1996) indicated that less treatment was as effective as more treatment in the same amount of time. Such findings suggest that a less intense treatment schedule might in fact be an appropriate scheduling decision rather than a more intense treatment schedule to preserve and extend limited financial resources available to patients in most clinical settings.

Dose Frequency Varied—Intervention Duration Varied—Cumulative Intervention Intensity Same

In examining Table 9.2, it is noted that a number of aphasia treatment studies varied both the dose frequency and the intervention duration in an attempt to maintain a constant cumulative intervention intensity, that is, they compared massed versus distributed practice schedules (Maas et al., 2008). To counter the concern of varying intervention duration, most of these studies were completed in individuals with chronic aphasia, where the influence of spontaneous recovery has mostly passed (Robey, 1998).

For example, two single-participant designs examined picture naming treatments delivered in contrasting dose frequency schedules. Raymer, Kohen, and Saffell (2006) examined the effects of a computerized word retrieval treatment delivered for 12 treatment sessions, one phase administered three to four sessions per week for 3 weeks and one phase completed one to two sessions per week for 6 weeks. The high dose frequency condition led to greater picture naming outcomes than the low dose frequency for all five participants, but no difference was noted for an auditory comprehension task administered to two participants. Ramsberger and Marie (2007) also delivered a computerized word retrieval treatment to two participants receiving 15 sessions of treatment and two receiving 20 sessions of treatment. Within each pair, one participant completed training in an intensive dose frequency schedule of five sessions per week, and one completed a nonintensive two sessions per week dose frequency schedule. Three of four participants increased picture naming abilities; two showed greater improvement in the intensive rather than the nonintensive schedule, and one showed greater improvement for the nonintensive over the intensive schedule. Finally, Harnish, Neils-Strunjas, Lamy, and Eliassen (2008) described a case study where their participant with aphasia received two 15-hour treatment phases, one scheduled at 7.5 hours per week for 2 weeks and one scheduled at 2 hours per week for 7.5 weeks. Again, better results were noted following the massed practice phase. Thus 8 of 10 participants in these three studies demonstrated greater improvements in word retrieval measures in the higher dose frequency schedule while holding cumulative intervention intensity constant.

In contrast, Sage, Snell, and Lambon Ralph (2011) reported a case series where all participants with aphasia completed 10 naming treatment sessions, one phase scheduled five times per week for 2 weeks and the other phase two times per week for 5 weeks. The group analysis showed little difference in dose frequency conditions immediately post-treatment and an advantage of the low dose frequency condition over high dose frequency at the 1 month follow up, an observation similar to findings in the motor learning literature where interventions delivered on a distributed schedule may have stronger retention of treatment effects (Dignam et al., 2016; Maas et al., 2008).

Pulvermüller et al. (2001) completed a controlled group trial that varied dose frequency with roughly comparable cumulative intervention intensity across conditions (31.5 hours versus 33.9 hours). Their high intensity group received Constraint-Induced Language Therapy (CILT) for 3 to 4 hours per day for 5 days per week for 2 weeks (higher dose frequency and longer session duration), and their low intensity group had standard speech therapy for 2 to 3 hours/week for 3 to 5 weeks. High intensity CILT surpassed low intensity standard treatment in scores for an overall aphasia battery, oral naming, auditory comprehension, and a communication activity log. Of note is that the advantage for high intensity in this study is confounded by the additional difference of treatment type administered during the high intensity treatment phase.

Two other controlled trials reported divergent results. Martins et al. (2013) compared two groups that received 100 hours of treatment in 2-hour sessions, one group scheduled five times per week for 10 weeks and another scheduled one time per week for 50 weeks. They reported no difference in the two groups on an aphasia quotient and a functional rating scale. Dignam et al. (2015) compared two groups that received 48 hours of treatment over 3 weeks (intensive: 16 hours/week) or 8 weeks (distributed: 6 hours/week). While there was no difference between groups for communication participation measures, there was an advantage of distributed training over intensive training for a standardized picture naming test both at treatment completion and at 1 month follow up. Although most of these dose frequency studies compared four to five sessions per week of training to one to two sessions per week, the cumulative intervention intensities varied greatly across studies, from 10 to 100 hours. Therefore, the differences in cumulative intensities may explain the divergent findings across studies. Immediately following a short course of treatment, some advantage may be evident in intensive dose frequency schedules, especially for naming outcomes. Yet those gains may not last, and less intensive treatment may have better results at follow up, as in the motor learning literature (Dignam et al., 2016; Maas et al., 2008) and as has been reported in the Dignam et al. (2015) aphasia trial. Over longer cumulative intervention intensities, it appears that results tend to equalize across dose frequencies.

Dose–Trial Relationship

In the complexities of aphasia treatment, few studies describe the dose of treatment considered in terms of the number of practice trials per session, optimally reported as dose per unit of time (Warren et al., 2007). Cumulative intervention intensity is a function of dose-by-dose frequency (sessions per week) by session duration (in hours) by intervention duration (in weeks). Baker (2012b) noted "dose may be particularly important to define and measure when trying to establish the optimal intensity of an intervention" (p. 481). Dose will be influenced by the dose form, that is, the type of task that is implemented in the treatment protocol, as some tasks take longer than others to complete, for example, sentence production versus picture naming, thereby lowering the dose within a given session. Terms related to dosage and their definitions appear in Table 9.1.

One domain where it is more practicable to report dose measurements is in the area of naming treatments for aphasic word retrieval difficulties. As an example, Harnish et al. (2014) carefully described dosing in their cued naming treatment for individuals with aphasia. Every participant took part in a picture naming task for 50 pictured nouns in an 8-step cueing hierarchy such that participants had 400 opportunities per 1 hour session to produce target words, an average dosage rate of 6.67 items per minute. The dose frequency of treatment was four times per week over 2 weeks leading to a cumulative intervention intensity of 3200 responses. This intervention intensity led to improvements in naming trained words for seven of eight participants. Understanding this base response will allow for future studies that systematically modify dose and cumulative intensity of treatment. Some recent studies have begun to explore the influence of different dosage parameters in picture naming treatment with respect to the numbers of exposures that take place within a session.

As a starting point, Snell, Sage, and Lambon Ralph (2010) completed a meta-analysis of the word retrieval treatment literature to examine the relationship between number of words trained across studies and outcomes reported. Although there was some indication of a negative correlation between number of items trained and naming outcomes, this finding was confounded by severity of impairment.

In an earlier study that directly examined dosage in an experimental manipulation, Laganaro, Di Pietro, and Schneider (2006) examined a computerized naming treatment and compared effects after five training sessions for 48 words per session versus 96 words per session. During the 48-item phase, participants completed 5 to 21 repetitions per item (mean dose 8.9 repetitions), whereas during the 96-item phase, participants completed 2.5 to 7.2 repetitions per item (mean dose 3.9 repetitions). The longer list (96 items) ultimately provided fewer opportunities for practice; that is, a lower dose and a lower cumulative intervention intensity (on average 1872 trials) than the shorter list (48 items) with higher dose practice (on average 2136 trials). Participants improved proportionally the same on the two lists as treatment was provided on a massed dose frequency schedule for both lists (five sessions/week). Yet significantly greater gains were noted on the longer list/lower dose than the shorter list/higher dose. Moreover, the low dose condition led to greater absolute gains because more words were relearned.

Snell et al. (2010) completed a systematic investigation of naming treatment in 13 individuals with aphasia in which they compared outcomes when treatment was administered for two 10-session phases, one for 20 nouns and one for 60 nouns. Each item was practiced three times per session (equal dose per item), yet cumulative intervention intensity varied because session durations were longer for the 60-item phase of training (1800 naming trials) than the 20-item phase (600 naming trials). The proportion of words learned did not differ by set size, as each word had the same dose of training, but the absolute number of words learned was greater in the 60-item set (average 39 words learned) than in the 20-item set (average 15 words learned).

While systematic investigations of dose in aphasia treatment are limited, the initial findings contrast somewhat with what might be predicted. There is no difference in the proportional gains based on set size. Therefore larger treatment sets, while receiving a lower or equal dose of treatment, may lead to greater treatment outcomes because more items are learned in treatment.

Cumulative Intervention Intensity

Cumulative intervention intensity (CII) is a singular value indicating the number of times a teaching episode, or active ingredient of treatment, is delivered in a treatment program, and it is a general indicator of intensity. Warren et al. (2007) defined the concepts of *teaching episode* and *dose form* (see Table 9.1) and the values of *dose, dose frequency,* and *total intervention,* using them to calculate cumulative intervention intensity. Multiplying the three values yields the number of teaching episodes delivered in a treatment program. For example, as noted previously, Harnish et al. (2014) defined the teaching episodes in their naming protocol and calculated the CII as 3200. One can then compare the CII of studies with similar protocols to evaluate differences in outcomes. Furthermore, the elements of CII, or CII itself, can be systematically varied to understand the effect of dosage. While counting is easy, determining the teaching episode is often more challenging as it requires the clinician to think about the therapeutic interaction—the stimulus and response—and determine how that interaction can be divided into components (Warren et al., 2007). Defining a teaching episode broadly (e.g., all steps in a cueing hierarchy) may lead to a diluted intervention effect. In contrast, using too narrow a definition may ignore important aspects of the interaction, such as nonverbal feedback.

Defining a teaching episode in an impairment-based treatment protocol is easier than defining a teaching episode in activity/participation–based treatment. However, even in the seemingly most straightforward treatment tasks, the teaching episode can become multifaceted through the clinician–client interaction, thus creating a challenge to clearly define what is being counted to calculate CII. Warren et al. (2007) noted several obstacles to clearly defining a teaching episode, such as the multiple small behaviors that may contribute to a single teaching episode, determining which of those behaviors is critical to quality in defining the teaching episode, or a treatment technique that is purposefully broad (e.g., a conversational period with content feedback). Furthermore, the variety of elements that contribute to CII makes the story a complex one to disentangle. This does not even take into consideration differences that may arise in the form that the treatment takes, the type and severity of aphasia, or the time post-onset and the etiology of the aphasia. Nonetheless, the effort to define a teaching episode so that it can be counted is required for this calculation to be useful. The conclusion to be drawn is that in some way, the type of intervention must be specified and the amount calculated to begin to understand the optimal dosage.

Therapeutic Intensity Ratio

Babbitt et al. (2015) proposed a method of understanding treatment dosage and quantifying treatment intensity that they termed the *therapeutic intensity ratio* (TIR). Recognizing that programs of intensive treatment, in this case ICAPs, may vary in the number of treatment hours delivered per week and the variety of treatment protocols offered, they sought to provide a value that could estimate what they call the "spread of treatment intensity" (Babbit et al., 2015, p. S860). The TIR is a ratio that represents the total number of therapy hours in which an intensive program, such as an ICAP, provides treatment, divided by the total number of potential hours available for therapy, assuming 40 hours are available for therapy in a week. For example, an ICAP may have 120 total therapy hours (6 hours/day x 5 days/week x 4 weeks) and total availability of 160 hours (40 hours/week x 4 weeks). Thus, 120 total therapy hours divided by 160 available hours produces a TIR of 75%. Other programs with more or fewer hours of treatment per week or weeks of treatment will produce different TIRs.

DELIVERING INTENSIVE APHASIA INTERVENTION IN CONTEMPORARY CLINICAL SETTINGS

We begin this section with an observation stated previously. In general, evidence shows that intensive speech-language intervention for people with aphasia is associated with positive behavioral change (Baker, 2012a; Cherney, 2012; Cherney et al., 2008, 2010, 2011; Lee et al., 2009; Snell et al., 2010). As with many aspects of life however, the story is not so simple. Cherney (2012) states "... intensity alone is insufficient without also considering the active ingredients of the teaching episode" (p. 424), and "... there may be an optimum combination of the parts of the treatment program that contribute to best outcomes ..." (p. 430). Baker (2012a) suggests that determining intensity does not have a simple answer, and a range of client-variables (e.g., amount of time available to participate in treatment), condition-related variables (e.g., concomitant diagnosis), clinician-related variables (e.g., expertise and experience), and service-related variables (e.g., caseload, third-party payment) also can influence the effect of an intervention and have an impact on how intensity of intervention results in behavior change. Warren et al. (2007) opine that identifying and clearly describing the teaching episode of an intervention can be complicated by many factors, yet it must be accomplished in order to calculate cumulative intervention intensity. Where does a clinician begin to sort out these influences? Some of the conclusions that can by drawn from the data surrounding the intensive intervention literature are:

- Short periods of intensive intervention or participation in an Intensive Comprehensive Aphasia Program can induce behavioral change in people with aphasia.

- Intensive treatment should be quantified in a manner that is appropriate for the delivery format.

- Intensive treatment can be beneficial at any point in the time course of aphasia. It may be that the initial phases of intervention are best scheduled using an intense, massed practice training schedule, with the schedule modifying to a more distributed form over time.

- Careful selection is required to best match intensive intervention with participant characteristics to ensure that an individual can tolerate intensive treatment and to maximize improvement.

- Resolution of workplace limitations in personnel, space, administrative support, and financial commitment is key to successful implementation of an intensive intervention program.

Guidance from the Evidence

The evidence surrounding treatment intensity or intensive treatment can be viewed from multiple perspectives. If treatment is a single technique (e.g., cueing hierarchy or PACE), in general, the evidence is favorable for intensive treatment delivered in short periods of time for acquisition of language behaviors in impairment-based outcome measures. Evidence also supports the advantage of intensive treatment for more complex treatments in which intensity is an integral component of the treatment (e.g., Constraint-Induced Language Therapy). If intensive treatment is the framework for a treatment program (e.g., ICAP), evidence supporting intensive treatment is also favorable. The conclusion drawn from these perspectives is that as long as the treatment parameters are clear, it is reasonable to expect that intensive treatment may induce behavioral change. That conclusion is moderated, however, by cautions from authors about variable outcomes depending in part on participant characteristics and on maintenance of those effects.

TIR (Table 9.1; Babbitt et al., 2015) and CII (Baker, 2012a; Warren et al., 2007) aid in determining the dosage and intensity. Both values are mathematically easy to calculate; however, they rely on different reference points. The TIR (Babbitt et al., 2015) references a 40-hour therapy week and does not consider individual elements of the daily treatment program, while the CII (Warren et al., 2007) references the number of times an intervention is delivered for the duration of the intervention. One aspect of the CII that makes it difficult to use is defining the teaching episode that comprises a dose.

Participants in most investigations of intensive treatment have been in the chronic stage of the course of aphasia. While the evidence for these individuals favors short periods of intensive treatment for some treatment techniques and some aphasia types, results are mixed when examining maintenance of those effects. Emerging evidence supports short periods of intensive, impairment-based intervention for individuals in the very early period of the course of aphasia (Godecke et al., 2014). The conclusion from these data is that intensive treatment, either an intensive delivery schedule of intervention or an ICAP, can induce behavioral change; however, it may be that the initial phases of intervention are best scheduled on an intense, massed practice training schedule, with the schedule being modified to a more distributed delivery over time to maximize maintenance of training effects.

Participant characteristics play an important role in the success of intensive treatment. Legh-Smith, Denis, Enderby, Wade, and Langton-Hewer (1987) reviewed data from 441 stroke patients, 71 of whom were referred for speech-language therapy. Of those 71, Legh-Smith et al. found that at 4 weeks post stroke, only five individuals were suitable for intensive speech therapy, defined as 4 hours per day/5 days per week. This determination was based on Functional Communication Profile scores (FCP; Sarno, 1969), the Barthel Activities of Daily Living Index (Granger, Dewis, Peters, Sherwood, & Barrett, 1979), the Raven's Coloured Progressive Matrices (Raven, 1965), and clinical rating by a speech-language pathologist. Among the reasons for excluding patients from intensive treatment at 4 weeks post stroke were severe comprehension deficit, severe confusion, physically too disabled to participate, fatigue from other treatments, transportation difficulties, or high FCP score indicating language skills that do not require treatment. Data from Godecke and others (Godecke, Hird, Lalor, Rai, & Phillips, 2012; Kirmess & Maher, 2010; Laska, Kahan, Hellblom, Murray, & von Arbin, 2011; Sickert, Anders, Münte, & Sailer, 2014) recast the suggestion by Legh-Smith et al. to delay intensive treatment until beyond 4 weeks post stroke, but acknowledge that participant characteristics play a role in suitability. People are complicated and messy in their behavior, thus inserting unpredictability into an otherwise clearly defined and well-planned intervention. Intrapersonal factors such as motivation, general health, attention, or concomitant disorders, and extrapersonal factors such as family life events or transportation, can influence an individual's participation in and success at intensive intervention, whether early or later in the recovery period. An important factor to address before beginning intensive intervention is the likelihood that an individual will be able to tolerate the intensive schedule and be able to sustain adherence to treatment protocols (Maas et al., 2008). Baker (2102b) noted the higher dropout rate for intensive treatment over nonintensive treatment and suggested that "although more intensive intervention for people with aphasia seems preferable, it may not always be suitable" (p. 479). The conclusion to be drawn is that, provided careful patient selection is carried out, intensive intervention can benefit people with aphasia at almost any stage of recovery.

Intensive treatment requires investment of resources from the clinical facility. Staff time devoted to delivering treatment and managing administrative details is time that is unavailable to serve patients not included in intensive treatment. A treatment protocol delivered on an intensive schedule requires detailed scheduling, but it should not require additional space for therapeutic events. In contrast, an ICAP requires both detailed scheduling and dedicated space for multiple and perhaps concurrent treatment activities. An administrative decision to support intensive treatment carries the obligation of financial commitment to resources such as staff, support personnel, space, and equipment. Even if participants self-pay, potential workplace limitations exist that must be acknowledged before beginning a treatment program (Baker, 2012b). These limitations might, in turn, be viewed as opportunities for innovation to influence future clinical practice (Rose, Attard, Mok, Lanyon, & Foster, 2013). The conclusion here is that implementing a program of intensive intervention requires attention to workplace limitations as well as treatment protocol requirements and participant characteristics.

Intensive Intervention Beyond the Face-to-Face Clinic Session

When an intensive intervention program is not easily available due to geographic, financial, family schedule, or other reasons, yet a clinician and person with aphasia would like to develop an intensive treatment program, creativity will be the guide. Clinical aphasiology has a rich history of recruiting human and other resources to supplement therapy. Reports have shown positive effects of programs incorporating volunteers (Worrall &

Yiu, 2000), speech-language pathology assistants (Wenke et al., 2014), computers (Lee, Fowler, Rodney, Cherney, & Small, 2010), telephone and television (Wertz et al., 1992), caregivers and family members (Purdy & Hindenlang, 2005), and pets (Macauley, 2006). Reports such as these provide foundations for expanding the positive effects of intensive intervention by means other than the traditional clinician–client, face-to-face interaction.

Training volunteers to deliver intensive treatment has been successfully demonstrated. Meinzer, Streiftau, and Rockstroh (2007) reported no differences in outcome of CIAT delivered by clinicians or lay persons, but limited their conclusion to delivery of structured programs for which lay persons can easily be trained and monitored. Marshall et al. (1989) compared individually designed intensive treatment (8–10 hours per week for 12 weeks) delivered by the speech-language pathologist or a trained volunteer supervised by a speech-language pathologist and found no difference in participant outcomes. Accordingly recruiting a volunteer lay person to deliver intensive treatment is a viable option. Meinzer et al. and Marshall et al. point out planning activities that will help ensure success of the program, including careful training, volunteer demonstration of competency, regular treatment fidelity checks, confirmation of participant/volunteer compatibility, and commitment to the program. Risk factors such as waning motivation or relationship strain may impede successful completion of the program, but can be mitigated through regular monitoring. Wenke et al. (2014) demonstrated feasibility of using speech-language pathology assistants to deliver intensive intervention. They measured client outcomes, consumer satisfaction (clinician, participant, and caregiver), and cost. There was no difference in outcome between participants in the speech-language pathologist group and the speech-language pathology assistant group, and none among consumer satisfaction scores in the three groups.

Self-management of an intensive treatment program is realistic for those individuals with a skill set sufficient to complete the treatment correctly, monitor their performance, and sustain adherence to the protocol (Enderby, 2012). Lee et al. (2009) demonstrated self-paced participant self-management using AphasiaScripts, a computer-based program. Participants were instructed to practice 30 minutes per day, a low dose of intensive treatment (30 minutes/day × 5 days = 150 minutes/week or 2.5 hours/week); however, most participants practiced more than that (mean = 5.2 hours per week). It is conceivable that many treatment protocols can be delivered via self-management (e.g., naming or sentence production) although most reports to date describe computer-based or tablet/ smartphone-based programs. Proof of concept for self-management through computer-delivered treatment protocols has been demonstrated; however, intervention intensity has not been the research focus (Mortley, Wade, Davies, & Enderby, 2004; Palmer et al., 2012; Palmer & Enderby, 2015). While it is clear that technology has an important place in intensive self-managed aphasia treatment, remaining immune to the glitz of the technology is important in order to build the protocol and establish conditions for successful use (Van de Sandt-Koenderman, 2011). Accordingly, self-managed protocols that can be monitored by a speech-language pathologist to assure adequate intervention intensity, such as AphasiaScripts are key.

A low-tech version of a self-managed intensive treatment protocol is a program of home practice. Baker (2012a, p. 406) provided a framework for measuring therapeutic inputs and client acts, which could be used to document intensive treatment in a home program. Two cumulative intervention intensity values are calculated, one for therapeutic inputs from the speech-language pathologist and one for client acts that occur in the home program. Using Table 9.1 as a guide, the teaching episode should be identified for the clinic-based treatment and separately for the home-based treatment (or only the home-based treatment if no clinic-based program is included). The teaching episodes may be the same or different, as may the dose, dose frequency, and total duration. For people with aphasia who have sufficient skills to engage in an entirely self-managed program, only regular check-ins with the client may be needed. In this case it would be prudent to build in a treatment fidelity check for the user as a way to confirm that he or she is correctly completing the program and providing the desired responses. If the self-managed treatment program has two components—clinic-based and home-based—the cumulative intervention intensities can be adjusted to achieve the overall desired intensity level. Johnson et al. (2014) describe Constraint-Induced Aphasia Therapy II (CIAT II), comprised of CIAT as originally described (Pulvermüller et al., 2001) plus a "transfer package" consisting of a behavioral contract, daily home diary, daily administration of the Verbal Activity Log, problem solving, home skills assignments, post-treatment practice, and post-treatment telephone contacts. Johnson et al. reported that their four participants made large gains on outcome measures. They could also have calculated cumulative intervention intensities for the clinic-based and home-based portions of CIAT II to examine the intensity of each treatment component. Beeson, Higginson, and Rising (2013) describe T-CART, a writing treatment based on texting that had both a clinic-based and home-based component. Activities in both were identical, making calculation of cumulative intervention intensity relatively easy.

Yet another way to increase intervention intensity is through the use of telehealth. Two very early demonstrations of the feasibility of telehealth were reported by Sanders (1977) and Wertz et al. (1992). In her Tele-communicology program, Sanders (1977) administered treatment techniques such as cued naming via telephone. The participant and clinician each had a notebook of stimulus items they mutually referred to during treatment. Wertz et al. (1992) compared aphasia appraisal in three conditions: face-to-face, closed circuit television, and video laser-discs with the telephone, and reported no differences in the outcome of appraisal for 72 participants. Telehealth has come a long way since then and several proof of concept papers demonstrate the utility of the Internet and telehealth in assessing and treating people with aphasia. Successful telehealth programs have been reported for anomia (e.g., Agostini et al., 2014; Dechêne et al., 2011; Palmer et al., 2012; Woolf et al., 2016), functional communication using virtual reality (Garcia, Rebolledo, Metthé, & Lefebvre, 2007), and videoconferencing (Hoenig et al., 2006; Taylor et al., 2009). Innovative telehealth applications have been developed such as iAphasia (Choi, Park, & Paik, 2016), and individualized interactive treatment books using iBooks Author installed on an iPad (Kurland, Willkins, & Stokes, 2014). We can expect to see increasingly more telehealth options become available that can be used to deliver intensive treatment. It is important to note that telehealth does not automatically change the amount of time the clinician devotes to treatment. In some cases it changes the delivery method and requirements for the participant to travel, but still requires the clinician's physical presence. In other cases, treatment intensity can be substantially increased if the participant can self-manage, relieving the clinician of the requirement of regular session attendance.

Three cautions are highlighted which, if addressed in treatment planning, will maximize the likelihood of success in delivering intensive treatment beyond the face-to-face clinic session. First, the participant must demonstrate skills and abilities appropriate to the technique. For example, the ability to text is required for T-CART, self-monitoring is required for a low tech self-management program, and the temperament to sustain an intense schedule is critical to all programs. Second, the appropriate equipment and supplies must be available, such as adequate bandwidth for telehealth videoconferencing. Finally an appropriate and sustainable support system is key to successful delivery of intensive treatment. That is, the clinician must be able to meet the timing needs, a family member or volunteer must be committed to the process, and the person with aphasia must feel invested in the enterprise.

EXEMPLARS OF IMPLEMENTING INTENSIVE TREATMENT FOR APHASIA

Two treatment methods have incorporated intensity as a crucial component in the treatment protocol. This is in contrast to treatment protocols that "add on" an intensive delivery schedule to the regular content of the protocol. One method is Constraint-Induced Language Therapy (CILT; Pulvermüller et al., 2001), which invokes intensive treatment as a principle in reducing learned non-use of speech and language skills. The second method, the Intensive Comprehensive Aphasia Program (ICAP; Rose et al., 2013), has emerged with the aim of delivering intervention in an intensive and multifaceted manner.

Constraint-Induced Language Therapy and Intensive Language Action Therapy

Treatment intensity became entwined with Constraint-Induced Aphasia (Language) Therapy (CIAT) following introduction of the technique by Pulvermüller et al. (2001). CIAT was introduced as a derivative of Constraint-Induced Movement Therapy (CIMT; Taub et al., 1993), and is also known as CILT (Maher et al., 2006), and more recently, as Intensive Language Action Therapy (ILAT; Berthier & Pulvermüller, 2011). Invoking the principles of constraint (verbal communication required), shaping (gradual transition to desired state of verbal communication), and intensive training (massed practice of verbal communication), Pulvermüller et al. (2001) compared changes in scores on standardized language tests and a communication activity log for two groups of patients with chronic aphasia. One group received CIAT for 3–4 hours per day for 2 weeks and one group received conventional therapy for an average of 34 hours over 4 weeks. Patients receiving CIAT improved significantly more than did patients receiving conventional therapy. Pulvermüller et al. (2001) observed that perhaps the "effective therapeutic factor" (p. 1621) is massed practice and constraint is adjunctive. Out of curiosity we calculated the TIR for this study (see **TABLE 9.3**) which ranged from 16.7% (fewest number of treatment hours in the conventional therapy group) to 41.3% (greatest number of treatment hours in the CIAT group). The TIR to achieve change for patients in the CIAT group ranged from 32.5% to 39.4%, suggesting that a TIR above 30% may be optimal to induce behavioral change. TIR values for the conventional therapy group were all below 30%.

By 2008 a sufficient number of studies had been published to warrant a systematic review (Cherney et al., 2008, 2010). Each study was evaluated for phase of treatment (discovery, efficacy, effectiveness, or cost-benefit) and subjected to quality ratings for elements such as assessor blinding and treatment fidelity. In completing the review, questions were posed examining both intensive treatment and CILT. Results showed modest support for intensive treatment and positive effects for CILT, particularly for impairment-based outcome measures for people with chronic, nonfluent aphasia.

Since the introduction of CILT, numerous studies have dissected it in search of the "active ingredient(s)" in the treatment, including treatment intensity. Pulvermüller et al. (2001) used pictured objects as stimulus items and compared CILT to a no-treatment group, with superior results for the CILT group. Meinzer, Djundja, Barthel, Elbert, and Rockstroh (2005) modified CILT by adding written materials and a home program, called CIATplus. While participants in both CIAT groups improved on impairment-based and activity/participation-based outcome measures, greater change was noted for the CIATplus group. Two examples of CILT modifications are additional constraints and generalization tasks. Faroqi-Shah and Virion (2009) introduced a morphosyntactic constraint on tense morphology to the required response creating the CILT-G condition

TABLE 9.3 Therapeutic Intensity Ratio (TIR; Babbit et al., 2013) for CIAT (Pulvermüller et al., 2001).

	CIAT			Conventional Therapy		
	Total Weeks	Total Hours	TIR	Total Weeks	Total Hours	TIR
Minimum hours	2	23	32.5%	3	20	16.7%
Maximum hours	2	33	41.3%	5	54	27%
Average hours	2	31.5	39.4%	4	33.9	21.2%

Data from TIR; Babbit et al., 2013 and Pulvermüller et al., 2001
TIR = number of hours of treatment divided by total number of hours available for treatment, assuming a 40-hour week. Pulvermüller et al. (2001) report CIAT delivered 3–4 hours per day and do not report hours per day for conventional therapy. CIAT was administered for 2 weeks to all patients and conventional therapy for ~4 weeks. Three weeks is assumed for the minimum hours value of conventional therapy and 5 weeks is assumed for the maximum hours value.

(CILT-Grammatical constraint) to contrast with the original CILT condition (CILT-O). Johnson et al. (2014) added more exercises and a transfer package for generalization and required more responses per session creating CIAT I and CIAT II. Two studies trained verbs (Bock & Ballard, 2003; Goral & Kempler, 2009). Berthier et al. (2009) conducted a randomized parallel group study of CIAT and pharmacological treatment using memantine, with the best outcome occurring when the two treatments were combined. Treatment delivery by a professional versus lay person has been investigated (Meinzer et al., 2007) as has dosage reduction (Mozeiko, Coelho, & Myers, 2015; Osborne & Nickels, 2012; Szaflarski et al., 2008). Several studies investigated neural changes following CIAT (e.g., Breier, Maher, Novak, & Papanicolaou, 2006; Meinzer, Paul, Weinbruch, Djundja, & Rockstroh, 2009; Richter, Miltner, & Straube, 2008). Studies compared CILT with other treatments such as Multi-Modality Aphasia Therapy (M-MAT; Rose et al., 2013), individual impairment-based treatment (Ciccone et al., 2015), semantic therapy (BOX; Wilssens et al., 2015), Model-Oriented Aphasia Therapy (MOAT; Barthel, Meinzer, Djundja, & Rockstroh, 2008) and Promoting Aphasics' Communicative Effectiveness (PACE; Kurland, Pulvermüller, Silva, Burke, & Andrianopoulos, 2012; Maher et al., 2006). Finally, recent studies investigated CILT delivered during acute or subacute rehabilitation (Aerts et al., 2015; Ciccone et al., 2015; Kirmess & Maher, 2010; Kristensen, Steensig, Pedersen, Pedersen, & Nielsen, 2015; Sickert et al., 2014).

Looking across these studies, one can draw the conclusion that CIAT/CILT/ILAT, broadly considered, is an efficacious treatment for aphasia, particularly for individuals with chronic nonfluent aphasia. Studies such as those noted here are pushing the envelope of CIAT in order to understand the contributions of its elements and the conditions under which it can be successfully delivered. Several questions remain, however, owing largely to the wide variety of treatment parameters present in these studies and the mixed results. For example, while several studies favorably compared CIAT and another treatment, that was not always the case (Mozeiko et al., 2015; Rose, 2013; Rose et al., 2013; Wilssens et al., 2015). The predominant administration time for CIAT has been 3 to 4 hours for 2 consecutive weeks. Studies are beginning to evaluate the intensity requirement for CIAT, for example, examining CIAT delivered over shorter periods in the acute care setting and CIAT delivered in distributed practice. Meinzer, Rodriguez, and Gonzalez Rothi (2012) nicely summarized the state of research in CILT after a decade. They suggested that while early studies of CILT report positive outcomes, subsequent research has not clearly substantiated the effect of constraint over intensive treatment. Furthermore, the optimal dosage is far from clear. In summary, CIAT/CILT/ILAT is a treatment with principles that are valid in aphasia therapy; however, with a definition that remains elusive, including disentangling the confound of constraint and intensity as well as determining optimal dosage in differing clinical settings.

Intensive Comprehensive Aphasia Program (ICAP)

The first program to meet the criteria of an ICAP, even before the term ICAP was coined, is the University of Michigan Residential Aphasia Program. Created in 1947 to serve veterans, it is still in existence today. Currently several programs identify themselves as offering intensive aphasia treatment but not all are an ICAP. Rose et al. (2013) define an ICAP as a service delivery model that incorporates several treatment techniques during a period of intensive service delivery. It is important to note that Rose and colleagues identify an ICAP as a service delivery model; it is not a treatment technique to be implemented in a prescribed format, nor does it mandate rigid adherence to a defined schedule. Rather, it is an attempt to address multiple domains in the International Classification of Functioning (ICF), Disability and Health (World Health Organization, 2001) principles of neural plasticity (Kleim & Jones, 2008), and intensive treatment in a defined-participation program.

Results of an international survey of ICAPs gathered information about existing programs that meet the criteria for an ICAP. Survey questions examined program staffing, philosophy and values, funding, admission criteria, structure and activities, family involvement, outcome measures, and factors important to success (Rose et al., 2013, p. 381; **TABLE 9.4**). Thirteen ICAPs were identified in four countries: United States of America, Canada, Australia, and United Kingdom, most of which were affiliated with university programs and funded through participant self-pay. Common themes in the ICAPs, whether formally written in a mission statement or identified in program materials, were emphasis on evidence-based practice, innovative clinical practice, education, and formation of a community of participants. As might be anticipated, the ICAPs differed in structural parameters. For example, contemporary ICAPs have existed for about five years and annually serve approximately 20 PWA. The number of PWA in each session is typically small, between five and ten, and they participate in about 100 hours of treatment during an ICAP session. Numerous and varied staff are involved in the ICAPS, including clinical professionals, support staff, and volunteers. Notably the ICAPs identified admission

TABLE 9.4 Characteristics of ICAPs, as reported by Rose et al. (2013).

ICAP Characteristic	Mean (Mode)
Years in existence	4.6 (2)
Number of ICAP sessions offered annually	3.13 (1)
Number of days per week ICAP meets	4.5 (5)
Duration of ICAP (in days)	21 (20)
Hours of therapy per day (individual, group, computer)	4.75 (3)
Total hours of therapy during ICAP session	101 (100)
Number of people with aphasia served annually	17.3 (15.5)
Number of people who attend each ICAP session	6 (6)

Reproduced from Rose, M. L., Cherney, L. R., & Worrall, L. E. (2013). Intensive comprehensive aphasia programs: An international survey of practice. Topics in Stroke Rehabilitation, 20(5), 379–387, p. 380.

criteria that included participant stamina and independence, and all ICAPs used tools to measure outcomes in linguistic behavior, cognitive skill, communication, quality of life, and client satisfaction.

Babbitt, Worrall, and Cherney (2013) reported perspectives of the clinicians involved with a subset of these ICAPs, and three themes emerged. Clinicians favored an intensive service delivery model, stating that it showed them a different view of the therapeutic process and it allowed them to delve deeply into planning, delivery, and documenting. The second theme described the rewards that clinicians experienced, such as learning opportunities, professional growth, collegial support, and relationships that developed within the intensive period. The third theme identified challenges the clinicians faced, such as time management for rapid paced treatment, documentation requirements and balancing patient and family expectations. Despite these challenges, clinicians' perspectives of their participation in an ICAP were generally positive.

ICAPs are a viable service delivery method; however, outcome measures that demonstrate participant improvement are important for understanding their role in promoting communicative change in people with aphasia. Outcome data from two ICAPs are reported in the following sections.

Residential ICAP—Pittsburgh VA PIRATE

The Program for Intensive Residential Aphasia Treatment and Education (PIRATE) was established within the Department of Veterans Affairs Pittsburgh Healthcare System in 2009 and annually serves 18 participants in 4-week programs (Winans-Mitrik et al., 2014). Six programs are offered each year, with three individuals in each program. Participants receive 5 hours of therapy daily in individual sessions, group and social activities, and education activities. Individual treatment respects principles of evidence-based practice and typically targets behavior at the impairment level. Group activities offer opportunities for generalization of learned behavior as well as improving social communication skills.

PIRATE outcome data are from two performance-based measures, the Comprehensive Aphasia Test (CAT; Swinburn, Porter, & Howard, 2004) and the Story Recall Procedure (Doyle et al., 2000), and from client and surrogate report via the Aphasia Communication Outcome Measure (ACOM; Hula et al., 2015). Across the United States, 73 individuals have participated in PIRATE programs (demographic data are available in Winans-Mitrik et al., 2013; Table 1, p. S334). The authors used statistical modeling to examine the four outcome measures in one analysis with respect to behavior change over time and measurement error (Winans-Mitrik et al., 2013, p. S334). Results showed a significant positive change on all outcome measures on average. For each outcome measure, some positive change was noted during the period between initial testing and treatment, with significantly greater change shown during the treatment period. Individual differences were noted in response patterns for participants, and not all participants improved on the selected outcome measures. Despite the lack of robust success for all participants,

Winans-Mitrik et al. (2013) demonstrated that an ICAP can result in positive behavioral change for some patients. A challenge to the clinicians in this and other programs is to carefully select participants who are most likely to benefit from an ICAP.

ICAP—Rehabilitation Institute of Chicago

Babbitt and colleagues (2015) report data from 74 individuals with aphasia who completed ICAP treatment in an urban setting. The ICAP offers two programs each year with 10 participants and six clinicians in each program. Individuals participate in 6 hours of treatment, for 30 hours of treatment per week in a 4-week program. Each day participants receive two individual therapy sessions of evidence-based treatments, such as Treatment for Underlying Forms (TUF; Thompson & Shapiro, 2005); a session of CILT (after Pulvermüller et al., 2001); a session of reading and writing activities; a computer group; and a conversation group. Treatment goals are individualized and carried though all activities of the day. A challenge in administering individualized goals within an ICAP is to maintain treatment fidelity, which this ICAP did though a detailed training and audit procedure for clinicians.

This report of ICAP outcome measures addressed two questions: (1) did first time ICAP participants demonstrate improvement on impairment and participation outcome measures; and (2) do factors such as aphasia type and severity, or time post-onset influence outcome. To address these questions, participants were administered the Western Aphasia Battery-Revised (WAB-R; Kertesz, 2006); the Boston Naming Test (BNT; Goodglass, Kaplan, & Weintraub, 2001); the Communicative Effectiveness Index (participant and family member) (CETI; Lomas et al., 1989); the American Speech-Language-Hearing Association Quality of Communicative Life (ASHA-QCL; Paul et al., 2004); and the Communication Confidence Rating Scale for Aphasia (CCRSA; Babbitt, Heineman, Semik, & Cherney, 2011). Pre- and post-treatment change scores were compared and Cohen's *d* effect sizes calculated. All measures showed positive change, with t-tests significant at < 0.001 and medium or large effect sizes (Babbitt et al., 2015). No effects of aphasia severity or type, or time post-onset were noted.

CONCLUSION

A good deal of research has centered on understanding principles of intensity in aphasia treatment. Evidence supports treatment delivered on an intensive schedule (high dose frequency) to incite therapeutic gains, which then moves toward a distributed schedule to promote maintenance of those gains. Clinical efforts have turned toward providing therapeutic programs in the form of CIAT or ICAPs that incorporate principles of treatment intensity to maximize treatment outcomes. Advances in technologies support these efforts to move treatment intensity from the clinic to self-managed home settings.

CASE ILLUSTRATION

Mrs. H., a 73-year-old female, sustained a left middle cerebral artery stroke approximately 8 weeks prior to beginning this course of treatment. She lived independently with her husband and successfully completed all aspects of daily living. She was initially diagnosed with mild Broca's aphasia (since resolved to anomic aphasia) and received speech-language therapy in the acute and subacute settings. The most recent standardized test scores were: Aphasia Quotient of 80.2 on the WAB and 35 on the BNT. During informal assessment, the topic of intensive treatment was discussed and Mrs. H. was enthusiastic about the possibility. The option of clinic-based intensive treatment was not available to Mrs. H. and the clinician, so they discussed the idea of intensive treatment delivered using a combination model of clinic-based plus home-based treatment. Positive confirmation in three practice areas was required for agreement of the suitability of this model for Mrs. H. at that point in her course of aphasia. Lack of positive confirmation in any one of the areas would lead to a decision against this combination model. It is important to note that Mrs. H. and her husband were equal partners with the clinician in these discussions in order to establish motivation to participate in treatment and increase the likelihood that, if implemented, this prog schedule could be sustained (see Chapter 13, this volume). This first decision point was to determine whether the behavioral goals of treatment and the selected treatment technique could conceivably be delivered in a self-managed home environment. In this case, a cueing treatment was selected to address the anomic symptoms (Harnish et al., 2014) and the clinician and Mr. and Mrs. H. determined that the treatment could be modified for home-based treatment. With careful attention to the theoretical and empirical requirements of the treatment, it is likely that many treatment protocols can be modified for home-based intensive delivery.

The second decision point was the perceived ability of the three individuals involved, Mr. and Mrs. H. and the clinician, to engage in the treatment enterprise. To arrive at this decision several factors were considered about each person. For example, for Mrs. H. these factors were her sensory abilities (in order to see and hear stimuli), how easily she may fatigue (clinic-based intensive treatment sessions would be 30 minutes of a 60-minute session and home-based treatment segments of 15 minutes each), her ability to sustain attention to the intervention throughout the intensive blocks, her ability to understand the elements of the treatment technique (e.g., instructions to reveal a cue or to repeat), her daily schedule that would provide opportunities to implement the intervention, and critically, her ability to self-monitor her responses. The design of this home-based delivery required Mrs. H. to judge her verbal responses, and if she cannot reliably demonstrate this ability then either the decision for this model is negative, or further modification must be made, such as having an intervention partner who will provide judgment. For Mr. H. two factors were important to consider. First was his support of the treatment in general ways, such as agreeing to the treatment schedule and assisting with logistics as needed. The second factor was his ability, if required, to judge Mrs. H.'s. naming attempts. This discussion is particularly important to have before beginning treatment to acknowledge the potential of relationship strain and, through education about the intervention activities, to maximize the likelihood that Mr. and Mrs. H. would adhere to the protocol and schedule. Factors considered for the clinician were largely time-based, such as time to create the materials for the home-based program and time for periodic check-ins, if needed. Clinicians have reported positive feelings toward intensive intervention (Babbitt et al., 2013); however, anecdotal information from clinicians suggests that the logistics of completing an intensive treatment schedule can be a challenge. In this case the clinician's role was to provide oversight for the intensive intervention but not to deliver it.

The third decision point was the logistics of the treatment program. The clinician determined that cued picture-naming treatment (Harnish et al., 2014) was a good match for Mrs. H. in terms of likelihood that she would respond favorably to it given her aphasia diagnosis (Harnish et al., 2014, p. S287), and that the "saturated practice schedule" used by Harnish et al. (p. S287), that is, incorporating a high density of teaching episodes, could be modified from clinic-based treatment to clinic-based plus self-managed treatment. In 1 hour sessions four times per week for 2 weeks, Harnish et al. delivered a dose of cued picture-naming treatment (50 pictures × 8 cues = 400 teaching episodes) at a dosage rate of 6.67 episodes per minute (400 teaching episodes per 60-minute period). This delivery schedule was appropriate for clinic-based treatment; however, Mrs. H. stated that she did not think she could sustain a 60-minute treatment session at home. Striving to maintain the dosage rate of 6.67 episodes per minute within the 15-minute self-managed treatment period Mrs. H. thought reasonable, the clinician modified the number of treatment items. **TABLE 9.5** shows the comparative information for Mrs. H. and Harnish et al. (2014). Dose form and active ingredients remain unchanged. The expectation was 30 minutes of cued picture-naming treatment per day delivered in two 15-minute time periods; the clinic-based treatment occurred during the 60-minute scheduled treatment session and the self-managed treatment occurred at Mrs. H.'s convenience. These modifications were jointly decided and considered logistically reasonable by Mrs. H. and the clinician. For the self-managed treatment, daily treatment time was reduced from 60 minutes to 30 minutes, the dose from 400 teaching episodes per day to 192 (two 15-minute treatment

TABLE 9.5 Comparison of treatment dosage for cued picture naming treatment from Harnish et al. (2014) and Mrs. H.

Dosage factor	Harnish et al. (2014)	Mrs. H.
Dose	400 teaching episodes (50 pictures × 8 cues)	96 teaching episodes (12 pictures × 8 cues)
Dose period	60 minutes	15 minutes
Dosage rate	6.67 teaching episodes/minute (400 teaching episodes/60 minutes)	6.4 teaching episodes/minute (96 teaching episodes/15 minutes)
Dose frequency	4 times per week (clinic-based)	8 times per week (two 12-item lists per day; clinic-based plus self-managed)
Total intervention duration	2 weeks	4 weeks
Cumulative intervention Intensity	3200 teaching episodes (400 teaching episodes × 4 times/week × 2 weeks)	3072 teaching episodes (96 teaching episodes × 8 times/week × 4 weeks)

Data from Harnish et al. (2014) and Mrs. H.

periods per day), and the total intervention duration increased from 2 weeks to 4 weeks. Despite these changes, the clinician believed that the cumulative intervention intensity was as equivalent as possible with respect to the clinical constraints (CII = 3072 for Mrs. H. and 3200 in Harnish et al., 2014). With this schedule the clinician was obligated to prepare four 12-item word lists to be used in both treatment settings as well as instructions for self-managed treatment. An important distinction here is that Harnish and colleagues delivered their treatment via a computer-controlled program using a laptop and Mrs. H.'s program was a low tech version using pictures and paper stimulus forms. Session time was controlled by computer in Harnish et al., by the clinician in the clinic-based treatment, and by the CD of verbal instructions in the self-managed treatment. Believing this treatment to be appropriate for Mrs. H., and recognizing the importance of session length to intervention intensity, the clinician made reasonable accommodations to ensure the dosage frequency would be comparable by carefully timing clinic-based sessions and controlling timing via CD instructions in the self-managed treatment. Assuring the clinician's agreement to preparation and management is critical to the success of the protocol.

The clinician prepared four 12-item word lists for this treatment. The same four lists were used in both treatment settings. In the clinic-based setting, the order of presentation was randomized and the clinician provided encouragement and feedback; in the self-managed setting, each target item was shown on an individual page, with written instructions below and verbal instructions on a CD (see **TABLE 9.6** for a sample page). Clearly, effort is required to prepare materials, first to

TABLE 9.6 Sample of a target item page for self-managed cued, picture naming treatment (adapted from Harnish et al., 2014).

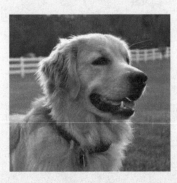

Cue Level* (Harnish et al., 2014)	Clinician Input (From Clinician or CD)	Correct/Incorrect (Marked by Clinician or Mrs. H.)
Independently name	"What is this?"	
Orthographic cue	DOG (See the printed word and the clinician asks, "What is this?")	
Repetition	"Say 'dog'"	
Name after a 3-second delay	Wait (mark 3 seconds) "What is this?"	
Semantic cue	"It barks and wags its tail. What is this?"	
Phonemic cue	"/dʌ/ What is this?"	
Repetition	"Say 'dog'"	
Name after a 3-second delay	Wait (mark 3 seconds) "What is this?"	

Data from Harnish et al., 2014.
*Cue levels are covered by a piece of paper and successively revealed. Mrs. H.'s expected response at each cue level is correctly saying "dog."

select picture stimuli and second to record the verbal cues for self-managed treatment. Harnish et al. (2014) created individual stimulus sets for each of their eight participants, with items selected from words named incorrectly on two naming trials. Items were not matched across participants. Considering this as well as the importance of maintaining Mrs. H.'s engagement throughout the intervention, the clinician selected the stimulus items from interest areas noted by Mrs. H. and from lists of nouns and verbs used in other treatment studies; no attempt was made to match lists.

Several risk factors that may undermine treatment success presented themselves for consideration before beginning treatment, chief among them, the potential that Mrs. H. may be unable to sustain the treatment program. To mitigate this risk, clear discussion occurred prior to treatment to ensure as much as possible that she understood the time and task requirements, and during treatment regular encouragement was offered. At each clinic-based session the clinician queried Mrs. H. about any difficulties she may have encountered in the self-managed intervention. The correct/incorrect responses on stimulus pages were graphed to demonstrate change. While clinician attitude is important to maintain adherence to the treatment protocol, ultimately Mrs. H. was responsible for her own level of engagement.

Another risk factor considered was that despite the best intentions to approximate as much as possible the CII identified in Harnish et al. (2014) and also meet Mrs. H.'s therapy goals and her ability to incorporate treatment into her daily life, the intensity may not be sufficient to induce change. Harnish et al. reported that all eight of their participants showed significant change after 3 hours of therapy of 1200 teaching episodes. Mrs. H. will have more sessions and more teaching episodes than 1200, giving the clinician confidence that this CII is reasonable.

A third risk that could undermine intervention was lack of treatment fidelity. Fidelity in the clinic-based treatment is relatively easy to monitor through audio- or videotaped samples or self-reflection. In the busy clinical setting, time did not permit reviewing session recordings on a regular basis, so the clinician used the treatment stimulus pages as a means to verify treatment fidelity. Self-managed treatment poses a much greater challenge in monitoring fidelity. While it was possible to ask Mrs. H. to audiotape her 15-minute sessions, that added an additional burden that may have created an inability to sustain engagement in treatment or would refocus Mrs. H.'s attention from the treatment to the recording procedure. As a substitute for session review, the clinician used the stimulus treatment pages, reviewing them with Mrs. H. to make sure she completed each step by checking her judgment responses. The weakness is evident—if Mrs. H. did not accurately monitor her responses, the treatment was not delivered appropriately.

To determine success of the treatment program the clinician examined three pieces of evidence, treatment compliance data, treatment performance data, and intervention review report. Mr. and Mrs. H. were committed to the treatment program and, according to treatment records, were compliant with the home-based portion. That is, Mrs. H. reported completing the treatment on a regular schedule and returned the treatment pages. While verification through observation was impossible, the clinician believed there was sufficient rapport established between herself and Mrs. H. to engage in honest discussion about treatment delivery and therefore accepted the response data as presented. Next the clinician reviewed graphs of probe data for trained and untrained nouns and verbs collected over the 4 weeks of treatment (see Chapter 11 for review of graphing treatment probe data). Effect sizes showed clinically meaningful change for all probe sets. Mr. and Mrs. H. both reported a perceptual change in functional communication, described as Mrs. H.'s increased engagement in communication activities (regardless of the presence of word-finding difficulties), and successful use of word retrieval strategies.

Finally, the clinician asked Mr. and Mrs. H. to describe their thoughts and experiences regarding this hybrid intervention program. Across the 4-week period, questions to Mr. and Mrs. H. included topics such as their opinions of how easy it was to adhere to the intervention schedule compared to what they anticipated, thoughts on the value of the intervention, recommendations for improvement, frustrations with any aspect of the program, and ease of use of the CD and response pages. They reported that compliance with some parts of the treatment program were more challenging than anticipated (e.g., judging responses); however, it was not onerous. They developed strategies for logistical management (e.g., to be sure they remembered to complete treatment).

In this case example the clinician embraced the theoretical foundation and delivery principles of cued picture-naming treatment, attempted to maximize the likelihood that the treatment would induce behavior change by keeping the CII relatively equivalent, and respected the principles of evidence-based practice by selecting a technique that is supported by empirical evidence and respecting Mrs. H.'s perspectives and clinical restrictions in implementation.

REFERENCES

Aerts, A., Batens, K., Santens, P., Van Mierlo, P., Huysman, E., Hartsuiker, R., ... De Letter, M. (2015). Aphasia therapy early after stroke: Behavioural and neurophysiological changes in the acute and post-acute phases. *Aphasiology*, *29*(7), 845–871.

Agostini, M., Garzon, M., Benavides-Varela, S., De Pellegrin, S., Bencini, G., Rossi, G., ... Tonin, P. (2014). Telerehabilitation in poststroke anomia. *BioMed Research International*, doi:10.1155/2014/706909

Babbitt, E. M., Heinemann, A. W., Semik, P., & Cherney, L. R. (2011). Psychometric properties of Communication Confidence Rating Scale for Aphasia (CCRSA): Phase 2. *Aphasiology, 25*(6–7), 727–735. doi:10.1080/02687038.2010.537347.

Babbitt, E. M., Worrall, L., & Cherney, L. R. (2013). Clinician perspectives of an intensive comprehensive aphasia program. *Topics in Stroke Rehabilitation, 20*(5), 398–408.

Babbitt, E. M., Worrall, L., & Cherney, L. R. (2015). Structure, processes, and retrospective outcomes from an intensive comprehensive aphasia program. *American Journal of Speech-Language Pathology, 24*, S854–S863.

Baker, E. (2012a). Optimal intervention intensity. *International Journal of Speech-Language Pathology, 14*(5), 401–409.

Baker, E. (2012b). Optimal intervention intensity in speech-language pathology: Discoveries, challenges, and unchartered territories. *International Journal of Speech-Language Pathology, 14*(5), 478–485.

Bakheit, A. M. O., Shaw, S., Barrett, L., Wood, J., Carrington, S., Griffiths, S., ... Koutsi, F. (2007). A prospective, randomized, parallel group, controlled study of the effect of intensity of speech and language therapy on early recovery from poststroke aphasia. *Clinical Rehabilitation, 21*, 885–894.

Barthel, G., Meinzer, M., Djundja, D., & Rockstroh, B. (2008). Intensive language therapy in chronic aphasia: Which aspects contribute most?" *Aphasiology, 22*(4), 408–421.

Basso, A., & Caporali, A. (2001). Aphasia therapy or the importance of being earnest. *Aphasiology, 15*, 307–332.

Beeson, P. M., Higginson, K., & Rising, K. (2013). Writing treatment for aphasia: A texting approach. *Journal of Speech, Language, and Hearing Research, 56*, 945–955.

Berthier, M. L., Green, C., Lara, J. P., Higueras, C., Barbancho, M. A., Dávila, G., & Pulvermüller, F. (2009). Memantine and constraint-induced aphasia therapy in chronic poststroke aphasia. *Annals of Neurology, 65*(5), 577–584.

Berthier, M. L., & Pulvermüller, F. (2011). Neuroscience insights improve neurorehabilitation of postroke aphasia. *Nature Reviews Neurology, 7*, 86–97. doi:10.1038/nrneurol.2010.201.

Bhogal, S. K., Teasell, R., & Speechley, M. (2003). Intensity of aphasia therapy, impact on recovery. *Stroke, 34*, 987–993.

Bock, E., & Ballard, K. J. (2003, May). A test of constraint-induced therapy for aphasia: Verb production. Paper presented at the Clinical Aphasiology Conference, Orcas Island, WA.

Breier, J. I., Maher, L. M., Novak, B., & Papanicolaou, A. C. (2006). Functional imaging before and after constraint-induced language therapy for aphasia using magnetoencephalography. *Neurocase, 12*, 322–331.

Cherney, L. R. (2012). Aphasia treatment: Intensity, dose parameters, and script training. *International Journal of Speech-Language Pathology, 14*(5), 424–431.

Cherney, L. R., Patterson, J. P., & Raymer, A. M. (2011). Intensity of aphasia therapy: Evidence and efficacy. *Current Neurology and Neuroscience Reports, 11*(6), 560–569.

Cherney, L. R., Patterson, J. P., Raymer, A., Frymark, T., & Schooling T. (2008). Evidence-based systematic review: Effects of intensity of treatment and constraint-induced language therapy for individuals with stroke-induced aphasia. *Journal of Speech, Language, and Hearing Research, 51*, 1282–1299.

Cherney, L. R., Patterson, J., Raymer, A., Frymark, T., & Schooling, T. (2010). Updated evidence-based systematic review: Effects of intensity of treatment and constraint-induced language therapy for individuals with stroke-induced aphasia. *ASHA's National Center for Evidence-Based Practice in Communication Disorders.* Rockville, MD: American Speech-Language-Hearing Association.

Choi, Y.-H, Park, H. K., & Paik, N.-J. (2016). A telerehabilitation approach for chronic aphasia following stroke. *Telemedicine and e-Health, 22*(5), 434–440.

Ciccone, H., West, D., Cream, A., Cartwright, J., Rai, T., Granger, A., ... Godecke, E. (2015). Constraint-induced aphasia therapy (CIAT): A randomised controlled trial in very early stroke rehabilitation. *Aphasiology, 30*(5), 566–584.

Darley, F. L. (1972). The efficacy of language rehabilitation in aphasia. *Journal of Speech and Hearing Disorders, 37*, 3–21.

Dechêne, L., Tousignant, M., Boissy, P., Macoir, J., Héroux, S., Hamel, M., ... Pagé, C. (2011). Simulated in-home teletreatment for anomia. *International Journal of Telerehabilitation, 3*(2), 3–10.

Denes, G., Perazzolo, C., Piani, A., & Piccione, F. (1996). Intensive versus regular speech therapy in global aphasia: A controlled study. *Aphasiology, 10*, 385–394.

Dignam, J., Copland, D., McKinnon, E., Burfien, P., O'Brien, K., Farrell, A., & Rodriguez, A. D. (2015). Intensive versus distributed aphasia therapy: A nonrandomized, parallel-group, dosage-controlled study. *Stroke, 46*, 2206–2211. doi:10.1161/STROKEAHA.115.009522.

Dignam, J., Rodriquez, A. D., & Copland, D. (2016). Evidence of intensive aphasia therapy: Consideration of theories from neuroscience and cognitive psychology. *Physical Medicine & Rehabilitation. 8*(3), 254–267. doi:10.1016/j.pmrj.2015.06.010.

Doyle, P. J., McNeil, M. R., Park, G., Goda, A., Rubenstein, E., Spencer, K. S., ... Szwarc, L. (2000). Linguistic validation of four parallel forms of story retelling procedure. *Aphasiology, 14*(5–6), 537–549. doi:10.1080/026870300401306.

Enderby, P. (2012). How much therapy is enough? The impossible question! *International Journal of Speech Language Pathology, 14*(5), 432–437. doi:10.3109/17549507.2012.686118.

Faroqi-Shah, Y., & Virion, C. R. (2009). Constraint-induced language therapy for agrammatism: Role of grammaticality constraints. *Aphasiology, 23*, 977–988.

Garcia, L. J., Rebolledo, M., Metthé, L., & Lefebvre, R. (2007). The potential of virtual reality to assess functional communication in aphasia. *Topics in Language Disorders, 27*(3), 272–288.

Godecke, E., Ciccone, N. A., Granger, A. S., Rai, T., West, D., Cream, A., ... Hankey, G.J. (2014). A comparison of aphasia therapy outcomes before and after a very early rehabilitation programme following stroke. *International Journal of Language and Communication Disorders, 49*(2), 149–161.

Godecke, E., Hird, K., Lalor, E. E., Rai, T., & Phillips, M. R. (2012). Very early poststroke aphasia therapy: A pilot randomized controlled efficacy trial. *International Journal of Stroke, 7*(8), 635–644. doi:10.1111/j.1747-4949.2011.00631.x

Godecke, E., Rai, T., Ciccone, N., Armstrong, E., Granger, A., & Hankey, G. J. (2013). Amount of therapy matters in very early aphasia rehabilitation after stroke: A clinical prognostic model. *Seminars in Speech and Language, 34*(3), 129–141.

Goodglass, H., Kaplan, E. G., & Weintraub, S. (2001). *Boston Naming Test.* Austin, TX: Pro-Ed.

Goral, M., & Kempler, D. (2009). Training verb production in communicative context: Evidence from a person with chronic non-fluent aphasia. *Aphasiology, 23*(12), 1383–1397.

Granger, C. V., Dewis, L. S., Peters, N. C., Sherwood, C. C., & Barrett, J. E. (1979). Stroke rehabilitation: Analysis of repeated Barthel index measures. *Archives of Physical Medicine and Rehabilitation, 60*(1), 14–17.

Harnish, S. M., Morgan, J., Lundine, J. P., Bauer, A., Singletary, F., Benjamin, M. L., ... Crosson, B. (2014). Dosing of a cued picture-naming treatment for anomia. *American Journal of Speech-Language Pathology, 23*, S285–S299.

Harnish, S. M., Neils-Strunjas, J., Lamy, M., & Eliassen, J. (2008). Use of fMRI in the study of chronic aphasia recovery after therapy: A case study. *Topics in Stroke Rehabilitation, 15*(5), 468–483.

Hinckley, J. J., & Carr, T. H. (2005). Comparing the outcomes of intensive and non-intensive context-based aphasia treatment. *Aphasiology, 19*, 965–974.

Hinckley, J. J., & Craig, H. K. (1998). Influence of rate of treatment on the naming abilities of adults with chronic aphasia. *Aphasiology, 12*, 989–1006.

Hoenig, H., Sanford, J. A., Butterfield, T., & Griffiths, P. C., Richardson, P., & Hargraves, K. (2006). Development of a teletechnology protocol for in-home rehabilitation. *Journal of Rehabilitation Research and Development, 43*(2), 287–298. doi:10.1682/JRRD.2004.07.0089.

Holland, A. L., Frattali, A. M., & Fromm, D. (1999). *Communication Activities of Daily Living* (2nd ed.). Austin, TX: Pro-Ed.

Huber, W., Poeck, K. & Willmes, K. (1984). The Aachen Aphasia Test. *Advances in Neurology, 42*, 291–303.

Hula, W. D., Doyle, P. J., Stone, C. A., Austermann Hula, S. N., Kellough, S., Wambauigh, J. L., …St. Jacque, A. (2015). The Aphasia Communication Outcome Measure (ACOM): Dimensionality, item bank calibration, and initial validation. *Journal of Speech, Language, and Hearing Research, 58*, 906–919.

Intensive. (n.d.). In *Oxford English Dictionary Online*. Retrieved May 25, 2016 from http://www.oed.com/view/Entry/97480?redirectedFrom=intensive

Johnson, M. L., Taub, E., Harper, L. H., Wade, J. T., Bowman, M. H., Bishop-McKay, S., … Uswatte, G. (2014). An enhanced protocol for constraint-induced aphasia therapy II: A case series. *American Journal of Speech-Language Pathology, 23*, 60–72.

Kagan, A., Simmons-Mackie, N., Victor, J., Carling-Rowland, A., Hoch J., Huijbregts M, et al. (2010). *Assessment for Living With Aphasia (ALA)*. Toronto, ON: Aphasia Institute.

Kay, J., Lesser, R., & Coltheart, M. (1992). *Psycholinguistic Assessment of Language Processing in Aphasia*. Mahwah, NJ: Erlbaum.

Kendall, D. L., Oelke, M., Brookshire, C. E., & Nadeau, S. E. (2015). The influence of phonomotor treatment on word retrieval abilities in 26 individuals with chronic aphasia: An open trial. *Journal of Speech, Language, and Hearing Research, 58*(3), 798–812. doi: 10.1044/2015_JSLHR-L-14-0131.

Kent, T. A., Rutherford, D. G., Breier, J. I., & Papanicoloau, A. C. (2009). What is the evidence for use dependent learning after stroke? *Stroke, 40*, S139–S140.

Kerr, A. L., Cheng, S.-Y., & Jones, T. A. (2011). Experience-dependent neural plasticity in the adult damaged brain. *Journal of Communicative Disorders, 44*(5), 538–548.

Kertesz, A. (2006). *Western Aphasia Battery-Revised*. San Antonio TX: PsychCorp.

Kirmess, M., & Maher, L. M. (2010). Constraint induced language therapy in early aphasia rehabilitation. *Aphasiology, 24*(6), 725–736.

Kleim, J. A., & Jones, T. A. (2008). Principles of experience-dependent neural plasticity: Implications for rehabilitation after brain damage. *Journal of Speech, Language, and Hearing Research, 51*, S225-S239. doi:10.1044/1092-4388(2008/018)

Kristensen, L. F., Steensig, I., Pedersen, A. D., Pedersen, A. R., & Nielsen, J. F. (2015). Constraint-induced aphasia therapy in subacute neurorehabilitation. *Aphasiology, 29*(10), 1152–1163.

Kurland, J., Pulvermüller, F., Silva, N., Burke, K., & Andrianopoulos, M. (2012). Constrained versus unconstrained intensive language therapy in two individuals with chronic, moderate-to-severe aphasia and apraxia of speech: Behavioral and fMRI outcomes. *American Journal of Speech-Language Pathology, 21*, S65–S87.

Kurland, J., Wilkins, A. R., & Stokes, P. (2014). iPractice: Piloting the effectiveness of a tablet-based home practice program in aphasia treatment. *Seminars in Speech and Language, 35*(1), 51–64.

Laganaro, M., Di Pietro, M., & Schnider, A. (2006). Computerised treatment of anomia in acute aphasia: Treatment intensity and training size. *Neuropsychological Rehabilitation*, *16*(6), 630–640.

Laska, A. C., Kahan, T., Hellblom, A., Murray, V., & von Arbin, M. (2011). A randomized controlled trial on very early speech and language therapy in acute stroke patients with aphasia. *Cerebrovascular Diseases Extra*, *1*, 66–74.

Lee, J. B, Fowler, R., Rodney, D., Cherney, L., & Small, S. L. (2010). IMITATE: An intensive computer-based treatment for aphasia based on action observation and imitation. *Aphasiology*, *24*(4), 449–465.

Lee, J. B., Kaye, R. C., & Cherney, L. R. (2009). Conversational script performance in adults with non-fluent aphasia: Treatment intensity and aphasia severity. *Aphasiology*, *23*(7), 885–897.

Legh-Smith, J. A., Denis, R., Enderby, P. M., Wade, D. T., & Langton-Hewer, R. (1987). Selection of aphasic stroke patients for intensive speech therapy. *Journal of Neurology, Neurosurgery, and Psychiatry*, *50*, 1488–1492.

Lomas, J., Pickard, L., Bester, S., Elbard, H., Finlayson, A., & Zoghaib, C. (1989). The communicative effectiveness index. *Journal of Speech and Hearing Disorders*, *54*, 113–124. doi:10.1044/jshd.5401.113.

Maas, E., Robin, D. A., Hula, S. N. A., Wulf, G., Ballard, K. J., & Schmidt, R. A. (2008). Principles of motor learning in treatment of motor speech disorders. *American Journal of Speech-Language Pathology*, *17*, 277–298.

Macauley, B. L. (2006). Animal-assisted therapy for persons with aphasia: A pilot study. *Journal of Rehabilitation Research & Development*, *43*(3), 357–366. doi:10.1682/JRRD.2005.01.0027.

Mackenzie, C. (1991). An aphasia group intensive efficacy study. *British Journal of Disorders of Communication*, *26*(3), 275–291.

Maher, L. M., Kendall, D., Swearengin, J. A., Rodriguez, A., Leon, S. A., Pingel, K., ... Gonzalez Rothi, L. J. (2006). A pilot study of use-dependent learning in the context of constraint induced language therapy. *Journal of the International Neuropsychological Society*, *12*, 843–852.

Marcotte, K., Adrover-Roig, D., Damien, B., de Préaumont, M., Généreux, S., Hubert, M., & Ansaldo, A. I. (2012). Therapy-induced neuroplasticity in chronic aphasia. *Neuropsychologia*, *50*(8), 1776–1786. doi:10.1016/j

Marcotte, K., Perlbarg, V., Marrelec, G., Benali, H., & Ansaldo, A. I. (2013). Default-mode network functional connectivity in aphasia: Therapy-induced neuroplasticity. *Brain and Language*, *124*(1), 45–55. doi:10.1016/j.bandl.2012.11.004.

Marshall, R. C. (2008). The impact of intensity of aphasia therapy on recovery [Letter to the editor]. *Stroke*, *39*, e49.

Marshall, R. C., Wertz, R. T., Weiss, D. G., Aten, J. L., Brookshire, R. H., Garcia-Bunuel, L., ... Goodman, R. (1989). Home treatment for aphasic patients by trained nonprofessionals. *Journal of Speech and Hearing Disorders*, *54*, 462–470. doi:10.1044/jshd.5403.462.

Martins, I. P., Leal, G., Fonseca, I., Farrajota, L., Aguiar, M., Fonseca, J., ... Ferro, J. M. (2013). A randomized, rater-blinded, parallel trial of intensive speech therapy in sub-acute post-stroke aphasia: The SP-I-R-IT study. *International Journal of Language and Communication Disorders*, *48*, 421–431.

McNeil, M. R., & Prescott, T. E. (1978). *Revised Token Test*. Austin, TX: Pro-Ed.

Meinzer, M., Djundja, D., Barthel, G., Elbert, T., & Rockstroh, B. (2005). Long-term stability of improved language functions in chronic aphasia after constraint-induced aphasia therapy. *Stroke*, *36*, 1462–1466.

Meinzer, M., Paul, L., Wienbruch, C., Djundja, D., & Rockstroh, B. (2009). Electromagnetic brain activity in higher frequency bands during automatic word processing indicates recovery of function in aphasia. *European Journal of Physical and Rehabilitation Medicine*, *45*(3), 369–378.

Meinzer M., Rodriguez, A. D., & Gonzalez Rothi, L. J. (2012). First decade of research on constrained-induced treatment approaches for aphasia rehabilitation. *Archives of Physical Medicine and Rehabilitation, 93*(Suppl. 1), S35–S45.

Meinzer, M., Streiftau, S., & Rockstroh, B. (2007). Intensive language training in the rehabilitation of chronic aphasia: Efficient training by laypersons. *Journal of the International Neuropsychological Society, 13,* 846–853.

Mortley, J., Wade, J., Davies, A., & Enderby, P. (2003). An investigation into the feasibility of remotely monitored computer therapy for people with aphasia. *Advances in Speech-Language Pathology, 5*(1), 27–36.

Mozeiko, J., Coelho, C. A., & Myers, E. B. (2015). The role of intensity in constraint-induced language therapy for people with chronic aphasia. *Aphasiology, 30,* 339–363.

Off, C. A., Griffin, J. R., Spencer, K. A., & Rogers, M. A. (2015). The impact of dose on naming accuracy with persons with aphasia. *Aphasiology, 30,* 1–29.

Osborne, A., & Nickels, L. (2012). Constraint in aphasia therapy. Is it important for clinical outcomes? [Abstract]. *International Journal of Stroke, 7*(Suppl. 1), 53–54.

Palmer, R., & Enderby, P. (2015). Volunteer involvement in the support of self-managed computerized aphasia treatment: The volunteer perspective. *International Journal of Speech-Language Pathology.* Published online 11 Nov 2015, 1–9. doi:10.3109/17549507.2015.1101160.

Palmer, R., Enderby, P., Cooper, C., Latimer, N., Julious, S., Paterson, G., ... Hughes, H. (2012). Computer therapy compared with usual care for people with long-standing aphasia poststroke: A pilot randomized controlled trial. *Stroke, 43,* 1904–1911.

Paul, D. R. Frattali, C. M., Holland, A. L., Thompson, C. K., Caperton, C. J., & Slater, S. C. (2004). *The American Speech-Language-Hearing Association Quality of Communication Life Scale (QCL): Manual.* Rockville, MD: American Speech-Language-Hearing Association.

Porch, B. E. (2001, 1981). *Porch Index of Communicative Ability.* Albuquerque, NM: PICA Programs.

Pulvermüller, F., Neininger, B., Elbert, T., Mohr, B., Rockstroh, B., Koebbel, P., & Taub, E. (2001). Constraint-induced therapy of chronic aphasia after stroke. *Stroke, 32,* 1621–1626.

Purdy, M., & Hindenlang, J. (2005). Educating and training caregivers of persons with aphasia. *Aphasiology, 19*(3–5), 377–388. doi:10.1080/02687030444000822/.

Ramsberger, G., & Marie, B. (2007). Self-administered cued naming therapy: A single-participant investigation of a computer-based therapy program replicated in four cases. *American Journal of Speech-Language Pathology, 16,* 343–358.

Raven, J. C. (1965). *Guide to using the colored progressive matrices, sets A, Ab, B.* Dumfries, Scotland: Grieve.

Raymer, A. M., Beeson, P., Holland, A., Kendall, D., Maher, L. M., Martin, N., ... Gonzalez Rothi, L. J. (2008). Translational research in aphasia: From neuroscience to neurorehabilitation. *Journal of Speech, Language, and Hearing Research, 51,* 259–275. doi:10.1044/1092-4388(2008/020).

Raymer, A. M., Kohen, F. P., & Saffell, D. (2006). Computerised training for impairments of word comprehension and retrieval in aphasia. *Aphasiology, 20,* 257–268.

Raymer, A. M., Maher, L. M., Patterson, J. P., & Cherney, L. R. (2007). Neuroplasticity and aphasia: Lessons from constraint-induced therapy. *SIG 2 Perspectives on Neurophysiology and Neurogenic Speech and Language Disorders, 17,* 12–17. doi:10.1044/nnsld17.2.12.

Richter, M., Miltner, W. H. R., & Straube, T. (2008). Association between therapy outcome and right-hemispheric activation in chronic aphasia. *Brain, 131,* 1391–1401.

Robey, R. R. (1998). A meta-analysis of clinical outcomes in the treatment of aphasia. *Journal of Speech-Language-Hearing Research, 41,* 172–187.

Rose, M. L. (2013). Releasing the constraints on aphasia therapy: The positive impact of gesture and multimodality treatments. *American Journal of Speech-Language Pathology, 22*, S227–S239.

Rose, M. L., Attard, M. C., Mok, Z., Lanyon, L. E., & Foster, A. M. (2013). Multi-modality aphasia therapy is as efficacious as a constraint-induced aphasia therapy for chronic aphasia: A phase 1 study. *Aphasiology, 27*(8), 938–971.

Rose, M. L., Cherney, L. R., & Worrall, L. E. (2013). Intensive comprehensive aphasia programs: An international survey of practice. *Topics in Stroke Rehabilitation, 20*(5), 379–387.

Sage, K., Snell, C., & Lambon Ralph, M. A. (2011). How intensive does anomia therapy for people with aphasia need to be? *Neuropsychological Rehabilitation, 21*(11), 26–41.

Sanders, S. B. (1977). The use of tel-communicology with the aphasic patient. In *Clinical Aphasiology Conference*. Amelia Island, FL (pp. 137–143). Minneapolis, MN: BRK Publishers.

Sarno, M. T. (1969). *The Functional Communication Profile*. New York University Medical Center, NY: Institute of Rehabilitation Medicine.

Sickert, A., Anders, L.-C., Münte, T. F., & Sailer, M. (2014). Constraint-induced aphasia therapy following sub-acute stroke: A single-blind, randomized clinical trial of a modified therapy schedule. *Journal of Neurology, Neurosurgery and Psychiatry, 85*, 51–55.

Snell, C., Sage, K., & Lambon Ralph, M. A. (2010). How many words should we provide in anomia therapy? A meta-analysis and a case series study. *Aphasiology, 24*, 1064–1094.

Swinburn, K., Porter, G., & Howard, D. (2004). *The Comprehensive Aphasia Test*. New York: Taylor & Francis.

Szaflarski, J. P., Ball, A. L., Grether, S., Al-fwaress, F., Griffith, N. M., Neils-Strunjas, J., ... Reichhardt, R. (2008). Constraint-induced aphasia therapy stimulates language recovery in patients with chronic aphasia after ischemic stroke. *Medical Science Monitor, 14*(5), CR243–CR250.

Taub, E., Miller, N. E., Novack, T. A., Cook, E. W., Fleming W. C., Nepomuceno, C. S., et al. (1993). Technique to improve chronic motor deficit after stroke. *Archives of Physical Medicine and Rehabilitation, 74*, 347–354.

Taylor, D. M., Cameron, J. I., Walsh, L., McEwan, S., Kagan, A., Streiner, D. L., & Huijbregts, M. P. J. (2009). Exploring the feasibility of videoconference delivery of a self-management program to rural participants with stroke. *Telemedicine and e-Health, 15*(7), 646–654.

Thompson, C., & Shapiro, L. (2005). Treating agrammatic aphasia within a linguistic framework: treatment of underlying forms. *Aphasiology, 19*(10–11), 1021–1036. doi:10.1080/02687030544000227.

Van de Sandt-Koenderman, W. M. E. (2011). Aphasia rehabilitation and the role of computer technology: Can we keep up with modern times? *International Journal of Speech-Language Pathology, 13*(1), 21–27. doi:10.3109/17549507.2010.502973

Wan, C. Y., Zheng, X., Marchina, S., Norton, A., & Schlaug, G. (2014). Intensive therapy induces contralateral white matter changes in chronic stroke patients with Broca's aphasia. *Brain & Language, 136*, 1–7.

Warren, S. F., Fey, M. E., & Yoder, P. J. (2007). Differential treatment intensity research: A missing link to creating optimally effective communication interventions. *Language and Communication, 13*(1), 70–77. doi:10.1002/mrdd.20139.

Wenke, R., Lawrie, M., Hosbon, T., Comben, W., Romano, M., Ward, E., & Cardell, E. (2014). Feasibility and cost analysis of implementing high intensity aphasia clinics within a sub-acute setting. *International Journal of Speech-Language Pathology, 16*(3), 250–259.

Wertz, R. T., Dronkers, N. F., Bernstein-Ellis, E., Sterling, L. K., Shubitowski, Y., Elman, R., ... Deal, J. L. (1992). Potential of telephonic and television technology for appraising and diagnosing neurogenic communication disorders in remote settings. *Aphasiology, 6*(2), 195–202.

Wertz, R. T., Weiss, D. G., Aten, J. L., Brookshire, R. H., Garcia-Buñuel, L., Holland, A. L., ... Goodman, R. (1986). Comparison of clinic, home and deferred language treatment for aphasia. *Archives of Neurology, 43*, 653–658.

Wilssens, I., Vandenborre, D., van Dun, K., Verhoeven, J., Visch-Brink, E., & Mariën, P. (2015). Constraint-induced aphasia therapy versus intensive semantic treatment in fluent aphasia. *American Journal of Speech-Language Pathology, 24*(2), 281–294.

Winans-Mitrik, R. L., Hula, W. D., Dickey, M. W., Schumacher, J. G., Swoyer, B., & Doyle, P. J. (2014). Description of an intensive residential aphasia treatment program: Rationale, clinical processes, and outcomes. *American Journal of Speech-Language Pathology, 23*, S330–S342.

Woolf, C., Caute, A., Haigh, Z., Galliers, J., Wilson, S., Kessie, A., ... Marshall, J. (2016). A comparison of remote therapy, face to face therapy and an attention control intervention for people with aphasia: A quasi-randomised controlled feasibility study. *Clinical Rehabilitation, 30*, 359–373.

World Health Organization. (2001). International Classification of Functioning, Disability and Health. Retrieved from http://www.who.int/classifications/icf/en/.

Worral, L., & Yiu, E. (2000). Effectiveness of functional communication therapy by volunteers for people with aphasia following stroke. *Aphasiology, 14*(9), 911–924.

CHAPTER 10

Selecting, Combining, and Bundling Different Therapy Approaches

Jacqueline Hinckley

INTRODUCTION

The process of selecting one or more therapies that match a particular client's language profile and personal goals is a complex one about which little is really known. As a result of active research in aphasia therapy over the last decades, multiple effective therapies are available from which to choose. The decision to select or combine interventions from among all of the possible options is dependent upon the clinician's knowledge of the client, the possible therapy options, the clinician's expertise or comfort with the possible appropriate interventions, and client preference.

Therapy selection is critical to the ultimate therapy outcome experienced by the client. A therapy that is not quite the best fit for the client's communication profile or personal values and needs may produce less effective results. The clinician's choice of therapy can either maximize a client's improvement, or limit potential improvement.

When and how should a clinician select one type of therapy or another? When and how should a clinician combine therapies that represent different approaches? A particular therapy might be selected because it is perceived as the best fit with the client's language profile, as determined by candidacy criteria. Or, a therapy might be selected because it targets a particular impairment that is perceived to be the most disabling for the client. Other ways to select therapies could be dependent on underlying theoretical approaches or on the long-term goal of the therapy. In the first section of this chapter, a simple additive model of combining therapies will be described, along with factors that affect therapy selection. The second section of the chapter will offer a theoretically based, integrative approach for combining different approaches with an emphasis on client-centered goals and values.

CURRENT APPROACHES TO SELECTING, COMBINING, AND BUNDLING THERAPIES

The easiest way to start thinking about how therapies are selected or combined is to consider options for a particular case.

CASE ILLUSTRATION: MR. F.—EPISODE 1

Mr. F. is a 63-year-old right-handed gentleman who was admitted to the hospital 3 days ago with a left hemispheric stroke. He had no previous medical history of stroke, brain injury, communication disability, or psychiatric condition. His wife is at his bedside most of the day.

Based on the administration of a standardized language assessment and consistent with informal observation, Mr. F. is diagnosed with a fluent, Wernicke's-type aphasia of moderate severity. Mrs. F. complains about the hospital food, indicating that if she is not there when the food service staff comes to take his order, he ends up with food he does not like and will not eat. She is worried that he is not getting enough to eat and that it will hamper his recovery.

There are three possible routes that a clinician might use to select therapies for this client. First, a clinician could choose to determine the impairments of greatest concern based on standardized testing and select one or more therapies that target those impairments. For example, a clinician might select therapy that focuses on auditory comprehension. A second approach is for the clinician to focus on the real-life, functional problem of not being able to order food preferences independently. In this case, the clinician is likely to focus therapy on using menus, using and understanding menu words, and recognizing menu items that the client strongly likes or dislikes. In addition, the clinician could train food service staff to apply supported conversation techniques to enable Mr. F. to order preferred items.

A third possible approach is for the clinician to spend the allocated treatment time on both of these approaches. For example, a clinician with about 30 minutes for therapy might use approximately 15 minutes to work on specific impairment-based therapy, and the remaining part of the session to practice words from the menu that are particular likes or dislikes, practice ordering, or training the dining staff to support communication.

In an informal show of hands at the ASHA 2015 Health Care Conference, nearly all of the audience members indicated that they would be likely to add one therapy to another and divide therapy time in some way between impairment-focused therapy and addressing an immediate, functional concern. Clinicians want to feel that they are targeting some generalizable skill that will help the client's overall language system, and thus they may feel compelled to incorporate an impairment-based therapy that they feel will have generalizable effects. Clinicians also want to address any immediate complaints or communication challenges, such as difficulty ordering food, and thus most clinicians are probably likely to add on some time dedicated to addressing the client's ability to participate in ordering preferred food

This third route, in which a portion of therapy time is allocated for impairment-focused therapy and another portion is allocated to participation-focused therapy, is depicted in **FIGURE 10.1**.

Figure 10.1 shows two different ways to select a particular treatment. The first approach, shown in the left column, is based on identifying impairments through standardized

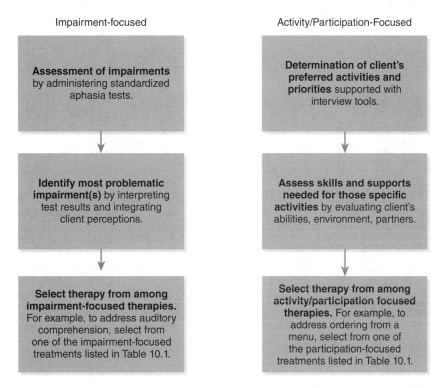

FIGURE 10.1 Selecting therapy approaches within either an impairment-focused or an activity/participation-focused approach. When both approaches are used for a single client or therapy session, this can be referred to as an additive model.

testing, and selecting a treatment based on one or more of the identified impairments. The second approach, shown in the right column, is based on identifying the values or priorities of the client and selecting therapy based on those factors. It is important to note that these two approaches are not mutually exclusive; they can be combined to respond to different needs, as perceived by the clinician.

In order to discuss this additive model, in which the two different approaches are combined, it is important first to consider the underlying elements of these two different approaches.

Categorizing Aphasia Therapies Based on WHO ICF

The International Classification of Functioning (ICF) of the World Health Organization (WHO, 2001) has organized our thinking about assessment, intervention, and outcomes in aphasia therapy for nearly 15 years. In this model, the impairment of specific body structures and functions correlates to specific cognitive-linguistic impairments, such as anomia, dyslexia, or agraphia. These impairments can have negative consequences on a person's ability to perform certain activities, such as answering the phone, filling out forms, or reading the newspaper. Other consequences may be on the person's participation in life goals and social roles, such as voting, working, riding a bus, or driving (Ashton et al., 2008; Graham, Pereira, & Teasell, 2011; Kane & Galbraith, 2013; Mackenzie & Paton, 2003). While impairments, consequences, and environmental and personal factors are all interrelated in the WHO ICF model, the model was not intended to be prescriptive, and it does not dictate how a clinician should select a particular therapy target or approach.

Assessments, interventions, and outcomes that target the underlying cognitive-linguistic functions can be characterized as impairment-focused (Papathanasiou & De Bleser, 2003). For example, a naming intervention whose outcome is measured by the improved ability to name pictures or objects fits into this category. Assessments, interventions, or outcomes that target the consequences of these impairments on activities and life participation can be characterized as participation-focused (Papathanasiou & De Bleser, 2003). For example, an intervention that aims to improve a person's ability to successfully use public transportation could be described as participation-focused. In this approach, the targets of the intervention can extend to important people in a person's life and the communication supports that make the activity accessible to the person with aphasia.

The Practice Portal of the American Speech-Language-Hearing Association (ASHA, n.d.) is one way for clinicians to access evidence and other resources that pertain to different therapy approaches for aphasia. The different aphasia therapy approaches included on ASHA's (n.d.) Practice Portal are listed in **TABLE 10.1**. ASHA categorizes these different therapy approaches based on whether the therapy targets the language impairment or the consequences of the impairment on activities and life participation according to definitions from the World Health Organization (WHO, 2001).

TABLE 10.1 Aphasia therapies listed on the ASHA Practice Portal categorized by WHO ICF definitions.

Impairment-Focused	Activity/Participation-Focused
Computer-Based Therapy targeting various language modalities (Brady et al., 2012)	Multi-Modal Therapy including: • Augmentative and Alternative Communication (Canadian Stroke Best Practices Advisory Committee, 2013) • Promoting Aphasics' Communication Effectiveness (PACE; Davis, 2005) • Oral Reading for Language in Aphasia (ORLA; Cherney, 2010)
Constraint-Induced Language Therapy (CILT) or Intensive Language Action Therapy (Allen et al., 2012)	Conversation Partner Training** (Simmons-Mackie et al., 2010) including: • Conversational Coaching • Supported Communication Intervention • Social and Life Participation Effectiveness
Melodic Intonation Therapy (van der Meulen et al., 2012)	Pragmatic Therapy targeting social communication deficits, including Reciprocal Scaffolding (da Fontoura et al., 2012)**
Reading Therapy (National Stroke Foundation [NSF], 2010)	Script Training (Cherney, Kaye, & van Vuuren, 2014)
Syntax Therapy (da Fontoura et al., 2012) including: • Therapy of Underlying Forms* (Thompson et al., 2010) • Verb Network Strengthening Therapy* (Edmonds et al., 2014) • Chaining (Sigurðardóttir & Sighvatsson, 2012) • Sentence Production Program for Aphasia (Helm-Estabrooks & Nicholas, 2000)	

(Continues)

TABLE 10.1 Aphasia therapies listed on the ASHA Practice Portal categorized by WHO ICF definitions. (Continued)

Impairment-Focused	Activity/Participation-Focused
Word-Finding Therapy (Wisenburn & Mahoney, 2009) including: • Word Retrieval Cueing Strategies (Semantic and Cueing Verbs; Wambaugh, Doyle, Martinez, & Kalinyak-Fliszar [2002])* • Gestural Facilitation of Naming (Rose et al., 2013) • Response Elaboration Training (Wambaugh, Martinez, & Alegre, 2001) • Semantic Feature Analysis (SFA; Maddy, Capiluoto, & Comas, 2014)	

* = examples of therapies that are typically described as neuropsychological
** = examples of therapies that are typically described as psychosocial

Impairment-focused therapy is defined by ASHA as "a therapy approach that addresses all communication modalities (spoken, written, and gestures) and focuses on training those areas in which a person makes errors" (ASHA, n.d.; see Table 10.1). What all of these therapies seem to have in common is the intention to improve an entire language domain, such as reading or word-finding, that would then generate broadly generalizable improvement across untrained targets in which that language domain is deployed.

Although ASHA does not provide a specific definition for "activities/participation-focused therapies," the therapies that are listed seem to be based on using methods to improve specific activities, such as conversation, or activities of daily living (see Table 10.1). Each of these therapies focuses on training broadly applicable compensatory strategies that can be used to participate in particular activities.

An alternative way to categorize therapies is to describe the underlying theoretical approach. Neuropsychological therapies have in common a psycholinguistic view of the language system, and these therapies address particular language components in the system. Some examples of therapies that are often categorized as neuropsychological are: specific cueing approaches, Therapy of Underlying Forms (Thompson, Choy, Holland, & Cole, 2010), and Verb Network Strengthening Therapy (Edmonds, Mammino, & Ojeda, 2014). Psychosocial interventions emphasize the individual's coping mechanisms and the important others in that person's environment. Examples of psychosocial approaches include conversation partner training and pragmatic approaches to social interaction.

In recent decades, categories of therapies have been developed based on different theoretical underpinnings. For example, neuropsychological therapies for aphasia have been the subject of entire textbooks (e.g., Hillis, 2015), and they share an understanding of the language system and a motivation to improve the language components that are disrupted. Psychosocial interventions share the goal of targeting aspects of the individual, such as motivation, coping, and adjustment, along with education and training for those who interact with the person with aphasia.

As can be seen in Table 10.1, therapies that can be categorized as neuropsychological fall into the "Impairment-Focused" category according to ASHA's Practice Portal. Psychosocial interventions fall into the "Participation-Focused" category of ASHA's Practice Portal. In order to facilitate profession-wide discourse, the categorization scheme adopted by ASHA for its Practice Portal will be used in the remainder of this chapter.

Approaches to Treatment Selection

The prevailing method for selecting a therapy for a given client is to match one or more of the predominant language impairments of the client with therapies that correspond to each of those impairments. In this approach, a therapy is selected based on what is most difficult for the client and provides the client with multiple opportunities to practice those tasks or skills on which the client makes the most errors (Holland, 1994).

This process is often driven by the assessments that are initially selected by the clinician. When these initial assessments are impairment-focused, then the corresponding goals and therapy selection are likely to be focused on the impairment as well (Hinckley, 2014). This approach can be characterized as "therapist controlled," because the clinician selects the formal assessment measures and determines the goals and therapy plan (Leach, Cornwell, Fleming, & Haines, 2010).

The clinician, in this case, would identify the language areas of greatest weakness based on the administration of a standardized aphasia battery. From that assessment, one or more areas of greatest impairment could be generated, for example, auditory comprehension and word-finding. The therapy selection process then is simply a match between any therapy that addresses that language domain and factors such as therapy time, delivery format, and therapy acceptability (see Figure 10.1).

An activity/participation-focused approach to therapy begins with the collaborative determination, between the clinician and the client, of activities that are of most importance to the client. In this approach, the client and family are asked first, before any formal assessment, about rehabilitation goals, activities, and life participation. Following that discussion, formal assessments that reveal aspects of the skills needed to perform those desired activities are administered. Thus, the client's desire to participate in one or more particular activities drives the remainder of the initial assessment, goal-setting, and therapy selection process (Hinckley, 2014; Hinckley & Holland, 2015).

Once the prioritized activities have been agreed upon, the next step in a participation-focused approach is to match formal assessments with the valued activities. This will require analyzing the activities based on skill and strategy requirements and identifying which assessments will be most closely linked to the activity to be targeted. For example, word-finding is likely to be a necessary skill in many possible activities. However, the performance of word-finding varies by context, so the assessment of word-finding on a picture naming test may not be an accurate or an adequate assessment of how the client's word-finding abilities will relate to the prioritized activity (see Figure 10.1).

Such a dichotomous categorization between impairment-focused and participation-focused can be convenient, but it can also be an oversimplification, for several reasons. Not all interventions clearly fit into one of these two categories, and some therapies might be applicable to both an impairment-focused and a participation-focused approach, depending on how the clinician chooses to implement the therapy.

Another reason that such a dichotomy is an oversimplification is that interventions that fit in one approach might produce an outcome typically associated with the other approach; for example, an impairment-focused therapy might affect participation in conversation, or a participation-focused therapy might have downstream effects on the language impairment, such as word-finding. Investigations of the effects of impairment-focused interventions frequently measure whether any improvement observed on an impairment-focused assessment also generalizes to untrained items or other, broader abilities. Although some impairment-focused interventions have shown generalization to non-trained, more contextualized tasks, the potential correlation between improvement in a component skill and improvement in its corresponding whole task is inconsistent and often weak (see Chapter 7, this volume). Although initial performance on impairment-focused assessments, such as standardized aphasia batteries, may be related to activity participation, change on impairment-focused assessments is not necessarily related to change on activity or participation (Ross & Wertz, 1999, 2002); however, this observation may vary depending on the therapy. For example, in a review of five aphasia therapy studies that investigated the conversational outcomes of an impairment-focused therapy, therapies that included semantic, phonological, orthographic, or gestural cueing strategies for lexical retrieval produced improved content and informativeness in conversation (Carragher, Conroy, Sage, & Wilkinson, 2012). There are mixed results about the generalizability of impairment-focused therapies to untrained items or across contexts.

When applying a participation-focused approach, generalization is often sought across contexts, because communication participation in various contexts is the conceptual goal of the approach. In a participation-focused approach, for example, we might be interested to know if learning the communication strategies and skills needed to ride the bus independently also generalize to other contexts, such as using a taxi or finding the way to a classroom at a particular time. Interestingly, using a discourse-based therapy (structured narrative or structured conversations) can result in downstream improvements in word-finding as measured by impairment-focused assessments (Boyle, 2011).

When an array of outcome measures, from impairment-focused word-finding tests to discourse, is collected from either an impairment-focused or a participation-focused therapy, different outcome patterns among all outcome types emerge relative to the two different treatment approaches (Hinckley, Patterson, & Carr, 2001). Importantly, those patterns of outcomes range from impairment to participation for either type of therapy. This suggests that adding an impairment-focused approach to a participation-focused approach, as described in the case of Mr. F. and shown in Figure 10.1, has potential for maximizing outcomes.

Although it can be convenient to characterize interventions as either impairment-focused or participation-focused, this type of categorization alone does not aid the clinician in the therapy selection process. Clinician knowledge and any applicable clinical decision-making model may provide the initial array of possible therapies from which to select. An individual clinician may not be equally knowledgeable or comfortable with every potential therapy, and clinicians will not select a therapy for which they do not have knowledge, comfort, or required materials. Finally, the setting in which the therapy is delivered will also affect which therapies are possible or can likely be expected to produce the desired outcome given the amount, intensity, or format of the available therapy.

Factors That Constrain Therapy Selection

From among the set of therapies for which a given client is a candidate, the clinician will have to select therapies for which reasonable benefit can be expected given the clinical setting and reimbursement policies. Thus, clinicians have to select from a set of therapies that not only match the client's needs, but also match the therapy time and delivery format that are available. In addition, the acceptability of the therapy, both by the client and the clinician, must be considered.

Therapy Time

In most clinical settings, therapy time is limited by a variety of factors, including reimbursement policies that often drive other institutional policies. Therapy can be limited in terms of the total number of sessions, the number of therapy sessions per week, or the duration of any given therapy session. This presents a challenge to clinicians because a large majority of the aphasia therapy evidence base is focused on therapy provided in ideal conditions, such as unlimited in total therapy time, or provide an amount of therapy that cannot often be replicated in actual practice conditions. For example, Constraint-Induced Language Therapy (CILT; Pulvermüller et al., 2001) is an example of a particular type of therapy that has intensity as one of its defining characteristics. This therapy typically has been provided in a schedule of 20 hours per week for 2 weeks or 15 hours per week for 3 weeks (Johnson et al., 2014). While this offers the opportunity to make progress in 2 or 3 weeks, it requires a large amount of therapy time during those weeks (see Chapter 9, this volume). For this reason, this particular type of therapy could only be used in particular types of clinical settings.

There is some evidence suggesting that participation-focused therapy can produce equally successful results with limited therapy time as it does with greater amounts of therapy time (Hinckley & Carr, 2005; Hopper & Holland, 1998). An intervention that focused on a particular activity was administered in either a nonintensive (4 hours per week) or an intensive (20–22 hours per week) therapy schedule to individuals with moderately severe aphasia. Accurate and durable performance on the targeted activity (ordering from a catalog) and transfer to similar activities or contexts that utilized similar strategies (such as ordering pizza) was achieved in only 1 to 10 hours of therapy. As therapy time increased, more widespread generalization to impairments (such as word-finding) was observed, but the initial improvement on a particular activity was achieved relatively quickly.

Delivery Format

Delivery format refers to individual or group therapy sessions. While some therapies, like CILT, are typically provided in a group format, other therapies have been provided in either individual or group settings. While some practice guidelines recommend that individuals with aphasia receive group therapy (NSF, 2010; New Zealand Ministry of Health, 2010), these practice guidelines are not necessarily implemented in a number of actual practice settings due to other policy constraints.

If group therapy can be offered, the clinician is faced with therapy selection from among various group therapies. Aphasia conversation groups, thematic language stimulation, and problem-solving groups are a few examples of different approaches that might be used in an aphasia group (Elman, 2006; Elman & Bernstein-Ellis, 1999; Marshall, 1993; Morganstein & Smith, 2001). A decision to follow any of these particular group approaches would most likely be guided by the clients' goals and the clinician's expertise.

Increasingly, alternatives to face-to-face treatment have been proposed, including computer programs, use of lay partners or volunteers, and telepractice. Each delivery format has advantages and disadvantages, and as with other delivery formats, must be carefully selected following the client's and clinician's review and discussion.

Therapy Acceptability

Therapy acceptability is defined as how well a therapy is perceived to be "fair, reasonable, appropriate for the given problem, and non-intrusive" (Kazdin, 1981; Mautone et al., 2009, p. 920). These perceptions could be those of the clinicians who are selecting a therapy or those of the clients who are to undergo the therapy.

Therapy acceptability is a critical perception of the clinician that will determine use of any given therapy. Therapy acceptability interacts not only with therapy effectiveness, but also with knowledge and understanding of the therapy procedures, time and effort required for use of the therapy, and therapy complexity (Briesch, Chafouleas, Neugebauer, & Riley-Tilman, 2013). The client's perception about the acceptability of the therapy could affect engagement in the therapy, which is often perceived by clinicians as motivation (see Chapter 12, this volume). Lack of acceptability of the clinician-selected therapy could also reduce the achieved outcome of the therapy. Finally, how acceptable the therapy is perceived to be by the client should be incorporated into any therapy selection process, because it bears on client rights and the collaborative process of client-centered care.

Therapy acceptability has rarely been studied in speech-language pathology, either as the perception of clinicians or of clients. Therefore, therapy acceptability remains a somewhat unknown factor in the therapy selection process. Although therapy acceptability relates to clinicians' knowledge of a particular therapy, it also pertains to the perceived effort required to administer the therapy, the perceived complexity of the therapy, or the number of different steps in the therapy program. These factors are undoubtedly incorporated into the therapy selection process, despite our lack of research on the topic.

CONSIDERATIONS FOR COMBINING OR BUNDLING THERAPIES

Care pathways (or clinical pathways) are management strategies that typically specify discipline-specific responsibilities, specific interventions, and a specific timeline or sequence of events or interventions. A clinical pathway is one way to combine or bundle different therapies to address a particular disorder. The general purposes of any care pathway are to improve efficiency, decrease healthcare costs, and improve patient care outcomes (Lanska, 1998). Typically, clinical pathways are multidisciplinary and span several different care activities, such as assessment, diagnosis, therapy, referral, and changes in care level. Over the last two decades, numerous clinical pathways have been developed, but the evidence for consistent positive outcomes of clinical pathways remains mixed (Kwan, 2007). Generally, though, clinicians perceive improved efficiency and consistency of care as a result of a care pathway. The Australian Aphasia Rehabilitation Pathway (n.d.) is an example of a care pathway for individuals experiencing aphasia due to stroke. It provides best-practice statements spanning the continuum of care from initial diagnosis of aphasia to goal-setting, assessment, and therapy.

A *care bundle* is defined as a group of evidence-based therapies that addresses a particular symptom or disorder (Fulbrook & Mooney, 2003). The intent is that when multiple evidence-based therapies are used in combination, the overall outcome will be greater than if only one of the therapies is used alone. Although each individual therapy in a care bundle is supported by evidence, the combination of the therapies has generally not been supported by evidence. Most care bundles contain a few evidence-based therapies that have been combined based on clinical reasoning and expertise.

The concept of bundling therapies was initially carried out in an effort to improve the quality of intensive care (Berenholtz, Dorman, Ngo, & Provonost, 2002). This work began by reviewing 35 years' worth of evidence in critical care and deriving from that review, a set of six interventions that were likely to make a substantial impact on intensive care outcome. The result of this work is the "ventilator care bundle," a set of four evidence-based therapies that improve outcome of patients on ventilators in the intensive care unit. At present, there are no formal care bundles for aphasia; however, it is likely that many clinicians use certain therapies together without considering them a formal bundle.

Summative Effects of Combining Therapies

Although some work has addressed combining pharmacological therapies with a behavioral therapy (for a review, see Berthier, Pulvermuller, Davila, Casares, & Guttierez, 2011), only a few aphasia therapy studies have explicitly addressed the outcomes of combining different types of behavioral therapies.

In one study, an impairment-focused practice—a semantic categorization task—was combined with PACE (Davis & Wilcox, 1985), a participation-focused therapy in which the person communicates information about a picture that is not visible to the listener, using any effective communication strategy (Springer, Glindemann, Huber, & Willmes, 1991). The combination of the semantic categorization task with the typical PACE practice was superior to PACE alone. In another study, the combination of an impairment-focused spelling practice with a participation-focused practice that focused on the everyday use of targeted words improved functional communication of an individual with jargon aphasia (Robson, Marshall, Pring, & Chiat, 1998). In a third example, gains were reported for a therapy combining an impairment-focused lexical therapy with communicative use of the targeted items (Herbert, Best, Hickin, Howard, & Osborne, 2003). None of these studies report a possible lessening of the effect of one of the therapies as a result of their combination.

In each of these examples, an activity/participation-focused therapy was combined with an impairment-focused therapy in an effort to facilitate the generalization of the impairment-focused therapy to a desired activity, such as the use of everyday words in conversation. It is reassuring to observe that, when this has been studied, the outcomes are positive and adding on an activity/participation-focused therapy to an impairment-focused therapy does indeed result in the desired gains.

The additive model described earlier and depicted in Figure 10.1 represents the way the interventions were combined in the preceding studies. A participation-focused treatment is added sequentially, either within a session or across sessions, to an impairment-focused treatment with the goal of facilitating generalization to the desired activity. It is possible to go beyond a simple additive model for selecting and combining therapies, and move toward an integrative model, in which different therapy approaches are woven together specifically in the service of one or more client-selected activities. This integrative model, the theory on which it is based, and the steps in the process will be discussed in the next section.

AN INTEGRATIVE APPROACH TO SELECTING AND COMBINING THERAPIES

Rather than simply adding one approach to another, we might be able to achieve desirable therapy outcomes even more efficiently by integrating the two approaches. An integrative approach to selecting and combining therapies begins with and completely depends on the client's prioritized activities, which serve as the context for any goal statement and are the basis for measurement of the therapy outcome. Assessment of impairments is only necessary inasmuch as the impairments directly bear on the ability to perform the desired activities. Therapy selection is also constrained by the targeted activities, given the context of the client's impairments. The clinician accomplishes this process through decomposition of the targeted task.

In an integrative model, either impairment-focused or activity/participation-focused therapies are selected because they address the specific aspect of the task that is prioritized by the client. Best practices for decomposing and training complex tasks can be derived from the literature in psychology and skill acquisition and can be applied to aphasia therapy, where they can make up the first step in an integrative model. Next, the clinician faces decisions about whether the prioritized activity should be trained in parts or as a whole. Should a complicated activity be broken down into specific parts? Should the whole task be trained completely, from start to finish, at the beginning of training? How should required skills for the activity be trained?

Therapy Selection in an Integrative Model

An integrative model for therapy selection must begin with the collaborative identification of client-centered goals. A number of tools are available to assist the clinician with identifying client-centered priorities and establishing collaborative goals (Hinckley, 2014). Once these goals have been determined, the clinician can apply principled task decomposition to identify important elements of the targeted activities (Fredericksen & White, 1989).

The process of task decomposition should progress in a top-down manner, preserving the ultimate goal of the task. For example, when ordering in a restaurant, the primary goal is to get one's preferred food. To find an optimal strategy to achieve the task goal, the clinician should ask three questions:

1. Does the strategy help achieve the goal without making it harder to achieve some other goal?
2. Does the execution of the strategy reduce or increase the cognitive load of achieving the goal?
3. Does the strategy require the acquisition of complex skills or concepts?

The key element in an integrative model is, that in all therapies, the ultimate goal of the client's selected activities is preserved. For an overview of this process, see **FIGURE 10.2**.

Mechanisms of Part- and Whole-Task Training

Directly training an activity selected by the client, such as in a role play or during a community outing, is analogous to what is described as whole-task training. Targeting component skills that are presumed to be necessary for the activity is more similar to part-task training (Fitts & Posner, 1967). In part-task training, tasks are reduced down to the most elemental parts, and these parts are trained separately from the actual task in which they might be used. In whole-task training, the sequence of steps and procedures required to complete a task is practiced in its entirety, in the appropriate order.

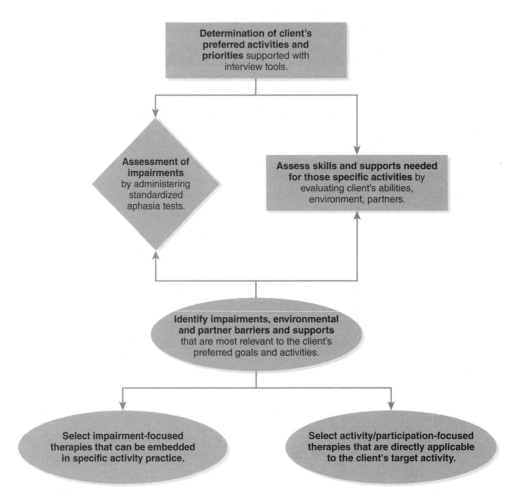

FIGURE 10.2 Integrating impairment-focused and activity/participation-focused therapies to best serve client goals and preferences. Rectangular boxes are linked to participation-focused approach as seen in Figure 10.1. The diamond-shaped box is linked to impairment-focused approach as seen in Figure 10.1. Ovoid boxes are unique to the integrated model.

Part-task training can be completed in different ways, by training the parts in different groupings or schedules (Wightman & Lintern, 1985). Simplification is a basic principle of part-task training, in which the whole task is either broken down into component parts, or trained in a context that reduces the stimuli or aspects of the task to be completed in order to make the training more accessible. Whole tasks can be subdivided based on temporal or spatial dimensions, in a procedure called segmentation. These segments or parts can be trained in different sequences. This latter process is called fractionation.

For example, script training is a type of aphasia therapy in which the whole script is broken down into component parts during training, and each phrase of the script is trained individually until mastery of that phrase is achieved based on a success criterion (e.g., Cherney et al., 2014). In this case the script is segmented and trained based on the order in which the phrases appear in the script. Another example of this might be practicing the ability to order for oneself in a restaurant. Each segment of the process could be practiced individually, such as the response to "What would you like to drink?"

In contrast to part-task training, whole-task training is typically composed of a complete, sequential practice of the target task. This type of training can be described as consistently mapped training, in which the learner is constantly confronting the stimulus or set of stimuli in the same manner during each training session. Whole-task training is based on the theoretical notion that repeated experiences in particular contexts result in the development of skills. These skills are context-specific, and only transfer to other contexts that are highly similar to the context that was trained.

Whole-task, or consistently mapped training, typically results in improvements in performance and the eventual development of automatic processing (Schneider & Shiffrin, 1977; Shiffrin & Schneider, 1977). In contrast, variably mapped training refers to those situations in which the learning contexts are inconsistent and the response or degree of attention requires changes from one stimulus to another. Typically, variably mapped training has been observed to result in little training effect (Fisk & Eboch, 1989).

Part-task only and whole-task only training have been compared in aphasia rehabilitation (Hinckley & Carr, 2005; Hinckley et al., 2001). The criterion whole-task training was a role play of ordering clothing from a catalog. Performance on this criterion task was reported for two groups of participants. One group received the equivalent of part-task training, in which specific vocabulary items or sentences that were necessary for the completion of the catalog ordering were trained, according to the specific impairments of each participant. The second group of participants practiced the whole task alone, repeating a role play of the entire catalog-ordering task with practice focusing on particular strategies that allowed the participant to complete the role play successfully.

Comparing the part-task only training to the whole-task only training showed different patterns of training outcomes. Participants with aphasia who underwent the whole-task, role-playing intervention were significantly better at performing that task than those who only underwent the part-task training. Participants in both groups showed transfer to other component skills, such as oral picture naming.

A similar pattern of training and results was obtained by Muñoz and Karow (2007), who reported the outcomes of an individual who underwent either whole-task or part-task script training. In this case, however, the whole-task was the production of an entire script, and the part-task training again related to production of vocabulary and sentence forms related to individual items of the targeted script. Outcomes paralleled those of Hinckley and colleagues (2001), in that the whole-task script training produced accurate performance of the script more quickly than the part-task training.

Part- and whole-task training are not mutually exclusive; that is, some of the most effective training includes both approaches. Indeed, combining whole-task and part-task training in particular ways, such as in integrated training, seems to produce robust performance that is less vulnerable to disruption or performance decrease when the task is completed under distracting or challenging conditions. In addition, integrated training has been associated with faster acquisition times and greater transfer to untrained contexts (Frederiksen & White, 1989).

Although the evidence is rather limited to date, these studies suggest that if the goal of intervention is for the client to be able to perform a particular task or activity, then the most effective therapy should be practicing that task as a whole. Alternatively, the whole task can be broken down in segments. In both of these approaches, however, a general skill domain is not trained. Whether whole-task or part-task practice, all training is embedded in the task context.

CASE ILLUSTRATION: MR. F.—EPISODE 2

In the case of Mr. F., the ultimate goal was to be able to order preferred food in the hospital environment despite his Wernicke's-type aphasia. Therefore, selected therapies would all link to the ultimate goal of being able to *express preferences or make requests*. To apply a whole-task practice approach to this goal, the clinician would obtain (or create) various meal menus or choice routines that exist in the client's targeted setting (hospital, nursing facility, restaurant). It is important to structure the routine as similarly as possible to the way it is normally presented. For example, in a hospital setting, the clinician can employ the same set of questions that the food service staff use when they present meal choices. Role play the typical exchange for ordering breakfast, lunch, and dinner. Visual and written supports should be used to support comprehension of the task. The client's most successful communication modalities should be targeted and practiced as the way for the client to express food and meal choices during the role play. At least three repetitions (breakfast, lunch, and dinner) should be incorporated into each therapy session.

This kind of whole-task, role-play practice is similar in structure regardless of the client's individual aphasia type or severity. Modalities used to support comprehension and expression will change depending on the individual abilities of the client, but the overall structure of the practice remains the same.

Table 10.1 lists five therapies that are most likely to preserve the goal of requesting preferred items. Two of these are listed in the "impairment-focused" category, CILT and Semantic Feature Analysis (SFA). Three more are included in the activity/participation-focused category: PACE, script training, and communication partner training. CILT is predicated on the use of pragmatic or language "games" that require the client to request particular items from other members in the group under various language conditions or constraints. Thus, this therapy maps on to the goal of the targeted activity, being able to request preferred items. SFA is a way of using organized semantic cues and features to facilitate naming. In the case of Mr. F., target items for SFA training could include the set of food items that he prefers or the items that he does not like (Olness, 2014). In both cases, improving his ability to name items he wants or items he does not want helps to meet his ultimate goal of ordering preferred food items. This is a direct route to integrating both impairment-focused and participation-focused therapies into a client-centered, client-chosen participation goal. In contrast, an indirect route would be to work on naming of any category of vocabulary items such as food, birds, household items, or tools. Such training might improve some generalized measure of word-finding that samples a number of different semantic categories, but is unlikely to quickly make a noticeable difference in Mr. F.'s ability to order his preferred food in the hospital.

PACE is a therapy approach in which the client can "request" certain items in a barrier game setting, and receive natural feedback from the clinician when the clinician is able to match the described and requested picture or item. Script training could also be appropriate as a means to train typically repeated phrases within the meal ordering routine. For example, script training could be used to train a strategy, such as requesting extra time from the wait staff and key phrases such as "more water, please" or other phrases that the client is likely to use repeatedly across events. Communication partner training focused on caregivers, such as the hospital food service staff, could also lead to achieving the client's goal of being able to order preferred food. In this case, hospital staff are trained to provide supports that will enable Mr. F. to successfully express his food preferences. In all of these examples, the therapy is selected because it matches the goal of the activity, and not because it matches an impairment of some linguistic domain.

Contrasting the Additive and Integrative Models of Treatment Selection

FIGURE 10.3 depicts the difference in ultimate therapy selection depending on whether the clinician is using an additive model or an integrative model to selecting and combining therapies. In an additive model, impairments are identified based on standardized testing, and that leads to selecting therapies that target those particular language domains. Using the menu of therapies available on the ASHA Practice Portal, four therapies are listed that specifically intend to target word-retrieval, for example. These are underlined in Figure 10.3 and include word retrieval cuing strategies, gestural facilitation of naming, response elaboration of naming, and SFA. In the additive model, the clinician might also select a participation-focused therapy designed to facilitate generalization to a desired context. The ultimate desired context would drive the selection of the participation-focused therapy.

Using an integrative model might result in a completely different selection of therapies. The first step will be to identify the client's valued activity that forms the basis of the therapy goal or goals, as shown in Figure 10.2. For example, in the case of Mr. F. the goal is

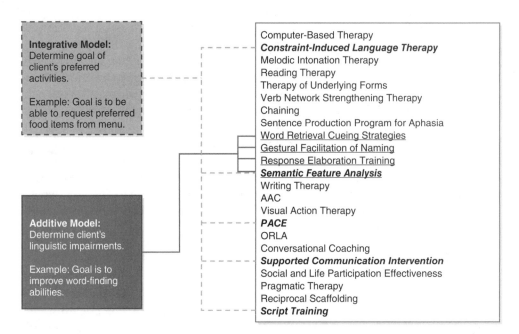

FIGURE 10.3 Therapy selection differs when activity goals or impairments are used as the primary characteristic for selection. a) In this example of an integrative model, five therapies are selected because they incorporate the same interactive goal as the targeted activity (dashed lines); b) In this example of an additive model, four therapies are selected because they intend to address the client's impairments (solid lines). One therapy (SFA) fits both examples.

to be able to order preferred food. Then, this activity is decomposed so that we identify the primary element, which is to be able to request desired items. We now look at the menu of treatments with a different view. We are looking for treatments that include requesting as a basic component of the treatment. As shown in Figure 10.3 and highlighted in dashed line, there are five treatments that would particularly focus on requesting: CILT, SFA, PACE, script training, and supported communication intervention.

When we start with the identification of impairments and match therapies to the impairment, we are likely to end up with a different selection or combination of therapies than we would if we began with the client's valued activity as the basis for goals and outcomes. We do not yet know how following different treatment selection strategies might affect ultimate outcomes or treatment efficiency, but these are important issues to address in the future.

CONCLUSION

Two broad categories of therapies have been identified: impairment-focused and activity/participation-focused. A simple additive model for clinical work describes the addition of activity/participation-focused goals and therapy as an adjunct to impairment-focused therapy under one of two different circumstances. First, adding an activity/participation-focused goal and therapy might be a response to a client-expressed preference or request. Second, activity/participation-focused therapy may be added on to impairment-focused therapy as a way to facilitate transfer and generalization.

In either case, treatment time is divided in some way between the two approaches, either within a single therapy session or across multiple sessions. In addition, therapy is selected by the clinician in different ways. To choose an impairment-focused therapy, the clinician administers a standardized assessment and selects a therapy that targets one or more particular language impairments. To choose a participation-focused therapy, the clinician responds to one or more priorities or requests made by the client and selects a treatment that will lead to participation in an activity that is valued by the client.

An integrative model starts with identifying the priorities of the client. After that, impairment-focused assessments may be incorporated, but only inasmuch as they directly bear on the client's valued activities. This is more specific than simply thinking that you need word retrieval skills to order menu items. Which words, exactly, do you need or want to retrieve? Can the client retrieve these words within the context of ordering, since in the context-driven integrative model, that is the only context of interest. The context-limited, impairment-focused assessment data are combined with the participation-focused performance data as a way to help the clinician determine goals and select treatments.

An integrative model for clinical work puts forward the notion that therapies are combined most effectively when the ultimate goal of the activity or task is preserved across all selected therapies. Therapies should be selected not because they map onto identified impairments, but because they map onto the primary goals of client-centered activities that have been collaboratively chosen as therapy goals.

This could result in the use of 30-minute outpatient sessions totally focused on ordering restaurant items, if that activity was important to the client. Thus the outcome of the therapy, in this case, would be simply the ability to order preferred food items.

Many clinicians might feel that they would be doing a potential disservice to the client if the entire therapy only led to being able to order at a restaurant. Most clinicians would want at least part of the therapy to target a language domain or skill that is assumed to become generalized across untrained items. However there are some reasons why a single participation outcome may be more powerful than working on a therapy that may only weakly generalize to untrained items.

First, if a client masters the ability to function in a particular context, in this case ordering for himself in a restaurant, the client is more likely to actually go out and do the activity. Doing the activity repeatedly will naturally foster reinforcement of the client's ability, and it is likely to facilitate generalization across contexts (ordering a pizza for the family, or ordering or requesting items at a store). Since the therapies were selected based on their focus on requesting items, the client is likely to be able to start requesting items across various contexts.

Second, since most impairment-focused therapies require a great deal of therapy time before generalization to untrained items is observed, current therapy settings do not provide sufficient therapy time to achieve generalization to untrained items. Therefore, delivering impairment-focused therapy in a time-limited setting may not result in any generalization. In addition, there may be very little to no improvement that is noticeable to the client. The kind of progress that can be made with this approach is unlikely to be self-sustaining.

Making one noticeable, valued change in a client's life is likely to be "worth it," both to the client and to the clinician. Applying an impairment-focused approach only inasmuch as it directly serves the decomposed goal of the valued activity can enhance the efficiency of our therapy and ensure that all of our therapy is targeting the priorities and values of our client.

CASE ILLUSTRATION: MR. F.—EPISODE 3

Mr. F. is now at home and receiving home healthcare services from another clinician. Therapy continues to focus on requesting preferences, including food preferences, at home. Transfer of skills to making other kinds of requests is also targeted, such as requesting TV volume changes, assistance making phone calls to his children, and assistance with his computer. The clinician creates a stack of picture stimuli that correspond to Mr. F.'s interests and typically requested items, and uses these stimuli in both SFA and PACE therapies. Outcomes are measured by percentage of successful requests during role plays, successfully communicated messages in PACE, and successfully named items during SFA. In addition, a measure such as the Communicative Effectiveness Index (Lomas et al., 1989) gathers the perceptions of Mrs. F. regarding his abilities.

REFERENCES

Allen, L., Mehta, S., McClure, J. A., & Teasell, R. (2012). Therapeutic interventions for aphasia initiated more than six months post stroke: A review of the evidence. *Topics in Stroke Rehabilitation, 19,* 523–535.

American Speech-Language-Hearing Association (ASHA). (n.d.). ASHA's Evidence Maps. Retrieved from http://www.asha.org/Evidence-Maps/.

ASHA. (n.d.). Practice Portal: Clinical Topics: Aphasia. Retrieved from http://www.asha.org/PRPSpecificTopic.aspx?folderid=8589934663&section=Therapy.

Ashton, C., Aziz, N. A., Barwood, C., French, R., Savina, E., & Worrall, L. (2008). Communicatively accessible public transport for people with aphasia: A pilot study. *Aphasiology, 22,* 305–320.

Australian Aphasia Rehabilitation Pathway. (n.d.). Australian Aphasia Rehabilitation Pathway. Retrieved from http://www.aphasiapathway.com.au.

Berenholtz, S. M., Dorman, T., Ngo, K., & Provonost, P. J. (2002). Qualitative review of intensive care unit indicators. *Journal of Critical Care, 17,* 12–15.

Berthier, L., Pulvermuller, F., Davila, G., Casares, N. G., & Gutierrez, A. (2011). Drug therapy of post-stroke aphasia: A review of current evidence. *Neuropsychology Review, 21*, 302–317.

Boyle, M. (2011). Discourse therapy for word retrieval impairment in aphasia: The story so far. *Aphasiology, 25*, 1308–1326.

Brady, M. C., Kelly, H., Godwin, J., & Enderby, P. (2012). Speech and language therapy for aphasia following stroke. *Cochrane Database of Systematic Reviews, 5*, CD000425.

Briesch, A. M., Chafouleas, S. M., Neugebauer, S. R., & Riley-Tilman, T. C. (2013). Assessing influences on intervention implementation: Revision of the Usage Rating Profile-Intervention. *Journal of School Psychology, 51*, 81–96.

Canadian Stroke Best Practices Advisory Committee and Writing Groups. (2013). *Canadian Best Practice Recommendations for Stroke Care* (4th ed.). Ottawa, ON: Heart and Stroke Foundation.

Carragher, M., Conroy, P., Sage, K., & Wilkinson, R. (2012). Can impairment-focused therapy change the everyday conversations of people with aphasia? A review of the literature and future directions. *Aphasiology, 26*, 895–916.

Cherney, L. R. (2010). Oral Reading for Language in Aphasia (ORLA): Evaluating the efficacy of computer-delivered therapy in chronic nonfluent aphasia. *Topics in Stroke Rehabilitation, 17*, 423–431.

Cherney, L. R., Kaye, R. C., & van Vuuren, S. (2014). Acquisition and maintenance of scripts in aphasia: A comparison of two cuing conditions. *American Journal of Speech-Language Pathology, 23*, S343–S360.

da Fontoura, D. R., Rodrigues, J., de Sa Carneiro, L. B., Moncao, A., & de Salles, J. (2012). Rehabilitation of language in expressive aphasia: A literature review. *Dementia & Neuropsychologia, 6*, 223–235.

Davis, G. A. (2005). PACE revisited. *Aphasiology, 19*, 21–38.

Davis, G. A., & Wilcox, M. J. (1985). *Adult Aphasia Rehabilitation: Applied Pragmatics*. San Diego, CA: Singular.

Edmonds, L. A., Mammino, K., & Ojeda, J. (2014). Effect of Verb Network Strengthening Treatment (VNeST) in persons with aphasia: Extension and replication of previous findings. *American Journal of Speech-Language Pathology, 23*, S312–S329.

Elman, R. J. (Ed.). (2006). *Group therapy of neurogenic communication disorders: The expert clinician's approach*. San Diego, CA: Plural Publishing.

Elman, R. J., & Bernstein-Ellis, E. (1999). The efficacy of group communication therapy in adults with chronic aphasia. *Journal of Speech, Language, and Hearing Research, 42*, 411–419.

Fisk, A. D., & Eboch, M. (1989). Application of automatic/controlled processing theory application to training component map reading skills. *Applied Ergonomics, 20*, 2–8.

Fitts, P. M., & Posner, M. I. (1967). *Human Performance*. Belmont, CA: Books/Cole Publishing Company.

Frederiksen, J. R., & White, B. Y. (1989). An approach to training based upon principled task decomposition. *Acta Psychologica, 71*, 89–146.

Fulbrook, P., & Mooney, S. (2003). Care bundles in critical care: A practical approach to evidence-based practice. *Nursing in Critical Care, 8*, 249–255.

Graham, J. R., Pereira, S., & Teasell, R. (2011). Aphasia and return to work in younger stroke survivors. *Aphasiology, 25*, 952–960.

Helm-Estabrooks, N., & Nicholas, M. (2000). *Sentence Production Program for Aphasia*. Austin, TX: Pro-Ed.

Herbert, R., Best, W., Hickin, J., Howard, D., & Osborne, F. (2003). Combining lexical and interactional approaches to therapy for word finding deficits in aphasia. *Aphasiology, 17*, 1163–1186.

Hillis, A. E. (Ed.). (2015). *Handbook of adult language disorders* (2nd ed.). New York, NY: Psychology Press.

Hinckley, J. J. (2014). Facilitating life participation in severe aphasia with limited therapy time. *SIG 2 Perspectives on Neurophysiology and Neurogenic Speech and Langauge Disorders, 24*, 89–99.

Hinckley, J. J., & Carr, T. H. (2005). Comparing the outcomes of intensive and nonintensive aphasia intervention. *Aphasiology, 19*, 965–974.

Hinckley, J. J., & Holland, A. L. (2015). A focus on life participation. In A. E. Hillis (Ed.), *Handbook of adult language disorders* (2nd ed.). New York, NY: Psychology Press.

Hinckley, J. J., Patterson, J. P., & Carr, T. H. (2001). Differential outcomes of context-based and skill-based intervention approaches: Preliminary findings. *Aphasiology, 15*, 463–476.

Holland, A. (1994). Cognitive neuropsychological theory and therapy for aphasia: Exploring the strengths and limitations. *Clinical Aphasiology, 22*, 275–282.

Hopper, T., & Holland, A. (1998). Situation-specific training for adults with aphasia: An example. *Aphasiology, 12*, 933–944.

Johnson, M. L., Taub, E., Harper, L. H., Wade, J. T., Bowman, M. H., Bishop-McKay, S., ... Uswatte, G. (2014). An enhanced protocol for Constraint-Induced Aphasia Therapy II: A case series. *American Journal of Speech-Language Pathology, 23*, 60–72.

Kane, S. K., & Galbraith, C. (2013). *Design Guidelines for Creating Voting Technology for Adults with Aphasia*. Washington, DC: Information Technology and Innovation Foundation.

Kazdin, A. E. (1981). Acceptability of child therapy techniques: The influence of therapy efficacy and adverse side effects. *Behavior Therapy, 12*, 493–506.

Kwan, J. (2007). Care pathways for acute stroke care and stroke rehabilitation: From theory to evidence. *Journal of Clinical Neuroscience, 14*, 189–200

Lanska, D. J. (1998). The role of clinical pathways in reducing the economic burden of stroke. *Pharmaeconomics, 14*, 151–158.

Leach, E., Cornwell, P., Fleming, J., & Haines, T. (2010). Patient-centered goal setting in a subacute rehabilitation setting. *Disability and Rehabilitation, 32*, 159–172.

Lomas, J., Pickard, L., Bester, S., Elbard, H., Finalyson, A., & Zoghaib, C. (1989). The Communicative Effectiveness Index: Development and psychometric evaluation of a functional communication measure for adult aphasia. *Journal of Speech and Hearing Disorders, 54*, 113–124.

Mackenzie, C., & Paton, G. (2003). Resumption of driving with aphasia following stroke. *Aphasiology, 17*, 107–122.

Maddy, K. M., Capilouto, G. J., & McComas, G. L. (2014). The effectiveness of semantic feature analysis: An evidence-based systematic review. *Annals of Physical Medicine and Rehabilitation, 57*, 254–267.

Marshall, R. (1993). Problem-focused group therapy for clients with mild aphasia. *American Journal of Speech-Language Pathology, 2*, 31–37.

Mautone, J. A., DuPaul, G. J., Jitendra, A. K., Tresco, K. E., Vilejunod, R., & Volpe, R. J. (2009). The relationship between therapy integrity and acceptability of reading interventions for children with attention-deficit/hyperactivity disorder. *Psychology in the Schools, 46*, 919–931.

Morganstein, S., & Smith, M. C. (2001). Thematic language stimulation therapy. In R. Chapey (Ed.). *Language intervention strategies in aphasia and related neurogenic communication disorders* (5th ed., pp. 450–468). Philadelphia, PA: Lippincott Williams & Wilkins.

Muñoz, M., & Karow, C. (2007). A comparison of therapy outcomes following whole-task and part-task methods for training scripts. In *Clinical aphasiology conference* (Vol. *37*). Scottsdale, AZ: Clinical Aphasiology Conference.

National Stroke Foundation. (2010). *Clinical guidelines for acute stroke management*. Melbourne, Australia: National Stroke Foundation.

New Zealand Ministry of Health. (2010). *New Zealand clinical guidelines for stroke management.* Wellington, New Zealand: Stroke Foundation of New Zealand.

Olness, G. (2014, June). Incorporation of emotion and salience into the design of psycholinguistic and psychosocial aphasia intervention: Proposals for evidence-based therapeutic adaptations. Paper presented at the International Aphasia Rehabilitation Conference, The Hague, Netherlands.

Papathanasiou, I., & De Bleser, R. (2003). *The sciences of aphasia: From therapy to theory.* Oxford, UK: Pergamon.

Pulvermüller, F., Neininger, B., Elbert, T., Mohr, B., Rockstroh, B., Koebbel, P., & Taub, E. (2001). Constraint-induced therapy of chronic aphasia after stroke. *Stroke, 32,* 1621-1626.

Robson, J., Marshall, J., Pring, T., & Chiat, S. (1998). Written communication in undifferentiated jargon aphasia: A therapy study. *International Journal of Language and Communication Disorders, 33,* 305-328.

Rose, M. L., Raymer, A. M., Lanyon, L. E., & Attard, M. C. (2013). A systematic review of gesture treatments for post-stroke aphasia. *Aphasiology, 27,* 1090-1127.

Ross, K. B., & Wertz, R. T. (1999). Comparison of impairment and disability measures for assessing severity of, and improvement in, aphasia. *Aphasiology, 13,* 113-124.

Ross, K., & Wertz, R. W. (2002). Relationships between language-based disability and quality of life in chronically aphasic adults. *Aphasiology, 16,* 791-800.

Schneider, W., & Shiffrin, R. M. (1977). Controlled and automatic human information processing I. Detection, search, and attention. *Psychological Review, 84,* 1-66.

Shiffrin, R. M., & Schneider, W. (1977). Controlled and automatic human information processing II. Perceptual learning, automatic attending and a general theory. *Psychological Review, 84,* 127-190.

Sigurðardóttir, Z. G. & Sighvatsson, M. B. (2012). Treatment of chronic aphasia with errorless learning procedures: A direct replication. *Journal of Speech-Language Pathology and Applied Behavioral Analysis, 5,* 47-58.

Simmons-Mackie, N., Raymer, A., Armstrong, E., Holland, A., & Cherney, L. R. (2010). Communication partner training in aphasia: A systematic review. *Archives of Physical Medicine & Rehabilitation, 91,* 1814-1837.

Springer, L., Glindemann, R., Huber, W., & Willmes, K. (1991). How efficacious is PACE-therapy when "Language Systematic Training" is incorporated? *Aphasiology, 5,* 391-399.

Thompson, C. K., Choy, J. J., Holland, A., & Cole, R. (2010). Sentactics®: Computer-automated treatment of underlying forms. *Aphasiology, 24,* 1242-1266.

Van der Meulen, I., van de Sandt-Koenderman, M. E., & Ribbers, G. M. (2012). Melodic intonation therapy: Present controversies and future opportunities. *Archives of Physical Medicine & Rehabilitation, 93*(Suppl. 1), S46-S52

Wambaugh, J. L., Martinez, A. L., & Alegre, M. N. (2001). Qualitative changes following application of modified response elaboration training apraxic-aphasia speakers. *Aphasiology, 15,* 965-976.

Wambaugh, J. L., Doyle, P. J., Martinez, A. L. & Kalinyak-Fliszar, M. (2002). Effects of two lexical retrieval cueing treatments in action naming in aphasia. *Journal of Rehabilitation Research and Development, 39,* 455-466.

Wightman, D. C., & Lintern, G. (1985). Part-task training for tracking and manual control. *Human Factors, 27,* 267-283.

Wisenburn, B., & Mahoney, K. (2009). A meta-analysis of word-finding treatments for aphasia. *Aphasiology, 23,* 1338-1352.

World Health Organization (WHO). (2001). *International Classification of Functioning, Disability, and Health.* Geneva, Switzerland: World Health Organization.

Integrating Principles of Evidence-Based Practice into Aphasia Rehabilitation

Janet Patterson
Patrick Coppens

INTRODUCTION

Evidence-based practice in aphasia treatment is a process designed to reach the best possible clinical decisions in order to achieve the best possible outcome for patients and family members during communication situations. This concept is not new, having philosophical origins in 19th-century medical practice (McDonald, 2001). In an oft-quoted definition, evidence-based medicine is described as "the conscientious, explicit and judicious use of current best evidence in making decisions about the care of individual patients. The practice of evidence-based medicine means integrating individual clinical expertise with the best available external clinical evidence from systematic research." (Evidence-Based Medicine Working Group, 1992; Sackett, Rosenberg, Gray, Haynes, & Richardson, 1996, p. 71). Evidence-based medicine (EBM), now commonly known as evidence-based practice (EBP), has become firmly entrenched in speech-language pathology practice, including in clinical aphasiology. Versions of the EBP model appear in the medical and rehabilitation literature, including publications in clinical aphasiology and by the American Speech-Language-Hearing Association (ASHA). These models identify three by now familiar contributors to EBP: *evidence* from the scholarly research literature; *experience and expertise* from clinicians engaged in patient care; and *perspectives* about the treatment process from patients and family members. Placing patient care at the center of EBP, **FIGURE 11.1** depicts the interrelationship of these three prongs to guide clinical decision making. While the

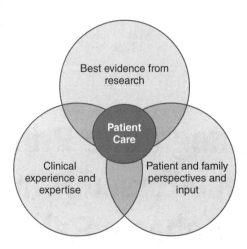

FIGURE 11.1 Prongs of evidence-based practice supporting patient care.

prongs are depicted as having equal contributions to EBP clinical decision-making, it is possible that, considering a patient's individual clinical and personal circumstances, the contribution from one of the prongs may figure more prominently into a particular clinical decision than contributions from the other prongs.

It is a safe bet that every graduate student trained in the United States (and many other countries) is knowledgeable about EBP (Zipoli & Kennedy, 2005). In fact, to achieve the ASHA Certificate of Clinical Competence, a student's training department must verify that he or she "has demonstrated knowledge of processes used in research and of the integration of research principles into evidence-based clinical practice. (Std. IV. F.)" (ASHA, 2016a). It is also a relatively safe bet that when students find themselves practicing in busy clinical settings, obstacles that interfere with consistent, active engagement in EBP begin to present themselves (Nail-Chiwetalu & Bernstein Ratner, 2007). Speech-language pathologists are not alone; occupational therapists (Dubouloz, Egan, Vallerand, & von Zweek, 1999) and nurses (Majid et al., 2011) share this dilemma. Chief among these obstacles is a lack of time, which may sometimes cause clinicians to resort to other less rigorous methods of gathering support for treatment decisions. Students and clinicians echo similar thoughts about EBP, praising its value yet voicing frustrations at its implementation.

In this chapter we address the hopes, frustrations, and realities of EBP in contemporary clinical aphasiology practice. In the first section of this chapter we examine the three EBP Prongs. We identify best practices and provide examples for clinicians to implement EBP into contemporary clinical aphasiology practice. In the second section we expand this foundation to view clinicians as researchers and consider ways in which clinicians can engage in EBP through practice-based evidence, practice-based research, practice-based networks, and implementation science.

THE THREE PRONGS OF EBP

Using evidence to make informed decisions is the ethical and right course of action in patient care (ASHA, 2005; Dollaghan, 2007). Through a series of steps, EBP facilitates clinical application of evidence that has been systematically gathered and thus avoids reliance on intuition and unsupported claims of clinical value (Lum, 2002). The clinical enterprise best serves patients when it is a thoughtful integration of information, grounded in theoretical and empirical evidence and framed in the context of good communication among the client, family, and clinician.

Two examples of the steps in the EBP process are shown in **TABLE 11.1**. Both examples respect the intent of EBP in identifying a clinical question, searching for and appraising evidence, and integrating the evidence into clinical practice. Variations between the examples are evident with the steps posited by Melnyk, Fineout-Overholt, Stillwell, and Williamson (2010) focusing on change to clinical practice, while the steps suggested by the Duke University Medical Center-University of North Carolina (DU-UNC; 2016) example are driven by individual patient care decisions. Both methods are valuable in contemporary clinical aphasiology.

Considering the perspective of the DU-UNC steps, one might broaden the definition of "resource" in step 3 and search additional resources beyond scholarly literature. For example, ASHA Special Interest Group 2—Neurophysiology and Neurogenic Speech

TABLE 11.1 Two views of the steps in the EBP process.

Step	DU/UNC	Melnyk et al., 2010
0		Cultivate a clinical culture of inquiry
1	Assess the patient to identify a clinical question that arose during their care	Ask clinical questions using the PICO or PICOT format
2	Ask well-built clinical questions derived from information obtained from the patient	Search for clinical evidence
3	Search for appropriate clinical evidence	Review and appraise the evidence for its validity and applicability to clinical practice
4	Appraise the evidence for its validity and applicability to clinical practice	Apply the evidence by integrating it with clinical expertise and experience, and patient preferences and values
5	Apply the evidence to practice by talking with the patient and integrating the evidence with clinical expertise and experience, and patient preference	Evaluate the outcomes of the practice decisions or changes based on evidence
6	Self-evaluate your clinical performance and the usefulness of the treatment with your patient	Share the EBP results with colleagues

Duke University Medical Center Library and Health Sciences Library at University of North Carolina Chapel Hill, 2016; Melnyk, Fineout-Overholt, Stillwell, & Williamson, 2010.

and Language Disorders has a community of clinicians who may have experience with a clinical question and who may be able to provide clinical expertise and experience to colleagues confronted with a challenging case. Similarly national, state, or local networks of speech-language pathologists are a source of information about practice decisions.

As a clinician gathers information from a search of resources, scholarly literature, or clinical expertise, it is critical to be mindful of the quality of the evidence and the recommendations that are based on that quality. Many groups have proposed systems to classify the quality of evidence and make recommendations for its clinical use. The Centre for Evidence-Based Medicine (CEBM; 2009) proposed a purpose-driven system of five levels of evidence, most of which also have sublevels. Purposes for gathering evidence include clinical decisions about treatment techniques, prognosis for change, diagnosis, and economic decision analysis. The highest level of evidence, 1a, is a systematic review or a randomized clinical trial, and the lowest, level 5, is expert opinion without critical appraisal. The American Academy of Neurology (AAN; 2011) proposed a four-tiered system to rate studies in five categories: therapeutic, causation, prognostic accuracy, diagnostic accuracy, and population screening. Ratings are based on the rigor of the study and the risk of bias in conducting and implementing a study. Class I studies are considered the highest quality evidence in each category. For example, in the therapeutic category a randomized controlled clinical trial (RCT) is considered the highest form of evidence while a case study, which is Class IV evidence, is the lowest quality. Class IV evidence also consists of consensus or expert opinion. **FIGURE 11.2** shows a hierarchical view of levels of evidence, with the highest level at the apex of the triangle. Recommendations that flow from these and other classification systems provide judgment on the effectiveness and usefulness of the evidence. Recommendation statements range from *strong and recommended*, supporting the use of the evidence based on Class I studies, to *inadequate or no evidence*, based on the presence of Class III and IV evidence or unsubstantiated expert opinion.

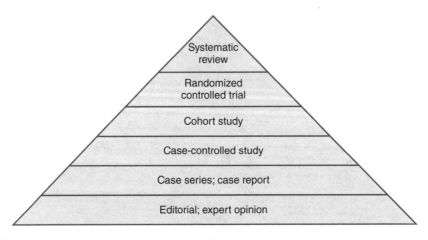

FIGURE 11.2 The EBP hierarchy of evidence.

Evidence class hierarchies such as those from CEBM and AAN have been criticized as being too rigid and only recognizing the highest class of study as the most important and informative. Two points moderate this view. First, several factors contribute to producing a high quality study, such as, assessor blinding, study methodology, and assessment and treatment fidelity. Even though a study uses a RCT methodology, its internal quality may be poor from factors other than study design, thus producing poor evidence that nonetheless is rated as Class I. If internal validity is not fully considered, for example, readers may be misled into placing value on the study based solely on the study design. Second, a Class I study may not be the design best suited to the research question (Petticrew & Roberts, 2003). Clinical aphasiology research is a good example of this, as a common study type used by researchers, the single-case experimental design (SCED), is considered a Class III study. If only Class I evidence is considered, the valuable evidence from a rigorous body of Class III evidence may be missed. When gathering external evidence a clinician must pay attention to the type of study, and just as importantly, evaluate the scientific rigor of the methods.

Clinicians should care about levels of evidence and strength of recommendations for use of the evidence (e.g., the evidence for treatment is strong and its use is recommended) because these recommendations form the foundation of clinical decisions. Most of the assessment and treatment protocols in clinical aphasiology do not have a strong evidence base of Class I studies, but there are many rigorous single-case experimental design studies that, when taken together, provide solid empirical support. Later we describe how to locate and use information about these studies. Clinicians should also recognize that expert opinion, while considered the weakest evidence by some, may be powerful if it reflects local knowledge and is critically appraised.

EBP is not without caveats (Steinberg & Luce, 2005). Straus and McAlister (2000) reviewed criticisms of EBP, grouping them into two categories: limitations of EBP and misperceptions of EBP. EBP limitations are either general in nature, such as shortage of consistent scientific evidence and difficulty applying evidence to individual patient care, or specific to the process of EBP itself, such as the need to develop new techniques and understand best practices in implementing them. In clinical aphasiology as in other fields of study, these limitations are addressed by programmatic research to develop or refine clinical assessment and treatment evidence and to examine how the evidence is translated to clinical practice. The latter topic is the focus of implementation science, which is discussed later. Misperceptions of EBP led Straus and McAlister (2000) to note three criticisms of EBP. First, that EBP promoted a cost-saving "cookbook" style of clinical treatment that could be delivered to patients without regard to individualized need, values, or preferences of patients or clinicians. Second, the EBP enterprise is limited to clinical research in controlled settings with insufficient application to daily clinical practice. Third, a misperception of EBP is that it fostered therapeutic nihilism, that is, the belief that no clinical trial or study can be believed because the rigor of the research does not match the reality of clinical practice (Mullen & Streiner, 2004; Straus & McAlister, 2000, p. 838). These criticisms have merit; however, each can be countered through individual and group actions.

Individually as clinicians, each of us is responsible for maintaining clinical vigilance so that in the face of workplace pressures we remain committed to the principles of EBP and principled clinical decision making rather than adopting a "one-size-fits-all" approach to treatment (see Chapter 10 for suggestions). Collectively, aphasia researchers have begun to bridge the gap between controlled research settings and the reality of clinical practice by using implementation science techniques and tools to examine assessment and treatment practices. In the following sections we look more closely at each of the three EBP prongs.

EBP Prong 1: Best Evidence from Research

The focus of EBP Prong 1 is to evaluate the efficacy of a treatment. A literature search is perhaps the most familiar method of gathering external scientific evidence to evaluate efficacy and support a clinical decision. Typically, data gathered through these resources represent treatment delivered in a controlled setting. In this digital age many databases are available to locate external evidence, and a few of the most popular databases are shown in **TABLE 11.2**. Some sites are freely available while others require an individual or institutional subscription. Some sites offer the most recent publications while others place an embargo of some number of months before studies are made available. University and medical center libraries provide access for employees; however, clinicians working in other settings may have to negotiate access. An old fashioned search, such as a review of the reference list of relevant papers can confirm that the search has been as exhaustive as possible.

A successful search for external evidence that is both scientifically rigorous and user friendly begins with a question that specifies the nature of the query. One type of

TABLE 11.2 Databases commonly used for gathering external evidence in communication disorders.

Database Title	URL	Brief Description
Academy of Neurologic Communication Disorders and Sciences	www.ancds.org/evidence-based-clinical-research	Resources and Systematic Reviews for EBP
Agency for Healthcare Research and Quality	www.guideline.gov/	Clinical guidelines and recommendations
ASHA Evidence-Based Practice page (N-CEP)	www.asha.org/Research/EBP/	Tools and information to incorporate EBP into clinical decision-making
Centre for Evidence-Based Medicine	www.cebm.net/	Systematic Reviews of rehabilitation topics

(Continues)

TABLE 11.2 Databases commonly used for gathering external evidence in communication disorders. (Continued)

Database Title	URL	Brief Description
CINAHL (Cumulative Index to Nursing & Allied Health Literature)	health.ebsco.com/products /cinahl-plus-with-full-text	Research database provides full text for nursing and allied health journals indexed in CINAHL Plus
Communication & Mass Media Complete	www.ebscohost.com/ academic/communication-mass-media-complete	Indexing and abstracts for journals covering communication, mass media, linguistics, discourse, rhetoric, sociolinguistics, communication theory, language, logic, organizational communication, and other closely related fields of study
ERIC (Educational Resources Information Center)	eric.ed.gov/	Education database
Google Scholar	scholar.google.com/	Provides a simple way to broadly search for scholarly literature
Linguistics & Language Behavior Abstracts (LLBA)	www.proquest.com/products-services/llba-set-c.html	Abstracts and indexes the international literature in linguistics and related disciplines in the language sciences
PsycBITE (Psychological Database for Brain Impairment Treatment Efficacy)	www.psycbite.com	Database for treatments for acquired brain injury; studies rated for quality
PsycInfo	www.apa.org/pubs/databases /psycinfo/index.aspx	Abstracts and citations of behavioral and social science research
PubMed	www.ncbi.nlm.nih.gov /pubmed	PubMed comprises more than 26 million citations for biomedical literature from MEDLINE, life science journals, and online books
speechBITE (Speech Pathology Database for Best Interventions and Treatment Efficacy)	speechbite.com/	Database of intervention studies across the scope of speech pathology practice
The Cochrane Collaboration	www.cochrane.org/	Global collaborative to produce systematic reviews of healthcare topics; primarily RCTs
Trip (Turning Research Into Practice)	tripdatabase.com	Clinical search engine with the motto, "Find Evidence Fast"

question could seek to understand the theoretical foundation and administration principles of a particular treatment technique. For example, "How do I administer semantic feature analysis in a clinic?" That type of question could be answered by reading the primary paper describing the technique or a recent paper if the treatment protocol is included in the appendix. The Academy of Neurologic Communication Disorders and Sciences (ANCDS, 2016) website (see Table 11.2) is an important source of papers describing individual study results. While an individual paper typically provides enough information to incorporate the technique into clinical practice, it may not provide sufficient evidence about success with a particular patient or in a specific practice setting. That is, this source of evidence may provide the "how" of delivering a treatment protocol but not the "why" it is the best match for a patient, or the recommendation from a critical review, or the flexibility of the treatment technique to undergo modification to some of its elements.

Another type of question examines the evidence supporting the success of a treatment technique. To answer this question, a clinician should look for a systematic review or meta-analysis. A systematic review uses explicit, systematic methods to collate empirical evidence that fits prespecified question criteria in order to answer a specific research question and provide the most reliable findings from which to draw conclusions (Higgins & Green, 2011). It is a high-level overview of primary research on a particular question that tries to identify, select, synthesize, and appraise all high quality research evidence relevant to a question. A meta-analysis is a "statistical technique for combining the findings from independent studies" (Crombie & Davies, 2009, p. 1; Sacks, Reitman, Pagano, & Kupelnick, 1996). Systematic reviews and meta-analyses are conducted when there is a sufficient amount of evidence to warrant a review. The outcome of these endeavors is typically a favorable answer to the question under review (e.g., yes, family members experience positive outcomes as a consequence of aphasia, despite the presence of third-party disability [Grawburg, Howe, Worrall, & Scarcini, 2012]) or insufficient evidence to draw a conclusion (e.g., little data exist to make a recommendation on communication partner training for people with acute aphasia on measures of language impairment, communication activity/impairment, psychosocial adjustment, or quality of life [Simmons-Mackie, Raymer, Armstrong, Holland, & Cherney, 2010; Simmons-Mackie, Raymer, & Cherney, 2016]). Through its evidence maps website, ASHA (2016b) maintains a compendium of systematic reviews and meta-analyses that clinicians may consult to find external evidence in these formats.

To estimate the likelihood of success in changing a communication behavior as a result of employing a technique, the clinical research question must be specific, preferably constructed in the PICO format (AAN, 2011; French & Gronseth, 2008; Schardt, Adams, Owens, Keitz, & Fontelo, 2007). PICO stands for *population, intervention, comparison,* and *outcome* (Huang, Lin, & Demner-Fushman, 2006) and each letter represents an element in a well-written, specific EBP question. Some authors favor the PICOTS format, with the added "T" representing *Time,* that is, the timing of the intervention in the patient management program or the time for the intervention to show effect (Melnyk et al., 2010), and "S" representing *Setting*, the location that is the focus of the question. Two examples of well-written PICO questions for aphasiology are, "For stroke-induced chronic aphasia, what is the influence of treatment intensity on measures of language impairment?" (Cherney, Patterson, Raymer, Frymark, & Schooling, 2008), and "In individuals with stroke-induced aphasia, do the effects of gesture training combined with verbal training surpass the effects of verbal training alone on measures of (a) language production abilities, (b) gestural expression abilities, (c) verbal communication activity/participation, and (d) nonverbal communication/activity/participation?" (Rose, Raymer, Lanyon, & Attard, 2013). An EBP literature search based on a PICOTS question with detailed but balanced information will have the greatest likelihood of returning clinically relevant evidence. PICOTS questions that are too specific will yield few results (e.g., what is the effect of phonological components analysis treatment [Leonard, Rochon, & Laird, 2008] versus phonomotor treatment [Kendall, Oelke, Brookshire, & Nadeau, 2015] delivered to patients with stroke-induced chronic aphasia using a distributed treatment schedule). Questions that are too vague (e.g., what is the best therapy for anomia) will return an inordinately large number of studies limiting the utility of the search result.

Critical Appraisal of External Evidence

Rating scales are commonly used to critically appraise the scientific rigor of a research report. Scales vary on criteria included; however, most include items examining patient characteristics, randomization, blinding and research design, procedural description, data analysis, and presentation (Coleman, Talati, & White, 2009; Evans, 2003; Reisch, Tyson, & Mize, 1989).

TABLE 11.3 contains select examples of tools for critical appraisal of evidence and five are described here. The first tool, The Strength of Recommendation Taxonomy (SORT; Ebell et al., 2004) is an example of a system that considers not only the study type (e.g., treatment, diagnosis) and quality (e.g., good or limited), but also the consistency of the evidence across studies. Importantly SORT emphasizes patient-oriented outcomes to derive three levels of recommendation. Level A, the highest level, is based on consistent, good quality, patient-oriented evidence, while level C, the lowest level recommendation is based on consensus, usual practice, opinion, or case series. Ebell et al. (2004) describe in detail how to grade studies.

The Scottish Intercollegiate Network Guidelines (SIGN; Harbour & Miller, 2001) is a series of checklists to evaluate research investigations that use various methodologies: systematic reviews and meta-analyses, randomized control trials, cohort studies, case-control studies, diagnostic studies, and economic studies. Each checklist comprises a series of questions relevant to the type of research investigation. For example, the checklist for case-control studies evaluates the quality of the research question, the internal validity (participants, assessment, confounding factors, and analysis), and overall assessment. Detailed notes assist the user in making a judgment for each item.

TABLE 11.3 Select systems to evaluate reports of research.

Rating System	Scale or Checklist
Appraisal Questions for Intervention Studies (Gillam & Gillam, 2008).	Eight categories (appraisal factors). The number of positive responses determines the strength of the evidence (0–8 score)
Checklist for Evaluating Research in the Practices of Audiology and Speech-Language Pathology (Meline, 2010, pp. 285–286).	Checklist follows the structure of an experimental study article (30 questions)
Critical Appraisal of Treatment Evidence (CATE) Critical Appraisal of Diagnostic Evidence (CADE) Critical Appraisal of Systematic Review or Meta-Analysis (CASM) Checklist for Appraising Patient/Practice Evidence (CAPE) Checklist for Appraising Evidence on Patient Preferences (CAPP) (Dollaghan, 2007)	Set of one-page appraisal documents to critically appraise clinical research and its application. Each document finishes with a Clinical Bottom Line statement which indicates whether or not the evidence supports change in practice.
EBP—Critically Appraised Article Summary Worksheet (Fanning & Lemoncello, 2010)	Checklist to appraise treatment article and identify the Clinical Bottom Line for usefulness of the treatment technique in clinical practice
Institute for Clinical Systems Improvement Evidence Grading System (ICSI; Greer, Mosser, Logan, & Halaas, 2000)	GRADE system (Grading of Recommendations Assessment, Development and Evaluation) Recommendations based on: (1) Balance between desirable and undesirable effects (2) Quality of evidence (3) Values and preferences (4) Costs
Preferred Reporting Items for Systematic Reviews and Meta-Analyses: The PRISMA Statement (Moher et al., 2009)	27-item checklist in seven categories (title, abstract, introduction, methods, results, discussion, and funding) Note presence and page report of item
Scottish Intercollegiate Guidelines Network (SIGN; Harbour & Milller, 2001) www.sign.ac.uk/guidelines/fulltext/50/annexoldb.html	Four levels of evidence (two with sublevels) Four grades of recommendation

(Continues)

TABLE 11.3 Select systems to evaluate reports of research. (Continued)

Rating System	Scale or Checklist
Single-Case Experimental Design Scale (SCED) (Tate et al., 2008)	11-item rating scale for single-subject research designs (10 items rate methodology; 1 item rates evidence for generalization)
Single-Case Reporting guideline In BEhavioral interventions (SCRIBE; Tate, Perdices, et al., 2016; Tate, Rosenkoetter, et al., 2016)	26-item checklist in 10 categories (title and abstract, introduction, design, participants, context, approval, measures and materials, analysis, results, discussion and documentation)
Strength of Recommendation Taxonomy (SORT; Ebell et al., 2004)	Three key elements in Agency for Healthcare Research and Quality (AHRQ) report: quality, quantity, consistency of evidence 1. Strength of recommendation—three levels 2. Study Quality—three levels 3. Type of study—three categories 4. Consistency across studies—two levels
Ten Questions for the Critical Appraisal of Research Studies (CARS; Meline, 2010, p. 61).	Checklist follows the structure of an experimental study article (10 questions)

A third example of a tool to critically appraise evidence is the Single-Case Experimental Design Scale (SCED; Tate et al., 2008). Recognizing the value of scientifically rigorous single-case experimental design studies yet finding no method of systematically appraising these studies, Tate et al. (2008) set out to create a tool. In clinical aphasiology single-case experimental designs are prevalent and contribute valuable data from a systematic observation of patient care in a clinical setting. Note that single-case experimental design studies are not to be confused with case reports in which no experimental control is evident. The SCED Scale is an 11-item checklist that has been validated and can be used in study design and evaluation.

The Preferred Reporting Items for Systematic Review and Meta-Analyses (PRISMA; Moher, Liberati, Tetzlaff, & Altman, 2009) is a checklist for transparent reporting of systematic reviews and meta-analyses. PRISMA offers a flowchart of the four phases of a systematic review, giving guidance for how information should flow from one phase to the next. For example, in the first phase, *identification*, the number of records located through all sources should be listed, then in the second phase, *screening*, duplicates should be removed. PRISMA also has a 27-item checklist with definitions of each item and a column to locate the page in the systematic review or meta-analysis where that information can be located. For example, the description for item 3, *rationale*, is "describe the rationale for the review in the context of what is already known." Although PRISMA was designed for authors to be transparent in reporting their work, it is useful to clinicians in evaluating a systematic review or meta-analysis.

Dollaghan (2007) developed a set of documents to aid clinicians in critical appraisal. Each clinician-friendly, easy-to-use checklist poses a series of questions based on the purpose of the appraisal—essentially the equivalent of the PICO question. For example, the question for the Critical Appraisal of Treatment Evidence (CATE) is: "For (specific patient/problem), is (specific treatment) associated with (specific outcome) as compared with (contrasting treatment or condition)" (Dollaghan, 2007, p. 153). A specific example is "For adults needing to generalize a speech skill is a wristband that issues tactile reminders associated with increased use of the skill as compared with an inert wristband?" (Dollaghan, 2007, p. 79). Similar formats are used for appraising diagnostic evidence (CADE), systematic reviews and meta-analyses (CASM), patient and practice evidence (CAPE), and patient preferences (CAPP). At the end of each of these appraisal tools the clinician completes a "clinical bottom line." This is a simple statement about the usefulness of the evidence for a clinician to consider changing a diagnostic or treatment approach, either generally or with a particular patient. The CAPE and CAPP checklists are particularly valuable in clinical practice to address EBP Prong 3—patient and family perspectives and input.

These five examples illustrate the range of tools available to critically appraise evidence. While the tools have different purposes, there are many common items among them, such as patient description and data analysis. Similar to individual research reports (e.g., RCT or SCED), a systematic review or meta-analysis may not be of the highest quality despite having passed peer review. Baylor and Yorkston (2007) offer suggestions on how to best use and understand systematic reviews. Clinicians are encouraged to use one of these scales or another from Table 11.3 to carefully evaluate the evidence as they translate it to their clinical practice. It is possible that a clinician may find that none of these scales is appropriate to the specific set of clinical circumstances for which critical appraisal is required, and thus they may wish to create a tool. While this action may increase local value to the clinician, unless the clinician attends to issues such as internal validity a new tool runs the risk of missing important information and thus frustrating the EBP enterprise and understating or overstating the quality of the evidence.

Barriers to Critical Appraisal of Evidence

Two sources of barriers present themselves as clinicians engage in EBP through the use of best evidence from research, characteristics of the literature and the evidence base and characteristics of the clinician. Each is addressed in turn.

Numerous treatment techniques have been described in the scientific literature, and even more papers report modifications to those techniques. While each of these techniques has evidence to support its utility, several questions emerge when examining the studies that report clinical use of a technique. First, many techniques have only one or two papers describing the treatment, thus creating a small body of literature that does not lend itself to systematic review or inspire confidence in robust application. Second, the literature base suffers from a reporting bias (Robey, 1998) as most published evidence is favorable and few studies report negative or disappointing outcomes. When selecting a treatment technique for a patient it is just as important to know what factors make the patient a poor candidate for that treatment as it is to know what factors make the patient a good candidate. If a particular client does not match well with the study population or if there are unreported contraindications to treatment candidacy, a clinician may use the technique but be unable to replicate the outcome. Third, replication of a study is not always eagerly accepted in scholarly journals, thus further limiting a potentially robust and unbiased view of a treatment technique. Fourth, and of critical importance to clinicians, patients, and funding sources, is that relatively little external scientific evidence exists regarding generalization of a learned behavior to a patient's daily life (see Chapter 7 for discussion of generalization). Finally, few techniques have sufficient evidence to move the treatment research into phases investigating treatment effectiveness in routine clinical practice (Robey, 2004; Robey & Schultz, 1998).

Other factors can also impede gathering external evidence. Some reports of clinical research may be poorly written or difficult to read and understand. For example, the participants or the treatment protocol may not be described in sufficient detail for a clinician to determine candidacy of an individual with aphasia for a particular technique. A treatment protocol may use complex methodology or equipment that is not readily available in routine clinical practice. Data analysis may use statistical techniques with which clinicians are not readily familiar.

In addition to obstacles from the literature itself, barriers may be clinician-related and appear as limited access to evidence or unwillingness to engage in EBP. For most contemporary clinicians keeping current with the vast literature is next to impossible considering the volume of published studies and the time limitations in a busy professional clinical life (Dodd, 2007; Nail-Chiwetalu & Bernstein Ratner, 2007). For example, the first systematic review in clinical aphasiology was published in 1997 and the trend line of systematic reviews published annually since then is steep, with the number in the double digits in recent years. Not all of these systematic reviews are of high quality, requiring clinicians to critically appraise the evidence, using CASM (Dollaghan, 2007) or PRISMA (Moher et al., 2009). Furthermore, many systematic reviews speak to the quality of the evidence but do not consider the delivery system for the treatment. For example, a systematic review of Constraint-Induced Aphasia Therapy (CIAT; Cherney et al., 2008, 2010) addressed questions of treatment effectiveness but not questions of the suitability of CIAT in a typical outpatient clinic that cannot support intensive treatment.

While clinicians have all had graduate-level training in research methods, that information may not be fresh in memory. Also, new ways of thinking (e.g., implementation science and patient-reported outcomes) regularly emerge, requiring acquisition of new knowledge

(Metcalfe et al., 2001). If clinicians are not conversant in the new knowledge, evidence that depends upon it cannot be fully utilized. The role of continuing education in reading the professional literature, participating in online events, and attending professional meetings cannot be understated as a way of updating one's knowledge base. Despite best efforts, the professional literature may not be readily available to a clinician, thus preventing optimal engagement. The Internet has increased availability of articles and the way we search the literature; however, not all articles are freely available to a clinician, thus blocking access to information that is potentially critical to EBP activities. While it is possible to travel to a university library or pay to rent or purchase a paper, those solutions are neither convenient nor expedient to clinicians and can interfere with use of evidence in clinical decision making. Clinicians may be able to develop working relationships with academic departments and be granted access to the university's library resources. For example, clinicians who supervise graduate students' internships can negotiate access to the library portal and interlibrary loan services.

Finally and regrettably, clinicians vary in their willingness to embrace new ways of thinking and clinical decision making. Some clinicians are unwilling to embrace change and remain unenlightened by best evidence from research. Furthermore, even the most ardent and impassioned clinician may be overwhelmed trying to overcome the obstacles related to the process of gathering external evidence (Zipoli & Kennedy, 2005), thus decreasing their motivation to remain engaged in seeking the best external and scientific evidence from research.

In summary, gathering, appraising, and using the best evidence from research is easier now than ever before, yet barriers remain in translating that evidence to clinical practice. Tools such as the SCED Scale and PRISMA aim to reduce the barriers and support translation of evidence.

EBP Prong 2: Practice-Based Evidence

As discussed previously, the purpose of EBP Prong 1 (best external evidence from research) is to find information about the *efficacy* of a specific therapy approach, that is, whether the approach has been found to improve a patient's symptoms in controlled environments and ideal circumstances. This process ideally includes a large sample size and a RCT research design. On the other hand, the results of therapy approaches arising from everyday clinical practice address *effectiveness* research, that is, the application of a rehabilitation method with intrinsic variability in patient characteristics and treatment administration parameters. In other words, efficacy research seeks to answer the following question: "Does this particular therapy technique work for a large number of similar patients?" Whereas effectiveness research is designed to answer the question: "Does this particular therapy technique work for this particular client?"

ASHA refers to this aspect of EBP as "clinical expertise" (ASHA, 2004, 2005). It denotes the clinician's "clinical expertise in making clinical decisions" (ASHA, 2005). Because of this concept's perceived vagueness, some authors have attempted to define this principle with more precision. For example, Dollaghan (2007) defines this concept as the "best available evidence internal to clinical practice" (p. 2) and Lof (2011) used this new definition to rechristen this principle as *practice-based evidence* (PBE). Hence, this EBP principle now represents the quality of the data gathered by the clinician during clinical interactions and how useful these data are to guide the clinical decision-making process. This revised interpretation of EBP Prong 2 has important consequences for clinicians, who should:

- Apply scientific principles to the clinical process.
- Treat the clinical interaction as a single-subject research design.
- Gather valid and reliable data.
- Ascertain that the therapy is the cause of the patient's behavioral improvement.

It may come as a surprise to clinicians that gathering data during therapy is considered research, but there should be very little difference between what researchers do and what clinicians do. In fact, Lum (2002) refers to "scientist-clinicians" as those individuals who successfully apply scientific thinking and critical thinking to clinical activities. The scientist-clinicians base their decisions on the available literature, test clinical hypotheses, measure behaviors accurately, and use the gathered data to inform subsequent clinical decisions (Lemoncello & Ness, 2013).

Clinicians tend to use ABA designs in clinical settings, where the first "A" is the baseline measurement, "B" is the therapy period, and the second "A" is the post-therapy measurement, or "withdrawal" phase (see **FIGURE 11.3**). Such a design is weak because if there is an improvement in the behavior measured, it is impossible to attribute the observed change to the therapy. Several confounding variables could have caused the change, such as spontaneous recovery, measurement error, or environmental influences. The only possible logical conclusion after an ABA design is that the patient improved, but not that the therapy caused the improvement. This is because such a design has poor internal validity. Internal validity can be thought of as a degree of certainty that variable X is the cause of the change in variable Y. In planning treatment and implementing a specific technique, clinicians need to strengthen the internal validity of their design to increase the certainty of their conclusion that the therapy caused the improvement. How is a clinician to achieve this? The answer is through systematic control of treatment variables in a single-case experimental design to strengthen internal validity. First, it should be stated that the internal validity of a single-case design will never be perfect; however, there are easy changes that clinicians can apply to their design to make internal validity significantly stronger. We will discuss the advantages of (a) improving measurement quality and (b) including control variables.

It is important to ascertain that the measurement of a specific behavior is valid and reliable; otherwise, the variability of measurement may be wrongly interpreted as improvement. For example, if the baseline stimuli for a naming objective consist only of items that a patient failed to name, subsequent measurement is likely to include successfully named items simply because of measurement variability. Such a measurement performed post-therapy could be misinterpreted as improvement in naming skills, or at the very

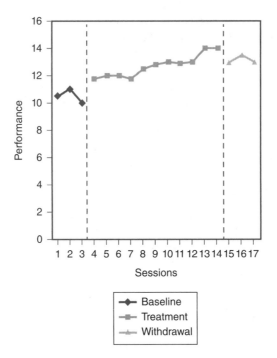

FIGURE 11.3 Example of an ABA design.

least an overestimation of the level of improvement. The solution is to select assessment stimuli pretherapy with a success rate of 20% to 50%, so that potential variability can be observed. Another potential risk is poor assessment fidelity (Richardson, Dalton, Shafer, & Patterson, in press) such as when the clinician scores a behavior differently across time because the scoring variables were not clearly defined *a priori*. For example, if the administration instructions do not clearly state how much time a clinician should allow before marking "error—no response" for an item, then the clinician may give a patient more time to name stimulus items in post-therapy testing than in pretherapy testing. This creates the potential that the accuracy score post-therapy is higher, not only as a result of treatment, but also because the patient was given more time for cognitive processing before responding. As a result, the report of behavior change will be artificially inflated. Thus, clinicians should define the parameters of the measurement task with precision and strictly adhere to the task administration criteria at all times. Richardson et al. (in press) offer a checklist for assessment fidelity that clinicians can use to self-examine their assessment procedures at the outset of treatment and during probe trials.

Another threat to internal validity is "observer drift," which can occur during measurement (Kazdin, 1977; Smith, 1986). Observer drift is the tendency to change the way behavioral definitions are applied over time. For example, a clinician may be well trained in administering an aphasia test during a graduate program but with the passage of time, his or her delivery of specific items changes and deviates, or drifts, from the original definition. One possible solution to this risk of observer drift is to maintain clinical vigilance to assure adherence to the behavioral definitions agreed upon in the assessment tool or at the outset of treatment. Another solution is to record the task and re-score it at a later time. The clinician should obtain the same score both times; this is referred to as *intrarater reliability*. A final threat to the quality of measurement is that the scoring may vary across time because of the clinician's increased familiarity with the patient. For example, when a clinician scores the word or sentence intelligibility of a patient with severe apraxia of speech it is possible that the post-treatment score will increase simply because the clinician has habituated to the patient's productions, independent of actual progress. The obvious solution in this case is to include a colleague unfamiliar with the client as an additional scorer. Both clinicians should obtain the same score; this is referred to as *interrater reliability*.

Another important way to improve internal validity is to control for confounding variables. A confounding variable has the potential to influence the results of therapy. For example, it could include factors such as mood, motivation, effects of medication, amount of home practice, and spontaneous recovery. Although it is hardly possible to control for all of these variables, one of the most influential variables in neurogenic communication disorders is spontaneous recovery, at least in the earlier stages of rehabilitation. It is easy to imagine that an ABA design during the spontaneous recovery period will show improvement even if therapy is unsuccessful. In other words, the sample ABA design in Figure 11.3 could readily represent the effect of spontaneous recovery without any clinician intervention. This is the reason why the ABA design never allows the clinician to conclude that therapy caused the change in patient behavior. Luckily, it is possible for clinicians to modify their design fairly easily in order to protect themselves against the influence of general confounding variables such as spontaneous recovery (or maturation in children, for example). The best thing to do is to collect baseline data for the target behavior several times and then add a control variable or set up a multiple baseline design.

As previously stated, the baseline period is the assessment of a specific clinical objective that takes place before the beginning of therapy. While demonstrating stable baseline performance is important, it is not clear how many probe trials are required to demonstrate stability (McNamara & MacDonough, 1972). Typically, it is recommended that the baseline measurement be taken at least three separate times (Barlow & Hersen, 1973), more if the baseline is not stable. Opinions differ on what constitutes baseline stability and certainly some variability in the data is to be expected, but data points should not fluctuate by more than 5% (Sidman, 1960). The presence of progressive improvement (i.e., an upward trend) represents a red flag for the possible influence of a general confounding variable such as spontaneous recovery. Finding this, the necessary next step is either to introduce a control variable or to set up a multiple baseline design. Logically, if spontaneous recovery (or any general confounding variable) is present, the patient's clinical symptoms should improve in all aspects of language. So, the clinician could simply measure a language skill that is not expected to change based on the clinical objectives chosen but that would show an improvement due to spontaneous recovery. For example, if the clinical objective is targeting anomia, the clinician could keep monitoring the patient's performance on nonword repetition or single-word reading. Importantly, the control variable selected should not be one that may be expected to change because of generalization. If the clinician attempts to measure generalization to related skills or exemplars, a separate generalization variable should be considered (see **FIGURE 11.4**).

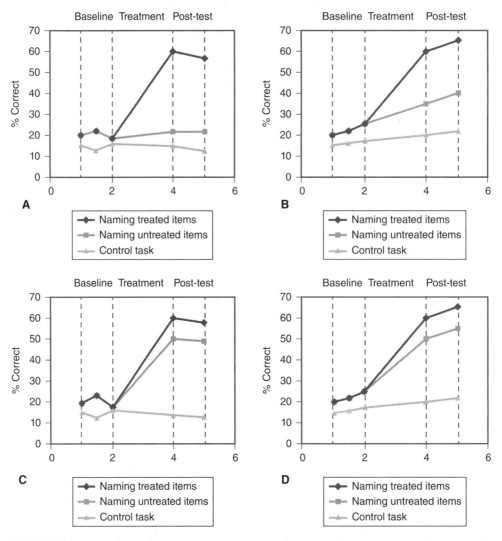

FIGURE 11.4 Examples of outcome measurements for trained items, a generalization variable (untrained items), and a control variable.

The examples displayed in Figure 11.4 illustrate various possible outcomes of the measurements. These types of data plots are useful for visual analysis of the data, even if no statistical comparisons are performed. Figure 11.4A depicts a stable baseline, a strong therapy effect, no generalization to untrained exemplars, and no change in the control variable. Therefore, it is unlikely in this case that a confounding variable influenced the results and the improvements in trained items are likely to be the result of the therapy. Figure 11.4B shows a positive slope in the baseline as well as a change in the control variable. This indicates that there is likely a general confounding variable at play, such as spontaneous recovery, that influenced the results. However, the larger improvement in the treated items also points to a positive therapy effect (and a minimal generalization effect) beyond the slope of the control variable. Figure 11.4C displays the ideal outcome of therapy. That is, there is a stable baseline, a strong therapy effect, a strong generalization effect, and no indication of a general confounding variable. Finally, Figure 11.4D shows the same situation as in 11.4C but with the presence of a confounding factor such as spontaneous recovery.

In conclusion, introducing a control variable allows the clinician to separate the therapy effects from the effects of the confounding variable. For example, if spontaneous recovery influences the results of the therapy, the clinician can still quantify the therapy effects over and above the changes due to spontaneous recovery.

Another option to control for confounding variables is to set up the therapy period as a multiple baseline design. **FIGURE 11.5** illustrates a multiple baseline design across variables. In this case, the clinician selects (usually) three variables to target in therapy. The variables are typically related, but generalization should not be expected from one variable to the others. For example, the first variable could be naming functional objects, the second variable action verbs, and the third variable functors (e.g., prepositions). Baseline probe data are collected for all three variables for 3 to 5 data points. If baseline stability is satisfactory, therapy begins on the first variable while the other two variables remain in the baseline phase. When a specific criterion is reached (either a minimum score on the first variable or a number of therapy sessions) therapy starts on the second variable. After a criterion is reached on the second variable, the third variable is targeted in therapy. By then, the therapy period is usually over for the first variable and post-treatment data is gathered. In other words, the start of the therapy phase is staggered across the variables. If there is a therapy effect, the improvement is limited to the therapy phase for each variable. But if a general confounding variable is present, all the variables would improve concurrently, even outside the therapy period.

In sum, EBP Prong 2 should be considered the evidence that derives from the clinical interaction measures. The clinician should strive to ascertain that the therapy implemented is the cause of the observed change in the behavior measured. To answer this question, some strengthening of internal validity is required, but some of these changes are actually relatively simple to implement in everyday clinical interactions.

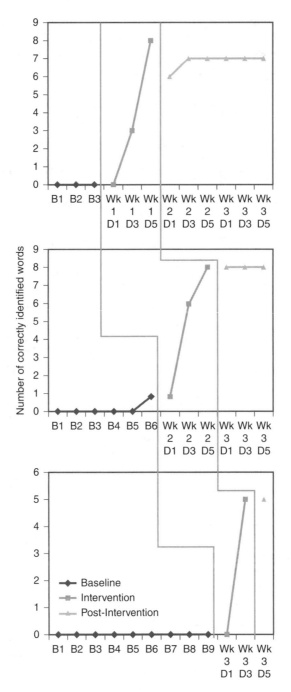

FIGURE 11.5 Example of a multiple baseline design. Wk = week; D = day

EBP Prong 3: Patient and Family Perspectives and Input

Prong 3 represents the role of the patient, family, and caregivers in clinical decision making. Various labels have been applied to Prong 3, using terms such as patient values, patient expectations, client/patient perspectives, and patient perspectives. Considering Prong 3, the Canadian Institutes of Health Research write, "by patient values we mean the unique preferences, concerns and expectations each patient brings to a clinical encounter and which must be integrated into clinical decisions if they are to serve the patient" (Knowledge Translation Clearinghouse, 2016). At face value this definition resonates with the idea of good clinical practice; however, looking beneath the surface there are many perspectives from which to approach integrating patient and family preferences and input into clinical decisions.

Prong 3 must represent a clinical partnership among the patient, clinician, and family members or caregiver. Like the prongs of the EBP diagram itself (see Figure 11.1) the partnership should be balanced but sometimes the influence of the clinician is greater and sometimes the influence of the patient or family is greater. Seeking the patient and family perspectives and input during treatment does not mean accepting without question the requirements, directions, or demands of a patient, nor does it mean that the patient is always right. Prong 3 does however require that the clinician seek to understand the clinical enterprise into which the patient and family are being drawn, to provide them with the best external and internal evidence available, and to engage in joint decisions about treatment. The previous sections on Prongs 1 and 2 describe how to gather, evaluate, and prepare evidence to present to a patient. Prong 3 considers how to put that information into a clinically usable format.

Before beginning treatment, it is important to determine whether a patient is a candidate for a specific treatment and is likely to respond positively to treatment. First, check the external evidence and judge if there is a match between the patient's clinical characteristics (e.g., aphasia type, time post-onset, severity) and those of the individuals with aphasia reported in the literature for whom the approach was successful. If this check is positive and there seems to be a good match indicating the patient may be a candidate for the treatment, then proceed to planning for the internal evidence. If the clinician has experience with administering this therapy approach and with prior patients who had similar characteristics, then the clinician can start developing a data gathering protocol and applying appropriate confounding variable controls. Finally, the clinician should check factors such as the patient's willingness to engage in the treatment program and the family members' belief that treatment can result in change, because these tend to contribute to potential treatment success. **TABLE 11.4** lists examples of these factors in three areas. The first area is an individual's attitude toward change in daily life, and specifically toward the behavior change that may accompany treatment success. Second is the ability and willingness to complete treatment activities that are both clinic-based and home-based. The third area is the individual's belief system in personal self-efficacy and the belief that change is possible.

TABLE 11.4 Personal characteristics of the patient, family member, and clinician that can assist in determining candidacy for treatment and readiness to engage in the therapy program.

Patient	Family Member	Clinician
1. Attitude toward change		
Motivation to change	Readiness to accept change in person with aphasia	Plan of evidence-based treatment to support likelihood of change
Readiness to change		
2. Treatment compliance		
Ability to complete treatment tasks	Ability to complete home program	Goals, methods, and measurement that are clearly written and understood by patient and family
Ability to complete home program	Willingness to support treatment protocol	
Willingness to complete treatment protocol		
3. Personal belief system		
Perceived self-efficacy	Belief that change is possible	Belief that change is possible

To maximize the likelihood of a patient responding positively to treatment, the clinician should assess whether the patient and family are ready, willing, and able to participate in treatment (see Chapter 12 for discussion on motivation). Patients may want a treatment they have read about; however, it may not be appropriate for them or they may not have the speech or language ability to complete the tasks required in that treatment. At a given point in a patient's recovery, the patient may not be ready for a particular treatment. For example, although studies have demonstrated the feasibility of delivering intensive treatment in the acute care setting (Godecke et al., 2014), the timing of treatment may not be optimal, considering other factors such as fatigue or general health (see Chapter 9 for discussion of intensive treatment). Finally treatment protocols, whether impairment-based or activity-participation-based, have response requirements that the patient and family must meet in order for the treatment to have the best chance of success. Maas et al. (2008) identified three prepractice considerations for successful treatment, (a) motivation to learn, (b) adequate understanding of the task including knowledge of a correct response, and (c) stimulability for acceptable response. Although Maas et al. applied these considerations to treatment for motor speech disorders, they noted that they are independent of a specific training program. Gathering input from the patient and family will assist in making a judgment about the patient's readiness for treatment.

Two other important aspects to consider when judging treatment candidacy are belief in the possibility of change—the patient's belief as well as that of the family members and clinicians, and perceived self-efficacy. Belief is a powerful tool in rehabilitation (Resnick, 1998). It cannot be directly measured and is not sufficient for predicting success, but it can support motivation and willingness to participate in treatment. Similarly, perceived self-efficacy (Bandura, 1977; Williams & Rhodes, 2014) has been shown to be valuable in motivating change. The supportive effects of a positive belief system and positive self-efficacy cannot be discounted, but act in concert with the planned treatment program rather than substitute for it. Nevertheless, understanding a patient's, family member's, and clinician's beliefs about aphasia, recovery, and treatment are important sources of input in clinical decision making.

Gathering Evidence of Patient and Family Member Perspective and Input

Two means of gathering information from patients and family members are questionnaire and interview. The Checklist for Appraising Evidence on Patient Preferences (CAPP; Dollaghan, 2007) as previously described, begins with a foreground question about the patient, treatment under consideration, and outcome. It has three sections and finishes with a clinical bottom line. The purpose of the first section is to establish common ground with the patient and family on such items as desired level of participation and treatment scheduling. In the second section clinical options, including costs, benefits, and risks of treatment are discussed. The third section is the synthesis of the external and internal evidence with patient preferences.

Conversations with patients and family members also provide valuable evidence on patient preference. The format of these conversations is individualized; however, the clinician should have both general and specific question areas in mind. Magasi and Heinemann (2009) conducted focus group interviews with individuals invested in the rehabilitation process—people with disabilities, caregivers, rehabilitation providers, funders, and policy makers. They reported three domains across which people participate in life activities: economic, social, and leisure. Across participants, they noted a set of core participation values: meaningful engagement in life, choice and control, access and opportunity, personal and societal responsibilities, supporting others, and social membership. From these items Magasi and Heinemann developed the community participation indicators (CPI; Rehabilitation Institute of Chicago, 2007). The CPI can be used in its checklist format or as the basis for an interview to understand a patient's perception of and values about participation.

In summary, gathering information about patient and family perspective and input is neither straightforward nor achieved in a single episode or conversation. It is however a critical piece to EBP Prong 3.

Patient-Reported Outcomes

Another way of viewing patient and family perspective and input is through patient-reported outcomes (Deshpande, Rajan, Sudeepthi, & Nazir, 2011). A *patient-reported outcome* (PRO) is any report of the status of a patient's health condition that comes directly from the patient, without interpretation of the patient's response by a clinician or anyone else

(The Patient-Reported Outcomes [PRO] Consortium, 2009). PROs can take many forms and be measured through interview or self-administration of a questionnaire or response scale. Fayer and Machin (2007) view PROs within the broad definition of healthcare quality of life and provide a detailed review of several instruments to measure outcomes as they are perceived by a patient. Clinical aphasiology has embraced the importance of PRO. For example, Eadie and colleagues (2006) reviewed six instruments that evaluated communication participation through patient self-report, including the American Speech-Language-Hearing Association Quality of Communication Life scale (ASHA-QCL; Paul et al., 2004) and the Burden of Stroke Scale (BOSS; Doyle, McNeil, Hula, & Mikolic, 2003). They described the vision and positive direction of these instruments and discussed three trends that will influence future work: (1) terminology and the conceptual framework about health, functioning, and disability to support measuring PRO; (2) acknowledgement of the importance of PRO in clinical management; and (3) advances in psychometric measurement (Eadie et al., 2006, p. 314). The cultural change surrounding PRO and its importance to EBP in speech-language pathology is apparent in many avenues. One example is work examining the patient-provider medical interaction, such as the interviews with individuals with aphasia and their family members conducted by Burns, Baylor, Dudgeon, Starks, and Yorkston (2015). Burns et al. (2015) reported several themes evident in participant interviews, (1) patients and family members are a team in communicating during medical interactions, (2) they want physicians to adjust their communication styles, and (3) physicians may not have the communication repertoire to easily adjust their style. Using evidence from these PROs, clinicians can facilitate medical interactions for their patients as Blackstone (2016) points out, identifying "curb cuts" or "communication ramps" that will assist patients.

Another example of the change in culture surrounding PROs is the NIH Patient-Reported Outcomes Measurement Information System (PROMIS, 2016). PROMIS "aims to provide clinicians and researchers access to efficient, precise, valid, and responsive adult- and child-reported measures of health and well-being." The PROMIS mission is to use measurement science to create a state-of-the-art assessment system for self-reported health. Three examples of instruments that embody the PROMIS mission and the goal of PRO are the Aphasia Communication Outcome Measure (ACOM; Hula et al., 2015), the Communication Confidence Rating Scale for Aphasia (CCRSA; Babbit, Heinemann, Senik, & Cherney, 2011), and the Communication Disability Profile (CDP; Swinburn & Byng, 2006). Although the focus of each of these instruments differs, they share the dual foundations of scientific rigor and value placed on PRO and can thus confidently be used by clinicians to document change (Irwin, 2012).

EBP AND JUSTICE

As EBP has become ingrained in mainstream clinical practice, the question of ethical application of the evidence has arisen. More specifically, the question has been framed as justice for persons within the framework of EBP. The Belmont Report (1979) identified three basic ethical principles in the treatment of human beings: (1) respect for persons,

(2) beneficence, and (3) justice. Applied to EBP these ethical principles suggest two avenues of thought that are relevant to clinical decisions. The first avenue is to what extent disadvantaged and underrepresented groups of people are included in production of research evidence, and the second avenue is the application of evidence in a clinical setting. Rogers (2004) suggested that when researchers adhere to the principles of EBP that require careful participant selection and data collection, their attention can be diverted from social and cultural factors that have an impact on how those data are used in clinical practice. For example, often participants in research are self-selected in that they value participation, can travel to the research site, and are aware of opportunities to participate in clinical research. In contrast, individuals who are considered disadvantaged through factors such as poverty or multiple comorbid health conditions, or who live far away from research centers, or are homebound, or who are unaware of research opportunities or uninterested in participation may not be included. Study participants may not include representation of population characteristics or social constructs such as race, ethnicity, or disability category. Conclusions drawn from research that excludes a diverse group of participants are less easily applied to individual patients in a clinical setting (Chabon, Morris, & Lemoncello, 2011).

The ability to draw clear and unambiguous conclusions from data and to statistically evaluate differences requires respect for the scientific parameters of empirical research. Among these parameters is participant selection so that study participants are homogeneous on as many factors as possible (e.g., population, neurology, social-cultural, demographic) in order to support accurate statistical analysis. In clinical aphasia research many studies report using "clean" participants, that is, individuals with a single left hemisphere stroke and no comorbidities, yet many patients have had multiple strokes and have other health conditions. This can lead to what Kent (1990) identified as fragmentation between clinical science (efficacy research) and clinical service (effectiveness research). Recommendations about treatment efficacy often do not come from studies that consider the breadth of human diversity, thus potentially limiting the expectations a clinician can offer through treatment.

Disadvantaged groups typically do not have a role in creating a research agenda. Hinckley, Boyle, Lombard, and Bartels-Tobin (2014) raised this question in aphasia research. In the context of person-centeredness in clinical practice, they used community-based participatory research in the form of questionnaire and interview to ask people with aphasia what research topics they thought were important. The group identified 22 potential research questions in five categories: best treatments; attitudes, emotions, and motivation; interaction with clinicians; personal relationships; and running an aphasia support group. While many questions could be answered through existing literature, others have no evidence base. This is one example of how clinicians can engage people with aphasia and create a consumer-informed research agenda rather than a researcher-initiated agenda.

Creating or using high quality research, implementing the evidence in clinical settings, and conducting ethical clinical practice are activities that pose scientific and ethical challenges. Returning to the prongs of EBP, meeting these challenges by balancing knowledge from the best external evidence, best clinical practice, and individual patient and family preferences and clinical needs is the goal of contemporary clinicians.

CLINICIAN AS RESEARCHER

So far in this chapter we have discussed how clinicians can embrace the principles of EBP and incorporate activities of the three prongs into their clinical routine and daily patient care. Other avenues are available for clinicians to further engage in EBP through collaborative efforts. These avenues, practice-based evidence, practice-based research, practice-based research network, participatory action research, and implementation science are discussed next.

Practice-based evidence (PBE) is the gathering of good quality data from routine practice (Margison et al., 2000, p. 123) or through qualitative inquiry (Leeman & Sandelowski, 2012). Previously we discussed PBE, Prong 2 of EBP, that is, the internal evidence related to the clinical management of a particular patient. However, in a wider sense, PBE can also incorporate cultural or community norms or traditions in diverse communities (Liebermann et al., 2010). It reflects the range of treatments and assists in judging candidacy for a treatment (Isaacs, Huang, Hernandez, & Echo-Hawk, 2005). One method to engage in PBE is Clinical Practice Improvement (CPI) research methodology (Gassaway et al., 2005). CPI recognizes the complexity of patient care that typically is not present in a RCT, the gold standard of clinical research (Horn & Gassaway, 2007). Four characteristic features of a CPI study are (1) comparison of clinically relevant alternatives, (2) inclusion of diverse participants, (3) inclusion of heterogeneous practice settings, and (4) reporting multiple outcome measures (Horn & Gassaway, 2007, p. S50). Each of these characteristics stands in sharp contrast to the characteristics of a RCT. While a practicing clinician may not initiate a CPI, it is not unrealistic to anticipate that a clinician may be invited to participate in a CPI and thus become a producer of evidence. As consumers of evidence, clinicians may look to PBE and CPIs to offer evidence about a treatment technique that is more closely related to their patient population than that found in a RCT (Wambaugh, 2007).

A clever approach to PBE is crowdsourcing (Birch & Heffernan, 2014). In crowdsourcing one puts out an "open call" for contributions on a topic, gathers information from many people acting in their regular daily lives, and makes that information widely available. Crowdsourcing is "the practice of obtaining participants, services, ideas, or content by soliciting contributions from a large group of people, especially via the Internet" (Swan, 2012, p. e46). In clinical research this means outsourcing the task of research to the clinicians who actually see the patients in real world environments (Cook, 2011). Crowdsourcing for clinical research is appealing because it uses ecologically valid data gathered in typical clinical settings and is a novel concept applied to health care and in particular to aphasia treatment (Rigney, 2014). Rigney (2014) surveyed speech-language pathologists about their clinical practice in aphasia treatment to explore the feasibility of using crowdsourcing to engage clinicians in EBP. While Rigney demonstrated proof of concept in this pilot study, as with other attempts at crowdsourcing several deterrents exist, such as methodological integrity, assurance of treatment fidelity, and cost to set up data gathering systems.

Practice-based research (PBR) is "the use of research-inspired principles, designs and information gathering techniques within existing forms of practice to answer questions that emerge from practice in ways that inform practice" (Epstein & Blumenfield, 2001, p.17). PBR can be used to identify problems in daily practice that "create a gap between recommended care and actual care" and demonstrate, as noted in the discussion of EBP Prong 2, whether efficacious treatments are also effective and sustainable in daily clinical practice (Chambers, 2014; Westfall, Mold, & Fagnan, 2007, p. 403). Epstein and Blumenfield (2001) used a mining metaphor and Westfall et al. (2007) used a highway map metaphor to illustrate PBR. In both cases the point to be made is that existing clinical data can provide insight to answer clinical research questions, such as identifying practice needs, monitoring service delivery, or measuring outcomes (Epstein & Tripodi, 1977). PBR is guided by four principles, (1) research questions that are relevant to practice, (2) retrospective or prospective research that is undertaken to understand correlation between practice and outcome, (3) data gathering through routine practice or clinical data mining, and (4) results that are expected to inform clinical practice (Epstein & Blumenfield, 2001). Crooke and Olswang (2015) illustrated PBR methodology in a retrospective study of social thinking (ST), a method of social communication and social learning for individuals with autism spectrum disorder. Results of this study were used to inform clinical practice of speech-language pathologists using ST. Furthermore, Crooke and Olswang (2015) exemplify PBR as a clinically useful tool. As with PBE, practicing clinicians may not initiate a PBR study; however, participating in data mining or using the results of PBR work will aid in bridging the research-practice gap.

A *practice-based research network* (PBRN), an extension of PBR, is defined as a sustained collaboration, often between clinicians and academics, to investigate a clinically relevant question in order to translate research into practice (Pearce, Love, Barron, Matheny, & Mahfoud, 2004). It is proposed as a means to organize PBR activities within a community context (Westfall et al., 2009). Westfall and colleagues (2007, 2009) thought about the real-life meanings of the words "community" and "engagement," the hallmarks of a PBRN, defining them in broad stroke and from multiple perspectives. The community in a PBRN might comprise a local geographical region or it might exist virtually, uniting individuals with a common clinical research interest. Engagement in a PBRN requires that work be focused within the community and that it uses institutional resources to address the clinical problems and questions within the community (Westfall et al., 2009). Participatory action research (PAR; Baum, MacDougall, & Smith, 2006) or partnership research (Frankham, 2009) are methodologies important to PBRNs. Both approaches require "user involvement," that is, the individuals in the "community" are directly involved in creating the clinical questions for the PBRN, gathering and analyzing data, and ultimately, being the recipients of changes to the system. PBRNs originated in primary care medicine as a way to bring together physicians engaged in family practice. The concept spread to other professions such as dentistry, and the Agency for Healthcare Research and Quality (AHRQ, 2016) currently reports 176 PBRNs in 25 countries; however, none address aphasia or speech-language pathology. Initiating a PBRN is a daunting task requiring organizational skills and institutional support (Frankham, 2009; Pearce et al., 2004; Westfall et al., 2009); however, a PBRN is not the only avenue to engaging in EBP through collaboration; a quick search of the literature reveals many collaborative partnerships in clinical aphasiology that span locations and focus on user involvement.

Implementation science (IS) is "the study of methods to promote the integration of research findings and evidence into healthcare policy and practice. It seeks to understand the behavior of healthcare professionals and other stakeholders as a key variable in the sustainable uptake, adoption, and implementation of evidence-based interventions." (NIH Fogarty International Center, 2016). IS research is the study of facilitators and barriers to bridging the research-practice gap leading to sustainable use of evidence-based techniques in clinical practice (Fixsen, Naoom, Blasé, Friedman, & Wallace, 2005). Douglas, Campbell, and Hinckley (2015) wondered if IS was a buzzword, a short-lived concept in speech-language pathology that would not gain traction in clinical practice or research, or if it represented a shift in thinking as we examine how evidence-based treatments are incorporated into routine clinical practice. Through clinical examples from the literature, they illustrated the process of applying an implementation science framework to achieve positive results for stakeholders (Douglas et al., 2015).

Olswang and Prelock (2015) described the steps of implementation science research as applied to evaluation of a treatment technique to teach eye gaze to young children with physical disabilities. At one point in their years-long research programs they recognized a "fork in the road." They realized that research could proceed to examine the intervention under controlled conditions or it could change direction and look at delivery under routine conditions (Olswang & Prelock, 2015, p. S1822). They chose the latter path and, guided by the Consolidated Framework for Implementation Research (CFIR; Damschroder et al., 2009), studied the acceptability, adoption, and fidelity of their treatment. Included in this new direction of study was the identification of barriers to implementing the treatment, for clinicians as well as for children and family members.

A final example of IS in clinical research is from Sohlberg, Kucheria, Fickas, and Wade (2015) who described their investigations of computer-delivered intervention and training of external tools for people with brain injury. Despite the differences in techniques in these two approaches, IS and CFIR guided Sohlberg et al. (2015) in clinical decisions. These three clinical examples have in common the use of an IS framework that includes the clients and other stakeholders as critical to the success of treatment. While practicing clinicians may not be in a position to independently initiate IS clinical research, implementing selected IS elements may be possible. For example, clinicians might follow Sohlberg et al. (2015) and early in treatment query the client, clinician, and family members regarding obstacles to implementing the treatment, including attitude toward the treatment and perceived self-efficacy in maintaining treatment fidelity or sustaining a home program (e.g., EBP Prong 3). The goal of such actions is implementing an evidence-based treatment technique in a manner that is responsive to client and clinician values.

CONCLUSION

The concept of EBP is now irrefutably intertwined with speech-language pathology in general and clinical aphasiology in particular, and it is for the better. When a clinician applies the three EBP prongs competently in his or her clinical practice, all parties benefit. The clinician provides an ethical service, the patients experience the best possible outcome, and the third-party reimbursement entity purchases the best service for their financial investment. Some clinicians came on board the EBP wagon slowly or reluctantly, but that was related more to perceived rather than true obstacles. This chapter has provided practical information on how to surmount these obstacles easily and effectively. In addition, the interested clinicians should consider contributing to one or more research communities described. This mechanism is invaluable in providing clinical application research to inform efficacy research.

CASE ILLUSTRATION

Jane worked as a speech-language clinician in the rehabilitation unit of a major metropolitan hospital. Her workload was demanding, but she enjoyed working with her assigned patients who tended to be almost exclusively left-hemisphere stroke patients. Jane completed her master's degree 6 years ago and considers herself well prepared to work with her population of interest. She received instruction on EBP principles while in her program and she is determined to apply these principles during her professional career. At the moment, her caseload contained several patients with global and Broca's aphasias with whom she developed rehabilitation programs built around techniques with which she was familiar and that she knew had strong evidence support in the literature. However, she was recently assigned two new patients, a woman with conduction aphasia and a man with Wernicke's aphasia, both disorders with which she has less experience. Jane was keenly aware of her limited available research time as well as the advice of Robey (2011) who stated that clinicians should select one disorder at a time for the sake of manageability. Jane has worked with a few cases of Wernicke's aphasia in the past and is familiar with some rehabilitation approaches with evidence support, but she has never encountered a case of chronic conduction aphasia. Therefore, she decided to focus her EBP efforts for the next few days on Mrs. Miller, her new patient with conduction aphasia.

Mrs. Miller is a 57-year-old woman who suffered a left middle cerebral artery infarct 2.5 weeks prior to admission into rehab. A CT scan indicated a cortical/subcortical lesion centered on the left supramarginal gyrus. The hospital discharge report revealed an AQ of 70 (Western Aphasia Battery-Revised; Kertesz, 2006) with functional auditory comprehension, moderately impaired naming, and severely impaired repetition. The errors were principally phonological, including many conduites d'approche.

Jane's first concern with all of her patients is to focus on Prong 3: patient and family perspectives and input. This allows Jane to understand the communicative and participation goals of the patient and her family, which influences the focus of her counseling, assessment, and rehabilitation objectives. Jane met with Mrs. Miller and her husband, Paul. Mrs. Miller was able to understand the conversation, but her output was marred by word-finding difficulties and phoneme errors leading to many conduites d'approche. Mrs. Miller tended to gesture toward her husband when she wanted him to answer the question. She then nodded in approval of his answer.

Mrs. Miller is the assistant manager of a grocery store. She and her husband have two grown children and one 2-year-old granddaughter with whom they have at least weekly contacts. She enjoys reading mysteries, playing bridge with her friends, and traveling. Mrs. Miller wants to resume her position at the grocery store, be able to find words more easily to converse, and be able to read books to her granddaughter.

Considering that information, Jane decided to assess Mrs. Miller's reading and writing skills. Based on her knowledge of conduction aphasia, Jane also decided to assess Mrs. Miller's auditory-verbal and nonverbal working memory, which are only slightly decreased. Finally, Jane informally assessed strategies that reduce phonological difficulties and improve repetition. Among those, Jane noted that unison speech did facilitate production. Based on all the gathered information, Jane decided to focus therapy objectives on (a) word-finding using phonological support strategies; (b) script training focusing on work environment, social situations involving card games, and travel; and (c) oral reading.

At this point, Jane's search for external evidence (Prong 1) began. A cursory review of the literature led Jane to phonological components analysis (PCA; Leonard et al., 2008) for the first goal, script training (Cherney, Halper, Holland, & Cole, 2008) for the second, and Oral Reading for Language in Aphasia (ORLA; Cherney, 2010) for the third. Jane generated the following external PICO questions to lead her searches:

1. For patients with conduction aphasia, does PCA improve word-finding skills as compared to no treatment?

2. For patients with conduction aphasia, does script training improve success of conversational turns as compared to no treatment?

3. For patients with conduction aphasia, does ORLA improve oral reading as compared to no treatment?

Jane's hospital library provides access to many databases, and accessing articles is not a problem for her at this point, but in a prior position, she had to access articles through a university (Jane negotiated library privileges as part of her role as externship supervisor) and by emailing the first author personally. When Jane entered "conduction aphasia" with any of the three therapy techniques selected into a Medline search, no hits appeared. Furthermore, neither the ASHA evidence maps page nor the ANCDS site revealed any review articles. This suggested that conduction aphasia has not been systematically studied in relation to these approaches and that there is no efficacy-level evidence. So, Jane decided to expand her search by ignoring the type of aphasia in her search strategy, at least for now. A search of "Phonological Components Analysis" revealed three articles, including a therapy study of 10 subjects (van Hees, Angwin, McMahon, & Copland, 2013); a search of "script training" and "aphasia" yielded nine articles, including several about a computerized program (Jane opted to put those articles on the side in case she and Mrs. Miller decided to start a home program for script training practice); and a search of "Oral Reading for Language in Aphasia" provided three hits but only with nonfluent aphasia patients.

For the first objective focusing on word-finding, Jane decided to review the most promising article (van Hees et al., 2013) which included two subjects with conduction aphasia. To do that, she filled out her research evidence form, based on the Critical Appraisal of Treatment Evidence form (CATE; Dollaghan, 2007). Her conclusion was that there is some evidence of effectiveness of the technique, particularly when looking at the two subjects with conduction aphasia. For the second objective focusing on script training, Jane reviewed several articles and filled out her evidence form. Her conclusion was that the technique itself shows good effectiveness, but only with nonfluent aphasia patients. Because Jane noted that Mrs. Miller improved her production with unison speech, Jane decided to run a trial therapy period using a modified script training program by inserting a unison speech step. Finally, for the third objective focusing on oral reading, Jane reviewed the evidence and concluded similarly that the technique has enough support to be tried with Mrs. Miller provided an additional step of unison reading be included in the strategy.

Jane had successfully established external evidence support for the objectives selected. The final EBP prong (i.e., Prong 2) now needed to provide support for the effectiveness of the therapy approach for Mrs. Miller specifically. In other words, Jane's data, gathered during the clinical rehabilitation process, need to answer the following internal PICO questions:

1. For this particular patient with conduction aphasia, does PCA improve word-finding skills as compared to no treatment?

2. For this particular patient with conduction aphasia, does modified script training improve success of conversational turns as compared to no treatment?

3. For this particular patient with conduction aphasia, does modified ORLA improve oral reading as compared to no treatment?

For all three objectives, Jane generated target items and various generalization probes. She further decided to use one control measure to protect herself against confounding variables such as spontaneous recovery. She opted for irregular word writing, which she did not expect to change based on the therapy objectives. She took three baseline data points of the therapy targets, the generalization probes, and the control variable. Baseline was stable within 5% variability in all instances. She then started rehabilitation work on the objectives while plotting the data over time. Because of her careful set-up of the variables, she will be able to distinguish between the therapy and generalization effects, as well as observe the potential influence of a general confounding factor (see Figure 11.4).

REFERENCES

Academy of Neurologic Communication Disorders and Sciences (ANCDS). (2016). Evidence-based clinical research. Retrieved from http://www.ancds.org/evidence-based-clinical-research#Aphasia and http://aphasiatx.arizona.edu/

Agency for Healthcare Research and Quality (AHRQ). (2016). Practice-based research networks: Research in everyday practice. Retrieved from https://pbrn.ahrq.gov/

American Academy of Neurology (AAN). (2011). *Clinical Practice Guideline Process Manual* (2011 ed.). St. Paul, MN: The American Academy of Neurology.

American Speech-Language-Hearing Association (ASHA). (2004). Report of the joint coordinating committee on evidence-based practice. Retrieved from http://www.asha.org/uploadedFiles/members/ebp/JCCEBPReport04.pdf

ASHA. (2005). Position statement: Evidence-based practice in communication disorders. Retrieved from http://www.asha.org/policy/PS2005-00221/

ASHA. (2016a). 2014 Standards and implementation procedures for the Certificate of Clinical Competence in speech-language pathology. Retrieved from http://www.asha.org/Certification/2014-Speech-Language-Pathology-Certification-Standards/

ASHA. (2016b). Evidence maps. Retrieved from http://www.asha.org/Evidence-Maps/

Babbit, E. M., Heinemann, A. W., Senik, P., & Cherney, L. R. (2011). Psychometric properties of the Communication Confidence Rating Scale for Aphasia (CCRSA). *Aphasiology, 25*(6–7), 727–735.

Bandura, A. (1977). *Self-efficacy: The exercise of control*. New York: W.H. Freeman.

Barlow, D. H., & Hersen, M. (1973). Single case experimental designs: Uses in applied clinical research. *Archives of General Psychiatry, 29*, 319–325.

Baum, F., MacDougall, C., & Smith, D. (2006). Participatory action research. *Journal of Epidemiology and Community Health, 60*(10), 854–857. doi:10.1136/jech.2004.028662

Baylor, C. R., & Yorkston, K. M. (2007). Using systematic reviews and practice guidelines: A how-to guide for clinicians. *Perspectives on Neurophysiology and Neurogenic Speech and Language Disorders, 17*, 6–10.

The Belmont Report: Ethical principles and guidelines for the protection of human subjects of research. (1979). Retrieved from hhs.gov/ohrp/humansubjects/guidance/belmont.html

Birch, K. E., & Heffernan, K. J. (2014). Crowdsourcing for clinical research: An evaluation of maturity. *Proceedings of the Seventh Australasian Workshop on Health Informatics and Knowledge Management, 153*, 3–11. Australian Computer Society, Inc.

Blackstone, W. W. (2016). What does the patient want? *ASHA Leader, 21*(3), 38.

Burns, M., Baylor, C., Dudgeon, B. J., Starks, H., & Yorkston, K. (2015). Asking the stakeholders: Perspectives of individuals with aphasia, their family members, and physicians regarding communication in medical interactions. *American Journal of Speech-Language-Pathology, 24,* 341–357. doi:10.1044/2015_AJSLP-14-0051

Centre for Evidence-Based Medicine (CEBM). (2009). OCEBM levels of evidence. Retrieved from http://www.cebm.net/ocebm-levels-of-evidence/

Chabon, S., Morris, J., & Lemoncello, R. (2011). Ethical deliberations: A foundation for evidence-based practice. *Seminars in Speech and Language, 32,* 298–308. doi:10.1055/s-0031-1292755

Chambers, D. A. (2014, March). *Advancing the science of sustainability: A dynamic perspective.* ASHA Clinical Research Education Library (CREd Library). doi:10.1044/cred-pvid-implscid2p4

Cherney, L. R. (2010). Oral reading for language in aphasia: Impact of aphasia severity on cross-modal outcomes in chronic nonfluent aphasia. *Seminars in Speech and Language, 31*(1), 42–52. doi:10.1055/s-0029-1244952

Cherney, L. R, Halper, A. S., Holland, A. L., & Cole, R. (2008). Computerised script training for aphasia: Preliminary results. *American Journal of Speech-Language Pathology, 17,* 19–34.

Cherney, L. R., Patterson, J. P., Raymer, A. M., Frymark, T., & Schooling, T. (2008). Evidence-based systematic review: Effects of intensity of treatment and constraint-induced language therapy for individuals with stroke-induced aphasia. *Journal of Speech-Language-Hearing Research, 51,* 1282–1299. doi:10.1044/1092-4388(2008/07-0206

Cherney, L. R., Patterson, J. P., Raymer, A. M., Frymark, T., & Schooling, T. (2010). Updated evidence-based systematic review: Effects of intensity of treatment and constraint-induced language therapy for individuals with stroke-induced aphasia. Rockville MD: National Center for Evidence-Based Practice in Communication Disorders, American Speech-Language-Hearing Association.

Coleman, C. I., Talati, R., & White, C. M. (2009). A clinician's perspective on rating the strength of evidence in a systematic review. *Pharmacotherapy 29*(9), 1017–1029.

Cook, C. (2011). Grassroots clinical research using crowdsourcing. *Journal of Manual and Manipulative Therapy, 19*(3), 125–126. doi:10.1179/106698111X12998437860767

Crombie, I. K., & Davies, H. T. O. (2009). What is meta-analysis? *Evidence-Based Medicine* (2nd ed., pp. 1–8). London: Hayward Medical Group.

Crooke, P. J., & Olswang, L. B. (2015). Practice-based research: Another pathway for closing the research-practice gap. *Journal of Speech, Language, and Hearing Research, 58,* S1871–S1882. doi:10.1044/2015_JSLHR-L-15-0243

Damschroder, L. J., Aron, D. C., Keith, R. E., Kirsh, S. R., Alexander, J. A., & Lowery, J. C. (2009). Fostering implementation of health services research findings into practice: A consolidated framework for advancing implementation science. *Implementation Research, 4,* 1–15.

Deshpande, P. R., Rajan, S., Sudeepthi, B. L., & Nazir, C. P. A. (2011). Patient-reported outcomes: A new era in clinical research. *Perspectives in Clinical Research, 2*(4), 137–144. doi:10.4103/2229-348586879

Dodd, B. (2007). Evidence-based practice and speech-language pathology: Strengths, weaknesses, opportunities and threats. *Folia Phoniatrica et Logopaedica, 59,* 118–129. doi:10.1159/000101770

Dollaghan, C. A. (2007). *The handbook for evidence-based practice in communication disorders.* Baltimore, MD: Paul Brookes.

Douglas, N. F., Campbell, W. N., & Hinckley, J. J. (2015). Implementation science: Buzzword or game changer? *Journal of Speech, Language & Hearing Research, 58*(6), S1827–S1836.

Doyle, P., McNeil, M., Hula, W., & Mikolic, J. (2003). The Burden of Stroke Scale (BOSS): Validating patient-reported communication difficulty and associated psychological distress in stroke survivors. *Aphasiology, 17*(3), 291–304. doi:10.1080/729255459

Dubouloz, C., Egan, M., Vallerand, J., & von Zweek, C. (1999). Occupational therapists' perceptions of evidence-based practice. *The American Journal of Occupational Therapy, 53*(5), 445–453. doi:10.5014/ajot.53.5.445

Duke University Medical Center-University of North Carolina (DU-UNC). (2016). Introduction to evidence-based practice. Retrieved from http://guides.mclibrary.duke.edu/ebmtutorial

Eadie, T. L., Yorkston, K. M., Klasner, E. R., Dudgeon, B. J., Deitz, J. C., Baylor, C. R., . . . Amtmann, D. (2006). Measuring communicative participation: A review of self-report instruments in speech-language pathology. *American Journal of Speech-Language Pathology, 15*(4), 307–320. doi:10.1044/1058-0360(2006/030)

Ebell, M. H., Siwek, J., Weiss, B. D., Woolf, S. H., Susman, J., Ewigman, B., & Bowman, M. (2004). Strength of recommendation taxonomy (SORT): A patient-centered approach to grading evidence in the medical literature. *Journal of the American Board of Family Medicine, 17*(1), 59–67. doi:10.3122/jabfm.17.1.59

Epstein, I., & Blumenfield, S. (2001). *Clinical data-mining in practice-based research: Social work in hospital settings.* New York and London: Routledge.

Epstein, I., & Tripodi, T. (1977). *Research techniques for program planning, monitoring, and evaluation.* New York: Columbia University Press.

Evans, D. (2003). Hierarchy of evidence: A framework for ranking evidence evaluating healthcare interventions. *Journal of Clinical Nursing, 12*(1), 77–84. doi:10.1046/j.1365-2702.2003.00662.x

Evidence-Based Medicine Working Group. (1992). Evidence-based medicine. A new approach to teaching the practice of medicine. *Journal of the American Medical Association, 268*, 2420–2425.

Fanning, J. L., & Lemoncello, R. (2010, October). Evidence-based practice and practice-based evidence in 2010: Declaring all clinicians as scientists. Presentation to the Oregon Speech-Language-Hearing Association (OSHA) annual meeting, Vancouver, WA.

Fayer, P. M., & Machin, D. (2007). *Scores and measurements: Validity, reliability, sensitivity, in quality of life: The assessment, analysis and interpretation of patient-reported outcomes.* Chichester, UK: John Wiley & Sons, Ltd.

Fixsen, D. L., Naoom, S. F., Blase, K. A., Friedman, R. M., & Wallace, F. (2005). *Implementation research: A synthesis of the literature.* Tampa, FL: University of South Florida, Louis de la Parte Florida Mental Health Institute, The National Implementation of Research Network (FMHI Publication #231).

Frankham, J. (2009). Partnership research: A review of approaches and challenges in conducting research in partnership with service users. *ESRC National Centre for Research Methods,* (NCRM/013).

French, J., & Gronseth, G. (2008). Lost in a jungle of evidence. We need a compass. *Neurology, 71,* 1634–1638.

Gassaway, J., Horn, S. D., DeJong, G., Smout, R. J., Clark, C., & James, R. (2005). Applying the clinical practice improvement approach, to stroke rehabilitation: Methods used and baseline results. *Archives of Physical Medicine and Rehabilitation, 86*(12), 16–33. doi:10.1016/j.apmr.2005.08.114

Gillam, S. L., & Gillam, R. B. (2008). Teaching graduate students to make evidence-based intervention decisions. *Topics in Language Disorders, 28*(3), 212–228.

Godecke, E., Ciccone, N. A., Granger, A. S., Rai, T., West, D., Cream, A., . . . Hankey, G. J. (2014). A comparison of aphasia therapy outcomes before and after a very early rehabilitation programme following stroke. *International Journal of Language and Communication Disorders, 49*(2), 149–161. doi:10.1111/1460-6984.12074

Grawburg, M., Howe, T., Worrall, L., & Scarinci, N. (2012). A systematic review of the positive outcomes for family members of people with aphasia. *Evidence-Based Communication Assessment and Intervention, 6,* 135–149. doi:10.1080/17489539.2012.739383

Greer, N., Mosser, G., Logan, G., & Halaas, G. W. (2000). A practical approach to evidence grading. *The Joint Commission Journal on Quality Improvement, 26*(12), 700–712.

Harbour, R., & Miller, J. (2001). A new system for grading recommendations in evidence based guidelines. *British Medical Journal, 323*, 334–336.

Higgins, J. P., & Green, S. (Eds.). (2011). *Cochrane handbook for systematic reviews of interventions.* Version 5.1.0 [updated March 2011]. The Cochrane Collaboration.

Hinckley, J. J., Boyle, E., Lombard, D., & Bartels-Tobin, L. (2014). Towards a consumer-informed research agenda for aphasia: Preliminary work. *Disability and Rehabilitation, 36*, 1042–1050.

Horn, S. D., & Gassaway, J. (2007). Practice-based evidence study design for comparative effectiveness research. *Medical Care, 45*(10), 50–57. doi:10.1097/MLR.0b013e318070c07b

Huang, X., Lin, J., & Demner-Fushman, D. (2006). Evaluation of PICO as a knowledge representation for clinical questions (pp. 359–363). *American Medical Information Association Symposium,* University of Maryland.

Hula, W. D., Doyle, P. J., Stone, C. A., Austermann Hula, S. N., Kellough, S., Wambaugh, J. L., . . . St. Jacque, A. (2015). The Aphasia Communication Outcome Measure (ACOM): Dimensionality, item bank calibration, and initial validation. *Journal of Speech, Language, and Hearing Research, 58*(3), 906–919. doi:10.1044/2015_JSLHR-L-14-0235

Irwin, B. (2012). Patient-reported outcome measures in aphasia. *Perspectives on Neurophysiology and Neurogenic Speech and Language Disorders, 22*, 160–166. doi:10.1044/nnsld22.4.160

Isaacs, M. R., Huang, L. N., Hernandez, M., & Echo-Hawk, H. (2005). The road to evidence: The intersection of evidence-based practices and cultural competence in children's mental health. *Report of the National Alliance of Multi-ethnic Behavioral Health Associations.* Washington, DC: National Alliance of Multi-ethnic behavioral health associations.

Kazdin, A. E. (1977). Artifact, bias, and complexity of assessment: The ABCs of reliability. *Journal of Applied Behavior Analysis, 10*(1), 141–150. doi:10.1901/jaba.1977.10-141

Kendall, D. L., Oelke, M., Brookshire, C. E., & Nadeau, S. E. (2015). The influence of phonomotor treatment on word retrieval abilities in 26 individuals with chronic aphasia: An open trial. *Journal of Speech-Language-Hearing Research, 58*, 798–812. doi:10.1044/2015_JSLHR-L-14-0131

Kent, R. D. (1990). Fragmentation of clinical service and clinical science in communicative disorders. *National Student Speech-Language-Hearing Association Journal, 17*, 4–16.

Kertesz, A. (2006). *Western Aphasia Battery-Revised.* San Antonio, TX: Pearson.

Knowledge Translation Clearinghouse. (2016). Introduction to EBM. Canadian Institutes of Health Research. Retrieved from http://ktclearinghouse.ca/cebm/intro/whatisebm

Leeman, J., & Sandelowski, M. (2012). Practice-based evidence and qualitative inquiry. *Journal of Nursing Scholarship, 44*(2), 171–179. doi:10.1111/j.1547-5069.2012.01449.x

Lemoncello, R., & Ness, B. (2013). Evidence-based practice & practice-based evidence applied to adult, medical speech pathology. *Perspectives on Gerontology, 18*(1), 14–26. doi:10.1044/gero18.1.14

Leonard, C., Rochon, E., & Laird, L. (2008). Treating naming impairments in aphasia: Findings from phonological components analysis treatment. *Aphasiology, 22*(9), 923–947. doi:10.1080/02687030701831474

Lieberman, R., Zubritsky, C., Martinez, K., Massey, O., Fisher, S., Kramer, T., . . . Obrochta, C. (2010). *Issue brief: Using practical-based evidence to complement evidence-based practice in children's mental health.* Atlanta: ICF Macro, Outcomes Roundtable for Children and Families.

Lof, G. L. (2011). Science-based practice and the speech-language pathologist. *International Journal of Speech-Language Pathology, 13*(3), 189–196. doi:10.3109/17549507.2011.528801

Lum, C. (2002). *Scientific thinking in speech and language therapy.* Mahwah, NJ: Lawrence Erlbaum Associates.

Maas, E., Robin, D., Hula, S. N. A., Freedman, S., Wulf, G., Ballard, K., & Schmidt, R. A. (2008). Principles of motor learning in treatment of motor speech disorders. *American Journal of Speech-Language Pathology, 17,* 277–298.

Magasi, S., & Heinemann, A. W. (2009). Integrating stakeholder perspectives in outcome measurement. *Neuropsychological Rehabilitation, 19,* 928–940.

Majid, S., Foo, S., Luyt, B., Zhang, X., Theng, Y., Chang, Y., & Mokhtar, I. A. (2011). Adopting evidence-based practice in clinical decision making: Nurses' perceptions, knowledge, and barriers. *Journal of the Medical Library Association, 99*(3), 229–236. doi:10.3163/1536-5050.99.3.010

Margison, F. R., Barkham, M., Evans, C., McGrath, G., Clark, J. M., Audin, K., & Connell, J. (2000). Measurement and psychotherapy. Evidence-based practice and practice-based evidence. *British Journal of Psychiatry, 177,* 123–130.

McDonald, L. (2001). Florence Nightingale and the early origins of evidence-based nursing. *Evidence Based Nursing, 4,* 68–69.

McNamara, J. R., & MacDonough, T. S. (1972). Some methodological considerations in the design and implementation of behavior therapy research. *Behavior Therapy, 3,* 361–378.

Meline, T. (2010). *A research primer for communication sciences and disorders.* Boston, MA: Pearson.

Melnyk, B. M., Fineout-Overholt, E., Stillwell, S. B., & Williamson, K. M. (2010). Evidence-based practice: Step by step: The seven steps of evidence-based practice. *American Journal of Nursing, 10,* 51–53.

Metcalfe, C., Lewin, R., Wisher, S., Perry, S., Bannigan, K., & Moffett, J. K. (2001). Barriers to implementing the evidence base in four NHS therapies. *Physiotherapy, 87*(8), 433–441.

Moher, D., Liberati, A., Tetzlaff, J., Altman, D. G., & the PRISMA Group. (2009). Preferred reporting items for systematic reviews and meta-analysis: The PRISMA statement. *Annals of Internal Medicine, 151*(4), 264–269.

Mullen, E. J., & Streiner, D. L. (2004). The evidence for and against evidence-based practice. *Brief Treatment and Crisis Intervention, 4,* 111–121.

Nail-Chiwetalu, B., & Bernstein Ratner, N. (2007). An assessment of the information-seeking abilities and needs of practicing speech-language pathologists. *Journal of the Medical Library Association, 95*(2), 182–188. doi:10.3163/1536-5050.95.2.182

NIH Fogarty International Center. (2016). Implementation science information and resources. Retrieved from http://www.fic.nih.gov/researchtopics/pages/implementationscience.aspx

Olswang, L. B., & Prelock, P. A. (2015). Bridging the gap between research and practice: Implementation science. *Journal of Speech, Language, and Hearing Research, 58,* S1818–S1826. doi:10.1044/2015_JSLHR-L-14-0305

Patient-Reported Outcomes Measurement Information System (PROMIS®). (2016). Retrieved from http://www.nihpromis.org/about/overview

Paul, D. R., Frattali, C. M., Holland, A. L., Thompson, C. K., Caperton, C. J., & Slater, S. C. (2004). *Quality of Communicating Life (ASHA-QCL) scale.* Rockville, MD: American Speech-Language-Hearing Association.

Pearce, K. A., Love, M. M., Barron, M. A., Matheny, S. C., & Mahfoud, Z. (2004). How and why to study the practice content of a practice-based research network. *Annals of Family Medicine, 2*(5), 425–428.

Petticrew, M., & Roberts, H. (2003). Evidence, hierarchies, and typologies: Horses for courses. *Journal of Epidemiology and Community Health, 57,* 527–529. doi:10.1136/jech.57.7.527

Rehabilitation Institute of Chicago. (2007). Community participation indicators. Retrieved from http://www.ric.org/research/research-centers--programs/cror/publications/cpi/

Reisch, J. S., Tyson, J. E., & Mize, S. G. (1989). Aid to the evaluation of therapeutic studies. *Pediatrics, 84*(5), 815–824.

Resnick, B. (1998). Efficacy beliefs in geriatric rehabilitation. *Journal of Gerontology Nursing, 24,* 33–44.

Richardson, J. D., Dalton, S. G. H., Shafer, J., & Patterson, J. P. (in press). Assessment fidelity in aphasia research. *American Journal of Speech-Language Pathology.*

Rigney, D. Y. (2014). *Pilot study of crowdsourcing evidence-based practice research for adults with aphasia.* (Unpublished doctoral dissertation). University of Texas, Austin, TX.

Robey, R. R. (1998). A meta-analysis of clinical outcomes in the treatment of aphasia. *Journal of Speech, Language, and Hearing Research, 41,* 172–187.

Robey, R. R. (2004). A five-phase model for clinical-outcome research. *Journal of Communication Disorders, 37,* 401–411. doi:10.1016/j.comdis.204.04.003

Robey, R. (2011). Treatment effectiveness and evidence-based practice. In L. L. Lapointe (Ed.), *Aphasia and related neurogenic language disorders* (pp. 197–210). New York, NY: Thieme.

Robey, R. R., & Schultz, M. C. (1998). A model for conducting clinical-outcome research: An adaptation of the standard protocol for use in aphasiology. *Aphasiology, 12,* 787–810. doi:10.1080/02687039808249573

Rogers, W. A. (2004). Evidence based medicine and justice: A framework for looking at the impact of EBM upon vulnerable or disadvantaged groups. *Journal of Medical Ethics, 30*(2), 141–145. doi:10.1136/jme.2003.007062

Rose, M. L., Raymer, A. M., Lanyon, L. F., & Attard, M. C. (2013). A systematic review of gesture treatments for post-stroke aphasia. *Aphasiology, 9,* 1090–1127.

Sackett, D. L., Rosenberg, W. M., Gray, J. A., Haynes, R. B., & Richardson, W. S. (1996). Evidence based medicine: What it is and what it isn't. *British Medical Journal, 312,* 71–72.

Sacks, H. S., Reitman, D., Pagano, D., & Kupelnick, B. (1996). Meta-analysis: An update. *The Mount Sinai Journal of Medicine, 63*(3/4), 216–224.

Schardt, C., Adams, M. B., Owens, T., Keitz, S., & Fontelo, P. (2007). Utilization of the PICO framework to improve searching PubMed for clinical questions. *BMC Medical Informatics and Decision Making, 7,* 1–6. doi:10.1186/1472-6947-7-16

Sidman, M. (1960). *Tactics of scientific research: Evaluating experimental design in psychology.* New York: Basic Books.

Simmons-Mackie, N., Raymer, A., Armstrong, E., Holland, A., & Cherney, L. (2010). Communication partner training in aphasia: A systematic review. *Archives of Physical Medicine and Rehabilitation, 91,* 1818–1837.

Simmons-Mackie, N., Raymer, A. M., & Cherney, L. (2016, May). Communication partner training in aphasia: An updated systematic review. Presentation to the Clinical Aphasiology Conference, Charlottesville, NC.

Smith, G. A. (1986). Observer drift: A drifting definition. *The Behavior Analyst, 9*(1), 127–128.

Sohlberg, M. M., Kucheria, P., Fickas, S., & Wade, S. L. (2015). Developing brain injury interventions on both ends of the treatment continuum depends upon early research partnerships and feasibility studies. *Journal of Speech-Language-Hearing Research, 58*(6), S1864-S1870. doi:10.1044/2015_JSLHR-L-15-0150

Steinberg, E. P., & Luce, B. R. (2005). Evidence based? Caveat emptor! *Health Affairs, 24*(1), 80–92. doi:10.1377/hlthaff.24.1.80

Straus, S. E., & McAlister, F. A. (2000). Evidence-based medicine: A commentary on common criticisms. *Canadian Medical Association Journal, 163*(7), 837–841.

Swan, M. (2012). Crowdsourced health research studies: An important emerging complement to clinical trials in the public health research ecosystem. *Journal of Medical Internet Research 14*(2), e46.

Swinburn, K., & Byng, S. (2006). *The communication disability profile*. London: Connect Press.

Tate, R. L., McDonald, S., Perdices, M., Togher, L., Schultz, R., & Savage, S. (2008). Rating the methodological quality of single-subject designs and n-of-1 trials: Introducing the single-case experimental design (SCED) scale. *Neuropsychological Rehabilitation: An International Journal, 18*(4), 385–401. doi:10.1080/09602010802009201

Tate, R. L., Perdices, M., Rosenkoetter, U., Shadish, W., Vohra, S., Barlow, D. H., & Wilson, B. (2016). The single-case-reporting guideline in behavioral interventions (SCRIBE) 2016 statement. *Aphasiology, 30*(7), 862–876. doi:10.1080/02687038.2016.1178022

Tate, R. L., Rosenkoetter, U., Togher, L., Horner, R., Barlow, D. H., Sampson, M., . . . Shamseer, L. (2016). The single-case reporting guideline in behavioural interventions (SCRIBE) 2016: Explanation and elaboration. *Archives of Scientific Psychology, 4*, 10–31.

The Patient-Reported Outcomes (PRO) Consortium. (2009). Retrieved from http://www.fda.gov /AboutFDA/PartnershipsCollaborations/PublicPrivatePartnershipProgram/ucm231129.htm

van Hees, S., Angwin, A., McMahon, K., & Copland, D. (2013). A comparison of semantic feature analysis and phonological components analysis for the treatment of naming impairments in aphasia. *Neuropsychological Rehabilitation, 23*(1), 102–132. doi:10.1080/09602011.2012.726201.

Wambaugh, J. L. (2007). The evidence-based practice and practice-based evidence nexus. *Perspectives on Neurophysiology and Neurogenic Speech and Language Disorders, 17*, 14–18. doi:10.1044 /nnsld17.1.14

Westfall, J. M., Fagnan, L. J., Handley, M., Salsberg, J., McGinnis, P., Zittleman, L. K., & Macaulay, A. C. (2009). Practice-based research is community engagement. *Journal of the American Board of Family Medicine, 22*(4), 423–427. doi:10.3122/jabfm.2009.04.090105

Westfall, J. M., Mold, J., & Fagnan, L. (2007). Practice-based research—"blue highways" on the NIH roadmap. *Journal of the American Medical Association, 297*(4), 403–406.

Williams, D. M., & Rhodes, R. E. (2014). The confounded self-efficacy construct: Conceptual analysis and recommendations for future research. *Health Psychology Review, 2*, 113–128. doi:10.1080 /17437199.2014.941998

Zipoli, R. P., & Kennedy, M. (2005). Evidence-based practice among speech-language pathologists: Attitudes, utilization, and barriers. *American Journal of Speech-Language Pathology, 14*(3), 208–220.

Understanding Motivation in Aphasia Rehabilitation

Mike Biel
Leslie Nitta
Catherine Jackson

INTRODUCTION

CASE ILLUSTRATION: MR. SMITH—EPISODE 1

Mr. Smith is a 70-year-old gentleman who had a left hemisphere stroke result-ing in moderate Broca's aphasia and mild to moderate apraxia of speech. After a brief course of acute rehabilitation, he was discharged home and continued to receive therapy as an outpatient. After 3 months of outpatient treatment, he was discharged from therapy because of lack of improvement and poor motivation. Encouraged by his wife, Mr. Smith came to our clinic for treatment 1 year later. During a phone conversation, his former clinician stated that she was puzzled by his lack of motivation. She stated that, while he appeared to be engaged in treat-ment early on and made some small improvements, he became progressively less adherent to his home practice assignments despite her attempts to encourage him or in response to changes she made to the treatment plan. During his first visit to our clinic, Mr. Smith acknowledged that he was less consistent with his home practice as time went on, but he was unsure why this was so. His wife believed it was because he was not improving as quickly as he had hoped.

The scenario above is not uncommon. Most clinicians, at one time or another, struggle with how to motivate their patients, particularly when improvements are slow and difficult to appreciate. Although there is a substantial body of evidence supporting the effectiveness of aphasia treatments, often clients do not experience the degree of improvement that these treatments seem to promise. Why is this so? We know that many factors influence the nature and extent of recovery and rehabilitation success, among them patient motivation. In our experience, when clinicians describe why a client is not making progress, it is not uncommon for poor motivation to be one of the reasons. Qualitative studies investigating the beliefs of rehabilitation professionals support this observation (Kaufmann & Becker, 1986; Maclean, Pound, Wolfe, & Rudd, 2002).

While some authors have acknowledged the importance of motivation during aphasia rehabilitation, exploration of this topic has, in general, been brief and/or not based upon theories of motivation (e.g., Eisenson, 1949; Fox, Sohlberg, & Fried-Oken, 2001; Haley, Womack, Helm-Estabrooks, Lovette, & Goff, 2013; Hersh, Worrall, Howe, Sherratt, & Davidson, 2012; Hopper & Holland, 2005). A notable exception is Wepman (1953) who believed that motivation was one of the main factors affecting treatment outcomes and who incorporated understanding and management of motivation into his model of aphasia treatment and recovery. Wepman's insights about the role of motivation appear to have been primarily guided by his intuitive perceptions and clinical experience. His focus on personally relevant goals and improving social and environmental supports for patients can be seen in most modern, theory-driven approaches to improving motivation. For Wepman, the rehabilitation process started with the clinician attempting to understand the patient's perspective and what motivated him or her.

Despite acknowledgement of the importance of motivation to the rehabilitation enterprise, to the best of our knowledge, the topic of motivation has not been the focus of research or discussion in the aphasia literature. There is, however, evidence that motivation plays a role in the treatment decisions that clinicians make. For example, Mackenzie et al. (1993) surveyed clinicians who treated adults with aphasia. Results of the survey showed that approximately 90% of reporting clinicians used "low motivation" as the most commonly reported discharge criterion, second only to "plateau reached." In another survey of clinicians, "low interest/motivation" was the most common reason for not prescribing home practice to a person with aphasia (PWA; Enderby & Petheram, 1992).

One of the reasons we decided to investigate this topic was the realization that, having no formal training in theories of motivation, we relied on our intuition when judging the motivation of our clients. This led us to wonder whether we could use a theoretical and evidence-based approach to assessing and managing our clients' motivation, much as we do when planning treatment for their language impairments. The intent of this chapter is to serve as an introduction to basic concepts of motivation and to illustrate how they may be applied in aphasia rehabilitation. It is not meant to be a comprehensive or critical review of theories of motivation and their clinical application, but rather it is intended as a springboard to the systematic application of theory and principles to the clinical enterprise.

WHAT IS MOTIVATION?

The concept of motivation has been criticized for being overly subjective, ill-defined, and of limited clinical utility (Drieschner, Lammers, & van der Staak, 2004; King & Barrowclough, 1989; Maclean & Pound, 2000; Maclean et al., 2002). This may be due to the broad range of behaviors associated with motivation and the innumerable variables that influence it. As Gorman (2004) noted, "In many ways the study of motivation is the study of psychology itself. It is concerned with explaining all forms of behavior" (p. 1). The description provided by Eccles and Wigfield (2002) is more relevant to clinical practice. They noted that modern theories of motivation tend to focus on "the relation of beliefs, values, and goals with action" (p. 110).

Despite the wide variety of definitions and conceptions of motivation, two features are highlighted in most authors' accounts (Drieschner et al., 2004). First, motivation is a force, energy, or drive that enables and sustains action. Second, this energy is directed in a specific way (e.g., toward a goal). Ryan and Deci (2000a) captured these two aspects in their succinct definition of motivation: "To be motivated means to be moved to do something" (p. 54).

Terms such as "force" or "drive" used to describe motivation suggest that its potential to initiate and sustain behavior is related to its strength. This belief is reflected in many theories of motivation (e.g., Bandura, 1997; Baumeister & Vohs, 2007) in which the intensity of motivation is considered the prime determiner of goal-directed behavior. That is, the more highly motivated patients are, the more likely it is that they will initiate and sustain goal-directed behaviors. The rehabilitation literature and clinicians' reports often echo this conception when qualifiers describe motivation, stating, for example, that a PWA is "highly motivated" or has "poor motivation." However, motivation can also be thought of qualitatively, with its effects determined as much by its nature as by its strength. Self-determination theory (SDT) takes this approach, proposing types of motivation that are based on the reasons that cause people to act (Deci & Ryan, 2008). In the next section, we will discuss these types of motivation and how motivation is promoted within SDT.

SELF-DETERMINATION THEORY

CASE ILLUSTRATION: MR. SMITH—EPISODE 2

During Mr. Smith's previous engagement in therapy, the main goal of treatment was to improve his ability to discuss the events of the day with his wife when she returned home from work. Mrs. Smith acknowledged that she recommended this goal partly from her desires and partly because Mr. Smith did not express a preference. When we asked Mr. Smith to rate the importance of this goal on a scale of 0 to 100, he rated it a "60." He rated the importance of improving his overall communication skills a "90." Noticing the difference in scores, and to encourage Mr. Smith to talk about the reasons he felt that improving his general communication ability was important, we asked him why he did not choose a lower rating, such as a 70. This form of questioning is common in motivational interviewing (MI; Miller & Rollnick, 2012,) and it tends to promote "change talk" (i.e., the reasons a person wishes to make a positive change or desires to accomplish a goal). Mr. Smith provided us with a few reasons—but one caught our attention more than the others. His face and the tone of his voice changed when he talked about how his difficulty speaking was causing him to lose his connection to his 10-year-old grandson. Later on, we learned more about his relationship with his grandson and the nature and depth of his concerns. Overall, our conversations with Mr. Smith revealed an accumulation of doubts about his ability to maintain relationships with people he cared about, the perception of a life that had shrunk in scope, and conflicted feelings about his increased dependence on others.

Broadly speaking, SDT categorizes motivation into three states/types: autonomous motivation, controlled motivation, and amotivation (Deci & Ryan, 2008). These motivational states and their subtypes lie on a continuum that is based on how self-determined they are (see **TABLE 12.1**). At one end of the continuum lie the *autonomous* forms of motivation, which are characterized by a sense of choice, volition, and self-endorsed reasons for action or behavioral regulation. The prototypical form of autonomous motivation is *intrinsic* motivation, a

TABLE 12.1 The self-determination continuum.

Type of Motivation	Amotivation	Controlled Motivation		Autonomous Motivation		
Type of Motivation		Extrinsic Motivation				Intrinsic Motivation
Type of Motivation/ Regulatory Style	Non-regulation	External regulation	Introjected regulation	Identified regulation	Integrated regulation	Intrinsic regulation
Perceived Locus of Causality	Impersonal	External	Somewhat external	Somewhat internal	Internal	Internal
Relevant Regulatory Processes	Non-intentional Non-valuing Incompetence Lack of Control	Compliance External rewards and punishments	Self-control Ego involvement Internal rewards and punishments	Personal importance Conscious valuing	Congruence Awareness Synthesis with self	Interest Enjoyment Inherent Satisfaction

Adapted from Ryan & Deci, 2000b.
Permission info at http://www.apa.org/about/contact/copyright/index.aspx.

state in which we are motivated to engage in an activity because the activity itself is enjoyable, interesting, and/or satisfies the need to feel competent and autonomous/self-determined. Attempting to increase a patient's engagement in therapy by offering a choice of which tasks to perform, including personally interesting content and providing optimally challenging tasks, are examples of common clinical practices that would be expected to promote intrinsic motivation. Intrinsic motivation is associated with a number of positive learning outcomes, such as deeper processing of information, greater engagement in learning activities, and more creativity (Vansteenkiste, Simons, Lens, Sheldon, & Deci, 2004). In *controlled* forms of motivation, the reasons for acting are external to the core self. Experientially, controlled forms of motivation are characterized by feeling pressured or coerced. As we describe in more detail later, the feeling of external control can emanate from the perceived demands placed on us by others or from demands that we place on ourselves. Controlled forms of motivation are thus associated with *extrinsic* motivation. In contrast to intrinsic motivation, in which the activity is inherently motivating, the motivating force in extrinsic motivation is outside, or separable from, the activity (e.g., rewards or threats of punishments are common extrinsic motivators). Finally, in the non–self-determined, amotivational state, individuals do not have the intention to act—they might abstain from treatment or simply participate out of politeness. *Amotivation* can occur when clients do not believe they are capable of performing the steps necessary to achieve a rehabilitation goal, do not believe their actions will result in achieving the goal, or do not value the goal (Ryan & Deci, 2000a).

In earlier theorizing about motivation (e.g., deCharms, 1968), intrinsic and extrinsic motivation were seen as dichotomous. Intrinsic motivation was associated with autonomously regulated behavior (i.e., freely choosing whether or not to engage in an activity), whereas extrinsic motivation was assumed to be controlling (i.e., engaging in an activity because one feels pressured to do so). This distinction did not take into consideration the fact that adults often engage in behaviors autonomously that are not necessarily intrinsically interesting or enjoyable, but represent an important value (e.g., doing one's duty) or lead to a valuable goal (Vansteenkiste, Niemiec, & Soenens, 2010). For example, health-related behaviors (e.g., abstaining from eating unhealthy foods) may not be inherently pleasurable, but people adopt them because the potential outcomes are personally significant (Ng et al., 2012; Ryan, Lynch, Vansteenkiste, & Deci, 2011).

According to SDT, extrinsic motivators, such as when patients feel the need to comply with the values, attitudes, beliefs, and behavioral regulations promoted by their clinicians, can be internalized, or "taken in," and integrated into the self to varying degrees (Deci & Ryan, 2000). The more internalized and integrated the value or regulation, the more autonomous/self-determined the motivation surrounding it. The most controlling and non–self-determined form of extrinsic motivation is *external regulation*. In this state, the motivating force is completely external and the patient's involvement in therapy is often contingent on his or her expectation of external punishments or rewards. For example, a patient may feel pressured to participate in therapy to avoid being discharged to a less desirable setting such as a nursing home or to ensure that he or she will continue to get careful, attentive care from the nurses and doctors. Patient behaviors that are dependent on these external contingencies tend to cease if the patient believes that the contingencies are no longer in effect (Deci & Ryan, 2000). For example, a patient who feels controlled by his or her clinician might only practice communication strategies when the clinician is present. Moving along the continuum, when extrinsic motives are partially internalized (i.e., taken in but not truly accepted as one's own), they can continue to exert a controlling influence and are often experienced internally in the form of "should" (e.g., I should do my home practice; I should be interested in therapy; Ryan et al., 2011). This type of extrinsic motivation is called *introjected regulation*. As in external regulation, behaviors are controlled by contingent consequences, but the consequences are self-imposed and typically affect feelings of self-worth (Deci & Ryan, 2000). For example, patients may experience pride or guilt/shame, depending on whether or not they adhere to their introjected *should* behaviors. Both external regulation and introjected regulation fall under the category of *controlled forms of motivation* (see Table 12.1).

The next two types of extrinsic motivation, *identified regulation* and *integrated regulation*, are *autonomous forms of motivation*. If a patient understands the rationale for adopting a behavior or committing to a goal, sees the value in it, and willingly subscribes to what is recommended, then the patient is said to be engaged in *identified regulation* (Deci & Ryan, 2000). Motivation is still extrinsic, because the patient's behavior is being driven by instrumental reasons (e.g., the attainment of specific speech goals) rather than out of the spontaneous enjoyment/satisfaction derived from therapy (i.e., intrinsic motivation). The transition on the SDT motivation continuum from introjected regulation to identified regulation can be characterized by the difference between a patient engaging in treatment because he or she *should* and willingly engaging in treatment because he or she understands and values the process and the potential outcome. The final, and most autonomous, form of extrinsic motivation is *integrated regulation*. This form of motivation arises when a treatment approach and associated values resonate with, and are integrated into, a patient's self-identity (Deci & Ryan, 1985). For example, this form of motivation is often evident in PWA who have completed individual therapy but continue to attend group therapy because patiently continuing to practice their communication skills and supporting other PWA have become part of who they are.

Intrinsic motivation and the most autonomous form of extrinsic motivation, integrated regulation, share important characteristics in that they both represent a total involvement of the self. Although intrinsic motivation is the ideal motivational state, all forms of autonomous motivation are associated with positive behavioral outcomes and, in the SDT literature, the different forms of autonomous motivation are sometimes combined into a composite measurement (Ryan & Deci, 2000b). Finally, SDT views motivation as a dynamic state. Different types of motivation may coexist for an activity (e.g., a mixture of an introjected "should" feeling for doing today's home practice but also an intrinsic interest in the practice task). From a clinical standpoint, what is most important is which form of motivation is predominant.

Promoting Autonomous Forms of Motivation

SDT is based on an organismic theoretical perspective; as such, it proposes that humans have an innate tendency to develop and grow. This desire to function more competently and with more self-determination is facilitated through a natural process called *internalization*, "the process through which an individual acquires an attitude, belief, or behavioral regulation and progressively transforms it into a personal value, goal, or organization" (Deci & Ryan, 1985, p. 130). Although the tendency to internalize and integrate external values and behaviors is innate, this process can be supported or thwarted by the social environment. During rehabilitation, clinicians may recommend different goals of treatment, communication strategies, and attitudes or beliefs to adopt (e.g., an attitude of patience and the belief that persistent effort will yield meaningful results). From an SDT perspective, whether or not patients internalize (i.e., genuinely adopt and self-endorse) our recommendations, and the degree to which they integrate these recommendations into their own sense of self, can be influenced by whether clinicians support three innate psychological needs proposed by SDT: *autonomy* (to act volitionally, to self-endorse one's actions), *competence* (to feel capable of affecting the outcomes of one's choosing), and *relatedness* (to feel a close connection with others) (Deci & Ryan, 2000; Sheldon, Elliot, Kim, & Kasser; 2001). Essentially, patients are more likely to adopt behaviors and values when they feel they have a choice in doing so (autonomy), they feel that the behavior or value will increase their experience of confidence in their capacity to affect outcomes (competence), and they receive help from clinicians they believe care about them unconditionally (relatedness). Aphasia rehabilitation may be unique in the rehabilitation domain, because satisfaction of these psychological needs is intimately tied to communication, which also happens to be the impaired function and focus of treatment. Depending on the degree of the aphasia, patients may have difficulty expressing their choices, demonstrating their competency, and establishing a relationship with their clinician. As such, having the skill to facilitate successful communication with PWA is important when assessing and promoting motivation. Before returning to the discussion of autonomy, competence, and relatedness, a word about communication is in order.

Supported Communication and Motivational Interviewing

Kagan (1998) provided a notable example of the benefit of learning how to improve communication with PWA. In her study, medical students who received training in supported conversation for adults with aphasia (SCA) demonstrated an improved ability to communicate with PWA, to establish rapport, and to reveal and acknowledge competency. We experienced similar improvements after learning SCA, even though we were licensed clinicians with some experience prior to training.

Because approaches such as SCA strive to improve communication with PWA, these approaches may naturally support a feeling of autonomy, competency, and relatedness. Clinicians can provide further support by adopting techniques and principles from motivational interviewing (MI). According to Miller and Rollnick (2012), MI is "a collaborative, goal-oriented style of communication with particular attention to the language of change. It is designed to strengthen personal motivation for and commitment to a specific goal by eliciting and exploring the person's own reasons for change within an atmosphere of acceptance and compassion" (p. 29).

MI is in conceptual harmony with SDT, has informed many SDT-based clinical interventions (Markland, Ryan, & Tobin, 2005; Miller & Rollnick, 2012; Patrick & Williams, 2012), and has a substantial evidence base supporting its use in health care (Burke, Arkowitz, & Menchola, 2003; Dunn, Deroo, & Rivara, 2001; Hettema, Steele, & Miller, 2005; Lundahl, Kunz, Brownell, Tollefson, & Burke, 2010). MI also provides a more plentiful and detailed description of clinical methods than one finds in the SDT literature. MI is a therapeutic approach, not a theory of motivation. It developed out of clinical experience in addiction counseling and has been influenced by a number of different theories (e.g., Bem, 1967; Festinger, 1957) and schools of psychotherapy, most notably Carl Roger's client-centered approach to counseling (1959). MI and SDT complement each other: SDT provides a theoretical framework for understanding MI and its outcomes; MI provides a detailed description for how to apply SDT-related concepts. An example of this integration was provided by a recent randomized controlled study comparing a standard weight-loss program with one that included MI (Gourlan, Sarrazin, & Trouilloud, 2013). The authors predicted that the addition of MI would result in important changes in SDT constructs, such as positive changes in subjects' perceived autonomy support and an increase in motivation, particularly autonomous forms of motivation. These predictions were confirmed after six MI sessions distributed over 6 months.

A core belief in MI, and one that is implicit in SDT, is that it is not the duty of the clinician to motivate patients or convince them to adopt a behavior. This stance falls under one of the principles of MI, which is to avoid the *righting reflex* (Miller & Rollnick, 2012). The righting reflex, as its name implies, is a natural response to the suffering of others. It occurs when clinicians attempt, usually out of good intentions, to solve patients' problems for them, or to convince them that they can achieve a desired change. During aphasia rehabilitation, the righting reflex commonly manifests when patients voice doubt about their progress. In response to these doubts, clinicians may attempt to convince patients of the utility of a rehabilitation approach and the value of adhering to treatment recommendations. According to Rollnick, Miller, and Butler (2008, pp. 8–9), patients are often ambivalent about treatment. That is, for any aspect of treatment, patients may have two opposing views or beliefs. For example, Mr. Smith (see Case Illustration: Episodes 1 and 2) was ambivalent about the treatment goal in his previous rehabilitation attempt. On the one hand, he wanted to improve his ability to communicate the day's events to his wife, but on the other hand, he also confided to us that the goal represented a lack of trust in his competency—it was a means of "checking up" on him. One risk of engaging in the righting reflex is that, by adopting one side of a patient's internal debate, we inadvertently encourage patients to defend the other side of the argument. In Mr. Smith's case, his clinician's or wife's attempts to convince him of the importance of the treatment goal did not appear to be effective and may have inadvertently strengthened his resistance (Rollnick et al., 2008). A more effective approach would have been to guide Mr. Smith to explore his ambivalence, that is, to describe the reasons the goal was or was not important. When it comes to the reasons for engaging in rehabilitation, MI and SDT focus on respecting patients' autonomy and adhering to the following sentiment expressed by the 17th-century Christian philosopher Blaise Pascal (1669/2003): "People are generally better persuaded by the reasons which they themselves discovered than by those which have come into the mind of others" (p. 4).

Although no empirical studies have investigated the utility of SDT for a neurogenic rehabilitation population, it is a macro theory intended to address universal human needs and thus applicable to our discussion of patient motivation. In SDT-based intervention studies, positive outcomes that are relevant to aphasia rehabilitation include improved academic engagement (Reeve, Jang, Carrell, Jeon, & Barch, 2004), higher quality learning (Deci, Ryan, & Williams, 1996), increased goal persistence and exercise adherence (Pelletier, Fortier, Vallerand, & Briere, 2001; Russell & Bray, 2010; Teixeira, Carraça, Markland, Silva, & Ryan, 2012), and improved mental health (i.e., depression, anxiety, somatization, and quality of life) (Ng et al., 2012). There is also evidence that improving autonomous motivation in one domain of functioning generalizes to other related domains (Patrick & Williams, 2012). We turn now to the discussion of how to support the three psychological needs that promote internalization and autonomous forms of motivation.

Autonomy Support

The need for autonomy is the desire to feel that one is free to choose what one wants to do. It is important to note that autonomy, as conceptualized in SDT, is not synonymous with independence (Deci & Ryan, 2000; Sheldon et al., 2001). For example, a PWA can choose to be dependent on his spouse by freely choosing to allow his wife to speak for him on a given occasion. In the SDT literature, autonomy support typically incorporates one or more of the following elements: taking the client's perspective, providing choice, and providing a meaningful rationale for engaging in non–intrinsically motivating behaviors (Sheldon, Williams, & Joiner, 2003). The first element, *taking the client's perspective*, is a prerequisite for any needs-supporting intervention and is similar to two important MI principles: *listening with empathy*, and *understanding and exploring the client's motivation* (Miller & Rollnick, 2012).

Adopting an empathic, perspective-taking mind-set encourages clinicians to set aside their ego and attend to what the patient is communicating, both verbally and nonverbally. In the SDT literature, autonomy support is often highly correlated with satisfaction of the need for competency and relatedness. One possible explanation for this tendency is that focusing on, and acknowledging, the client's internal frame of reference leads to more accurate and personalized support for the other psychological needs (Sierens, Vansteenkiste, Goossens, Soenens, & Dochy, 2009; Vansteenkiste et al., 2010). Given the communication difficulties of the PWA, consciously adopting a perspective-taking mind-set can help reduce any misunderstandings during different phases of treatment and subsequent tension in the patient-clinician relationship (Worrall, Davidson, et al., 2010).

One method for confirming and demonstrating understanding of a patient's perspective is to use what MI calls *reflective listening* (Miller & Rollnick, 2012), a technique similar to Carl Rogers' (1959) accurate empathy approach. Reflective listening involves repeating or paraphrasing key statements made by patients with the intention of confirming or acknowledging their subjective experiences or the meaning of their statements. Reflective listening is a useful way to express empathy, demonstrate understanding of the patient's concerns, and ensure that the conversation remains patient-driven (Patrick & Williams, 2012; Resnicow & McMaster, 2012). Even occasional use of simple reflections has been found to have a positive effect on patients' sense of autonomy and satisfaction with their healthcare provider (Pollak et al., 2011). Reflective listening can be particularly useful in helping clinicians avoid what MI calls the *expert trap* (Miller & Rollnick, 2012). When consultations begin with a litany of questions designed to catalogue a patient's symptoms and complaints, this tends to reinforce the clinician's controlling role as the expert who, after gathering enough information, will have the solution to the patient's problem and will tell him or her what to do. Patients may find this approach, and a premature movement to expose impairments via formal testing, demotivating and demeaning—an exacerbation of the already existing patient-professional power imbalance (Hersh et al., 2012; Wade, 2009). At any point in the rehabilitation process, interactions that reinforce our "expert" role in a controlling manner can engender patient passivity (Simmons-Mackie & Damico, 2007).

The second element, *providing choice,* is another means of satisfying patients' need for autonomy and of fostering autonomous forms of motivation. However, choice is not always motivating. For example, providing overly difficult, complex, or important choices may be depleting to patients and diminish the motivating effects of choice (Patall, Cooper, & Robinson, 2008). Individuals facing such options, particularly if they lack confidence in their ability to make a choice, may abstain from choosing or may make a random choice (Katz & Assor, 2007). There appears to be a motivational "sweet spot" for the number of choices provided to people. In their meta-analysis of the effects of choice on intrinsic motivation in normal subjects, Patall and colleagues (2008) concluded that three to five choices may be optimal. However, we assume that, during rehabilitation, factors such as fatigue, depression, and cognitive-communicative impairments can reduce the number of optimal choices that a patient can manage. The manner in which choices are provided can also affect motivation. If clinicians overtly or covertly communicate a preference for one of the choices offered, patients may feel pressured (controlled) and the motivating effect of choice will be undermined (Patall et al., 2008).

The final element, *providing a meaningful rationale,* also supports the process of autonomous motivation. When choices are, by necessity, very limited or uninteresting, acknowledging this fact and providing a meaningful rationale for the choices is autonomy supportive and can promote autonomous forms of motivation and increased effort (Deci, Eghrari, Patrick, & Leone, 1994; Reeve, Jang, Hardre, & Omura, 2002). Take, for example, the new patient with severe aphasia who produces only recurrent nonlexical utterances. The patient has been in therapy in the past and has made no improvement toward volitional speech production, but has some writing and gesturing ability that can be capitalized on. The patient may want to continue to work on his speech, but the clinician does not believe that is a viable option, at least not in the short term, and recommends that therapy start with a focus on nonspeech methods of communication (e.g., writing, gesture, AAC). The clinician could make acceptance of the recommended therapy plan a prerequisite for accepting the patient into treatment or she could assume the expert role and attempt to convince the patient about why he should accept her plan. Both of these approaches may motivate the patient to accept the clinician's recommendations, but they do so in a way that pressures the patient, either through denial of service or by making it clear that the clinician's positive regard for the patient is contingent on his compliance. An autonomy-supportive solution to this dilemma would be to make an attempt to understand the patient's perspective and then ask permission to provide the clinician's rationale. Rationales that acknowledge patients' feelings and avoid using controlling or guilt-inducing language (e.g., "ought to," "have to," "should") have been shown to support autonomous forms of extrinsic motivation for uninteresting activities (Deci et al., 1994; Reeve et al., 2002).

Competence Support

The need for competence refers to the desire to feel effective; it does not refer to actual ability per se, but to the desire for the feeling of effectiveness (Deci & Ryan, 2000; Sheldon et al., 2001). In SDT, three factors are relevant to supporting the need for competency (Deci & Ryan, 1985). First, tasks or goals should be neither too easy nor too difficult, but should be set at an optimal level of challenge. Second, patients should get feedback about their performance, either from the task itself or from another person. Third, feedback should not be evaluative or controlling (e.g., "good, you did it just the way you should have" or "good, you are doing it just the way I want you to") but should provide objective and useful information about progress or adjustments that could be made.

Clinicians can also support the need for competency by helping patients feel more in control of the rehabilitation process. On the basis of interviews with PWA and their families, Hersh and colleagues (2012) found that, particularly in the acute stage of recovery, PWA and their families may feel overwhelmed by their situation and condition and may not feel competent to make decisions about treatment. Referring to the rehabilitation process, Hersh and colleagues noted, "clients need to be orientated as if to a new job" (p. 226). Preparing PWA and their families for rehabilitation can include orienting them to the rehabilitation setting, reviewing the rehabilitation schedule, discussing the roles of different healthcare professionals, and so forth. Discussing what the patient believes to be potential barriers to participating in rehabilitation and beginning to form plans to manage these barriers can also satisfy the need for competency in being able to meet the demands of rehabilitation (Sierens et al., 2009). Of course, the kinds of information and support needed by PWA and their families are different at different stages of recovery (Avent et al., 2005).

Relatedness Support

The need for relatedness refers to the desire to have the experience of caring for and being cared for by other people—both individuals and communities, such as aphasia therapy/support groups (Deci & Ryan, 2000; Sheldon et al., 2001). A number of aphasiologists have written about the important and unique role the patient-clinician relationship plays during rehabilitation (e.g., Hersh et al., 2012; Worrall, Davidson, et al., 2010). In a discussion of the importance of the therapeutic relationship to the motivation of PWA, Cyr-Stafford (1993) expressed her belief that a genuine therapeutic relationship can exist only in an atmosphere of trust, which is based, in part, on a clinician's ability to communicate empathy, concern, and unconditional acceptance. Cyr-Stafford states that a PWA's belief in the clinician's expertise is also a necessary component for trust to occur; however, the clinician's role is not to "spoon-feed" patients but to be a "companion" who fosters the maximum amount of autonomy during each stage of the recovery process. Cyr-Stafford's ideas about how to establish a good relationship with patients are consistent with SDT. In SDT, clinicians establish a close relationship with patients and satisfy the need for relatedness by demonstrating a sincere involvement in promoting their patients' welfare and through an unconditional positive regard and acceptance (Deci & Ryan, 1991; Roth, Assor, Niemiec, Deci, & Ryan, 2009). Although it is unlikely that clinicians regularly engage in conditional regard in blatant ways, such as when parents withhold affection from children who do not behave as desired (Roth et al., 2009), a degree of mindfulness is required to refrain from the many subtle ways, both verbal and nonverbal, that clinicians can send a PWA the message that he is only a "good" patient when he acts in prescribed ways. For example, a clinician who disapproves of a patient's behavior or is dissatisfied with a patient's perceived level of engagement may adopt a colder, more distant demeanor in response. Part of satisfying the need for relatedness is letting patients know that our positive regard toward them is secure and stable (Baumeister & Leary, 1995); we do not want them to feel that they have to sacrifice some of their autonomy to maintain the relationship.

SDT Summary and Aphasia Therapy

SDT is a macro theory that attempts to describe the innate, universal influences affecting motivation and motivated behavior. It proposes three universal psychological needs: autonomy, competence, and relatedness. The satisfaction or thwarting of these needs influences whether people perceive their motivation to be truly volitional and self-endorsed or controlled by external factors. Support for all three of these needs helps to fully nourish the innate internalizing and integrating processes that give rise to autono-mous forms of motivation. Although some patients may want clinicians to take a more controlling approach, this does not preclude supporting their needs for autonomy, competence, and relatedness. There is no significant evidence supporting a "matching hypothesis," wherein clients who appear to want to be controlled benefit from a con-trolling approach (Sheldon et al., 2003; Vansteenkiste, Lens, & Deci, 2006). Even small, seemingly inconsequential gestures toward autonomy support, such as providing choice for the order of tasks to be completed, can have a positive impact on behavior (Wulf, Freitas, & Tandy, 2014).

We believe that there is a great deal of overlap between SDT and person-centered approaches to intervention described in the aphasia literature, such as the social model (Byng & Duchan, 2005) or the life participation approach to aphasia (Chapey et al., 2008), and collaborative goal-setting approaches, such as the SMARTER goal-setting framework (Hersh et al., 2012). Difficulties establishing a sense of autonomy, competence, and relat-edness are some of the most common issues faced by PWA. To one degree or another, person-centered approaches to aphasia intervention attempt to satisfy these basic psy-chological needs. SDT, to the best of our knowledge, is the only theory of motivation to directly address autonomy, competence, and relatedness and therefore seems to be a useful approach to understanding and supporting the motivation of PWA. In the next section, we discuss other motivational constructs that are relevant to aphasia rehabilitation and that are commonly found in prominent theories of motivation and health behavior change.

MOTIVATIONAL CONSTRUCTS

In 2009, Scobbie, Wyke, and Dixon completed a systematic review of empirical studies and review papers from the rehabilitation and health self-management literature that proposed the use of theories of motivation and behavior change. Their purpose was to identify psychological constructs that could be applied to setting and achieving goals during rehabilitation. After analyzing the key constructs, clinical application, and empiri-cal evidence of these papers, they concluded that social cognitive theory (Bandura, 1997), the health action process approach (Schwarzer, Lippke, & Luszczynska, 2011), and goal-setting theory (Locke & Latham, 2002) provided the most potential for the development of their clinical framework for goal setting and action planning. Within these theories, Scobbie and colleagues (2009) identified the following psychological constructs that cli-nicians could incorporate into goal setting and treatment to enhance the motivation and participation of patients during stroke rehabilitation:

- Self-efficacy: belief in one's ability to perform actions toward achieving a goal
- Outcome expectancies: belief about what the likelihood and consequences of achieving a goal will be
- Goal attributes: characteristics of the goal, such as goal specificity and difficulty

- Action planning: specifying when, where, and how to implement action toward reaching a goal
- Coping planning: anticipating potential barriers and establishing plans to manage them
- Appraisal: assessment of performance in carrying out the plan and progress toward the goal
- Feedback: feedback about performance in carrying out the plan and progress toward the goal

In the remainder of this chapter, we focus our discussion on three of these psychological constructs: self-efficacy, outcome expectancies, and goal attributes. These constructs represent the most commonly discussed psychological/motivational constructs in the healthcare literature and in other settings, such as education and sports.

Self-Efficacy

Of the seven psychological constructs Scobbie and colleagues (2009) identified, self-efficacy is the most researched; it is a principal construct in social cognitive theory (SCT; Bandura, 1986, 1997) and it plays an important role in many current theories and models of motivation and health behavior change (Rothman & Salovey, 2007). Self-efficacy "refers to beliefs in one's capabilities to organize and execute the courses of action required to produce given levels of attainments" (Bandura, 1998, p. 624). The terms *self-efficacy*, as used in SCT, and *competence*, in SDT, are related in that both refer to a subjective sense of ability. SCT focuses on self-efficacy beliefs, which are essentially predictions about one's ability to perform specific tasks. SDT, on the other hand, focuses on the innate need for competency; that, when satisfied, leads to a positive affective experience.

In general, self-efficacy beliefs are task and situation specific. Some authors have further divided self-efficacy into *task self-efficacy*, *coping self-efficacy*, and *scheduling self-efficacy* (Kirsch, 1995; Rodgers, Wilson, Hall, Fraser, & Murray, 2008). Task self-efficacy refers to people's beliefs about their abilities to perform specific tasks in specific contexts; for example, a PWA might have high self-efficacy that he or she can name a set of pictured objects with help from the clinician but not with help from a spouse. Coping self-efficacy refers to people's beliefs in their ability to manage barriers/challenges while performing a task; for PWA, barriers/challenges might include fatigue, anxiety, time pressure, noisy environments, and so forth. In the context of aphasia rehabilitation, scheduling self-efficacy refers to PWA, beliefs in their ability to schedule and manage the tasks necessary to attend therapy and complete home practice sessions on a regular basis—common issues include beliefs about the ability to arrange transportation, schedule speech therapy around other healthcare appointments, or secure assistance from caregivers in order to perform home exercises.

In SCT, self-efficacy beliefs are a crucial determiner of motivation because, in general, people do not feel motivated to engage in behaviors unless they believe they can do so successfully. Self-efficacy beliefs also play an important regulatory role in motivation and behavior. For instance, whether people believe they can organize and perform certain actions will affect the goals they choose (Locke & Latham, 2002), the effort and persistence toward those goals (Bagwell & West, 2008; Luszczynska, Tryburcy, & Schwarzer, 2007; Payne et al., 2012), and how they respond to failures and manage obstacles during their goal pursuit (Bandura, 1997; Scobbie et al., 2009). People with low self-efficacy tend to avoid challenging goals or abandon them in the face of obstacles. When failures occur, as they inevitably will during rehabilitation, people with low self-efficacy tend to interpret their failures as a confirmation of their lack of ability. People with high self-efficacy, on the other hand, tend to interpret failure as a lack of applying the necessary amount of effort or the correct strategy (Bandura, 1997). An important consideration during neurorehabilitation is the effect that deficit awareness can have on self-efficacy beliefs and motivation (Lequerica & Kortte, 2010). Underestimating the nature and degree of one's impairments, which is common in traumatic brain injury, can distort self-efficacy beliefs and result in negative reactions to unexpected failures (Toglia & Kirk, 2000). Although impaired deficit awareness in aphasia may not be as common or pronounced as it is in other neurogenic conditions, it can co-occur with aphasia (Kertesz, 2010; see Chapter 3, this volume) and should be taken into consideration when assessing a PWA's self-efficacy beliefs (Cocchini & Della Sala, 2010). In our experience, PWA may also overestimate their impairments, leading to unreasonably low self-efficacy beliefs and a tendency to avoid tasks and situations in which successful performance is possible.

Within SCT, self-efficacy beliefs are one of multiple determiners of motivation and, depending on the situation, influence behavior to varying degrees. Although there are no studies investigating the relationship between self-efficacy beliefs and rehabilitation or quality of life outcomes for PWA, the support for the importance of self-efficacy is broad, covers multiple domains, and does include some neurogenic populations. For example, meta-analyses support the contention that self-efficacy beliefs contribute to accomplishments and performance in contexts such as education (Multon, Brown, & Lent, 1991), sports (Moritz, Feltz, Fahrbach, & Mack, 2000), and the workplace (Stajkovic & Luthans, 1998). Self-efficacy beliefs also influence adherence to a wide range of health-related behaviors (Amireault, Godin, & Vézina-Im, 2013; Holden, 1991) and are associated with quality of life, depression, and performance of activities of daily living after stroke (Jones & Riazi, 2011; Korpershoek, van der Bijl, & Hafsteinsdóttir, 2011). In a study of 97 community-dwelling subjects after a traumatic brain injury, Cicerone and Azulay (2007) investigated the contribution of community functioning, activity-related satisfaction, and perceived self-efficacy to global life satisfaction. They found that self-efficacy beliefs, particularly for self-management of cognitive symptoms, were a stronger predictor of global life satisfaction than were community functioning, activity-related satisfaction, and injury-related variables such as severity.

Promoting Self-Efficacy

According to Bandura (1997), self-efficacy beliefs are based upon and continuously influenced by four sources of information: past successes or failures (mastery experiences), watching others perform similar acts (vicarious experiences), encouragement from others (verbal persuasion), and interpretations of physiological and affective states. In this section, we describe each of these sources of information and how they can be used to influence self-efficacy beliefs during aphasia rehabilitation. **TABLE 12.2** presents a list of self-efficacy enhancing strategies focusing on the different sources of self-efficacy information.

TABLE 12.2 Strategies to enhance self-efficacy based on the four sources of self-efficacy information.

Mastery experience
• Ensure early experiences of success in order to build a reservoir of self-efficacy before addressing more challenging goals.
• Encourage patient participation toward setting a level of task and goal difficulty that is challenging and achievable.
• Address long-term goals through a progression of achievable short-term goals.
• Break complex skills into treatable subskills.
• Practice strategies and skills in progressively more challenging contexts (e.g., moving from role playing in clinic to spontaneous use with familiar people).
• Promote the use of self-regulatory skills (e.g., self-monitoring, pacing, planning) to manage barriers to successful performances.
• Frame gradual improvements as expected and as a sign of good rehabilitation potential.
• Encourage attribution of success to the patient's efforts and abilities and not the skill of the clinician.

Vicarious experience
• Early in treatment, or when a new behavior is introduced, vicarious experiences may play a significant role in shaping self-efficacy beliefs.
• Vicarious experiences are most effective when the model is perceived to be similar to the patient in important ways (e.g., type of injury, shared history of aphasia severity at onset, age).
• Incorporate audio or video self-modeling of successful performances.
• Provide exposure to realistic and positive recovery role models, either via group therapy or individual peer mentoring.
• Role play the use of different skills and strategies during group therapy.

(Continues)

TABLE 12.2 Strategies to enhance self-efficacy based on the four sources of self-efficacy information. (Continued)

Verbal persuasion
• Verbal persuasion is most effective after clinicians have established rapport and trust with a patient.
• Verbal persuasion and feedback should be genuine, objective, and bring attention to successes—avoid the habit of frequent knee-jerk praise.
• Include verbal encouragement/feedback that highlights self-regulatory efforts (e.g., self-monitoring, patience).
• Arrange for positive feedback to be given by other credible sources (e.g., MDs, OTs, PTs, RNs, family members, and friends).

Physiological and affective experiences
• Guide patients away from the misattributions of negative states (e.g., fatigue or anxiety) with a lack of ability.
• Encourage reflection on physiological and affective states and their influence on communication performance.
• Identify physiological and affective barriers to performance and develop strategies to manage them.
• Consider stress management techniques (e.g., progressive relaxation, mindfulness-based stress reduction).
• Communicate with the patient's physician about any suspected physiological or affective issues that may interfere with the patient's confidence to succeed in rehabilitation (e.g., sleep disturbance, pain, mood disorder).

Mastery experiences.   The main influences on the development and strength of self-efficacy beliefs are past experiences of success or failure (Bandura, 1997; Usher & Pajares, 2008; Welch & West, 1995). Repeated success in performing an activity strengthens patients' beliefs that they can perform a similar activity in the future, whereas repeated failures weaken their confidence. It is important to understand that self-efficacy beliefs are not based upon objective performances per se; they are based on people's cognitive interpretations of their performances (Bandura, 1997). For example, in an early study examining the effects of mastery experiences on self-efficacy beliefs in subjects with snake phobias, Bandura (1982) found that subjects who had achieved the same level of performance in addressing their fears had different degrees of confidence in their ability to regulate these fears. Some subjects had self-efficacy beliefs that were roughly commensurate with their recent accomplishments, some had significantly less belief in their abilities compared with their performances, and some had much higher levels of confidence in their ability to approach and handle snakes than they had demonstrated. Overall, Bandura found that self-efficacy beliefs were a greater predictor of future behavior than the level of performance achieved. The subjective nature of people's self-appraisal of their performances draws attention to the need for clinicians to be sensitive to how patients judge their experiences during rehabilitation (Jones, 2006). For example, a clinician may believe a patient is doing well on the basis of the speech and language data she collected, but her patient may have a different interpretation. The patient may discount success on tasks perceived to be easy or on tasks in which success is attributed to assistance received from the clinician.

The goal of an intervention incorporating mastery experience is to configure treatment so that a patient has frequent experiences of meaningful success, and that the patient interprets successes as being due to his or her own effort and ability (Bandura, 1997; Jones, 2006). Many of the typical practices used by clinicians are forms of guided mastery building: for example, using cueing hierarchies that fade cues as performance improves, breaking down complex skills and focusing on subskills, practicing strategies and skills in progressively more challenging settings, and using a series of short-term goals to achieve a long-term goal. For any task or goal, clarity about what constitutes success will help patients correctly interpret their performances and adjust their behavior as needed. In a qualitative study investigating the perceptions of self-efficacy among neurological rehabilitation patients, recognizing progress in therapy was a vital source of encouragement and hope for the patients (Dixon, Thornton, & Young, 2007). Recognizing improvements was reported to be difficult, particularly when gains were small and gradual. Setting and achieving goals helped patients recognize their progress, and this process was aided by dismantling the goals into manageable steps.

Although graded mastery tasks are often described as a means of building self-efficacy, two meta-analyses of interventions designed to improve self-efficacy for physical activity in healthy adults found that progressively increasing the difficulty of tasks resulted in lower self-efficacy reports than did interventions that did not include this technique (Ashford, Edmunds, & French, 2010; Williams & French, 2011). It is unclear why graded mastery tasks were ineffective in this context. Williams and French recommended caution when using graded tasks at the beginning stages of behavior change (ensuring, instead, that a stable foundation of self-efficacy for initial tasks was established) and suggested that progression to more challenging tasks be done in consultation with the participant. Early in rehabilitation, failures are less likely to diminish self-efficacy if they are accompanied by a high proportion of confidence-building successes. In addition to the frequency of successes experienced, the difficulty of tasks should also be considered. In self-efficacy interventions, the aim is to provide patients with a degree of challenge that allows them to experience how their efforts translate into improvements in performance. Because a patient's perception of the difficulty of a task is subjective, choosing a level of challenge that is satisfying is best done through frequent feedback from the patient. Although not intended to be a study of self-efficacy beliefs, a study by Conroy, Sage, and Lambon Ralph (2009) provides an example of how different degrees of challenge can affect the treatment satisfaction that different PWA experience at different stages of treatment. Conroy and colleagues compared errorless and errorful naming treatments among subjects who had mild, moderate, and severe anomia. After an initial period of success in the errorless condition, PWA with mild and moderate naming impairments felt more satisfied by an errorful approach; PWA with severe naming difficulties continued to prefer an errorless approach.

Vicarious experiences.   Observing other people perform an activity successfully can strengthen a patient's belief that she can perform similar actions if the patient judges the model to be like herself in relevant ways (e.g., severity of aphasia, time post-onset, age, etc.) (Bandura, 1997). In much the same way, observing a model much further along in the recovery process can give a patient confidence in his or her ability to attain comparable results. Vicarious experiences can be particularly informative for patients in the early stages of recovery or if the activity in question is novel and the patient has little past experience to inform his or her self-efficacy beliefs (Bandura, 1997; Dixon et al., 2007). Inviting PWA who are positive models of recovery to participate in group therapy and share their experiences with other members is one way to provide vicarious experiences. Gonzalez, Goeppinger, and Lorig (1990) emphasized the need to choose models who are not "super patients" but realistic examples of patients who have struggled with their disability, persisted in their rehabilitation efforts, made meaningful improvements, and adjusted to their disability. Qualitative studies of neurological and orthopedic rehabilitation patients (Dixon et al., 2007; Resnick, 2002) support the importance of patients having the opportunity to observe successful models of recovery and to share experiences of how they have managed their disability. In the aphasiology literature, the importance of positive role models for PWA has been discussed in first-person accounts of aphasia (e.g., Green & Waks, 2008) and a report describing an aphasia peer-mentoring program (Coles & Snow, 2011). Providing realistic and positive role models to PWA who are in the acute phase of recovery, either via peer mentoring or support/therapy groups, can not only strengthen self-efficacy but also help PWA begin to form realistic outcome expectations and prevent unnecessary levels of disappointment when improvements are occurring slowly.

Self-modeling, via audio or video recordings, is another form of vicarious experience. In general, the aim is to show patients performances they are capable of but have not yet mastered (Bandura, 1997). Self-modeling can consist of recordings of emerging skills that were performed successfully or viewing edited performances where errors and facilitatory cues have been removed. For complex activities, clinicians can capture a patient performing elements of an activity and then construct a successful depiction of the total activity (Dowrick, 1999). For example, early in script training (e.g., Youmans, Holland, Muñoz, & Bourgeois, 2005; see Chapter 10, this volume), the clinician could focus on capturing the correct production of the individual phrases making up a script, splicing those performances together, and providing them to the patient as an illustration of successful performance of the whole script. Poor performances can also be used in self-modeling, but this is best done after the patient has developed adequate self-efficacy beliefs and when the recordings provide the kind of information that would clearly result in a solution to the observed difficulty. Care should be taken when using self-modeling. It is possible for patients to have a negative reaction to recordings, even if they are positive portrayals of ability. This may be more likely with patients who are in the acute stage of recovery or who have poor deficit awareness. Whenever one uses self-modeling, it is always a good idea to respect patients' autonomy by providing a rationale and asking permission.

In speech-language pathology, self-modeling has been used in the treatment of stuttering (Cream & O'Brian, 2012), voice (van Leer & Connor, 2012), autism (Wilson, 2013), and childhood language (Buggey, 1995). In a broad review of the self-modeling research, Dowrick (1999) identified seven aspects of self-modeling that contribute to learning, self-efficacy, and well-being:

- Clarification of goals and outcomes
- Demonstration of a positive self-image
- Reminders of previous competence in the case of a skill level that has decreased because of disuse
- Repetition of the observation of competent role play
- Observation of one's skills applied to a new setting
- Experience of anxiety-free behavior or successful outcomes despite anxiety
- Demonstration of new skills composed of pre-existing subskills (p. 36)

Verbal persuasion.   Verbal persuasion is another means of increasing self-efficacy by encouraging patients to believe that they are capable of success or by using feedback to influence how they interpret their performances. Although verbal persuasion is one of the more frequently used methods to improve patients' confidence, by and large, it is not as effective as mastery experiences or vicarious experiences and should not be relied upon as a primary means of improving self-efficacy (Bandura, 1997). Verbal persuasion is most effective when it comes from a credible and trusted source and when it is used in conjunction with other sources of self-efficacy information, particularly mastery experiences in which patients' attention can be directed toward their successes (Bandura, 1997). Whether feedback or praise should highlight ability, effort, or both is unclear. In reviews of the educational and developmental literature on feedback and praise, attributing successes to ability has been found to improve self-efficacy and motivation, but it may not prepare individuals to manage failures or obstacles over the long term (Hattie & Timperley, 2007; Henderlong & Lepper, 2002). It appears that attributing successes to self-regulatory control (e.g., acknowledging successful error detection, practicing patience during word-finding blocks, or making use of a compensatory strategy when needed) may be a more effective means of building stable and resilient self-efficacy beliefs and motivation. In the SDT literature, praise or positive verbal reinforcement can either promote or thwart autonomous forms of motivation depending on how the feedback is perceived by the patient. According to Ryan (1982)

". . . the more we interpret what someone says as pressure to achieve a particular outcome (e.g., because we are being evaluated) the less likely we are to be intrinsically motivated to perform that activity. On the other hand, verbalizations that do not imply pressure to attain particular outcomes and that convey positive effectance information are likely to enhance interest in the activity." (p. 451)

Providing even simple feedback, such as praise for a job well done, in a way that is not subtly controlling requires some vigilance. Miller and Rollnick (2012, p.65) suggest avoiding the word "I" when giving praise/affirmations. For example, statements such as "good, that's just the way I wanted you to do it!" or "I am proud of you" may be well intentioned and well received but they may also have parental/controlling overtones and imply that one of the purposes of therapy is to satisfy the clinician. If a patient perceives that our positive regard for them is contingent upon how well they perform or follow our instructions, there is a risk that the patient's motivation will shift from a focus on learning (i.e., intrinsic motivation) to securing our approval (i.e., extrinsic, controlling motivation). Rather, phrases that emphasize the patient's performance or achievement are preferred. For example, in response to a patient recognizing an error the clinician might say, "You caught the mistake and changed your answer; good work. How do you think that went?"

Physiological and affective states.   People tend to interpret physiological and affective states experienced before, during, or after an activity as a comment on their ability to manage the demands of that activity (Bandura, 1997). For example, heightened arousal before speaking to a group of strangers may diminish a PWA's confidence that he or she can communicate successfully. In terms of aphasia, fatigue (Le Dorze & Brassard, 1995; Lerdal et al., 2009), anxiety (Cahana-Amitay et al., 2011), and depression (Kauhanen et al., 2000) are among the most common experiences that may have a negative effect on self-efficacy. Depression, in particular, appears to be as strong a predictor of subjective cognitive complaints after stroke as the presence of objective cognitive impairments (van Rijsbergen, Mark, de Kort, & Sitskoorn, 2014). In a review of the literature concerning anxiety and language as a stressor in aphasia, Cahana-Amitay and colleagues (2011) concluded that the frequent stress associated with language use could result in "linguistic anxiety." A PWA with linguistic anxiety "is one in whom the deliberate, effortful production of language involves anticipation of an error, with the imminence of linguistic failure serving as the threat" (Cahana-Amitay et al., 2011, p. 603). There is often a reciprocal relationship between unpleasant physical and affective states and self-efficacy beliefs (Bandura, 1997); for example, low self-efficacy may exacerbate anxiety, which then reinforces or further weakens low self-efficacy, etc.

In the stroke rehabilitation and chronic disease self-management literature (which usually addresses self-efficacy beliefs related to exercise or activities of daily living) interventions aimed at managing the effects of negative physical and affective states usually consist of (1) identifying barriers to performance posed by negative states and creating strategies to manage them, (2) correcting the misattribution of symptoms to a lack of capability, and (3) pacing activities to reduce the buildup of fatigue, pain, and anxiety (Lorig & Holman, 2003; Robinson-Smith & Pizzi, 2003; Shaughnessy & Resnick, 2009). An example of applying these approaches to a patient who misattributes or overattributes their experience of fatigue to difficulty in speaking might include educating the patient about the biological nature and prevalence of post-stroke fatigue and encouraging the patient to monitor his energy level and take short breaks during therapy, home practice, or social interactions. In addition to the approaches mentioned above, stress management techniques, such as mindfulness and relaxation-based training programs, show promise in their ability to reduce anxiety and symptoms associated with low mood (Hofmann, Sawyer, Witt, & Oh, 2010). In the aphasia literature, stress management techniques have been suggested as a means of managing linguistic anxiety (Cahana-Amitay et al., 2011) and improving self-efficacy (Murray, 2008). Pharmacological treatments to reduce depression (Small & Llano, 2009) and linguistic anxiety (Cahana-Amitay, Albert, & Oveis, 2014) in PWA have also been proposed.

Summary of self-efficacy interventions.   "As health professionals, our job is to determine what and why people believe as they do and, when possible, help them change or reinterpret those beliefs" (Gonzalez et al., 1990, pp. 134–135). Interventions to improve self-efficacy focus on shaping and strengthening patients' beliefs about their abilities by providing self-efficacy–enhancing information. Systematic reviews in the stroke literature have concluded that interventions based on the sources of self-efficacy information hold promise, but that the results, both for clinical outcomes and enhancing self-efficacy beliefs, are mixed (Jones & Riazi, 2011; Korpershoek et al., 2011). In addition to having a variety of methodological issues, the self-efficacy intervention programs in the reviewed studies did not include all four sources of information in their interventions, which has been recommended by Bandura (1997). Self-efficacy interventions that have targeted all four sources of information have been found to improve self-efficacy beliefs, treatment adherence, and/or performance in cardiac rehabilitation (Millen & Bray, 2009), physical activity promotion (Lee, Arthur, & Avis, 2007), and memory training (West, Bagwell, & Dark-Freudeman, 2008). Finally, generic self-efficacy intervention programs may not address the unique set of self-efficacy beliefs that patients have about their abilities or the challenges they face.

Assessing Self-Efficacy

CASE ILLUSTRATION: MR. SMITH—EPISODE 3

Because Mr. Smith had been discharged by his previous clinician for poor treatment adherence and a lack of significant progress, our initial focus was to understand the reasons for his struggle to remain motivated and how his previous experiences in therapy may have affected his beliefs about his ability to improve

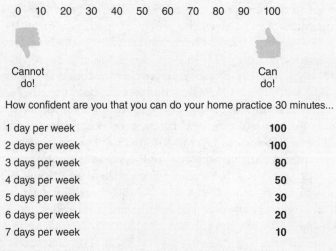

FIGURE 12.1 A self-efficacy scale measuring confidence in the ability to adhere to a home practice schedule. Mr. Smith's responses are shown in bold.

his communication skills. Our early conversations with Mr. Smith and his wife resulted in the identification of three factors that may have hampered his motivation and engagement in therapy: (1) His previous goal in therapy did not appear to be sufficiently motivating, (2) he was disappointed by his slow progress, and (3) he had chronic pain due to degenerative disc disease and complained of post-stroke fatigue, both of which affected his motivation and ability to adhere to his home practice schedule. **FIGURE 12.1** shows a self-efficacy scale that we created to measure Mr. Smith's confidence in his ability to adhere to a home practice schedule.

Self-efficacy measures are easy to construct and can be used at any point in the rehabilitation process. They can consist of single-item measures of confidence that are used as needed during the course of treatment, or more planned and systematic investigations of the patient's beliefs (e.g., pre-post measures after implementing a plan to improve self-efficacy). In our practice, we focus on the use of simple, ad hoc self-efficacy scales created by the clinician to meet the individual needs of the patient. Figures 12.1–12.3 show variations of an ad hoc self-efficacy scale created for use with Mr. Smith. Each scale assesses his confidence to perform a behavior or task at various stages of his treatment. For example, Figure 12.1 assesses his confidence in adhering to a home program while Figure 12.3 assesses the behavior under challenging conditions or barriers.

Published self-efficacy measures, which are often general, domain-level self-efficacy scales, may be useful for measuring the generalization of self-efficacy beliefs over the course of treatment. However, given the potential specificity of self-efficacy beliefs, domain-level scales may not address the unique activities patients wish to pursue or all the barriers they are likely to meet (Miller, McCrady, Abrams, & Labouvie, 1994); as such, their usefulness in guiding self-efficacy interventions in communicative rehabilitation are limited (Maddux & Lewis, 1995). An example of a published self-efficacy–related measurement developed for PWA is the Communication Confidence Rating Scale for Aphasia (CCRSA; Babbitt & Cherney, 2010; Babbitt, Heinemann, Semik, & Cherney, 2011). The CCRSA was developed after its authors noted that subjects completing an experimental treatment reported improved confidence in their ability to communicate and that these improvements were meaningful, even when significant improvements in language scores were not evident. The CCRSA is a 10-item self-report questionnaire that measures general communication confidence. Babbitt and colleagues (2011) defined *communication confidence* as "a feeling about one's power to participate in a communication situation, one's sense about one's own skills and/or ability to express oneself and to understand the communications of others" (pp. 727–728). Although the authors do not expressly call the CCRSA a self-efficacy measure, it appears to address similar beliefs. A Rasch analysis, which is designed to evaluate the characteristics of rating scales, has shown the CCRSA to have high person and item reliability (Babbitt et al., 2011). The CCRSA is still a fairly new tool and additional psychometric analyses are planned.

Bandura (2006) has provided detailed instructions for constructing self-efficacy scales; the discussion that follows covers some of the guidelines that are most relevant to clinicians interested in creating custom scales for individual patients. The primary consideration when creating a self-efficacy scale is recognizing that questions addressing a specific task and situation are usually more predictive of future behavior than are more general questions (Beaudoin & Desrichard, 2011; Moritz et al., 2000; Pajares, 1996). In aphasia rehabilitation, the content and level of detail of self-efficacy questions will often be determined by the goals of treatment and the internal and external challenges patients may face when attempting to achieve those goals. For instance, if one is interested in a patient's beliefs about her ability to successfully engage in a conversation, then questions might be organized around a specific topic and different situational challenges that are relevant to the client (e.g., conversing with strangers versus friends, speaking under time pressures, managing anomic blocks).

Measurement of self-efficacy beliefs takes into consideration three dimensions: strength, level, and generality (Bandura, 1997, p. 43). *Strength* corresponds to the degree of confidence patients have in their ability to perform an activity. For example, on a scale of 0 to 100, a PWA may be confident that he can exchange social greetings with strangers and rate his confidence at 90. *Level* refers to the amount of challenge a person anticipates. For a PWA, the level of challenge may refer to the complexity of the communication exchange (e.g., social greetings versus carrying on a conversation about politics), or the magnitude of different perceived barriers to successful communication (e.g., engaging in a conversation when relaxed or anxious). *Generality* refers to the degree to which self-efficacy beliefs are positively related, either within a domain or between related domains. Bandura has outlined some of the conditions under which self-efficacy beliefs are predicted to generalize (Bandura, 1997, p. 51). Generalization is expected across domains of activity that share similar subskills. Generalization may also occur after the development of self-regulatory skills and strategy usage. For example, we incorporated self-monitoring exercises (Whitney & Goldstein, 1989) into the treatment plan of one of our recent patients; these exercises helped the patient notice and self-correct his paraphasic errors when speaking. After he developed some skill at self-monitoring his speech we noticed that, not only did his confidence in his ability to speak improve, but he also gained confidence in his ability to self-monitor for errors and write understandable emails to his friends.

When constructing self-efficacy scales, Bandura (2006) recommends phrasing questions in terms of *can do* (which addresses capability) rather than *will do* (which addresses intention). Response scales can be based on 100- or 10-point scales and should span from 0 ("cannot do at all") to 10 or 100 ("highly certain can do"). To improve reading comprehension, we have simplified our scale descriptors to read "cannot do!" and "can do!" (e.g., see Figure 12.1).

A Demonstration of Applying Principles of Self-Efficacy to Treatment

Goal-setting and treatment planning that aim to improve a patient's self-efficacy should take into account both the clinician's assessment of the patient's abilities and prognosis and the patient's subjective self-efficacy beliefs. When we started working with Mr. Smith, we believed that his prognosis for making significant improvements was good. The copies of progress reports we received from his previous clinician suggested that he made improvement early on when he was adhering to his home practice schedule. We wanted Mr. Smith to become confident that he could adhere to his new treatment plan, manage any obstacles along the way, and realize the benefits of his efforts. In the early weeks of treatment, building up Mr. Smith's self-efficacy was as much our focus as improving his speech and language skills.

Many options and combinations exist for incorporating the four sources of self-efficacy information into a treatment plan and approach (See Table 12.2). The following is an example of the options we selected for Mr. Smith.

1. Mastery experiences: Begin with a meaningful and achievable short-term goal and provide graded mastery experiences working toward that goal; break complex, long-term goals into achievable subgoals.

2. Vicarious experiences: Create self-modeling videos to provide information on how to complete home practice exercises correctly and to build self-efficacy through presenting ideal performances; offer group therapy with other PWA who can serve as informative and encouraging role models.

3. Verbal persuasion: Use motivational interviewing to guide Mr. Smith toward acknowledging his successes and strengths and correctly interpreting failures and slow progress.

4. Physiological and affective states: Educate Mr. Smith about how negative physiological and affective states can affect communication performance; improve his awareness and understanding of potential physiological and affective barriers and preemptively develop strategies to manage them.

CASE ILLUSTRATION: MR. SMITH—EPISODE 4

In the following four sections, we describe how we used measures of self-efficacy to guide some of our treatment decisions and how we incorporated the four sources of self-efficacy information into Mr. Smith's treatment. To illustrate these practices clearly, we will focus on one of the short-term goals that we addressed early in treatment.

1. Mastery experiences. Recognizing the central role that mastery experiences play in the formation of self-efficacy beliefs (Bandura, 1997), we thought it best to start with a meaningful short-term goal that was achievable and would provide Mr. Smith with an early experience of success. Because Mr. Smith had yet to experience any meaningful improvement through therapy, we wanted to increase his confidence in his abilities before we addressed a more complex goal. After consulting with Mr. Smith and providing him with our rationale, he agreed to this approach. The first goal that Mr. Smith chose to address was his ability to order a grande cappuccino at his local Starbucks. For years, Mr. Smith met his friends every Tuesday morning for coffee but, since his stroke, his friends have ordered his drink for him. Although he appreciated their help, he disliked feeling dependent on others for such a basic task. Treatment for this goal focused on graded mastery tasks, which progressed from repetition of the target utterance (i.e., "I would like a grande cappuccino"), to role playing with the clinician and unfamiliar people, and finally, to ordering in the medical center's Starbucks with his clinician present. After each treatment session, we administered an informal self-efficacy scale that addressed the next level of mastery under varying conditions. We asked Mr. Smith to choose a confidence rating for the most challenging item on the scale that he would like to achieve before moving to the next level; he chose 80. In the goal-setting and action planning framework, a score of 70 or greater is considered adequate self-efficacy (Scobbie, McLean, Dixon, Duncan, & Wyke, 2013). **FIGURE 12.2** shows the scale that we used when practicing at the medical center's Starbucks—it

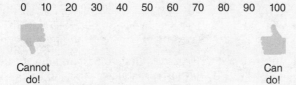

0 10 20 30 40 50 60 70 80 90 100

Cannot   Can
do!   do!

How confident are you that you can order a grande cappuccino at Starbucks when...

There is no pressure to order quickly	**60**
You feel pressured by the Starbucks employee	**40**
You feel pressured by the people in line behind you	**50**
You feel pressured by the Starbucks employee and the people in line behind you	**20**

FIGURE 12.2 A self-efficacy scale measuring confidence in the ability to order a coffee at Starbucks. Mr. Smith's responses are shown in bold.

addresses Mr. Smith's confidence to perform at the next challenge level, which was to order at his local Starbucks by himself.

2. Vicarious experiences. After mastery experiences, vicarious experiences are considered to be the most influential form of self-efficacy information (Bandura, 1997). In this regard, one of our main focuses was to provide Mr. Smith confidence building vicarious experiences through video self-modeling. Mr. Smith had mild apraxia of speech and responded well to integral stimulation (i.e., "watch me, listen to me, repeat along with me"; Rosenbek, Lemme, Ahern, Harris, & Wertz, 1973). By video recording his correct productions of the target script on his smartphone, the videos served as both a support for home practice and a source of self-efficacy reinforcement. After accuracy of the production of the target script stabilized, we included videos of successful role-playing encounters in his home practice.

3. Verbal persuasion. As mentioned previously, verbal persuasion, in general, is not considered to be a strong source of self-efficacy information, particularly when it is relied upon to the exclusion of other sources of information (Bandura, 1997). Our approach to verbal persuasion with Mr. Smith differed from how it is typically described in the self-efficacy literature. Although we used direct verbal encouragement and feedback, directing Mr. Smith's attention to his successes, we also used MI a great deal. Our rationale for this approach was that guiding Mr. Smith to describe his successes and the logical reasons for his failures may have been a more powerful form of verbal persuasion than what we could offer. At the beginning of treatment, it was

particularly important that Mr. Smith reflected upon how his physical pain, fatigue, and lack of commitment to his goal in his previous therapy experience may have contributed to his lack of treatment adherence and poor progress.

4. Physiological and affective states. Negative physiological and affective experiences can distort or diminish self-efficacy beliefs and can also serve as barriers to goal-directed behavior (Bandura, 1997; Shaughnessy & Resnick, 2009). Physical pain and fatigue were two physiological experiences that both shaped Mr. Smith's self-efficacy beliefs about what he was capable of doing and served as outright barriers to fully engaging in rehabilitation. Through MI, we were able to raise Mr. Smith's awareness of how his physical pain and fatigue could affect his engagement in therapy. We took these physiological barriers and other potential obstacles that Mr. Smith had suggested and created a scale addressing his self-efficacy to manage them (see **FIGURE 12.3**). The scale helped us identify the conditions that Mr. Smith was least confident he could manage, develop strategies to address them, and measure whether the strategies improved his self-efficacy. For instance, we identified the time of day that Mr. Smith typically had the most energy (morning) and was in the least pain (morning). In addition, Mr. Smith identified how long it took for him to reach his optimal pain relief from his morning pain medication. With this information, Mr. Smith was able to determine the best time to schedule his home practice. After we guided Mr. Smith to solve problems to get past these barriers (i.e., coping planning), his confidence in his ability to complete his home practice, at least 4 days per week, improved from a 50 to a 70.

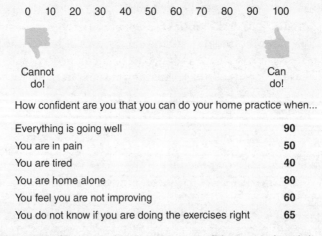

| 0 | 10 | 20 | 30 | 40 | 50 | 60 | 70 | 80 | 90 | 100 |

Cannot do!   Can do!

How confident are you that you can do your home practice when...

Everything is going well	**90**
You are in pain	**50**
You are tired	**40**
You are home alone	**80**
You feel you are not improving	**60**
You do not know if you are doing the exercises right	**65**

FIGURE 12.3 A self-efficacy scale measuring confidence in the ability to manage potential barriers to home practice. Mr. Smith's responses are shown in bold.

Outcome Expectancy

Clinicians tend to have a broad definition of the term "outcome," which usually reflects any positive change that results from treatment. In SCT, *outcome* has a narrower definition; it refers to the consequence of a performance (Bandura, 2006), such as feeling proud or embarrassed after giving a speech. Many speech-language therapy goals, such as improving the ability to hold a conversation or write, do not represent outcomes as defined by SCT. They are *performance attainments,* and patients' confidence in their ability to achieve these goals reflects self-efficacy expectations. *Outcome expectancies* are beliefs about the likelihood that certain consequences (outcomes) will flow from the actions people take or the performance attainments they reach. According to Bandura (1997), outcome expectancies take three forms: *physical, social,* or *self-evaluative.* Examples of physical outcomes are pleasure/ wellness or pain. Social outcomes concern the social reactions of others. Social outcomes can be positive, such as expressions of approval, caring, interest, or social recognition, or negative, such as disapproval, disinterest, or rejection. Finally, self-evaluative outcomes refer to the self-satisfaction or disappointment one has with one's performance. Often, both positive and negative outcome expectancies exist for any particular goal/activity. For example, a patient may believe that regular home speech therapy practice will result in experiencing a certain amount of stress and frustration while, at the same time, expecting a lessening of social anxiety as a result of improved communication skills.

In general, there is a limited amount of research in the healthcare field on the role that Bandura's outcome expectancy construct has on motivation and behavior (Williams, 2010). Although outcome expectancies are a central component of SCT, an emphasis is placed on the influence of self-efficacy beliefs on motivation because, generally speaking, people do not expect to achieve outcomes if they do not believe they can perform the actions necessary to realize them (Bandura, 1997). Whether outcome expectancies will influence motivation depends on a number of factors, the relative weighting of positive and negative outcome expectancies, the importance of the outcome, and the perceived likelihood of the outcome (Bandura, 1997).

CASE ILLUSTRATION: MR. SMITH—EPISODE 5

As mentioned previously, one of Mr. Smith's concerns was his inability to converse with his grandson and maintain their relationship. We helped Mr. Smith think of specific communication acts he could engage in and which he believed would draw them closer together. After discussing ways to achieve this, Mr. Smith decided that improving his ability to discuss topics that his grandson was interested in might strengthen their bond. Before pursuing this goal with Mr. Smith, we wanted to understand the nature of the topics and his self-efficacy in relation to them. We

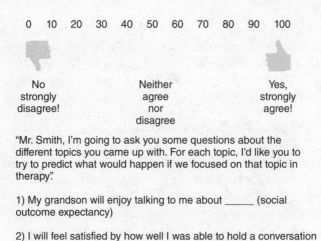

FIGURE 12.4 Outcome expectancy scale for conversational topics.

asked Mr. Smith what topics of conversation he believed would strengthen his bond with his grandson and he identified four topics that would engage his grandson: Little League Baseball, fishing, comics, and computer games. Then we asked how strong his self-efficacy beliefs were for being able to converse on those topics. **FIGURE 12.4** shows a simple ad hoc scale we devised to probe his outcome expectancies for each topic; **TABLE 12.3** shows his self-efficacy and outcome expectancy self-ratings for each topic (only the social and self-evaluative aspects of outcome expectancies were measured).

TABLE 12.3 Mr. Smith's self-efficacy and social and self-evaluative outcome expectancy self-ratings for conversational topics.

Topic	Self-Efficacy	Social	Self-Evaluative
Baseball	70	90	90
Fishing	70	80	80
Comics	60	70	70
Computer games	40	70	60

Note. Mr. Smith's self-efficacy ratings were based on the following instructions and question: "We want to know how confident you are that you could talk about each of these topics after you practiced them in therapy. How confident are you that you will be able to carry on a conversation with your grandson about . . . ?"

Mr. Smith was not very familiar with computers or computer games and this was reflected in his low self-efficacy and outcome expectancy self-ratings. We asked him why his outcome expectancy ratings for baseball were higher than "fishing" or "comics," particularly since the self-efficacy ratings were not significantly different. He told us that he was an avid baseball fan and played on teams up until he was an adult. This simple process—quickly creating informal outcome expectancy and self-efficacy scales—provided a context for Mr. Smith and his clinician to explore his goals and the beliefs surrounding them; it helped ensure that Mr. Smith was choosing the most motivating topic and that he reflected upon and self-endorsed the reasons for choosing it.

Hope

Although the concept of hope is not directly addressed in the theories reviewed in this chapter, it is related to self-efficacy and outcome expectations. Hope tends to reflect a more general desire for idealized outcomes, whereas self-efficacy and outcome expectations are driven by a sense of probability and are situation specific (Bright, Kayes, McCann, & McPherson, 2011; Leung, Silvius, Pimlott, Dalziel, & Drummond, 2009). Bright, Kayes, McCann, and McPherson (2013) interviewed five PWA in the post-acute phase of recovery and identified two distinct experiences of hope. The first, *simply having hope*, was the primary form of hope that the PWA experienced. It was a generalized form of hope that waxed and waned but remained relatively stable. The second form, *actively hoping*, involved identifying and working toward broad, meaningful hopes and/or more focused stroke-related hopes. When subjects felt uncertain about their future and had a difficult time engaging in active hoping, they tended to rely on simply hoping as a coping mechanism. Simply hoping was nurtured through the support of others, spiritual beliefs, experiencing progress, and hearing stories of others' progress. Actively hoping was supported by developing and acting on plans for improvement. In this study and other qualitative studies involving PWA and/or their family members (Avent et al., 2005; Worrall, Brown, et al., 2010; Worrall, Davidson, et al., 2010), participants emphasized the need for clinicians to support and promote a sense of hope during the rehabilitation process. In a systematic review of the stroke literature, Bright and colleagues (2011) found that hope was often described as a motivator during recovery and that it helped stroke survivors cope with obstacles and slow improvement. Clinicians are often concerned about giving PWA false hope while, at the same time, being aware that hope is a motivator and necessary during rehabilitation (Hersh, 2003; Worrall, Davidson, et al., 2010). PWA with high hopes generally understand that some of their hopes are improbable, but whether clinicians should accept or even encourage distorted beliefs about ability and recovery is a difficult question to navigate during rehabilitation. Snyder, Rand, King, Feldman, and Woodward (2002) have argued that unattained high hopes, as long as they are not the product of denial, do not result in negative psychological reactions and can serve a positive motivational role. When discussing self-efficacy interventions, Maddux and Lewis (1995) recommended encouraging minor, overly optimistic self-efficacy beliefs, because there is a reciprocal relationship between self-efficacy beliefs and behavior (i.e., high self-efficacy encourages goal pursuit and effort, and positive performances strengthen self-efficacy beliefs). Overall, when it comes to hopes and aspirations, in our experiences more PWA are harmed by setting the bar too low than too high. We should also remember that there is a difference between setting a high bar for measurable language performance and setting a high bar for what PWA can do, or are willing to try to do, with the language skills they currently have.

Goal Attributes

In goal-setting theory (Locke & Latham, 2002) and in SCT (Bandura, 1997), goals emerge from an internal discrepancy between one's current condition and what one wants to achieve. The dissatisfaction that results from this negative discrepancy motivates people to form goals and to act upon them. If a goal is compelling and a person has confidence in his abilities, it promotes effort, resilience in the face of obstacles, and the development and use of whatever strategies and knowledge are needed (Bandura, 1997; Locke & Latham, 2002). In goal-setting theory, two primary goal attributes influence motivation and performance: goal *specificity* and *difficulty*. Summarizing 35 years of research in goal-setting theory, Locke and Latham highlighted the repeated finding that setting specific and difficult goals results in higher performance than do easy or vague "do your best" type goals (Locke & Latham, 2002). Goals that specify the exact behavior, performance level, and outcome to work toward help to focus people's efforts. For Mr. Smith, a vague or "do your best" goal may have been "Mr. Smith will use his practiced script when ordering coffee at Starbucks." A goal that is both specific and difficult might state "Mr. Smith will use his practiced script to order coffee at Starbucks, without noticeable errors, in the context of a high degree of perceived time pressure." Goals that are difficult (but achievable) improve performance by encouraging people to increase and sustain their effort. The positive effect of goal difficulty on performance is most apparent on goals that are simple and can be accomplished in a short period (Levack et al., 2006). For complex distal goals, patients may be better served by setting a number of smaller proximal goals that provide mastery experiences and build up the skills and knowledge necessary to achieve the complex goal (Bandura, 1997).

To the best of our knowledge, there are no published guidelines for determining what constitutes an appropriately difficult goal in a rehabilitation-like setting. In laboratory studies assessing the effect of goal setting on the motor and cognitive performance of subjects with acquired brain damage, Gauggel and colleagues (Gauggel & Billino, 2002; Gauggel, Leinberger, & Richardt, 2001) set difficult goals for a trial by adding 20% to subjects' baseline performance. In another laboratory experiment addressing the memory beliefs and performance of older adults, West and Yassuda (2004) provided subjects with a list of words to remember. Subjects were given a range of goal options to strive toward (i.e., recalling 10% to 100% of the words on the list) and asked to choose a performance level that was difficult but achievable.

CASE ILLUSTRATION: MR. SMITH—EPISODE 6

For Mr. Smith's goal to discuss baseball with his grandson, we set a series of short-term goals addressing vocabulary and phrase acquisition, using a similar format and instructions to those of West and Yassuda (2004). For instance, we provided Mr. Smith with a list of baseball terms to target during naming treatments and asked him to choose the number of words he could learn in 2 weeks that was both challenging and achievable. To increase Mr. Smith's confidence that he could adhere to a home practice schedule, we recommended adherence as a goal of intervention, hoping that it would increase his focus and effort on this aspect of his treatment.

When targeting the number of days per week that Mr. Smith would attempt to do his home practice, we took into consideration his home practice self-efficacy scores (see Figure 12.1). As we mentioned earlier, Mr. Smith's self-efficacy rating for practicing 4 days per week improved from 50 to 70 after we engaged him in formulating plans to manage the impact of his pain and fatigue. After consulting Mr. Smith, we agreed that targeting home practice 4 days per week was both challenging and achievable.

Other factors that moderate the relationship between goals and performance include feedback, self-efficacy, and goal commitment (Locke & Latham, 2002). In the context of difficult and specific goals, periodic feedback that summarizes progress can serve as a motivational inducement to continue putting forth effort, or it can help a person understand what adjustments he needs to make in the level or direction of his effort (Ashford & De Stobbeleir, 2013). In a study of the effects of feedback and goal setting on the memory performance of older adults, West, Bagwell, and Dark-Freudeman (2005) found that either objective feedback (e.g., feedback that performance had improved, but the goal had not yet been reached) or positive feedback (e.g., simply telling subjects they are improving and expressing confidence that they can do better on subsequent trials) improved memory performance compared with no feedback and that positive feedback resulted in the highest levels of goal commitment and motivation.

In goal-setting theory, goal commitment is considered to be the most important moderator, particularly during the pursuit of difficult goals (Locke & Latham, 2002); as such, a focus on goal commitment during aphasia rehabilitation seems warranted, given the perplexing and protracted nature of recovery. According to Locke and Latham (2002), the key factors that contribute to goal commitment are the importance of the goal and the belief that one can attain it (i.e., self-efficacy). In MI, goal importance is measured using a one-item scale called an "importance ruler" (Miller & Rollnick, 2012, p. 174). For example, we used this method to ask Mr. Smith to rate the importance of being able to carry on a conversation about baseball with his grandson (i.e., from 0 ["not important!"] to 100 ["very, very important!"]). From our discussions with Mr. Smith, we never questioned the strength of his commitment to this goal. However, the importance ruler gave us the opportunity to reinforce his commitment (e.g., by asking why he did not choose a lower rating). To do this, we blended techniques from MI with recommendations from the SDT literature on *goal framing* (Vansteenkiste et al., 2006). Goal framing involves providing someone with a rationale for why they should pursue a goal. In SDT, the focus is on providing rationales that frame goals in terms of their intrinsic values. Broadly speaking, intrinsic goals satisfy the need for autonomy, competence, and relatedness. They may be goals that address personal growth or interests, building relationships, or community involvement. In Mr. Smith's case, conversing with his grandson was an intrinsic goal that addressed his need for autonomy, competency, and relatedness. Extrinsic goals are concerned with securing external markers of self-worth, such as approval from others, positive comparisons against other people, or material gain. Multiple studies have found that subjects who are given rationales focusing on the intrinsic value of a goal are more autonomously motivated, demonstrate deeper learning, experience more achievement, and are more goal persistent than subjects who receive extrinsic goal framing (Vansteenkiste et al., 2006). In the SDT literature, goal framing is usually provided by a clinician, teacher, or researcher. We chose to use MI to guide Mr. Smith toward self-describing the intrinsic values and needs that his goal addressed.

Summary of Motivational Constructs

In the goal-setting and action planning framework of Scobbie, Dixon, and Wyke (2011) and Scobbie and colleagues (2013), as well as the theories it is based upon, patients' initial intention/motivation for therapy is influenced by the perceived positive and negative outcomes that they expect and the confidence they have in their ability to perform the actions necessary to reach valued outcomes and levels of performance. Once the initial motivation to address a problem is established, setting specific and challenging goals focuses and enhances this energy. Setting specific plans for how goals will be pursued (i.e., action planning), along with preemptively identifying and forming plans to manage obstacles (i.e., coping planning), has been described as a means of overcoming the *intention-behavior gap* (Schwarzer et al., 2011). The intention-behavior gap refers to the common experience of being motivated to pursue a goal but not acting on that intention. The motivational constructs described in the preceding sections, particularly self-efficacy, continue to exert an influence over behavior once patients become engaged in treatment.

CASE ILLUSTRATION: MR. SMITH—EPISODE 7

Applying motivational constructs during rehabilitation is a dynamic process and requires sensitivity to changes in a patient's beliefs and needs. For example, Mr. Smith made what we thought was good progress toward his goal to hold a conversation about baseball with his grandson. He recognized the improvements he made and that his steady adherence to his home practice was influential; however, it became clear after a while that he was expecting to improve faster and to a greater degree. According to Scobbie and colleagues (2013), rehabilitation patients may be disappointed and frustrated by not achieving goals—but goal nonattainment is also an opportunity to disengage from unrealistic expectations, develop acceptance, and reapply one's efforts in different ways or in a different direction. We continued to use self-efficacy–enhancing approaches to support Mr. Smith's confidence in his abilities and MI to explore the sense of ambiguity he had about his progress. Vicarious sources of self-efficacy information began to play an even more important role than mastery experiences (which Mr. Smith was experiencing, but not fast enough). Video self-modeling helped Mr. Smith see past his word-finding hesitations and speech errors and recognize the growing amount of content he was able to express. Equally important at this stage were the stories that group therapy members shared about how their patience and persistence over long periods resulted in meaningful improvements. It also became apparent to us—and this is perhaps something we should have incorporated from the start—that Mr. Smith needed to engage in other ways of satisfying his need to feel autonomous, competent, and close to others. We explored this approach with Mr. Smith, and one of the solutions we arrived at was for Mr. Smith to attempt to get his driver's license reinstated. Mr. Smith believed that if he was able to drive again and prove himself safe, he would be able to interact with his grandson without others being involved, such as driving his grandson to baseball practice and going fishing together.

CONCLUSION

Over time, there has been movement toward integrating different theories of motivation and health behavior change in order to develop more effective motivational interventions that address the challenges posed by specific medical conditions (Hagger, 2009; Noar & Zimmerman, 2005; Scobbie et al., 2009). Combining SDT and components of SCT is one such proposed integrated approach (e.g., Sweet, Fortier, Strachan, Blanchard, & Boulay, 2014). Constructs such as self-efficacy and outcome expectancies are useful because they address the situation-specific and goal-specific beliefs and expectations of patients, while SDT addresses some of the more global concerns of PWA, such as the need to feel autonomous, competent, and connected to other people. SDT also acknowledges the need for autonomous forms of motivation, which SCT and goal-setting theory do not address. Finally, SDT and the closely related MI approach are particularly useful because they provide clinicians with a set of principles and techniques that guide interaction with PWA in a manner that fosters a positive therapeutic relationship and helps both clinicians and patients integrate critical rehabilitation values and practices.

The theories and constructs discussed in this chapter have been applied across diverse domains of human behavior and settings and, although little has been written about the motivational needs of PWA, we believe that these theories and constructs can also be applied to aphasia rehabilitation. Until studies exploring the application of theories of motivation during aphasia rehabilitation are conducted, clinicians will need to rely on evidence from related fields and their clinical judgment when choosing and applying different theories and their components.

Understanding our patients' beliefs, experiences, values, and hopes and incorporating this understanding into treatment is consistent with the principles of evidence-based practice (American Speech-Language-Hearing Association, 2005) and person-centered approaches to healthcare and rehabilitation (Worrall, 2006). Theories of motivation help describe why these practices are important and why they may result in better treatment outcomes. The approaches to supporting motivation outlined in this chapter have helped us fill a gap in our clinical skill set and the scope of our evidence-based practice. That is, we understood the available communication treatments and the evidence supporting them but were often unsure about how to help our patients stay engaged long enough and consistently enough to reap the benefits of those treatments.

REFERENCES

American Speech-Language-Hearing Association (ASHA). (2005). *Evidence-based practice in communication disorders.* Retrieved from http://www.asha.org/policy/PS2005-00221.htm

Amireault, S., Godin, G., & Vézina-Im, L.-A. (2013). Determinants of physical activity maintenance: A systematic review and meta-analyses. *Health Psychology Review, 7,* 55–91.

Ashford, S. J., & De Stobbeleir, K. E. (2013). Feedback, goal setting, and task performance revisited. In E. A. Locke & G. P. Latham (Eds.), *New developments in goal setting and task performance* (pp. 51–64). New York, NY: Routledge.

Ashford, S., Edmunds, J., & French, D. P. (2010). What is the best way to change self-efficacy to promote lifestyle and recreational physical activity? A systematic review with meta-analysis. *British Journal of Health Psychology, 15,* 265–288.

Avent, J., Glista, S., Wallace, S., Jackson, J., Nishioka, J., & Yip, W. (2005). Family information needs about aphasia. *Aphasiology, 19,* 365–375.

Babbitt, E. M., & Cherney, L. R. (2010). Communication confidence in persons with aphasia. *Topics in Stroke Rehabilitation, 17,* 214–223.

Babbitt, E. M., Heinemann, A. W., Semik, P., & Cherney, L. R. (2011). Psychometric properties of the communication confidence rating scale for aphasia (CCRSA): Phase 2. *Aphasiology, 25,* 727–735.

Bagwell, D. K., & West, R. L. (2008). Assessing compliance: Active versus inactive trainees in a memory intervention. *Clinical Interventions in Aging, 3,* 371–382.

Bandura, A. (1982). Self-efficacy mechanism in human agency. *American Psychologist, 37,* 122–147.

Bandura, A. (1986). *Social foundations of thought and action: A social cognitive theory.* Englewood Cliffs, NJ: Prentice-Hall.

Bandura, A. (1997). *Self-efficacy: The exercise of control.* New York, NY: W.H. Freeman.

Bandura, A. (1998). Health promotion from the perspective of social cognitive theory. *Psychology and Health, 13,* 623–649.

Bandura, A. (2006). Guide for constructing self-efficacy scales. In F. Pajares & T. C. Urdan (Eds.), *Self-efficacy beliefs of adolescents* (pp. 307–337). Greenwich, CT: Information Age Publishing.

Baumeister, R. F., & Leary, M. R. (1995). The need to belong: Desire for interpersonal attachments as a fundamental human motivation. *Psychological Bulletin, 117,* 497–529.

Baumeister, R. F., & Vohs, K. D. (2007). Self-regulation, ego depletion, and motivation. *Social and Personality Psychology Compass, 1,* 115–128.

Beaudoin, M., & Desrichard, O. (2011). Are memory self-efficacy and memory performance related? A meta-analysis. *Psychological Bulletin, 137,* 211–241.

Bem, D. J. (1967). Self-perception: An alternative interpretation of cognitive dissonance phenomena. *Psychological Review, 74,* 183–200.

Bright, F. A. S., Kayes, N. M., McCann, C. M., & McPherson, K. M. (2011). Understanding hope after stroke: A systematic review of the literature using concept analysis. *Topics in Stroke Rehabilitation, 18,* 490–508.

Bright, F. A. S., Kayes, N. M., McCann, C. M., & McPherson, K. M. (2013). Hope in people with aphasia. *Aphasiology, 27,* 41–58.

Buggey, T. (1995). An examination of the effectiveness of videotaped self-modeling in teaching specific linguistic structures to preschoolers. *Topics in Early Childhood Special Education, 15,* 434–458.

Burke, B. L., Arkowitz, H., & Menchola, M. (2003). The efficacy of motivational interviewing: A meta-analysis of controlled clinical trials. *Journal of Consulting and Clinical Psychology, 71,* 843–861.

Byng, S., & Duchan, J. F. (2005). Social model philosophies and principles: Their applications to therapies for aphasia. *Aphasiology, 19,* 906–922.

Cahana-Amitay, D., Albert, M. L., & Oveis, A. (2014). Psycholinguistics of aphasia pharmacotherapy: Asking the right questions. *Aphasiology, 28,* 133–154.

Cahana-Amitay, D., Albert, M. L., Pyun, S. B., Westwood, A., Jenkins, T., Wolford, S., & Finley, M. (2011). Language as a stressor in aphasia. *Aphasiology, 25,* 593–614.

Chapey, R., Duchan, J. F., Elman, R. J., Garcia, L. J., Kagan, A., Lyon, J. G., & Simmons-Mackie, N. (2008). Life-participation approach to aphasia: A statement of values for the future. In R. Chapey (Ed.), *Language intervention strategies in aphasia and related neurogenic communication disorders* (5th ed., pp. 279–289). Baltimore, MD: Lippincott Williams & Wilkins.

Cicerone, K. D., & Azulay, J. (2007). Perceived self-efficacy and life satisfaction after traumatic brain injury. *Journal of Head Trauma Rehabilitation, 22,* 257–266.

Cocchini, G., & Della Sala, S. (2010). Assessing anosognosia for motor and language impairments. In G. P. Prigatano (Ed.), *The study of anosognosia* (pp. 123–146). New York, NY: Oxford University Press.

Coles, J., & Snow, B. (2011). Applying the principles of peer mentorship in persons with aphasia. *Topics in Stroke Rehabilitation, 18,* 106–111.

Conroy, P., Sage, K., & Lambon Ralph, M. A. (2009). Errorless and errorful therapy for verb and noun naming in aphasia. *Aphasiology, 23,* 1311–1337.

Cream, A., & O'Brian, S. (2012). Self-modelling for chronic stuttering. In S. J. Jakšić & M. Onslow (Eds.), *The science and practice of stuttering treatment: A symposium* (pp. 159–170). Chichester, United Kingdom: Wiley-Blackwell.

Cyr-Stafford, C. (1993). The dynamics of speech therapy in aphasia. In D. LaFond (Ed.), *Living with aphasia: Psychosocial issues* (pp. 103–116). San Diego, CA: Singular Publishing Group.

deCharms, R. (1968). *Personal causation: The internal affective determinants of behavior*. New York, NY: Academic Press.

Deci, E. L., Eghrari, H., Patrick, B. C., & Leone, D. R. (1994). Facilitating internalization: The self-determination theory perspective. *Journal of Personality, 62*, 119–142.

Deci, E. L., & Ryan, R. M. (1985). *Intrinsic motivation and self-determination in human behavior*. New York, NY: Plenum Press.

Deci, E. L., & Ryan, R. M. (1991). A motivational approach to self: Integration in personality. In R. Dienstbier (Ed.), *Nebraska Symposium on Motivation* (Vol. 38, Perspectives on Motivation, pp. 237–288). Lincoln, NB: University of Nebraska Press.

Deci, E. L., & Ryan, R. M. (2000). The "what" and "why" of goal pursuits: Human needs and the self-determination of behavior. *Psychological Inquiry, 11*, 227–268.

Deci, E. L., & Ryan, R. M. (2008). Facilitating optimal motivation and psychological well-being across life's domains. *Canadian Psychology, 49*, 14–23.

Deci, E. L., Ryan, R. M., & Williams, G. C. (1996). Need satisfaction and the self-regulation of learning. *Learning and Individual Differences, 8*, 165–183.

Dixon, G., Thornton, E. W., & Young, C. A. (2007). Perceptions of self-efficacy and rehabilitation among neurologically disabled adults. *Clinical Rehabilitation, 21*, 230–240.

Dowrick, P. W. (1999). A review of self modeling and related interventions. *Applied and Preventive Psychology, 8*, 23–39.

Drieschner, K. H., Lammers, S. M. M., & van der Staak, C. P. (2004). Treatment motivation: An attempt for clarification of an ambiguous concept. *Clinical Psychology Review, 23*, 1115–1137.

Dunn, C., Deroo, L., & Rivara, F. P. (2001). The use of brief interventions adapted from motivational interviewing across behavioral domains: A systematic review. *Addiction, 96*, 1725–1742.

Eccles, J. S., & Wigfield, A. (2002). Motivational beliefs, values, and goals. *Annual Review of Psychology, 53*, 109–132.

Eisenson, J. (1949). Prognostic factors related to language rehabilitation in aphasic patients. *Journal of Speech and Hearing Disorders, 14*, 262–264.

Enderby, P., & Petheram, B. (1992). Self-administered therapy at home for aphasic patients. *Aphasiology, 6*, 321–324.

Festinger, L. (1957). *A theory of cognitive dissonance*. Stanford, CA: Stanford University Press.

Fox, L. E., Sohlberg, M. M., & Fried-Oken, M. (2001). Effects of conversational topic choice on outcomes of augmentative communication intervention for adults with aphasia. *Aphasiology, 15*, 171–200.

Gauggel, S., & Billino, J. (2002). The effects of goal setting on the arithmetic performance of brain-damaged patients. *Archives of Clinical Neuropsychology, 17*, 283–294.

Gauggel, S., Leinberger, R., & Richardt, M. (2001). Goal setting and reaction time performance in brain-damaged patients. *Journal of Clinical and Experimental Neuropsychology, 23*, 351–361.

Gonzalez, V. M., Goeppinger, J., & Lorig, K. (1990). Four psychosocial theories and their application to patient education and clinical practice. *Arthritis & Rheumatism, 3*, 132–143.

Gorman, P. (2004). *Motivation and emotion*. New York, NY: Routledge.

Gourlan, M., Sarrazin, P., & Trouilloud, D. (2013). Motivational interviewing as a way to promote physical activity in obese adolescents: A randomised-controlled trial using self-determination theory as an explanatory framework. *Psychology and Health, 28*, 1265–1286.

Green, C., & Waks, L. (2008). A second chance: Recovering language with aphasia. *International Journal of Speech Language Pathology, 10*, 127–131.

Hagger, M. S. (2009). Theoretical integration in health psychology: Unifying ideas and complementary explanations. *British Journal of Health Psychology, 14,* 189–194.

Haley, K. L., Womack, J., Helm-Estabrooks, N., Lovette, B., & Goff, R. (2013). Supporting autonomy for people with aphasia: Use of the life interests and values (LIV) cards. *Topics in Stroke Rehabilitation, 20,* 22–35.

Hattie, J., & Timperley, H. (2007). The power of feedback. *Review of Educational Research, 77,* 81–112.

Henderlong, J., & Lepper, M. R. (2002). The effects of praise on children's intrinsic motivation: A review and synthesis. *Psychological Bulletin, 128,* 774–795.

Hersh, D. (2003). "Weaning" clients from aphasia therapy: Speech pathologists: Strategies for discharge. *Aphasiology, 17*(11), 1007–1029.

Hersh, D., Worrall, L., Howe, T., Sherratt, S., & Davidson, B. (2012). SMARTER goal setting in aphasia rehabilitation. *Aphasiology, 26*(2), 220–233.

Hettema, J., Steele, J., & Miller, W. R. (2005). Motivational interviewing. *Annual Review of Clinical Psychology, 1,* 91–111.

Hofmann, S. G., Sawyer, A. T., Witt, A. A., & Oh, D. (2010). The effect of mindfulness-based therapy on anxiety and depression: A meta-analytic review. *Journal of Consulting and Clinical Psychology, 78,* 169–183.

Holden, G. (1991). The relationship of self-efficacy appraisals to subsequent health related outcomes. *Social Work in Health Care, 16*(1), 53–93.

Hopper, T., & Holland, A. L. (2005). Aphasia and learning in adults: Key concepts and clinical considerations. *Topics in Geriatric Rehabilitation, 21,* 315–322.

Jones, F. (2006). Strategies to enhance chronic disease self-management: How can we apply this to stroke? *Disability and Rehabilitation, 28,* 841–847.

Jones, F., & Riazi, A. (2011). Self-efficacy and self-management after stroke: A systematic review. *Disability and Rehabilitation, 33,* 797–810.

Kagan, A. (1998). Supported conversation for adults with aphasia: Methods and resources for training conversation partners. *Aphasiology, 12,* 816–830.

Katz, I., & Assor, A. (2007). When choice motivates and when it does not. *Educational Psychology Review, 19,* 429–442.

Kaufman, S., & Becker, G. (1986). Stroke: Health care on the periphery. *Social Science and Medicine, 22,* 983–989.

Kauhanen, M. L., Korpelainen, J. T., Hiltunen, P., Maatta, R., Mononen, H., Brusin, E., . . . Myllyla, V. (2000). Aphasia, depression, and non-verbal cognitive impairment in ischaemic stroke. *Cerebrovascular Diseases, 10,* 455–461.

Kertesz, A. (2010). Anosognosia in aphasia. In G. P. Prigatano (Ed.), *The study of anosognosia* (pp. 113–122). New York, NY: Oxford University Press.

King, P., & Barrowclough, C. (1989). Rating the motivation of elderly patients on a rehabilitation ward. *Clinical Rehabilitation, 3,* 289–291.

Kirsch, I. (1995). Self-efficacy and outcome expectancy: A concluding commentary. In J. E. Maddux (Ed.), *Self-efficacy, adaptation, and adjustment: Theory, research, and application* (pp. 331–346). New York: Plenum Press.

Korpershoek, C., van der Bijl, J., & Hafsteinsdóttir, T. B. (2011). Self-efficacy and its influence on recovery of patients with stroke: A systematic review. *Journal of Advanced Nursing, 67,* 1876–1894.

Le Dorze, G., & Brassard, C. (1995). A description of the consequences of aphasia on aphasic persons and their relatives and friends, based on the WHO model of chronic diseases. *Aphasiology, 9,* 239–255.

Lee, L. L., Arthur, A., & Avis, M. (2007). Evaluating a community-based walking intervention for hypertensive older people in Taiwan: A randomized controlled trial. *Preventive Medicine, 44,* 160–166.

Lequerica, A. H., & Kortte, K. (2010). Therapeutic engagement: A proposed model of engagement in medical rehabilitation. *American Journal of Physical Medicine and Rehabilitation, 89,* 415–422.

Lerdal, A., Bakken, L. N., Kouwenhoven, S. E., Pedersen, G., Kirkevold, M., Finset, A., & Kim, H. S. (2009). Poststroke fatigue—a review. *Journal of Pain and Symptom Management, 38,* 928–949.

Leung, K. K., Silvius, J. L., Pimlott, N., Dalziel, W., & Drummond, N. (2009). Why health expectations and hopes are different: The development of a conceptual model. *Health Expectations, 12,* 347–360.

Levack, W. M. M., Taylor, K., Siegert, R. J., Dean, S. G., McPherson, K. M., & Weatherall, M. (2006). Is goal planning in rehabilitation effective? A systematic review. *Clinical Rehabilitation, 20,* 739–755.

Locke, E. A., & Latham, G. P. (2002). Building a practically useful theory of goal setting and task motivation. A 35-year odyssey. *American Psychologist, 57,* 705–717.

Lorig, K. R., & Holman, H. (2003). Self-management education: History, definition, outcomes, and mechanisms. *Annals of Behavioral Medicine, 26,* 1–7.

Lundahl, B. W., Kunz, C., Brownell, C., Tollefson, D., & Burke, B. L. (2010). A meta-analysis of motivational interviewing: Twenty-five years of empirical studies. *Research on Social Work Practice, 20,* 137–160.

Luszczynska, A., Tryburcy, M., & Schwarzer, R. (2007). Improving fruit and vegetable consumption: A self-efficacy intervention compared with a combined self-efficacy and planning intervention. *Health Education Research, 22,* 630–638.

Mackenzie, C., Le May, M., Lendrem, W., McGuirk, E., Marshall, J., & Rossiter, D. (1993). A survey of aphasia services in the United Kingdom. *European Journal of Disorders of Communication, 28,* 43–61.

Maclean, N., & Pound, P. (2000). A critical review of the concept of patient motivation in the literature on physical rehabilitation. *Social Science and Medicine, 50,* 495–506.

Maclean, N., Pound, P., Wolfe, C., & Rudd, A. (2002). The concept of patient motivation: A qualitative analysis of stroke professionals' attitudes. *Stroke, 33,* 444–448.

Maddux, J. E., & Lewis, J. (1995). Self-efficacy and adjustment: Basic principles and issues. In J. E. Maddux (Ed.), *Self-efficacy, adaptation, and adjustment: Theory, research, and application* (pp. 37–68). New York, NY: Plenum Press.

Markland, D., Ryan, R. M., & Tobin, V. J. (2005). Motivational interviewing and self–determination theory. *Journal of Social and Clinical Psychology, 24,* 811–831.

Millen, J. A., & Bray, S. R. (2009). Promoting self-efficacy and outcome expectations to enable adherence to resistance training after cardiac rehabilitation. *Journal of Cardiovascular Nursing, 24,* 316–327.

Miller, K. J., McCrady, B. S., Abrams, D. B., & Labouvie, E. W. (1994). Taking an individualized approach to the assessment of self-efficacy and the prediction of alcoholic relapse. *Journal of Psychopathology and Behavioral Assessment, 16,* 111–120.

Miller, W. R., & Rollnick, S. (2012). *Motivational interviewing: Helping people change* (3rd ed.). New York, NY: Guilford Press.

Moritz, S. E., Feltz, D. L., Fahrbach, K. R., & Mack, D. E. (2000). The relation of self-efficacy measures to sport performance: A meta-analytic review. *Research Quarterly for Exercise and Sport, 71,* 280–294.

Multon, K. D., Brown, S. D., & Lent, R. W. (1991). Relation of self-efficacy beliefs to academic outcomes: A meta-analytic investigation. *Journal of Counseling Psychology, 38,* 30–38.

Murray, L. (2008). The application of relaxation training approaches to patients with neurogenic disorders and their caregivers. *Perspectives on Neurophysiology and Neurogenic Speech and Language Disorders, 18*(3), 90–98.

Ng, J. Y. Y., Ntoumanis, N., Thogersen-Ntoumani, C., Deci, E. L., Ryan, R. M., Duda, J. L., & Williams, G. C. (2012). Self-determination theory applied to health contexts: A meta-analysis. *Perspectives on Psychological Science, 7*, 325–340.

Noar, S. M., & Zimmerman, R. S. (2005). Health behavior theory and cumulative knowledge regarding health behaviors: Are we moving in the right direction? *Health Education Research, 20*, 275–290.

Pajares, F. (1996). Self-efficacy beliefs in academic settings. *Review of Educational Research, 66*, 543–578.

Pascal, B. (2003). *Pensées* [Thoughts] (W. F. Trotter, Trans.). Mineola, NY: Dover Publications (Original work published 1669).

Patall, E. A., Cooper, H., & Robinson, J. C. (2008). The effects of choice on intrinsic motivation and related outcomes: A meta-analysis of research findings. *Psychological Bulletin, 134*, 270–300.

Patrick, H., & Williams, G. C. (2012). Self-determination theory: Its application to health behavior and complementarity with motivational interviewing. *The International Journal of Behavioral Nutrition and Physical Activity, 9*, 18. Retrieved from http://www.ijbnpa.org/content/9/1/18

Payne, B. R., Jackson, J. J., Hill, P. L., Gao, X., Roberts, B. W., & Stine-Morrow, E. A. L. (2012). Memory self-efficacy predicts responsiveness to inductive reasoning training in older adults. *The Journals of Gerontology, Series B: Psychological Sciences and Social Sciences, 67*, 27–35.

Pelletier, L. G., Fortier, M. S., Vallerand, R. J., & Briere, N. M. (2001). Associations among perceived autonomy support, forms of self-regulation, and persistence: A prospective study. *Motivation and Emotion, 25*, 279–306.

Pollak, K. I., Alexander, S. C., Tulsky, J. A., Lyna, P., Coffman, C. J., Dolor, R. J., . . . Ostbye, T. (2011). Physician empathy and listening: Associations with patient satisfaction and autonomy. *Journal of the American Board of Family Medicine, 24*, 665–672.

Reeve, J., Jang, H., Carrell, D., Jeon, S., & Barch, J. (2004). Enhancing students' engagement by increasing teachers' autonomy support. *Motivation and Emotion, 28*, 147–169.

Reeve, J., Jang, H., Hardre, P., & Omura, M. (2002). Providing a rationale in an autonomy-supportive way as a strategy to motivate others during an uninteresting activity. *Motivation and Emotion, 26*, 183–207.

Resnick, B. (2002). Geriatric rehabilitation: The influence of efficacy beliefs and motivation. *Rehabilitation Nursing, 27*, 152–159.

Resnicow, K., & McMaster, F. (2012). Motivational interviewing: Moving from why to how with autonomy support. *International Journal of Behavioral Nutrition and Physical Activity, 9*(1), 19. Retrieved from http://www.ijbnpa.org/content/9/1/19

Robinson-Smith, G., & Pizzi, E. R. (2003). Maximizing stroke recovery using patient self-care self-efficacy. *Rehabilitation Nursing, 28*, 48–51.

Rodgers, M., Wilson, M., Hall, R., Fraser, N., & Murray, C. (2008). Evidence for a multidimensional self-efficacy for exercise scale. *Research Quarterly for Exercise and Sport, 79*(2), 222–234.

Rogers, C. R. (1959). A theory of therapy, personality, and interpersonal relationships as developed in the client-centered framework. In S. Koch (Ed.), *Psychology: The study of a science* (Vol. 3, Formulations of the person and the social context, pp. 184–256). New York, NY: McGraw-Hill.

Rollnick, S., Miller, W. R., & Butler, C. (2008). *Motivational interviewing in health care: Helping patients change behavior.* New York, NY: Guilford Press.

Rosenbek, J. C., Lemme, M. L., Ahern, M. B., Harris, E. H., & Wertz, R. T. (1973). A treatment for apraxia of speech in adults. *Journal of Speech and Hearing Disorders, 38*, 462–472.

Roth, G., Assor, A., Niemiec, C. P., Deci, E. L., & Ryan, R. M. (2009). The emotional and academic consequences of parental conditional regard: Comparing conditional positive regard, conditional negative regard, and autonomy support as parenting practices. *Developmental Psychology*, *45*, 1119–1142.

Rothman, A. J., & Salovey, P. (2007). The reciprocal relation between principles and practice: Social psychology and health behavior. In A. W. Kruglanski & E. T. Higgins (Eds.), *Social psychology: Handbook of basic principles* (2nd ed., pp. 826–849). New York, NY: Guilford Press.

Russell, K. L., & Bray, S. R. (2010). Promoting self-determined motivation for exercise in cardiac rehabilitation: The role of autonomy support. *Rehabilitation Psychology*, *55*, 74–80.

Ryan, R. M. (1982). Control and information in the intrapersonal sphere: An extension of cognitive evaluation theory. *Journal of Personality and Social Psychology*, *43*(3), 450–461.

Ryan, R. M., & Deci, E. L. (2000a). Intrinsic and extrinsic motivations: Classic definitions and new directions. *Contemporary Educational Psychology*, *25*, 54–67.

Ryan, R. M., & Deci, E. L. (2000b). Self-determination theory and the facilitation of intrinsic motivation, social development, and well-being. *American Psychologist*, *55*, 68–78.

Ryan, R. M., Lynch, M. F., Vansteenkiste, M., & Deci, E. L. (2011). Motivation and autonomy in counseling, psychotherapy, and behavior change: A look at theory and practice. *The Counseling Psychologist*, *39*, 193–260.

Schwarzer, R., Lippke, S., & Luszczynska, A. (2011). Mechanisms of health behavior change in persons with chronic illness or disability: The health action process approach (HAPA). *Rehabilitation Psychology*, *56*, 161–170.

Scobbie, L., Dixon, D., & Wyke, S. (2011). Goal setting and action planning in the rehabilitation setting: Development of a theoretically informed practice framework. *Clinical Rehabilitation*, *25*, 468–482.

Scobbie, L., McLean, D., Dixon, D., Duncan, E., & Wyke, S. (2013). Implementing a framework for goal setting in community based stroke rehabilitation: A process evaluation. *BMC Health Service Research*, *13*, 190. Retrieved from http://www.biomedcentral.com/1472-6963/13/190

Scobbie, L., Wyke, S., & Dixon, D. (2009). Identifying and applying psychological theory to setting and achieving rehabilitation goals. *Clinical Rehabilitation*, *23*, 321–333.

Shaughnessy, M., & Resnick, B. M. (2009). Using theory to develop an exercise intervention for patients post stroke. *Topics in Stroke Rehabilitation*, *16*, 140–146.

Sheldon, K. M., Elliot, A. J., Kim, Y., & Kasser, T. (2001). What is satisfying about satisfying events? Testing 10 candidate psychological needs. *Journal of Personality and Social Psychology*, *80*, 325–339.

Sheldon, K. M., Williams, G., & Joiner, T. E. (2003). *Self-determination theory in the clinic: Motivating physical and mental health*. New Haven, CT: Yale University Press.

Sierens, E., Vansteenkiste, M., Goossens, L., Soenens, B., & Dochy, F. (2009). The synergistic relationship of perceived autonomy support and structure in the prediction of self-regulated learning. *The British Journal of Educational Psychology*, *79*, 57–68.

Simmons-Mackie, N., & Damico, J. (2007). Access and social inclusion in aphasia: Interactional principles and applications. *Aphasiology*, *21*, 81–97.

Small, S. L., & Llano, D. A. (2009). Biological approaches to aphasia treatment. *Current Neurology and Neuroscience Reports*, *9*, 443–450.

Snyder, C. R., Rand, K. L., King, E. A., Feldman, D. B., & Woodward, J. T. (2002). "False" hope. *Journal of Clinical Psychology*, *58*, 1003–1022.

Stajkovic, A. D., & Luthans, F. (1998). Self-efficacy and work-related performance: A meta-analysis. *Psychological Bulletin*, *124*, 240–261.

Sweet, S. N., Fortier, M. S., Strachan, S. M., Blanchard, C. M., & Boulay, P. (2014). Testing a longitudinal integrated self-efficacy and self-determination theory model for physical activity post-cardiac rehabilitation. *Health Psychology Research, 2,* 30–37.

Teixeira, P. J., Carraça, E. V., Markland, D., Silva, M. N., & Ryan, R. M. (2012). Exercise, physical activity, and self-determination theory: A systematic review. *The International Journal of Behavioral Nutrition and Physical Activity, 9,* 78. Retrieved from http://www.ijbnpa.org/content/9/1/78

Toglia, J., & Kirk, U. (2000). Understanding awareness deficits following brain injury. *NeuroRehabilitation, 15,* 57–70.

Usher, L., & Pajares, F. (2008). Sources of self-efficacy in school: Critical review of the literature and future directions. *Review of Educational Research, 78,* 751–796.

van Leer, E., & Connor, N. P. (2012). Use of portable digital media players increases patient motivation and practice in voice therapy. *Journal of Voice, 26,* 447–453.

van Rijsbergen, M. W., Mark, R. E., de Kort, P. L., & Sitskoorn, M. M. (2014). Subjective cognitive complaints after stroke: A systematic review. *Journal of Stroke and Cerebrovascular Diseases, 23,* 408–420.

Vansteenkiste, M., Lens, W., & Deci, E. L. (2006). Intrinsic versus extrinsic goal contents in self-determination theory: Another look at the quality of academic motivation. *Educational Psychologist, 41,* 19–31.

Vansteenkiste, M., Niemiec, C. P., & Soenens, B. (2010). The development of the five mini-theories of self-determination theory: An historical overview, emerging trends, and future directions. *Advances in Motivation and Achievement, 16,* 105–165.

Vansteenkiste, M., Simons, J., Lens, W., Sheldon, K. M., & Deci, E. L. (2004). Motivating learning, performance, and persistence: The synergistic effects of intrinsic goal contents and autonomy-supportive contexts. *Journal of Personality and Social Psychology, 87*(2), 246–260.

Wade, D. (2009). Adverse effects of rehabilitation—an opportunity to increase quality and effectiveness of rehabilitation. *Clinical Rehabilitation, 23,* 387–393.

Welch, D. C., & West, R. L. (1995). Self-efficacy and mastery: Its application to issues of environmental control, cognition, and aging. *Developmental Review, 15,* 150–171.

Wepman, J. M. (1953). A conceptual model for the processes involved in recovery from aphasia. *Journal of Speech and Hearing Disorders, 18,* 4–13.

West, R. L., Bagwell, D. K., & Dark-Freudeman, A. (2005). Memory and goal setting: The response of older and younger adults to positive and objective feedback. *Psychology and Aging, 20,* 195–201.

West, R. L., Bagwell, D. K., & Dark-Freudeman, A. (2008). Self-efficacy and memory aging: The impact of a memory intervention based on self-efficacy. *Aging, Neuropsychology, and Cognition, 15*(3), 302–329.

West, R. L., & Yassuda, M. S. (2004). Aging and memory control beliefs: Performance in relation to goal setting and memory self-evaluation. *The Journals of Gerontology: Psychological Sciences, 59B,* P56–P65.

Whitney, J. L., & Goldstein, H. (1989). Using self-monitoring to reduce disfluencies in speakers with mild aphasia. *Journal of Speech and Hearing Disorders, 54*(4), 576–586.

Williams, D. M. (2010). Outcome expectancy and self-efficacy: Theoretical implications of an unresolved contradiction. *Personality and Social Psychology Review, 14,* 417–425.

Williams, S. L., & French, D. P. (2011). What are the most effective intervention techniques for changing physical activity self-efficacy and physical activity behaviour—and are they the same? *Health Education Research, 26,* 308–322.

Wilson, K. P. (2013). Incorporating video modeling into a school-based intervention for students with autism spectrum disorders. *Language, Speech, and Hearing Services in Schools, 44,* 105–117.

Worrall, L. (2006). Professionalism and functional outcomes. *Journal of Communication Disorders, 39,* 320–327.

Worrall, L., Brown, K., Cruice, M., Davidson, B., Hersh, D., Howe, T., & Sherratt, S. (2010). The evidence for a life-coaching approach to aphasia. *Aphasiology, 24,* 497–514.

Worrall, L., Davidson, B., Hersh, D., Ferguson, A., Howe, T., & Sherratt, S. (2010). The evidence for relationship-centred practice in aphasia rehabilitation. *Journal of Interactional Research in Communication Disorders, 1,* 277–300.

Wulf, G., Freitas, H. E., & Tandy, R. D. (2014). Choosing to exercise more: Small choices increase exercise engagement. *Psychology of Sport and Exercise, 15,* 268–271.

Youmans, G., Holland, A., Muñoz, M. L., & Bourgeois, M. (2005). Script training and automaticity in two individuals with aphasia. *Aphasiology, 19,* 435–450.

CHAPTER 13

Operationalizing Informal Assessment

Patrick Coppens
Nina Simmons-Mackie

INTRODUCTION

It is traditional for speech-language pathologists to administer standardized tests to their patients with aphasia. The main purpose of such formal assessments is twofold: to quantify communicative behaviors (such as for diagnosis or classification) and to provide pretherapy measurements for future comparisons. However, the data generated by these formal measures contribute only minimally to clinical decisions. Although these data may provide general information about the patient's relative strengths and weaknesses, they do not allow clinicians to determine which skills are the most functional for the patient, which strategy is most likely to facilitate the patient's successful communication, which specific underlying mechanism is at the root of the patient's difficulties, or which outcome goals are most important to the person with aphasia and his or her family. To maximize the success of the clinical process, these questions must be answered, and they are best addressed during informal assessment procedures. It follows then, that the informal assessment process is a necessary step between the formal assessment and the articulation of appropriate clinical goals.

Master clinicians may be adept at selecting the most relevant therapeutic objectives from information gathered informally, but they may be hard-pressed to put into words the procedure they use to carry out these important steps, let alone be able to teach this process to clinicians-in-training. Conceptualizing the informal assessment process into an organizational structure of purposes and associated procedures may help clinicians apply informal assessment methods more effectively and may assist clinicians-in-training in applying informal assessment more systematically and logically. It is the intent of this chapter to operationalize the process of informal assessment

BACKGROUND AND DEFINITIONS

Informal Assessment

There is relatively little research specifically focused on informal assessment, particularly in adult neurogenic communication disorders. However, there is universal agreement that standardized test results are not the be-all and end-all of assessment. For example, Muma (1978) states "behavior simply cannot be reduced to numbers without losing essential information" (p. 215). Few authors provide a definition of informal assessment; and furthermore, the concept is usually described rather than defined. For example, Haynes and Pindzola (2012) include the following goals in their assessment protocol: identify the type of error, response to cueing, and compensatory strategies (p. 232). For Muma (1978), informal assessment is *contextualized* and formal assessment is *decontextualized* (p. 226). The former makes use of any contextual cues to assist communication, while the latter seeks to isolate the patient's language knowledge from its use.

Most clinicians are familiar with the concept of *dynamic assessment*, and most authors implicitly equate dynamic assessment with informal assessment. As will become clear in this chapter, we believe that dynamic assessment is only one element of the informal assessment process, and the latter concept is broader in scope. Regardless of which of the two labels is used, most authors describe the informal assessment process as seeking answers to specific questions. Haynes and Pindzola (2012) list a series of appropriate questions that bear on the types of errors, compensatory and facilitation strategies, multimodal approaches to facilitate communication, and cueing strategies. They also emphasize the importance of observation in this process. According to Lidz and Peña (1996), the clinician generates hypotheses that are answered by the client's behavior, which they define as a "mini-experiment in intervention" (p. 368). Rosenbek, Lapointe, and Wertz (1989) suggest that investigating the underlying cause of a patient's anomia is akin to making "the clinic a laboratory" (p. 187). Tomblin, Morris, and Spriestersbach (2000) equate informal assessment to a "problem-solving process" (p. 5). ASHA (2004) appears to use the term *dynamic assessment* interchangeably with *informal assessment*, describing it as "using hypothesis-testing procedures." Similarly, Coelho, Ylvisaker, and Turkstra (2005) state that "dynamic assessment is experimental" (p. 224), is geared toward therapy planning, and is a "hypothesis-testing assessment" (p. 231). They conclude that "without experimentation it is never possible to know with certainty how to interpret failure on a test or other task or what recommendation would be most effective in improving performance" (p. 232). Whitworth, Webster, and Howard (2005) also recommend a "hypothesis-testing approach" (p. 25) specifically to identify the underlying mechanism of impairment, but they highlight observation as a necessary component of the process. Murray and Coppens (2017) think of informal assessment as "a fluid exercise in critical thinking" (p. 77). Finally, informal assessment can also be viewed as a process of discovery with an emphasis on capturing the perspective of the patient and significant others. The collaborative skill of the clinician is required to enlist the patient as a partner in testing hypotheses related to personally relevant lifestyle changes and social consequences of aphasia. From these examples, it is clear that the informal assessment process requires a clinician to generate hypothesis-testing questions by relying on their background knowledge, observation skills, interactive skills, and critical thinking skills.

If formal tests are seen as *quantitative*, informal assessment is seen as *qualitative*. For example, Murray and Clark (2015) recommend that a clinician observe the manner in which a patient executes a task for clues to possible compensatory strategies that might be developed in treatment (p. 133). However, informal assessment can also yield quantitative results. In the child language domain, McCauley (1996) describes informal criterion-referenced measures that yield a score. She considers these measures a way to answer clinical questions (i.e., hypothesis-testing questions), and offers a flow chart delineating a stepwise process from asking a hypothesis (clinical) question, to the administration of a clinician-generated informal testing tool, leading to a quantification of the behavior. For example, a clinician wonders whether a client is able to produce a particular morpheme. The clinician devises a series of stimuli and a success criterion and runs the trial. The quantitative results answer the original question.

If formal tests are seen as *static*, nonstandardized testing procedures are perceived as *dynamic*. Dynamic assessment is expressly addressed in an American Speech-Language-Hearing Preferred Practice document (ASHA, 2004). ASHA's stated goals for dynamic assessment are to "identify potentially successful interventions and support procedures." The concept of dynamic assessment was developed in the context of the child language development literature (e.g., Butler, 1997; Peña, Summers, & Resendiz, 2007) and borrowed from Vygotsky's work on *zone of proximal development* (Vygotsky, 1978), which ultimately morphed into the concept of *zone of instructional sensitivity* (Butler, 1997). In that context, dynamic assessment is part of informal assessment and focuses on modifying children's responses based on the clinician's manipulation of the support context. For example, Lidz and Peña (1996) describe dynamic assessment as applying a therapy-based interaction into the assessment process with an emphasis on how the child is processing the task. This requires a much more active interaction between child and examiner compared to the passive role the examiner plays when administering a formal test. More specifically, the authors identify three purposes of dynamic assessment as the examiner attempts (a) to observe how the child performs the tasks, (b) to identify what can prompt a modification of the observed behavior, and (c) to identify the approach with the best potential for rehabilitation. For all intents and purposes, dynamic assessment is used to "determine a client's range of performance, given help by the clinician" (Haynes & Pindzola, 2012, p. 9). Butler (1997) highlighted the collaborative aspect of dynamic assessment where the clinician becomes the child's "knowledgeable partner" (p. 48) to maximize the child's language performance and emergent knowledge. Implicit in such an interaction is its naturalness, that is, the assessment is now contextualized. These elements of active and collaborative interaction—noting processing style and determining a client's range of performance—are directly applicable while performing an informal assessment with an adult with aphasia.

Dynamic assessment has been extended beyond the initial sessions and into the therapy period per se. In the child language literature, the child's language is manipulated, helped, and scaffolded; the child's metacognitive skills are recruited to aid learning and ultimately generalization and carry-over; and data are gathered by the clinician before and after the intervention phase. As such, the application of dynamic assessment is reminiscent of an ABA experimental design where a baseline period of no treatment-A is followed by a period of treatment-B, and then a second period of no treatment-A. This description (Butler, 1997) underscores the importance of an organized data-gathering practice (hence inclusion of assessment in the therapy phase) and of a flexible, adaptive therapy procedure based on constant informal observation of the patient's behavior. In sum, as presented in this model from child language assessment, the components and the objectives of informal assessment should not only be used to articulate appropriate therapy goals at the onset of therapy, they also must be constantly used to adapt the therapy to the effected changes in the patient's abilities. This logic applies to the adult population with aphasia. For example, Hersh et al. (2013) describe "therapeutic assessment" as a dynamic assessment process that is embedded in the identification and the attainment of rehabilitation goals.

In conclusion, the development of appropriate clinical objectives at any time during aphasia rehabilitation must rely on the informal rather than the formal assessment process. For the purpose of this chapter, we will define *formal* assessment as the administration of standardized tests or subtests and *informal* assessment as any additional measures, data gathering, or observations performed by the clinician. In keeping with this definition, informal assessment can be contextualized (e.g., the clinician investigates which multimodal combination maximizes the patient's communicative effectiveness) or decontextualized (e.g., the clinician asks a client to write a series of functional words without assistance). Similarly, informal assessment results could be quantitative (e.g., percentage correct) or qualitative, in the case of a functional observation procedure. Our definition of informal assessment does encompass dynamic assessment and is similar to the nonstandardized assessment described by Coelho, Ylvisaker, and Turkstra (2005).

Psychosocial Approach

Starting in the late 1960s, some researchers began advocating for a more functional, contextualized approach to aphasia assessment and therapy (Holland, 1980; Sarno, 1969). This change heralded movement toward the *psychosocial* school, which emerged in parallel to the traditional *neuropsychological* approach. In the 1990s, the disability movement and social theory contributed to an expansion of the psychosocial model. Thus, social models of aphasia intervention (Simmons-Mackie, 1998) and Life Participation Approach to Aphasia (LPAA, 2000) were introduced. The proponents of the psychosocial/social model tend to focus assessment and rehabilitation efforts on conversational partners, communicative and social environments, and quality of life. This approach has relied heavily on the International Classification of Functioning, Disability and Health (ICF) of the World Health Organization (WHO, 2001), as applied to aphasia therapy by the Living with Aphasia: Framework for Outcome Measurement model (A-FROM, Kagan et al., 2008; see **FIGURE 13.1**). A-FROM provides an organizational framework for identifying assessment and intervention priorities.

Although there are formal assessment tools available for each category in the A-FROM model (Kagan et al., 2008), because the psychosocial approach has focused on informal assessment than the more traditional neuropsychological method (Simmons-Mackie, 2008), informal assessment tools play a significant role in the assessment process. Outcomes in the area of participation, personal factors, and quality of life often require subjective perspectives or reports from the client. For example, Simmons-Mackie (2008) describes the Social Network Analysis, which is a qualitative representation of a patient's socialization pattern derived from client and caregiver interviews. Similarly, interviews are often useful in determining personally relevant goals in the domain of participation. Not surprisingly, in the psychosocial/social approach the emphasis falls on dynamic assessment. As is the case in the child language literature (e.g., Lidz & Peña, 1996), dynamic assessment is seen as contextualized, functional, embedded in the rehabilitation process, and providing a more positive experience for the client than static assessment (Hersh et al., 2013). Informal assessment allows the clinician to partner with the client in the shared goal of improving communication; this is requisite to fulfilling the values inherent in the movement in medicine toward relationship or patient-centered practices (see for example Worrall et al., 2010) and has the potential to affect motivation positively (see Chapter 12, this volume).

The respective proponents of the neuropsychological and the psychosocial schools have come to the agreement that their methods contain more commonalities than disagreements (Martin, Thompson, & Worrall, 2008) and that their respective approaches to aphasia assessment and therapy differ in focus but not in substance. Contemporary aphasia rehabilitation has reconciled the psychosocial and the neuropsychological viewpoints into a *biopsychosocial* approach (Worrall, Sherrat, & Papathanasiou, 2017). It is thus necessary that this extended view of aphasia therapy be encompassed in a thorough informal assessment process.

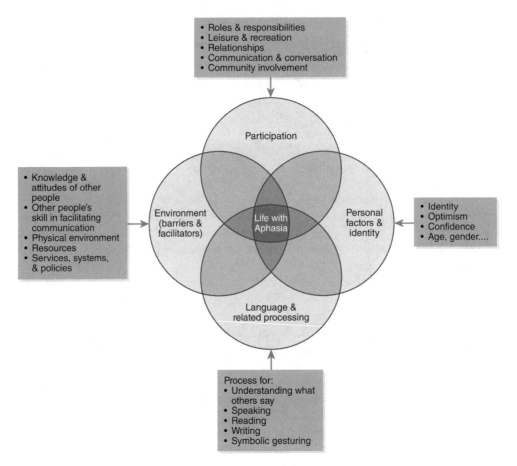

FIGURE 13.1 Examples of categories that make up the four key domains in the Living with Aphasia: Framework for Outcome Measurement (A-FROM).

Kagan, A. Simmons-Mackie, N., Rowland, A., Huijbregts, M., Shumay, E., McEwen, S.,...Sharp, S. [2008] Counting what counts: A framework for capturing real-life outcomes of aphasia intervention. Aphasiology, 22, 258-280; adapted by permission of Aphasia Institute.

THE INFORMAL ASSESSMENT

The informal assessment process described here should not be construed as a sequence of ordered steps. Rather, the successful application of this process hinges on important elements, all of which should contribute to an effective and thorough analysis of the patient's clinical abilities and maximize the pertinence and importance of the clinical objectives eventually selected. In our view, these crucial components of the process include the clinical acumen of the clinician, the appropriateness of the hypothesis-testing questions generated, and the thoroughness of the answers to specific goal-oriented questions (see **FIGURE 13.2**).

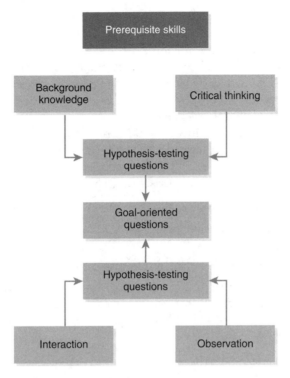

FIGURE 13.2 The informal assessment process: pre-requisite skills.

Prerequisite Clinician Skills

As stated previously, researchers have recognized that an effective informal assessment process starts with asking hypothesis questions designed to illuminate an area of the client's abilities or experience that was not addressed in the formal assessment procedures. This exercise is indispensable to reach appropriate clinical objectives. In order to formulate the most relevant questions, clinicians must possess (a) good background knowledge of the specific clinical population, (b) good critical thinking skills, (c) good observation skills, and (d) good interactive skills in order to work with the patient as a partner in the assessment process.

First, a thorough knowledge of the aphasia type and its relevant literature will help clinicians suspect potential associated difficulties and anticipate potential facilitation strategies. For example, knowing that some clients with aphasia following a lesion in the left postero-superior temporal lobe have significant auditory-verbal working memory impairments (Leff et al., 2009) should prompt an investigation of that skill to evaluate its impact on the clinical picture. Also, being able to disambiguate phonemic paraphasias from apraxia of speech errors in a client with Broca's aphasia will help clinicians focus therapy on the most impaired skill. Another example with a functional focus would be to ask the patient and spouse specific questions about the family roles the person with aphasia was fulfilling premorbidly and hopes to fulfill in the future. This information will assist in establishing functional objectives, in an attempt to prevent or minimize negative social and emotional consequences of aphasia. These kinds of hypothesis-testing questions rely on the clinicians' accumulated knowledge about similar cases in the literature and/or in their previous clinical experience.

Second, critical thinking skills are essential in order to ask the most pertinent clinical questions. While these skills are hard to teach and usually not directly addressed in the professional training of clinicians, they are nevertheless intertwined in everything clinicians do. According to the Foundation for Critical Thinking (2013), a critical thinker:

- Raises vital questions and problems, formulating them clearly and precisely
- Gathers and assesses relevant information, using abstract ideas to interpret it effectively
- Comes to well-reasoned conclusions and solutions, testing them against relevant criteria and standards
- Thinks openmindedly within alternative systems of thought, recognizing and assessing, as need be, their assumptions, implications, and practical consequences

This definition clearly implies that critical thinking is a tool that should help formulate questions and answers based on a logical and methodical interpretation of information. Applied to clinical assessment, this definition emphasizes that appropriate questions be asked, that they be clear, and that they be answered thoughtfully and without bias. In addition, it requires that clinicians consciously evaluate and reflect on their thinking process.

Third, good observation skills will help clinicians glean precious information from a client's behavior. A savvy clinician is constantly dissecting a patient's responses, spontaneous compensatory strategies, communication breakdown, and conversation repairs to seek relevant clinical information, in the event that one of these behaviors may become a useful add-on to the therapeutic armamentarium. Observation permeates all levels of assessment and therapy and may trigger hypothesis-testing clinical questions that may require further informal measurement. For example, during an interaction with his spouse, a person with aphasia showed very limited attempts at initiation, whereas his responses were mostly communicative, albeit agrammatic. The clinician suspected particular difficulty with questions, and informally assessed production of "wh-" words. The results were poor, and it was decided to add question asking as a therapy objective. Skillful observation also includes the ability to observe or listen for deeper meanings in clients' behavior and communication—meanings that provide insight into the personal, emotional, and social consequences of aphasia for each individual. For example, the client who explains his lack of social interactions as follows: "seeing people ... don't want to ... can't talk ... embarrass" provides important clues to the loss of self-esteem associated with his aphasia. For this client, issues of self-confidence and self-esteem are barriers to generalization of language gains; thus, treatment will need to simultaneously address communication and communicative confidence.

A fourth critical prerequisite is interactive skill, including the ability to engage the client in the assessment process and collaborate with the client as a partner. The skilled clinician views the assessment process as teamwork between two adults (client and clinician) who share the ultimate goal of improving the communicative life of the person with aphasia. Respect for the client as a partner is inherent in a relationship-centered approach to assessment (Worrall et al., 2010). Simmons-Mackie and Damico (2011) suggest that the success of assessment and therapy relies on the clinician's successful management of the social interaction with the client. The skilled clinician is able to enlist the cooperation of the client and the family while simultaneously crafting and managing interactions that provide insight into the client's communicative abilities and the impact of aphasia on their communicative life.

These four crucial prerequisite skills—background knowledge, critical thinking, observation, and interactive skill—are indispensible for clinicians to generate pertinent clinical hypothesis questions during informal assessment and ultimately to maximize the quality of their rehabilitation objectives.

Goals and Strategies

Informal assessment serves as the investigative period during which the clinician seeks all the useful clinical information needed to design the most appropriate objectives and strategies for the rehabilitative effort. In this section we propose a framework of goal-oriented questions that can help clinicians approach informal assessment more systematically. All of the goal-oriented questions address important information that will influence therapy objectives, and each main question may in turn require further hypothesis-testing questions. The first goal-oriented question focuses on understanding the breadth of the clinical picture and its consequences, and consideration of "big picture" outcomes, whereas the three subsequent questions address different aspects of a specific behavior; respectively its severity, its potential as a compensatory strategy, and finally its cause (see **FIGURE 13.3**).

Goal-Oriented Question 1: What Is the Scope of the Clinical Symptomatology and Its Impact on the Client's Life?
In order to identify the target areas with the most pressing need of rehabilitation, one of the clinician's responsibilities is to have a thorough understanding of the client's total clinical picture. The formal assessment process may have included an aphasia battery (e.g., Western Aphasia Battery-Revised [WAB-R]; Kertesz, 2007) and/or a more contextualized

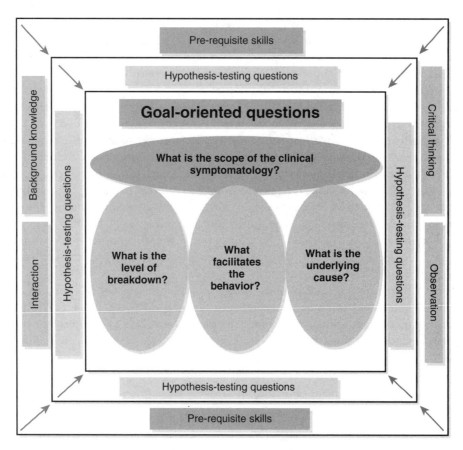

FIGURE 13.3 The informal assessment process: goal-oriented questions.

test (e.g., Communication Abilities of Daily Living-2 [CADL-2]; Holland, Frattali, & Fromm, 1999). Although these tools reveal pertinent information about the client's linguistic abilities and functional communicative skills, there are many unexplored domains that have the potential to significantly influence therapeutic decisions. For example, what do we know about written language ability, any type of apraxia, conversational breakdowns with caregivers, communication needs in social activities, or any other language and communicative behaviors? When clinically relevant, these additional areas should be further examined. It is possible for the clinician to investigate these domains using additional formal tests such as an apraxia battery, a questionnaire measuring quality of life, or an assessment tool measuring life participation. It is just as likely, and frequently more efficient, for the clinician to rely on informal assessment procedures.

The functional areas with potential impairment can be rather numerous, and it is unrealistic to expect any kind of real-world assessment to be exhaustive. So, the clinician must rely on knowledge of aphasia symptomatologies and observation skills to select the most clinically relevant behaviors to investigate. For example, dyscalculia is a symptom frequently encountered following left hemisphere strokes. However, assessing this ability may only be necessary if there is a recognized functional need for it. On the other hand, if the clinician observes articulatory struggle behavior in her patient with Broca's aphasia, assessing apraxia of speech informally may be important for the development of therapy objectives. Knowledge of symptomatology and its potential impacts on communicative life also help the clinician ask questions that are focused and relevant to functional interventions. For example, if the client wants to use email to communicate with his adult children, various factors must be considered, such as written language processing, mechanical problems due to right hemiparesis, or prior skill using email. Using this information as a guide, the clinician focuses on questions that are relevant to potential intervention for each client.

In fact, part of this goal-oriented question procedure requires considering the ultimate goal of aphasia treatment, which is successful participation in personally relevant communicative situations. Improved communicative participation might be accomplished through recovery of language, compensatory strategies used by the person with aphasia, or supports provided in the external environment. Because degree of life participation is highly correlated with life satisfaction and perceived life quality (Cruice, Hill, Worrall, & Hickson, 2010; Cruice, Worrall, & Hickson, 2003, 2006), consideration of potential participation goals helps the clinician determine how to bridge the gap from specific treatment tasks (or change in specific behaviors) to re-engagement in communicative life. Kagan and Simmons-Mackie (2007) describe this process as setting goals by "beginning with the end" in mind. The authors contrast this approach to the linear focus on administering a test *then* deciding on treatment goals and designing treatment based on the test results. Rather, informal assessment is cyclical and dynamic, evolving from an overview of the case and big picture goals, and evolving towards an ever-narrowing focus on individually relevant behaviors or skills. Determination of participation goals will vary depending on factors such as severity of aphasia, personal preferences and lifestyles, time post-onset, and/or any additional influencing factor deemed relevant (McClung, Gonzalez Rothi, & Nadeau, 2010). For example, a client with very severe aphasia who was recently admitted to a long-term care facility would likely need to communicate basic needs and thoughts to staff members. Informal assessment would initially focus on the most effective supports for immediate communication with the staff in the facility. A client who sustained a moderate aphasia 1 year ago might identify reading for pleasure as an important functional goal, which would justify an informal assessment of reading.

Determining relevant participation goals follows naturally from an understanding of a client's clinical symptoms and the impact of these symptoms on the client's daily life. Once the clinician has some understanding of what a client hopes to be doing in the near and distant future, the clinician can craft hypothesis-testing questions that home in on behaviors that have a positive or negative impact on the relevant communication functions.

The four prerequisite skills described above are instrumental in assisting the clinician in generating appropriate hypothesis-testing questions, such as: "Is apraxia of speech impeding expressive functional communication in this patient?" In addition, critical thinking skills are further needed to devise informal assessment tasks that isolate the behavior under investigation and allow for a reliable measurement scheme by clearly defining a success criterion, thereby providing an accurate answer to the hypothesis-testing question. For example, if a clinician decides to measure auditory-verbal working memory in a client with severe conduction aphasia, a nonverbal (i.e., pointing) response could be implemented (Martin & Saffran, 1992) to ascertain that the severity of the expressive language output does not confound the results of the working memory assessment.

Goal-Oriented Question 2: What Is the Level of Breakdown for Each Behavior?

Once the clinician has determined behaviors that constitute potential therapy objectives, it is important to have a detailed understanding of the severity level of each of these skills. Answering this question will allow each therapy objective and materials to be tailored to a level that fits the client's current performance and is neither too easy nor too difficult. It is true that formal testing can render this severity level in quantitative terms (e.g., the client is able to name 46% of pictured objects), but this goal-oriented question focuses on a more molecular analysis of the behavior for clinical purposes. If naming ability is limited, are all the items equally affected? Is verb naming better or worse than noun naming? What word factors are affected: word length, word frequency, or concreteness? If the client has agrammatism, at which syntactic complexity level does the performance break down? If the person with aphasia has a reduced level of social contacts, the clinician may seek to compare this situation to the premorbid social involvement by generating a social network analysis (Simmons-Mackie, 2008) and qualitatively judging the severity of the loss. Once again, the clinician must use the prerequisite skills to generate hypothesis-testing questions and run a "mini-experiment" (Lidz & Peña, 1996) in order to answer them appropriately.

Goal-Oriented Question 3: What Facilitates the Behavior?

After the clinician has identified the client's level of competence for each skill, it is essential for therapy objective planning to investigate which strategies, resources, or cues improve the behavior. Although the conceptualization of informal assessment described here is broader than dynamic assessment per se, this goal-oriented question clearly encompasses the traditional concept of dynamic assessment (Haynes & Pindzola, 2012; Hersh et al., 2013). (See earlier discussion.)

It is second nature to most clinicians to use cueing and other strategies to facilitate patients' communicative attempts. However, such an approach is experimental in nature and relies on the four important prerequisite skills we identified and described earlier.

For example, drawing on background knowledge (and clinical experience), the clinician may suspect that a particular cue may be effective when associated with a specific clinical symptomatology. In another instance, relying on good observation skills, the clinician may have noticed the client's attempt to trace a letter with her finger while attempting to name an object. An informal direct comparison of written and oral naming may reveal a useful multimodal compensatory mechanism. Further, the clinician may want to assess whether the client can self-cue by producing the phoneme corresponding to the grapheme she can access. In each of these cases, the clinician needs to generate a hypothesis-testing question (e.g., Can the client point to written functional words to express basic needs? Would the client be able to type as opposed to write a functional word?), isolate the behavior to investigate, and measure the results.

It should be emphasized that facilitatory strategies such as cueing are different than compensatory mechanisms. If phonemic cueing helps the patient's production of lexical items, it is only when the patient can self-cue that it becomes compensatory. A compensatory mechanism implies that the communicative attempt was successful, but through a modified process. When a clinician notes that a given cue can be successful or that a patient is able to generate single words in writing slightly better than orally, it is to identify strategies that have the *potential* to become compensatory, rather than state that the strategy is currently used in a compensatory manner.

These compensatory mechanisms can be multimodal, focus on the client and/or the conversation partners, or involve external or internalized strategies. First, multimodality is an important source of help for most patients with aphasia. If the objective is to maximize communication, the channel of delivery becomes less important than the eventual success of the communicative attempt. The informal process seeks to identify the easiest modality (or combination of modalities) for the client to successfully get the point across. Written materials, gestures, drawings, voice output devices, and tablet applications, are a few examples of the available multimodal strategies at one's disposal (see Chapter 8, this volume). Client-specific spontaneous strategies can be identified by observation (Simmons-Mackie & Damico, 1997) or by hypothesis testing. Informal assessment (i.e., in this case dynamic assessment) requires the clinician to develop a hypothesis-testing question, measure the results, and form a conclusion regarding the clinical usefulness of the strategy (see McCauley [1996] for a similar process focusing on child language development).

Second, although this example describes informal assessment focusing on the client's performance, the same logic can be utilized with external supports within the environment (e.g., "aphasia-friendly" written material, pictographic signage; Simmons-Mackie, King, & Beukelman, 2013). One effective form of environmental support is the availability of trained or skilled communication partners. It has been established that training conversational partners provides communicative, participation, and possibly psychosocial benefits (Kagan, Black, Duchan, Simmons-Mackie, & Square, 2001; Simmons-Mackie, Raymer, Armstrong, Holland, & Cherney, 2010; Turner & Whitworth, 2006). It logically follows that clinicians may want to extend dynamic assessment to familiar conversational partners of people with aphasia to determine whether a modification of partners' communicative behaviors can impact positively on the quality of a functional exchange of information and social interaction. For example, starting with the observation of an interaction between the person with aphasia and the spouse, the clinician and conversation partner can explore various modifications of the partner's turns (i.e., rate, syntax, type of questions, etc.) and see which facilitates the interaction.

Finally, compensatory methods can involve a different way for the patient to process language internally and/or use external supports, such as paper and pencil or communication aids. The clinician must rely on both types during the informal assessment process to maximize the client's communicative attempts. In some instances, the client may be able to self-cue the production of a word by consciously processing semantic or phonological elements related to the target word, such as in semantic feature analysis (Boyle & Coelho, 1995) or phonological components analysis (Leonarda, Rochon, & Laird, 2008). In such cases, the client must be able to internalize the cueing strategy. Conversely, the client may be better served by relying on external tools to support communication, such as writing material, using a communication book, or an assistive device. In all instances, the clinician is responsible for assessing the potential success of such approaches during dynamic assessment.

Importantly, these facilitatory strategies must be revised over time lest they become maladaptive as the client's needs change. Therefore, the dynamic assessment aspect of informal testing should be addressed during the therapy phase as well. Hersh and colleagues (2013) have recently argued in favor of integrating dynamic assessment at all levels of therapy, an approach echoing the same argument found in the child language literature (Jeltova et al., 2007).

Goal-Oriented Question 4: What Is the Underlying Cause of the Behavior?

This goal-oriented question attempts to get to the root cause of the observed behavior or communication barrier. Muma (1978) states "the most important issue—the nature of the problem—is not broached by a quantitative procedure" (p. 215). Anomia, for example, can stem from a variety of causes, such as attention impairments, phonological problems, semantic difficulties, or any combination of those processes. Communication breakdowns between a person with aphasia and a caregiver may arise because the spouse uses complex syntax, because the patient's communication book contains too many items, because the caregiver uses too many open questions, or from numerous other possible causal factors. It is important for the clinician to understand the root cause of the symptom in order to focus therapy objectives to the actual impaired mechanism. Such an approach is more likely to generalize than focusing on a task-specific therapy target.

The clinician must rely on observation and on hypothesis-testing questions to address this goal-oriented question. A good starting point is an analysis of the error types or presenting difficulty during or after the task at hand. For example, with regard to lexical retrieval, the distribution of phonemic versus semantic paraphasias may help establish the source of the linguistic difficulty, as well as the nature of the most effective cues. Using a neuropsychological perspective, the analysis can be carried out with more depth (Martin, 2017; Whitworth et al., 2005) by posing, for example, the following hypothesis-testing question: "Are the client's naming skills affected by imageability?" The answer may indicate a breakdown between the semantic system and the phonological output lexicon. Whitworth et al. (2005) provide a helpful review of these strategies for word-finding, comprehension, reading, and writing. Because such an analysis must depend on a theoretical model, the authors rely on a current cognitive neuropsychological model of language production and comprehension. Such a model helps clinicians conceptualize the underlying mechanism or mechanisms that explain the client's symptoms. It is the reliance on such models that enable the clinician to generate the most focused and appropriate hypothesis-testing questions. This also requires the clinician to possess sufficient relevant background knowledge.

From a psychosocial perspective, observation is also relevant to a root-cause behavioral analysis. For example, the clinician has established that the social network of a patient with aphasia is significantly decreased. In particular, the contacts with the client's best friend have been reduced. In collaboration with the client, the clinician has organized a visit and is observing the interaction between the two individuals. The purpose is to observe where the communicative difficulties occur and pinpoint possible causal factors. Then, dynamic assessment may offer some potential solutions and therapy can focus on the source of the breakdown.

CONCLUSION

This conceptualization of the informal assessment process is designed to provide clinicians with a logical structure of goals and procedures; it should not be construed as a flow chart (see **FIGURE 13.4**).

Although the goal-oriented questions appear sequential, their application usually is not. The only exception is the first goal-oriented question, addressing the scope of the client's clinical symptomatology and the impact of aphasia on communicative life. Habitually, the clinician seeks an overall perspective of the clinical picture before focusing on individual symptoms. The subsequent three goal-oriented questions, however, address specific behaviors and can be confronted at any point during assessment. Yoder and Kent (1988) provided detailed flowcharts highlighting the steps necessary for assessment and therapy decisions for a variety of communication disorders. The authors readily acknowledged that a decision tree must not be followed rigidly lest it becomes a cookbook approach. Still, the steps involved in such an approach address "what to do next" rather than *how* to do it or *why*. Particularly with informal assessment,

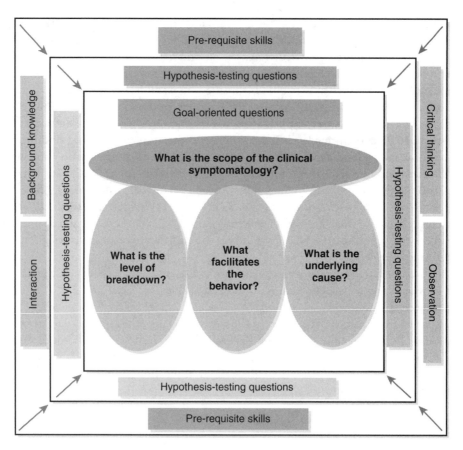

FIGURE 13.4 The informal assessment process.

the thinking process behind clinical decisions is the challenge. In other words, listing a sequence of things to do "focuses your attention on doing something rather than the process of problem solving" (Tomblin et al., 2000, p. 5), which is the heart of informal assessment. Therefore, in our view, an approach focusing on pertinent, thoughtful clinical questions is more useful than an assessment process presented as a series of distinct and sequential phases.

Another indication that the lines between the phases of the assessment process are blurred is that elements of informal assessment can be addressed during formal test administration and the information transferred to informal assessment results. During the administration of formal assessment tools, the clinician should note which items may be particularly easy or difficult for the client and heed the type of errors committed. These observations may lead to clinical hypotheses addressing Goal-Oriented Questions 2 (level of breakdown) and 4 (underlying cause). In addition, the clinician should observe the patient's behavior closely at any point during the rehabilitation period for possible spontaneous compensatory behaviors (Goal-Oriented Question 3). These hypothesis-testing questions can later be investigated informally when the clinician seeks to answer them by conducting a "mini-experiment" (Lidz & Peña, 1996). According to McCauley (1996), this consists of designing a basic ad hoc procedure, appropriate stimuli, and a success criterion. For example, a patient with aphasia and agrammatism has not used any verbs spontaneously (other than copulas) in the conversational and expository speech section of the Boston Diagnostic Aphasia Examination (BDAE-3; Goodglass, Kaplan, & Baresi, 2001). The clinician decides to assess verb naming informally in order to determine whether the client is able to produce verbs in isolation. Twenty action pictures are gathered from the web, including items of varying frequency and length. Because the client reached a 35% success rate on the noun naming portion of the formal test, for comparison purposes, the success criterion for this task was also set at 35%. The clinician also built in a cueing paradigm to be able to compare its effectiveness with that used during the formal noun naming test. Carrying out the task will provide the clinician with potential information about (a) the level of breakdown because of the inclusion of items of different length and frequency (Goal-Oriented Question 2), (b) the effectiveness of phonemic cueing (Goal-Oriented Question 3), and possibly (c) the underlying cause of the anomia (Goal-Oriented Question 4) if one type of cueing is significantly more powerful than another or if a length and/or frequency effect is observed.

In conclusion, formal and informal assessments have very different objectives. Whereas formal assessment is considered helpful for differential diagnosis and behavior quantification, informal assessment is a crucial procedure for developing appropriate clinical objectives. Formal assessment is clearly understood and easily applied by clinicians because its application is carefully scripted and each step is predetermined. On the other hand, informal assessment is amorphous, unstructured, and left to interpretation. The literature does not provide an organized script to assist clinicians in this process; what is more, the objectives of the process itself are ill defined. We have proposed an organizational structure of objectives, components, and procedures in an attempt to circumscribe informal assessment and operationalize its application. Although the procedures discussed are not linear or sequential, the mere articulation of such a framework should provide some support to clinicians in the difficult but important task of articulating the most relevant clinical goals for their clients.

CASE ILLUSTRATION

Kate, a 58-year-old woman, sustained a left hemisphere stroke 5 days prior to being seen by Dan, a clinician on an inpatient rehabilitation unit. Dan had read Kate's medical chart and noted that Kate had sustained a thrombotic stroke affecting Broca's area and extending slightly posteriorly towards the parietal lobe. She had right hemiparesis and was medically stable. During his initial bedside visit to Kate, Dan introduced himself, explained his role and engaged Kate in a conversation, including questions about what brought her into the hospital, what problems she was having, and basic information about her life. While this informal conversation helped to establish rapport important to the therapeutic relationship, it also marked the beginning of informal assessment.

During the conversation Dan made *observations* of Kate's language and communication, as well as her affect and interactive style. Kate appeared to understand his simple questions, but she had significant difficulty expressing herself. She tended to use one-word utterances, and most of these were unintelligible. Her attempts were replete with hesitations, attempted self-corrections, and articulatory posturing and groping. Kate interacted socially and appropriately although she was significantly frustrated and tearful early in the interaction (Goal-Oriented Question 1). Based on his observations and data from the medical chart, Dan used his *knowledge* of and *experience* with aphasia to hypothesize a potential diagnosis of Broca's aphasia and apraxia of speech (AOS).

Based on these hypothesized diagnoses, Dan asked pertinent clinical questions (i.e., applied *critical thinking*). He asked Kate to follow simple instructions, repeat words and phrases of increasing complexity, read simple instructions, and provide a written picture description. Kate followed one-step auditory commands accurately, but had difficulty with two-step instructions or more complex auditory commands (e.g., put the pen under the tablet; Goal-Oriented Question 2). Kate performed 4 out of 5 simple written instructions. Verbal repetition resulted in significant difficulty, including visible groping and attempted self-correction. Attempts to write a picture description resulted largely in content words that were correctly spelled, thereby possibly offering a compensatory strategy for communication (Goal-Oriented Question 3). Dan's *observations* during these informal tasks (mini-experiments) supported his working hypothesis regarding Kate's communication disorders (Goal-Oriented Question 1).

Throughout the informal assessment Dan kept Kate engaged in the process in spite of her considerable frustration and emotional reactions to failed attempts to communicate (i.e., *interactive skill*). In fact, Dan's skill in tempering difficult tasks with counseling and positive information alleviated many of Kate's fears, and over the course of the session her frustration markedly decreased. Unlike formal assessment, where Dan would be less free to provide feedback and elicit Kate's opinions, informal assessment allowed Dan to collaborate with Kate in identifying information that would help with intervention planning. Dan's interactive style made Kate feel like a respected adult; she felt more hopeful and looked forward to working in partnership with Dan.

In addition, Dan spoke to Kate's husband and the unit staff, and he found that Kate was extremely frustrated by her inability to get her needs and ideas across verbally. The staff noted that on two occasions she became "nearly hysterical" when staff did not understand her, resulting in dangerous blood pressure spikes. Furthermore, Dan noted that Kate's husband and the staff did not appear knowledgeable regarding methods of facilitating Kate's communication. As Dan collected information through this initial informal assessment a more complete picture of Kate's communication emerged (see **FIGURE 13.5**; Goal-Oriented Question 1).

In order to quantify Kate's linguistic symptoms, Dan administered the WAB-R. Kate obtained an AQ of 51, which indicates a moderate level of aphasia severity. The breakdown of subtest scores confirmed Dan's clinical impressions. Kate had functional language comprehension and more severe difficulties with spontaneous speech (i.e., agrammatism), repetition, and word-finding. During the formal test administration, Dan noted that Kate was benefiting from phonemic but not semantic cues (Goal-Oriented Questions 3 and 4) and that her picture description contained mostly nouns but hardly any verbs (Goal-Oriented Question 2). Dan decided to investigate Kate's verb processing by designing three simple tasks: matching action pictures with oral presentation of verbs, matching SVO reversible sentences with action pictures, and naming action pictures. Kate was able to name 50% of actions, which was comparable to her word-finding score for nouns. She was able to understand 100% of the orally presented verbs; however, she had significant difficulties understanding reversible sentences. From these results, Dan concluded that Kate had difficulty mapping thematic roles onto the verb's argument structure (Marshall, 2017; Goal-Oriented Question 4). In terms of Kate's word-finding process, Dan knew that Kate had similar difficulty with nouns and verbs, that her repetition and her reading of single lexical items was better than her oral word-finding, and that her word-finding errors were inconsistent. Dan decided to investigate the frequency effect and the length effect in two balanced word lists. Kate showed a frequency effect but not a length effect. Taken together, these results led Dan to diagnose a particular difficulty accessing the phonological and orthographic output lexicons from a well-preserved semantic system (Goal-Oriented Question 4). Finally, Dan decided against further evaluation of AOS, because his informal clinical observations were sufficient to assess the presence and severity of AOS.

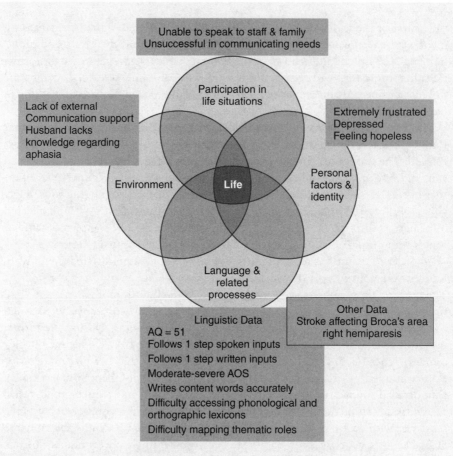

FIGURE 13.5 Initial observations regarding Kate's communication status.

Dan's knowledge of aphasia and AOS suggested to him that the expressive language impairment might be the most significant communication barrier for Kate at this stage of her recovery. To pursue this hypothesis, Dan used supported communication to converse with Kate (e.g., Kagan et al., 2001; Simmons-Mackie et al., 2013); that is, Dan modified his manner of speaking with Kate (e.g., slower speaking rate, simple syntax) and simultaneously used multimodality resources such as gestures, pictographs, and written key words. The goal of this conversation was to find out what Kate considered her biggest challenges at present. After collecting initial data and talking with Kate, Dan identified the most immediate goals as (1) identifying compensatory strategies and external supports that would help Kate communicate with unit staff and family and (2) improving spoken language/speech to meet future communication needs. In addition, secondary goals including reducing Kate's frustration and depression as well as increasing external communicative support in the environment. These goals were mapped onto a framework for outcome measurement to help organize intervention plans (see **FIGURE 13.6**).

Informal assessment required Dan to rely on his knowledge of aphasia, his critical thinking skills, his observational abilities, and his skill in enlisting Kate as a partner in planning and implementing treatment. The process of informal assessment was cyclical and ongoing, allowing Dan to identify general behaviors that would influence treatment, hone in on relevant goals, and then define specific behaviors to target in treatment.

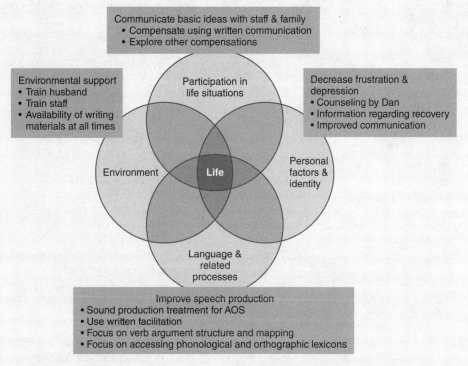

FIGURE 13.6 Identified goals & treatments based on informal assessment.

REFERENCES

American Speech-Language-Hearing Association (ASHA). (2004). *Preferred practice patterns for the profession of speech-language pathology (Preferred practice document)*. Rockville, MD: Author.

Boyle, M., & Coelho, C. A. (1995). Application of a semantic feature analysis as a treatment for aphasic dysnomia. *American Journal of Speech-Language Pathology, 4*, 135–138.

Butler, K. G. (1997). Dynamic assessment at the millennium: A transient tutorial for today! *Journal of Children's Communication Development, 19*(1), 43–54.

Coelho, C., Ylvisaker, M., & Turkstra, L. S. (2005). Nonstandardized assessment approaches for individuals with traumatic brain injuries. *Seminars in Speech and Language, 26*(4), 223–241.

Cruice, M., Hill, R., Worrall, L., & Hickson, L. (2010). Conceptualising quality of life for older people with aphasia. *Aphasiology, 24*(3), 327–347.

Cruice, M., Worrall, L., & Hickson, L. (2003). Finding a focus for quality of life with aphasia: Social and emotional health, and psychological well-being. *Aphasiology, 17*(4), 333–353.

Cruice, M., Worrall, L., & Hickson, L. (2006). Perspectives of quality of life by people with aphasia and their family: Suggestions for successful living. *Topics in Stroke Rehabilitation, 13*(1), 14–24.

Foundation for Critical Thinking. (2013, September 25). Defining critical thinking. Retrieved from http://www.criticalthinking.org/pages/defining-critical-thinking/766

Goodglass, H., Kaplan, E., & Baresi, B. (2001). *Boston Diagnostic Aphasia Examination* (3rd ed.). Philadelphia, PA: Lippincott, Williams, & Wilkins.

Haynes, W. O., & Pindzola, R. H. (2012). *Diagnosis and evaluation in speech pathology*. Boston, MA: Pearson.

Hersh, D., Worrall, L., O'Halloran, R., Brown, K., Grohn, B., & Rodriguez, A. D. (2013). Assess for success: Evidence for therapeutic assessment. In N. Simmons-Mackie, J. M. King, & D. R. Beukelman (Eds.), *Supporting communication for adults with acute and chronic aphasia* (pp. 145–164). Baltimore, MD: Paul Brookes.

Holland, A. L. (1980). *Communicative Abilities in Daily Living*. Baltimore, MD: University Park Press.

Holland, A., Frattali, C., & Fromm, D. (1999). *Communication Abilities of Daily Living-2*. Austin, TX: Pro-Ed.

Jeltova, I., Birney, D., Fresine, N., Jarvin, L., Sternberg, R. J., & Grigorenko, E. L. (2007). Dynamic assessment as a process-oriented assessment in educational settings. *Advances in Speech-Language Pathology, 9*(4), 273–285.

Kagan, A., Black, S. E., Duchan, F. J., Simmons-Mackie, N., & Square, P. (2001). Training volunteers as conversation partners using "Supported Conversation for Adults with Aphasia" (SCA): A controlled trial. *Journal of Speech, Language, and Hearing Research, 44*(3), 624–638.

Kagan, A., & Simmons-Mackie, N. (2007). Beginning with the end: Outcome driven assessment and intervention with life participation in mind. *Topics in Language Disorders, 27*, 309–317.

Kagan, A., Simmons-Mackie, N., Rowland, A., Huijbregts, M., Shumway, E., McEwen, S., ... Sharp, S. (2008). Counting what counts: A framework for capturing real-life outcomes of aphasia intervention. *Aphasiology, 22*(3), 258–280.

Kertesz, A. (2007). *Western Aphasia Battery-Revised*. San Antonio, TX: PsychCorp.

Leff, A. P., Schoffield, T. M., Crinion, J. T., Seghier, M. L., Grogan, A., Green, D. W., & Price, C. J. (2009). The left superior temporal gyrus is a shared substrate for auditory short-term memory and speech comprehension: Evidence from 210 patients with stroke. *Brain, 132*, 3401–3410.

Leonarda, C., Rochon, E., & Laird, L. (2008). Treating naming impairments in aphasia: Findings from a phonological components analysis treatment. *Aphasiology, 22*(9), 923–947.

Lidz, C. S., & Peña, E. D. (1996). Dynamic assessment: The model, its relevance as a nonbiased approach, and its application to Latino American preschool children. *Language, Speech, and Hearing Services in Schools, 27*, 367–372.

LPAA Project Group (Chapey, R., Duchan, J., Elman, R., Garcia, L., Kagan, A., Lyon, J., & Simmons-Mackie, N.). (2000, February). Life Participation Approach to Aphasia: A statement of values for the future. *ASHA Leader, 5*, 4–6. Retrieved from http://www.asha.org/Publications/leader/2000/000215/Life-Participation-Approach-to-Aphasia—A-Statement-of-Values-for-the-Future.htm

Marshall, J. (2017). Disorders in sentence processing in aphasia. In I. Papathanasiou & P. Coppens (Eds.), *Aphasia and related neurogenic communication disorders* (pp. 245–267). Burlington, MA: Jones & Bartlett Learning.

Martin, N. (2017). Disorders of word production. In I. Papathanasiou & P. Coppens(Eds.), *Aphasia and related neurogenic communication disorders* (pp. 169–194). Burlington, MA: Jones & Bartlett Learning.

Martin, N., & Saffran, E. M. (1992). A computational account of deep dysphasia: Evidence from a single case study. *Brain and Language, 43*(2), 240–274.

Martin, N., Thompson, C. K., & Worrall, L. (2008). Aphasia rehabilitation: The impairment and its consequences. San Diego, CA: Plural Publishing.

McCauley, R. J. (1996). Familiar strangers: Criterion-referenced measures in communication disorders. *Language, Speech, and Hearing Services in Schools, 27*, 122–131.

McClung, J. S., Gonzalez Rothi, L. J., & Nadeau, S. E. (2010). Ambient experience in restitutive treatment of aphasia. *Frontiers in Human Neuroscience, 4*, 1–19.

Muma, J. R. (1978). *Language handbook. Concepts, assessment, intervention.* Englewood Cliffs, NJ: Prentice Hall.

Murray, L. L., & Clark, H. M. (2015). *Neurogenic disorders of language and cognition. Evidence-based clinical practice* (2nd ed.). Austin, TX: Pro-Ed.

Murray, L., & Coppens, P. (2017). Formal and informal assessment of aphasia. In I. Papathanasiou & P. Coppens (Eds.), *Aphasia and related neurogenic communication disorders* (pp. 81–108). Burlington, MA: Jones & Bartlett Learning.

Peña, E. D., Summers, C., & Resendiz, M. (2007). Language variation, assessment, and intervention. In A. Kamhi, J. Masterson, & K. Apel (Eds.), *Clinical decision making in developmental language disorders* (pp. 99–118). Baltimore, MD: Paul Brookes.

Rosenbek, J. C., Lapointe, L. L., & Wertz, R. T. (1989). *Aphasia. A clinical approach.* Austin, TX: Pro-Ed.

Sarno, M. T. (1969). *The functional communication profile.* New York, NY: New York University Institute of Rehabilitation Medicine.

Simmons-Mackie, N. (1998). A solution to the discharge dilemma in aphasia: Social approaches to aphasia management. *Aphasiology, 12*, 231–239.

Simmons-Mackie, N. (2008). Intervention for a case of severe apraxia of speech and aphasia: A functional-social perspective. In N. Martin, C. K. Thompson, & L. Worrall (Eds.), *Aphasia rehabilitation. The impairment and its consequences* (pp. 75–108). San Diego, CA: Plural Publishing.

Simmons-Mackie, N., & Damico, J. S. (1997). Reformulating the definition of compensatory strategies in aphasia. *Aphasiology, 11*(8), 761–781.

Simmons-Mackie, N., & Damico, J. S. (2011). Exploring clinical interaction in speech language therapy: Narrative, discourse and relationships. In R. Fourie (Ed.). *Therapeutic processes for communication disorders* (pp. 35–52). Hove, England: Psychology Press.

Simmons-Mackie, N., King, J., Beukelman, D. (Eds.). (2013). *Supporting communication for adults with acute and chronic aphasia.* Baltimore, MD: Paul Brookes Publishing.

Simmons-Mackie, N., Raymer, A., Armstrong, E., Holland, A., & Cherney, L. R. (2010). *Communication partner training in aphasia: A systematic review.* Archives of Physical Medicine and Rehabilitation, 91(12), 1814–1837.

Tomblin, J. B., Morris, H. L., & Spriesterbach, D. C. (2000). *Diagnosis in speech-language pathology.* San Diego, CA: Singular.

Turner, S., & Whitworth, A. (2006). Conversational partner training programmes in aphasia: A review of key themes and participants' roles. *Aphasiology, 20,* 483–510.

Vygotsky, L. S. (1978). *Mind in society: The development of higher psychological processes.* Cambridge, MA: Harvard University Press.

Whitworth, A., Webster, J., & Howard, D. (2005). *A cognitive neuropsychological approach to assessment and intervention in aphasia.* Hove, England: Psychology Press.

World Health Organization (WHO). (2001). International Classification of Functioning, Disability and Health. Geneva, Switzerland: Author.

Worrall, L., Davidson, B., Hersh, D., Howe, T., Sherratt, S., & Ferguson, A. (2010). The evidence for relationship-centered practice in aphasia rehabilitation. *Journal of Interactional Research in Communication Disorders, 1,* 277–300.

Worrall, L., Sherratt, S., & Papathanasiou, I. (2017). Therapy approaches to aphasia. In I. Papathanasiou & P. Coppens (Eds.), *Aphasia and related neurogenic communication disorders* (pp. 109–127). Burlington, MA: Jones & Bartlett Learning.

Yoder, D. E., & Kent, R. D. (1988). Decision making in speech-language pathology. Toronto, Canada: B.C. Decker.

Index

Note: Page numbers followed by "*f*", "*n*" or "*t*" indicate figure, note, or table respectively.